Management of Hypertension

Vasilios Papademetriou
Emmanuel A. Andreadis
Charalampia Geladari
Editors

Management of Hypertension

Current Practice and the Application of Landmark Trials

Springer

Editors
Vasilios Papademetriou
Georgetown University and
VA Medical Center
Washington, DC
USA

Emmanuel A. Andreadis
Fourth Internal Medicine Department
Evangelismos State General Hospital
Athens
Greece

Charalampia Geladari
Fourth Internal Medicine Department
Evangelismos State General Hospital
Athens
Greece

ISBN 978-3-319-92945-3 ISBN 978-3-319-92946-0 (eBook)
https://doi.org/10.1007/978-3-319-92946-0

Library of Congress Control Number: 2018957847

This Springer imprint is published by the registered company Springer Nature Switzerland AG
The registered company address is: Gewerbestrasse 11, 6330 Cham, Switzerland

Dedication to Edward David Freis

By Vasilios Papademetriou, MD

Professor of Medicine, Georgetown University

It is with a great deal of gratitude and pride that I write this dedication to Edward D. Freis, the man, the teacher, the mentor, the giant, my boss. I had the good fortune of knowing Edward D. Freis as a man, as a physician, as a scientist, and as a human being. Ed Freis was a good man, a great scientist, and a great philanthropist. He had a good life and a great career, and he died happy, fulfilled by his achievements, surrounded by his children, and covered by appreciation and respect by his peers.

I first met him in 1981, when I walked into his office looking for a job. I was a research fellow then at the National Institutes of Health, investigating the role of murine macrophages on immunoreactivity, but I had had enough and decided that I wanted to deal with patients. Having heard about Dr. Freis and his work, I called and made an appointment for an interview. It did not take long. After a brief conversation, he said "So, you are interested in clinical research? Ha, and what have you done so far?" When I told him about my experience working with mice, that my group had published 11 papers in 18 months, and that I was more interested in humans, he said "You've got the job, when can you start? And by the way, how much money do you make?" After I explained that I was making only $13,000 a year, he said, "We can do better than that: we'll pay you $18,000." We had a deal, and I started working with him. Ed Freis was a fair and a generous man. He was fair to his science and supportive *to those who worked for him. By the time I joined his group in June 1981, his landmark work had had a big impact on patient care and the medical community. The treatment of hypertension was widespread, and many other outcome trials were in press or in progress. His work was mostly focused on the treatment of hypertension using diuretic-based regimens. He always held the position that these regimens were safe and effective, but his competitors tried in many different ways to undermine his work. Soon after I joined his group, Dr. Freis attended the American Heart Association's annual meeting, at which Dr. Bryan Holland presented data from a small study suggesting that diuretics cause arrhythmias and sudden death. This became very controversial and dominated research on hypertension throughout the 1980s and into the 1990s. No wonder Dr. Freis asked me to design a protocol to assess the effect of diuretic-induced hypokalemia on cardiac arrhythmias. The initial study was designed and carried out in patients treated with high-dose diuretics who developed severe hypokalemia. Yet our data indicated no harm from diuretics to our patient population. Even severe hypokalemia had no effect on arrhythmias. After that, we carried out several other studies that repeatedly proved the safety of diuretics. Ed Freis found great satisfaction in these results and continued commenting and writing about them for two decades. Our team and Marvin Moser were the lone defenders of diuretics in the 1980s and part of the 1990s and had several debates and arguments both from the podium and through the literature, but at the end, we were proved correct.*

Ed Freis enjoyed life immensely. He prided himself on knowing every good restaurant in town, particularly every good deal (cost-effectiveness). Confidentially, he told me that the best deal was a Greek restaurant called Ambrosia, where one could dine on good food for $15. On numerous occasions, he commented on how much he enjoyed Greek food and in particular my wife's cooking. Long after he retired, Ed continued coming to the clinic, and in fact, we shared office space for another decade. He authored more than 400 original papers, editorials, book chapters, and reviews. I could write a lot more anecdotal encounters about Ed Freis, but instead I prefer to present a brief outline of his life and commentaries from his students and colleagues following his death.

Edward David Freis was the pioneer researcher who designed and spearheaded the landmark, VA Cooperative studies that revolutionized the treatment of hypertension. He was born in Chicago on May 13, 1912, and died in Washington on February 1, 2005. He was the youngest of four sons of Roy Freis, a real estate developer, and his wife Rose. Freis grew up in Chicago and graduated from Nicholas Senn High School in 1930. He hoped to become an actor and took time off from college to train at the Pasadena Playhouse. (A sympathetic uncle supported this endeavor, in defiance of his father who vowed to disown his son if he stayed at Hollywood, but later relented.) Freis soon decided that he was not tall enough to succeed in show business and returned to the university, where he got his BS in 1936. Later, he showed great zeal for golf and wanted to become a professional golfer.

Freis had been inspired to pursue a career in medicine after reading Paul De Kruif's popular books, Microbe Hunters and Hunger Fighters. He received his MD from the College of Physicians and Surgeons at Columbia University in 1940. He completed his internship and residency at Massachusetts Memorial Hospital and the Boston City Hospital, briefly joined the US Army Air Forces (now the US Air Force) and served as assistant chief, and then became chief of the laboratory service at Lincoln Air Force Base in Lincoln, Nebraska, from 1942 to 1944. From 1944 to 1945, he headed the laboratory service for the USAAF Rheumatic Fever Research Program at Gowen Field in Boise, Idaho. After the war, Ed Freis returned to Boston for a cardiology residency at Evans Memorial Hospital, followed by a research fellowship there. Under the supervision of Robert Wilkin, Ed Freis began his clinical research, in hemodynamics and the drug treatment of hypertension, an area that he later revolutionized.

After experimenting with ganglionic blockers, snake venom and hemapheresis, and drugs such as pentaquine, veratrum viride, and hexamethonium, that were effective, but with intolerable side effects, he came across the first diuretic – chlorothiazide – that he studied in a small group of patients and found to be effective and well tolerated. At that time, hypertension was thought to be a normal part of aging, except in severe or in malignant forms.

In 1949, Freis was appointed Assistant Chief of the Medical Service at the Veterans Administration (VA) Hospital in Washington, DC, with a joint appointment as Adjunct Clinical Professor of Medicine at Georgetown University School of

Medicine. He also served as director of Georgetown's Cardiovascular Research Laboratory (1949–1965) and Chief of the Hypertension Clinic there (1950–1960). In 1954, he became Chief of the VA Medical Service and, in 1959, was named Senior Medical Investigator. During this period, he continued his investigations into the mechanisms and control of hypertension. New antihypertensive drugs were gradually developed, including the ganglion blockers, such as hexamethonium, reserpine, and hydralazine and of course, the first thiazide diuretic, chlorothiazide (in 1956).

At about the same time, the researchers at the VA began a controlled clinical trial to evaluate the growing arsenal of antihypertensive drugs. Controlled clinical trials were something of a novelty at the time, but the VA had done a similar study to evaluate the effectiveness of drugs for treating tuberculosis several years earlier. Although many drugs had been developed during the 1950s for treating hypertension, there was no proof that they provided long-term benefits.

In 1962, Freis formed the VA Cooperative Study Group and designed the landmark VA Cooperative Studies aiming to assess whether treatment of hypertension would help prevent death and cardiovascular complications of hypertension such as stroke, congestive heart failure, kidney damage, and heart attack. The study ran from January 1964 through December 1969, and it was the first randomized, placebo-controlled, double-blind, multi-institutional clinical trial ever done in the United States. The study group included two distinct subgroups of patients: with severe or mild to moderate hypertension. Patients were randomized to either active treatment or placebo. In only 18 months, adverse events in patients with severe hypertension were reduced by more than 90% (21 vs 1 events) and in the mild to moderate groups by more than 50%.

The study results were published in 1969 and 1972, to relatively little fanfare. They attracted more attention the following year, when Ed Freis was honored with a Lasker Award for his leadership of the VA study. Philanthropist and health policy advocate, Mary Lasker, head of the Lasker Foundation, believed that the study revealed a major public health problem that should – and could – be remedied. She asked Elliot Richardson, Secretary of Health, Education, and Welfare, to establish a hypertension education program to alert physicians and the general public about this "silent killer."

The National High Blood Pressure Education Program was started in 1972 and launched a successful nationwide campaign for hypertension awareness, screening, and treatment. During the next two decades, public awareness of hypertension's role in heart disease and stroke increased threefold, and the mortality rates from those diseases dropped dramatically. The wide spread interest in the United States and around the word in hypertension diagnosis treatment and control can be traced back to the work of Ed Freis.

Freis continued to direct cooperative studies on hypertension and to advocate the treatment of the condition, becoming recognized as one of the world's foremost authorities. In 1979, with science writer Gina Kolata, he wrote The High Blood Pressure Book, a guide for patients and their families, which won the American Heart Association's Howard Blakeslee award in 1980. Freis broadened his research into various aspects of hypertension treatment, including the role of race in treatment outcomes and the use of medications for elderly patients. He conducted clinical trials on new hypertension drugs, such as the beta-blockers (which slow the heart rate) and angiotensin-converting enzyme (ACE) inhibitors (which block the production of angiotensin II, a hormone that causes blood vessels to narrow) as they were developed. He also participated in many discussions about how and whether to treat mild hypertension.

By the mid-1980s, there were growing concerns about the use of diuretics in hypertension treatment, specifically the danger that they might cause potassium depletion and induce dangerous cardiac arrhythmias and sudden death. Some critics argued that with all the new antihypertensive drugs available there was no need to use "obsolete" drugs like diuretics in any case. He asked me to design and carry out control studies to assess the effect of diuretic-induced hypokalemia on cardiac arrhythmias. Our studies indicated that diuretics were safe and effective and remained the cornerstone of hypertension treatment and control. Freis had long recommended diuretics – which were safe and inexpensive – as the first step in hypertension treatment, alone or in combination with other drugs. Later our position was vindicated by the Antihypertensive and Lipid-Lowering Treatment to prevent Heart Attack Trial (ALLHAT) study (1994–2002), which showed that treatment with diuretics controlled blood pressure better and was significantly better for preventing cardiovascular disease events, when compared to treatment with ACE inhibitors, calcium channel blockers, or alpha-adrenergic blockers.

Freis retired in 1987 and was named distinguished physician by the VA Medical Center and professor emeritus by Georgetown University School of Medicine. He continued to advise ongoing clinical studies and to publish about hypertension for nearly two decades. At the time of his death on February 1, 2005, he was working on a second hypertension book for a popular audience. That book remained unfinished and given by his daughter to the National Library of Medicine.

Freis mentored a lot of fellows, many of whom later became authorities in the field of hypertension and cardiovascular disease:

***Comments by Edward D. Frohlich**: "Several years ago, while I was Editor-in-Chief of Hypertension, I invited Ed to summarize for the journal some of his more well-known studies emanating from his cardiovascular research laboratory. He reviewed his other work on the hemodynamics of congestive heart failure and myocardial infarction, advancing a new concept of 'unloading the heart.' How taken back most investigators were at the thought of administering a ganglion blocking agent in these circumstances to reduce left ventricular preload! He first tried out this concept using a mechanical model of the heart that demonstrated improved cardiac performance when venous return was reduced, using his specially constructed venous reservoir. To my more recent (and personal) thinking and amazement were his studies on blood flow velocity that provided more fundamental support to the earlier clinical reports of Alton Ochsner, who used leg compression by an elastic stocking as a prophylaxis against phlebothrombosis in surgical patients by diverting flow from the more superficial veins to deep veins, thus accelerating deep venous flow. His studies on blood pressure in small arteries, on the velocity of red blood cells and other elements in circulating blood compared with plasma, as well as his work on transcapillary migration of other constituents in the circulation were truly innovative.*

No doubt these experiences allowed him to conceive the concept of combination therapy. Each of these various areas of investigation gave great impetus to those of us who trained with him as well as those who were his research fellows or on our own who later follow through on the foregoing areas as well as with 'cardiogenic hypertension', vascular compliance, plasma volume expansion, and aging. It is remarkable, indeed, to see the beginnings of their studies forecasted in Freis' classic review of the hemodynamics of hypertension in Physiological Reviews in 1960. I still suggest this review as the first reference to be read by fellows in training."

Comments by Jay Cohn*: "What I learned from Ed Freis' mentorship more than 40 years ago was the virtue of critical, incisive thinking and care in research design. Ed was incredibly disciplined in his life and in his work. His daily routine left little room for spontaneity, from daily naps on his office couch to afternoon golf practice on the field adjacent to the VA Hospital. He tried to teach me a better golf swing, which was his passion. We played rain or shine. One hot day, when I almost collapsed on the 13th tee, he left me lying on the grass with a comment that he would come back for me after he finished the back nine. In scientific discussions he cut to the chase. His desktop was always clear because he dealt immediately and efficiently with all mail and messages. I never learned to discipline my life, which is cluttered with books and papers that I never find time to deal with. But the research integrity and intellectual discipline that Ed demonstrated in our daily encounters have had a profound effect on my career."*

Comments by Edward G. Lakatta*: "Ed Freis was my first research mentor. While a medical student at Georgetown University, I had not previously been exposed to research and wished to find out what it was like. Ed's genuine zeal for research rubbed off on me! We spent substantial periods of time planning experiments, interpreting results, and, subsequently, writing up the findings. He instilled in me the confidence needed to deliver my first paper describing our results at an American Heart Association Meeting, a rare experience for a medical student. Because of my interaction, I developed a passion for research that has never dwindled. Following my training in internal medicine, I spent 2 years at NIH studying cardiac muscle changes with aging. Later, when I was a fellow in cardiology, Ed made another substantial impact on my career. He and others at the Washington VA Hospital had made remarkable contributions to hemodynamics research, and I was* *poised to commit to this area of research as well. Ed advised me, however, that the door toward understanding the mysteries of the cardiovascular system was not via hemodynamics but in heart cell research, (ie, the type of stuff I had explored at NIH). I heeded this advice and have enjoyed a challenging 30-year career doing so, and following in his footsteps."*

Many other fellows credit their work and interests to Ed Freis, to name a few:

***Robert Tarazi**, fellow at the Cleveland Clinic, would credit Ed Freis' concept of cardiogenic hypertension for his personal interests in that area.*

***John Rose**, who became the Chairman of Physiology at Georgetown and later Dean of the Medical School, in reflecting about Ed Freis, said that he became a research fellow after his internship in 1951 and "I was a close personal friend ever since. He was a remarkable guy, a great teacher: gentle, kind, and prodding. But, in the experimental laboratory of the early 1950s, he was also compulsive, having all of the qualities of a true scientist, intensity and stress when things were not going well!" As a former Dean of the School of Medicine, Rose was justly proud to say that Ed donated his Lasker Awards to the university for display.*

***Dr. Larry Lillienfield**, another research fellow of Freis, succeeded John Rose as Chairman of Physiology and commented, "Ed was a wonderful guy who made a tremendous impact on the fundamentals of cardiovascular physiology as well as the more widely known contributions in the area of clinical hypertension."*

***Barry Materson** wrote the following: "I owe him big and I remember telling him that every time that whenever I spoke with him. He was a great mentor even though I never worked directly for him. I enjoyed playing golf with him, and he not only tolerated playing with me but also gave me some lessons in the process. Ed Freis was never swayed by the dogma of the moment unless it was thoroughly back by valid data. He demanded databased opinions long before evidence-based medicine was popularized."*

***Ed Frohlich** writes: Another successor to Freis' work was Vasilios Papademetriou at the VA Hospital in Washington. At Ed's funeral, Vasilios commented in his warm and thoughtful* *eulogy that "Ed Freis was a good man, someone who served science religiously but also someone who enjoyed life tremendously.*

He was a great man, and had a good life, a brilliant career, and passed away quietly."

Ed Freis had an impact in medicine like only few others. His work on hypertension changed the course of history and saved untold hundreds of thousands of lives. His name and his work will remain imprinted in the literature forever.

"He was a good man, a great scientist, and an amazing mentor. He was one of the giants, he was my boss."

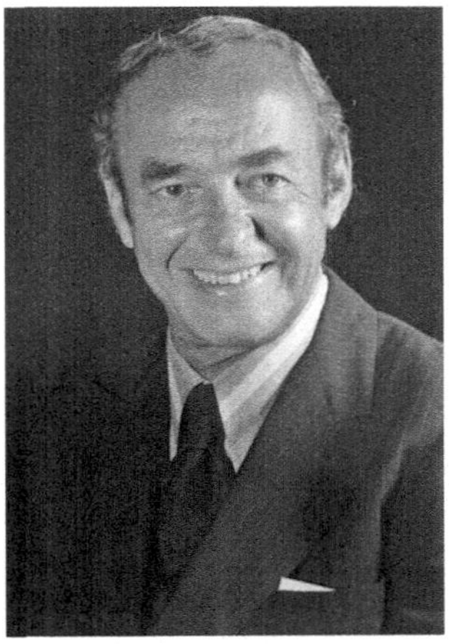

Edward D. Freis (1912–2015)

Preface

It is with great pleasure and excitement that we publish this book, entitled *Management of Hypertension: Current Practice and the Application of Landmark Trials*. Hypertension is indeed a major public health problem worldwide and the most widely recognized modifiable risk factor for cardiovascular disease, with an estimated overall prevalence in adults, aged 25 and over, around 40% in 2008. As such, it is a subject that gathers a special interest among physician-scientists involved in cardiovascular research. With the completion of this project, we aim to offer to young physicians and other scientists engaged in the clinical cardiovascular field a book that reviews the milestone hypertension trials that changed the false belief that was dominating at the dawn of the twentieth century and which supported that blood pressure was essential for the perfusion of vital organs and, therefore, it should not be treated. The studies of Irvine Page, who first observed that despite lowering blood pressure using colloidal sulfur injections, kidney function was well maintained and the first who described the famous mosaic theory of hypertension, as well as the first randomized controlled trials conducted by the farsighted physician, Edward D. Freis, were pivotal in changing the "medieval" understanding of this devastating condition, once and for all.

This book is organized into five major parts. The first part is an introduction to medical research. Its objective is to help scientists and hypertension specialists understand the importance of applying evidence-based medicine in clinical practice, and become familiar with the basic concepts in biostatistics, which will assist them in interpreting the results of scientific papers – it helps them, in particular, to recognize the strengths and weaknesses of a published work. We believe it is of critical importance for a scientist involved in the cardiovascular field to understand deeply the process of analyzing and interpreting medical data.

The second part that comprises 11 chapters review some of the major landmark studies which answered some of the most important questions that altered the course of the investigation and treatment of high blood pressure and influenced the lives of many hypertensives around the world: Is arterial hypertension linked to increased cardiovascular risk? Should we treat higher levels of diastolic blood pressure in adults? Should we treat isolated systolic hypertension in older persons? What is the best way to treat high blood pressure? The VA Cooperative studies – the first randomized controlled trials anywhere in the world – the DASH, the SHEP, the AASK, the ASCOT, the ACCOMPLISH, the MRC, the HDFP, the HOT, the ACCORD, the SPRINT, and the HOPE3 are only some of the major hypertension trials discussed in this part. How did they influence the management of hypertension? This part also reviews the recently updated 2017 ACC/AHA Guidelines for the management of hypertension and tries to examine the advantages and disadvantages of clinical trials.

In the third part of this book, there is only one chapter that reviews the methods of blood pressure assessment used in milestone hypertension trials.

The fourth part is dedicated to three of the most important and pioneer researchers in hypertension research: Dr. Irvine Page, Dr. Edward D. Freis, and the legendary Stevo Julius who is still actively involved in hypertension research. We cordially want to thank Dr. Brent Egan who willingly accepted to review his major scientific contributions in the field of hypertension.

The last part of this book takes a look into the future of cardiovascular medicine with the advent of microfluidics. How these could be applied in hypertension research is a subject discussed thoroughly in the last chapter of this part.

For the completion of this project, we did invite as authors hypertension experts who are widely recognized as global leaders in the field of cardiovascular research. We deeply appreciate their time and work to expertly and concisely review the milestone hypertension trials discussed in this book. Each chapter merits multiple reads and can be read as a unique manuscript, and therefore, any overlapping in the mention of some of the landmark studies was inevitable. These chapters can act as a starting point for anyone seeking an up-to-date and scientifically accurate review regarding the hypertension landmark clinical trials. Their outstanding work has given this book the opportunity to succeed as an educational resource for the scientific community and to enhance the clinical skills of practicing physicians. Most importantly, we would also like to give special thanks to Professor Costas Tsioufis, the President of the European Society of Hypertension and the President of the Hellenic Society of Cardiology, our friend and collaborator, who supported our work by endorsing our book as an ESH endorsed book and contributed a valuable chapter to this book.

We would also like to thank Grant Weston, the Editor of Springer International Publishing, who believed in this project and gave us the green light to publish this book.

Washington, DC, USA — Vasilios Papademetriou
Athens, Greece — Emmanuel A. Andreadis
Athens, Greece — Charalampia Geladari

Special Thanks

Dr. Andreadis and I, on behalf of all contributors, wholeheartedly want to thank Dr. Charalampia (Chara) Geladari, for all she has done to make this book possible. Chara has been the heart and soul of this publication, took care of every little detail, and put bright colors on every page of this book. We all thank you Chara!

I also want to thank all my good friends and colleagues from the United States, Greece, and Europe for their great contributions, time, and effort that made this book possible.

Last but not least, I want to thank my family for putting up with me, despite my frequent travels and long leave of absence.

I thank you all.

Vasilios Papademetriou, MD, PhD

I would like to thank my associates, Professor Vasilios Papademetriou and Dr. Charalampia (Chara) Geladari for the accomplishment of this great book. Professor Papademetriou and I are especially grateful to Chara, my dedicated colleague, for her enthusiasm, creativity, and commitment and for her exhaustive and thorough work. This book could not have been written without her generous assistance.

I would like to express my immense gratitude to my wife for her help and, of course, to my daughter for her encouragement in my clinical and research activities. To all of them, I extend my deep appreciation.

Emmanuel A. Andreadis, MD, PhD.

I would like to express my deepest gratitude to my mentor Emmanuel A. Andreadis for believing in me and for being my inspiration to pursue my goals with hard work and dedication. I cordially thank you, Dr. Andreadis, for your sincere support, commitment, time, and mentorship! You have made an impact on my life. To me, you are absolutely family!

I would also like to thank Professor Vasilios Papademetriou for this great opportunity, to be one of the editors of this book, and for his support and trust. Dr. Papademetriou, it is truly an honor to work with you!

My warmest thanks to my family for their unconditional support, encouragement, and love!

Charalampia Geladari, MD.

Contents

Contributors

Emmanuel A. Andreadis Hypertension and Cardiovascular Disease Prevention Center, Evangelismos General Hospital, Athens, Greece

Fourth Internal Medicine Department, Evangelismos State General Hospital, Athens, Greece

George L. Bakris Comprehensive Hypertension Center, Department of Medicine, University of Chicago, Chicago, IL, USA

Konstantinos I. Bougioukas Department of Hygiene, Social-Preventive Medicine and Medical Statistics, Medical School, Aristotle University of Thessaloniki, Thessaloniki, Greece

Yi Chen Department of Hypertension, Shanghai Key Laboratory of Hypertension, Centre for Epidemiological Studies and Clinical Trials, The Shanghai Institute of Hypertension, Ruijin Hospital, Shanghai Jiao Tong University School of Medicine, Shanghai, China

Annise K. Chung Georgetown University Hospital, Washington, DC, USA

Renata Cifkova Center for Cardiovascular Prevention, Charles University in Prague, First Faculty of Medicine and Thomayer Hospital, Prague, Czech Republic

Department of Medicine II – Cardiology and Angiology, Charles University in Prague, First Faculty of Medicine and General University Hospital, Prague, Czech Republic

Kyriakos Dimitriadis 1st Academic Department of Cardiology, Athens, Greece

Jeanne M. Dobrzynski Cardiovascular Institute, Rutgers Robert Wood Johnson Medical School, New Brunswick, NJ, USA

Michael Doumas Second Propedeutic Department of Internal Medicine, Aristotle University, Thessaloniki, Greece

Veteran Affairs Medical Center and George Washington University, Washington, DC, USA

Brent M. Egan University of South Carolina School of Medicine–Greenville, Care Coordination Institute, Greenville, SC, USA

Charles Faselis Veterans Affairs Medical Center, and George Washington University School of Medicine, Washington, DC, USA

Keith C. Ferdinand Tulane Heart and Vascular Institute, Tulane University School of Medicine, New Orleans, LA, USA

Christina Filippou Clinical Dietician-Nutritionist. First Cardiology Clinic, Hippokration Hospital, University of Athens, Athens, Greece

Takeshi Fujiwara Division of Cardiovascular Medicine, Department of Medicine, Jichi Medical University School of Medicine, Shimotsuke, Japan

Higashiagatsuma-machi National Health Insurance Clinic, Gunma, Japan

Charalampia V. Geladari Fourth Internal Medicine Department, Evangelismos State General Hospital, Athens, Greece

Department of Medicine, Division of Cardiology, Beth Israel Deaconess Medical Center, Harvard Medical School, Boston, MA, USA

Anna-Bettina Haidich Department of Hygiene, Social-Preventive Medicine and Medical Statistics, Medical School, Aristotle University of Thessaloniki, Thessaloniki, Greece

Pedro A. Jose Division of Renal Diseases & Hypertension, The George Washington University School of Medicine & Health Sciences, Washington, DC, USA

Department of Medicine and Department of Pharmacology and Physiology, The George Washington University School of Medicine & Health Sciences, Washington, DC, USA

Thomas Karagiannis Hippokration General Hospital, Thessaloniki, Greece

Clinical Research and Evidence-Based Medicine Unit, Aristotle University of Thessaloniki, Thessaloniki, Greece

Athanasia Kapota Hipporcration General Hospital of Athens, Athens, Greece

Kazuomi Kario Division of Cardiovascular Medicine, Department of Medicine, Jichi Medical University School of Medicine, Tochigi, Japan

John B. Kostis Cardiovascular Institute, Cardiovascular Research, John G. Detwiler Professor of Cardiology, Medicine and Pharmacology, Rutgers Robert Wood Johnson Medical School, Biomedical Engineering, Rutgers University, New Brunswick, NJ, USA

William J. Kostis Cardiovascular Institute, Rutgers Robert Wood Johnson Medical School, New Brunswick, NJ, USA

Medicine at Massachusetts General Hospital, Boston, MA, USA

Lei Lei Department of Hypertension, Shanghai Key Laboratory of Hypertension, Centre for Epidemiological Studies and Clinical Trials, The Shanghai Institute of Hypertension, Ruijin Hospital, Shanghai Jiao Tong University School of Medicine, Shanghai, China

Ping Li Washington Veterans Affairs Medical Center, Washington, DC, USA

Georgetown University Hospital, Washington, DC, USA

George Washington University School of Medicine, Washington, DC, USA

Nikolaos Magkas First Cardiology Clinic, Medical School, National and Kapodistrian University of Athens, Hippokration Hospital, Athens, Greece

Samar A. Nasser Department of Clinical Research & Leadership, School of Medicine and Health Sciences. The George Washington University, Washington, DC, USA

Jason V. Papademetriou Department of Mechanical Engineering, Boston University, Boston, MA, USA

Vasilios Papademetriou Georgetown University and VA Medical Center, Washington, DC, USA

Samir S. Patel George Washington University School of Medicine, Washington, DC, USA

Washington Veterans Affairs Medical Center, Washington, DC, USA

Spyros I. Siakavellas National and Kapodistrian University of Athens, Medical School, Academic Department of Gastroenterology, Laikon General Hospital, Athens, Greece

Costas Tsioufis VA Medical Center and Georgetown University, Washington, DC, USA

1st Academic Department of Cardiology, Athens, Greece

Van Anthony M. Villar Division of Renal Diseases & Hypertension, Department of Medicine, The George Washington University School of Medicine & Health Sciences, Washington, DC, USA

Ji-Guang Wang Centre for Epidemiological Studies and Clinical Trials, Shanghai Key Laboratory of Hypertension, The Shanghai Institute of Hypertension, Ruijin Hospital, Shanghai Jiaotong University School of Medicine, Shanghai, China

Part I

Introduction to Medical Research

The Importance of Applying Evidence-Based Medicine in Clinical Practice

1

Thomas Karagiannis

What Is Evidence-Based Medicine?

The first scientific origins of evidence-based medicine (EBM) can be traced back to mid-nineteenth century in the works of John Snow and Pierre Charles Alexandre Louis [1], or even earlier in James Lind's study on scurvy [2]. Despite these innovative attempts, clinical practice in medicine was still largely based on expert opinion, driven by physiological rationale and individual clinician's expertise. It was not until mid-twentieth century that the medical community began to realize that reliance on uncontrolled clinical experience and pathophysiological reasoning alone, was flawed [3]. In fact, in 1962 the Food and Drug Administration passed the Kefauver-Harris Amendment in the United States, which required evidence from rigorous clinical trials in order to determine drug efficacy [4]. Later, in the 1970s and 1980s, the seminal works of Archie Cochrane [5], David Eddy [6] and David Sackett [7] further highlighted the need for strengthening the empirical practice of medicine and established the key concepts behind evidence-based practice.

The first published use of the term "evidence-based" in medical literature appeared in a series of articles by D. Eddy in 1990 [8]. These papers discussed the limitations of expert opinion in medical decision making, but focused mainly on the development of clinical guidelines, arguing that these should be based on substantial evidence, rather than subjective judgment or consensus. In 1991, G.H. Guyatt introduced the term "evidence-based medicine", which differed from the definition proposed by D. Eddy, as it had a more clinical orientation, promoting the careful assessment of existing research evidence by physicians and its application in their daily decisions about individual patients [9]. A more comprehensive article, published a year later by the EBM Working Group, presented EBM as a novel paradigm in the teaching and practice of medicine [10], while the User's Guides to the Medical Literature series in JAMA brought the underlying concepts of EBM to the attention of a wider medical community [11]. Subsequently, the influence of EBM has been constantly growing worldwide, resulting in its recognition as one of the most important medical milestones since 1840 [12].

The Principles of Evidence-Based Medicine

In its most commonly cited definition, EBM is described as "the conscientious, explicit, and

T. Karagiannis (✉)
Clinical Research and Evidence-Based Medicine Unit, Aristotle University Thessaloniki, Thessaloniki, Greece
e-mail: tkaragian@auth.gr

V. Papademetriou et al. (eds.), *Management of Hypertension*,
https://doi.org/10.1007/978-3-319-92946-0_1

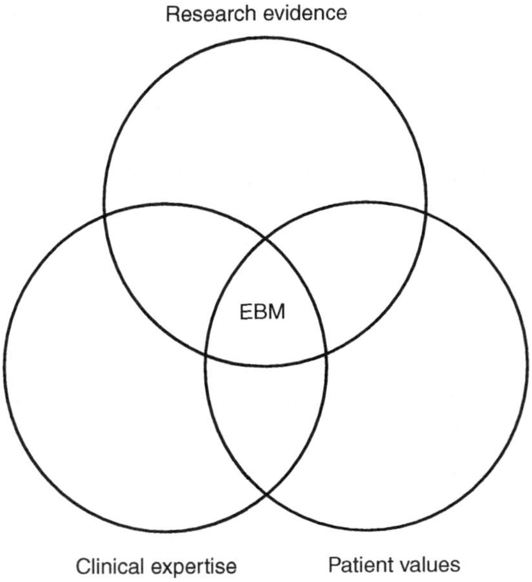

Fig. 1.1 The key principles of evidence-based medicine (EBM)

judicious use of current best evidence in making decisions about the care of individual patients. The practice of evidence based medicine means integrating individual clinical expertise with the best available external clinical evidence from systematic research" [13]. Later, this definition was refined, emphasizing the importance of patients' values and preferences in optimal clinical decision making. As a result, EBM can more accurately be described as the "integration of best research evidence with clinical expertise and patient values" [14], as depicted in Fig. 1.1. A variation of this characterization has also incorporated the clinical state and circumstances within the context of clinical expertise [15], while in a broader definition, that of evidence-based practice, health care resources are also considered an important parameter for optimal decision making [16]. Regardless of the exact definition used, the principles of EBM emphasize that all medical decisions about a therapeutic or diagnostic procedure should be based on high quality, up-to-date research evidence, acknowledge the importance of clinical expertise and intuition and highlight that patient value and preference judgements are implicit in every clinical decision.

Best Research Evidence

Research evidence originates from various types of studies, including laboratory observations, pathophysiologic studies, case reports, observational studies, or more advanced applied clinical research from randomized controlled trials (RCTs). EBM acknowledges that not all research is created equal and that some study designs are more suitable than others in answering specific research questions [1]. Therefore, EBM, from its early inception, has suggested a hierarchy for ranking the quality of evidence [17]. Figure 1.2 illustrates such a hierarchy framework of evidence. The pyramid shape is used to represent the decrease in risk of bias (or increase in quality) associated with each study type as one goes up the pyramid.

In this hierarchy, RCTs are placed at the highest level of the pyramid, thus represent the most reliable evidence for determining the effectiveness of medical interventions, as opposed to observational studies or other study designs. Notably, since the first documented report of an RCT in 1948 (streptomycin treatment for pulmonary tuberculosis [18]), the RCT has been considered as the most scientifically rigorous method for hypothesis testing [19]. In a typical RCT, participants are randomly allocated to one or another intervention and are followed for a specific period. At the end of the study, any differences observed in predefined outcomes are attributed solely to the trial intervention [19].

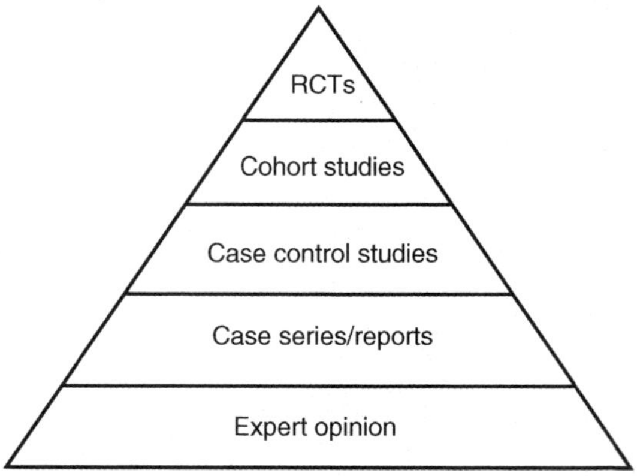

Fig. 1.2 The evidence-based medicine pyramid

However, it is now recognized that evidence from RCTs is not necessarily always of high quality and that not all research questions can be answered through an RCT [1]. For example, the diagnostic accuracy of a medical test can be answered from a well-conducted cross-sectional study, while an observational study is required for a question about prognosis [13]. On this account, a revised form of the traditional evidence pyramid has been proposed, in which the straight lines separating study types have been converted to wavy lines, suggesting that there is overlap in study quality among different designs [20]. For instance, it is possible that for a specific research question observational studies provide more reliable information than RCTs. Furthermore, quality of evidence does not depend solely on study type, but on other parameters as well, such as bias in study implementation, imprecision, inconsistency and indirectness. As a result, a more sophisticated approach to rating evidence quality has been developed, termed the Grades of Recommendation Assessment, Development and Evaluation (GRADE) system [21]. In the GRADE framework, non-RCTs begin as low-quality evidence, but can be rated up based on the parameters mentioned above, as opposed to RCTs, that start at high level and can be rated down.

Systematic reviews and meta-analyses are an additional important tool of EBM [22]. A systematic review provides a summary of all primary studies about a specific clinical question, using predefined methods for identifying, critically appraising and synthesizing all available research evidence. Due to their explicit methodology and cumulative data synthesis, systematic reviews are considered to provide more reliable and accurate conclusions compared to individual studies [22].

Clinical Expertise

The practice of EBM dictates that research evidence alone is inadequate for optimal decision making if the information is not efficiently combined with clinical expertise. Clinical expertise includes the general basic skills and proficiency acquired through clinical practice, as well as the experience of the individual practitioner [23]. Clinical expertise can be reflected in many ways, including obtaining the right diagnosis, determining relevant treatment options and placing research evidence within the context of the individual patient's clinical state and circumstances [23, 24].

Obtaining a history and conducting a physical examination are essential skills for getting the right diagnosis, that come only from thorough background training and clinical experience [24]. In addition, many diagnostic tests may differ in their accuracy depending on the skill of the practitioner [10]. In a similar manner, the effectiveness and complications associated with therapeutic interventions, particularly surgical interventions, can also depend on individual clinician's experience and skills [10]. Finally, after obtaining the best relevant research evidence, the clinician, using sound clinical judgement, must determine whether the external evidence can be applied to the individual patient. In doing so, the clinician must consider all relevant comorbidities that may influence the treatment effect, in addition to research-related factors, such as whether the available studies have measured all important outcomes, included relevant comparators and have a reasonable follow up period [24, 25]. Additional features of clinical expertise are related to the ability to provide patients with the information they need in a manner that facilitates informed decision making and developing values such as integrity, compassion, respect and sustained professional curiosity [15, 26].

A concise definition summarizing all the essential characteristics that constitute clinical expertise, has been given by W.S. Richardson: "Clinical expertise includes the deliberate practice of communication skills, clinical skills, and decision skills, as well as the experiential learning that comes through the care of sick persons, with the development of clinical judgment" [26].

Patient Values and Preferences

Clinical expertise and knowing the best research evidence are necessary, but insufficient for delivering the highest quality of care. The third key principle of EBM advocates that clinical decisions and recommendations must attend to the values and preferences of the informed patient. This patient centered approach means that it is not the clinician who should exclusively decide what will happen to the patient, but it is also the patient's right to participate in decision making about their treatment options or diagnostic procedures [27].

Values and preferences refer to patient characteristics that can variably affect decision making during the clinical encounter. These may include experience of former and current illnesses or other relevant life experiences, health habits, goals and expectations, social or family support, and personal beliefs about medical interventions [26]. Depending on these factors, patients may have either no views or unchangeable views on how to proceed with their treatment or diagnostic options. Of note, research has shown that considerable variation exists between physicians' and patients' preferences when it comes to weighting the benefits and drawbacks of therapeutic options [28]. Moreover, patients' actions may differ not only from their clinician's advice, but also from the preferences and views they expressed during the clinical consultation [15]. Thus, in addition to exploring patients' perceptions and values, a clinician should ideally be able to understand the procedures individuals use to consider their treatment options, in order to assess whether patients are likely to adhere to their prescriptions and therapeutic recommendations [29, 30].

From an ethical point of view, respecting patients' preferences should be justified on moral grounds alone [31]. Patient centered care has a theoretical foundation in the principle of patient autonomy, a belief that originates from the patients' rights movement in the 1960s [32]. Since then, several medical associations, institutions and health planners have endorsed and incorporated patient centered care in their guidelines, recommendations and policies. In fact, the National Health Service Constitution in the United Kingdom advocates patient participation in decision making [33], while in the United States, the Institute of Medicine, in its "Quality Chasm" report, has designated evidence-based patient centered care as one of six key elements of high quality care [34].

Applying Evidence-Based Medicine in Clinical Practice

The practice of EBM involves a multi-stage process [35]. First, the clinical problem must be translated into an answerable question. Subsequently, one needs to retrieve the best evidence that answers this question and critically appraise the findings with respect to their validity and usefulness. The fourth step involves implementing the results of the appraisal into clinical practice, while the final step is related to evaluating the effectiveness and efficiency in executing previous steps and seeking ways to improve them [35].

It has been suggested that clinicians can incorporate this five-step process into their practices in three different ways [35]. First, in the "doing" mode, at least the four first steps are followed before a medical decision is made. In the "using" mode, step 3 is skipped by restricting the search to evidence that has already undergone critical appraisal, such as databases of guidelines or pre-appraised information. Finally, in the "replicating" mode, decisions are based on respected leaders' opinion, thus both steps 2 and 3 are omitted. Ideally, the "doing" mode should be followed in most cases, however depending on the specific clinical problem they encounter, physicians can move back and forth between the three modes [35].

Formulating an Answerable Question

The practice of EBM should begin with a well formulated clinical question. Several times a day, physicians are asked to come up with answers to various clinical problems in order to make medical decisions. Questions that arise for most clinical situations are typically divided into two broad categories [36]:

- Quantitative questions, which aim to discover cause and effect relationships by comparing two or more individuals or groups based on differing outcomes associated with exposures or interventions.
- Qualitative questions, which aim to discover meaning or gain an understanding of a phenomena.

A more detailed categorization of clinical questions, based on their type and the respective study design that is most appropriate to provide answers, is presented in Table 1.1.

The questions that arise may be unstructured and complex at first, but it is important that they are translated in a clear form before proceeding to literature search. A good clinical question should be directly focused on the problem at hand and structured in a form that can be answered by searching the medical literature [37]. Without a well-formulated question, it can be impractical and very time consuming to search for and identify relevant evidence. Practitioners of EBM often use a specialized framework, called PICO, to form more focused and relevant questions [38]. PICO stands for Patient (or condition), Intervention (or diagnostic test or exposure), Comparison, and Outcome (or diagnosis/development/prevention of a condition). The PICO format can be expanded to PICOT, adding information about the Type of question being asked (for example therapy, diagnosis, prognosis) or the most appropriate study design for that particular question [39]. Notably, research has shown that the PICO format can help clinicians formulate more precise questions and develop more detailed search strategies [40, 41].

Identifying the Best Evidence

After having formulated an answerable and clinically relevant question, the next step is to track down the best available research evidence. In years past, searching for answers in the medical literature was a very daunting process, but nowadays the development of internet and large electronic databases has made searching and retrieval of information much easier. To further facilitate the identification of high quality evidence for a particular clinical problem, the EBM Working Group, in its guidance series, originally proposed a 4S model for ranking the quality and validity of various sources of evidence [24]. This 4S model has now been refined to a 6S pyramid that represents a hierarchy of six literature sources [42]. Similarly to the hierarchy based on study design, the quality of evidence increases as one goes up the pyramid. As illustrated in Fig. 1.3, the 6S pyramid begins with original primary studies and builds up to synopses of studies, syntheses (systematic reviews), synopses of syntheses, evidence summaries and systems [42].

When using the 6S model to retrieve research evidence, one should begin their search at the highest layer. Ideally this would be the "systems" layer, placed at the peak of the pyramid. "Systems" refer to computerized decision support systems, in which individual patient's characteristics are automatically linked (through

Table 1.1 Types of clinical questions and appropriate study designs

Type of question	Interpretation	Type of study
Treatment	How do we select among different treatments?	Randomized controlled trial
Diagnosis	How do we identify whether a person has a specific condition?	Randomized controlled trial or cross-sectional study
Prognosis	What is a patient's likely clinical course over time?	Cohort study
Etiology/prevention	How do we identify/prevent the causes of a specific condition?	Cohort study
Experiences	How does it feel to have a specific condition?	Qualitative study

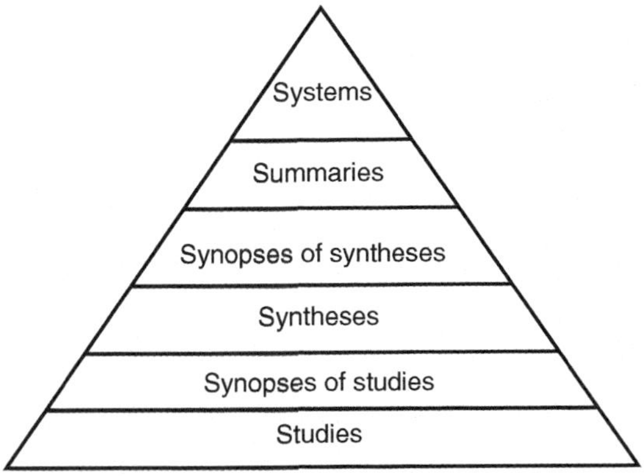

Fig. 1.3 The 6S pyramid of evidence sources

an electronic health record) to all important research evidence that are relevant to a specific clinical problem [43]. Subsequently, all key information is concisely summarized for clinicians in the form of patient-specific assessments or recommendations. However, to date few such systems are available, therefore one would need to look for "summaries" as the next best source. These "summaries" include pre-appraised resources of evidence that are regularly updated and integrate evidence-based information about specific clinical problems [42]. Such sources include DynaMed [44], UpToDate [45], BMJ Clinical Evidence [46] and BMJ Best Practice [47]. An additional type of pre-appraised summaries are clinical practice guidelines, provided they are based on comprehensive search and appraisal of the literature and report levels of evidence for each recommendation.

If a clinical question cannot be answered through a "summary", then a synopsis of a synthesis (systematic review) is the next stop. A good synopsis summarizes the main methods and findings of a high quality systematic review, providing sufficient information to support clinical action [42]. Such synopses are available in the Database of Abstracts of Reviews of Effects (DARE) [48] and in specific journals, including ACP Journal Club [49] and Evidence-Based Medicine [50]. Notably, other than systematic review summaries, these evidence-based abstraction journals also provide summaries of individual primary studies.

If more detail is needed or no synopsis is available, one should look for original systematic reviews or primary studies. These can be identified through search of electronic databases, such as PubMed, EMBASE and the Cochrane Library, by using relevant keywords (based on the PICO format of the clinical question) and specific study type search filters [51]. Finally, search engines like TRIP [52] or Epistemonikos [53] sort evidence across a broad range of various sources, including guidelines, structured summaries, systematic reviews and primary studies.

Critically Appraising the Evidence

Not all published research is good or even transferable to a particular patient. Therefore, the evidence retrieved from the literature search during step 2 must be critically appraised in terms of its quality (internal validity) and generalizability or applicability (external validity) [54]. Assessment of external validity of research findings is an issue regardless of the source of evidence, as it is related to whether the patient of interest differs significantly with the reference population, in terms of clinical or demographic characteristics, such as comorbidity, age, stage of disease, overall health status or concomitant medications. With regards to internal validity, it is reasonable to assume that evidence from most pre-appraised literature sources has been adequately peer-reviewed beforehand; however, this is not the case with primary research, such as individual studies, systematic reviews or even some guidelines. On this account, expert committees have issued formal guidance for optimal reporting for different types of studies. These are available at the EQUATOR website [55] and include CONSORT [56], STROBE [57], PRISMA [58] and RIGHT [59] statements for RCTs, observational studies, systematic reviews and clinical practice guidelines, respectively. In addition, useful tools for critical appraisal covering a wide range of research designs have been developed by the Critical Appraisal Skills Programme (CASP) and are freely available online [60].

Implementing the Results in Clinical Practice

The fourth step is perhaps the most complex, as it involves adjusting the evidence findings to the unique clinical circumstances, personal values and preferences of an individual patient. Under this premise, all relevant key evidence should be fully discussed during the clinical consultation, allowing for a therapeutic alliance to be formed between the patient and the clinician [37]. In particular, information should be tailored to patients' needs in order to permit meaningful deliberation and ideally facilitate shared decision making [31]. The shared decision making model has been seen as a mechanism of decreasing the informational and power asymmetry between patient and physician, by increasing patients' knowledge, enhancing their sense of autonomy and engaging them in making decisions, insofar as they wish to participate [61]. Shared decision making is increasingly advocated as an ideal model for most medical encounters and several countries have adopted policies that support its implementation within their healthcare systems [62]. It should be noted however, that shared decision making does not mean merely presenting the patient with a series of decision options alongside their respective advantages and drawbacks. Instead, real shared decision making involves introducing research evidence in a way that informs a dialogue about what matters to the patient, what is the best course of action and how this may affect the patient's well-being [63].

To facilitate this patient centered approach, a variety of tools for use during the clinical consultation have been developed for several medical conditions. According to a Cochrane systematic review, these decisions aids are "interventions that support patients by making their decisions explicit, providing information about options and associated benefits/harms, and helping clarify congruence between decisions and personal values" [64]. Two distinct types of decision aids have been described, patient decision aids (PtDAs) and conversation aids. Both types include a concise description of current research evidence about a medical condition and relevant treatment (or diagnostic) options, in a manner that can be easily understandable by patients [65]. However, while PtDAs aim is to improve patient knowledge and encourage patient involvement in decision making, conversation aids take this process one step further, by directly supporting and improving the quality of conversations that patients and clinicians have when making decisions together [66].

Evaluating the Overall Process

The fifth and final step involves evaluation our overall approach at frequent intervals in order to decide whether we need to improve any of the four steps. During this process, we need to ask whether we have formulated answerable questions, effectively identified and critically appraised the literature and integrated best available evidence with our clinical expertise and patient's values in the decision making [37]. In addition, it is also important to assess whether our overall approach has had a favorable effect on patient important outcomes. Interestingly, self-evaluation tools in practicing EBM are available online [67], while, according to a Cochrane systematic review, external audit and feedback on the practice of healthcare professionals can improve their performance [68].

The Importance of Evidence-Based Medicine

Despite its widespread recognition, EBM has also received criticism both by clinicians and researchers. However, as explained below, most of these criticisms are misperceptions, either of the definition of EBM or the way it should be practiced. Once cleared up, these misinterpretations highlight the benefits and importance of EBM.

Evidence-Based Medicine Is Superior to Experience-Based Medicine

Given that clinical practice has long been dominated by expert opinion and many guideline committees have used, and probably still use, expert consensus to make recommendations, one could argue that physiological reasoning and expert opinion should be the main drivers in clinical decision making. It has also been claimed that EBM does not represent a scientific approach to medicine and that reliance research evidence when making medical decisions, is problematic [69].

However, there are many examples where EBM, through the use of either RCTs or systematic reviews, has rightfully questioned unsubstantiated therapeutic claims of interventions that were later proven to be ineffective or even harmful [24]. It was only after the completion of RCTs, that administration of growth hormone in critically ill patients [70], ibopamine [71] and epoprostonol [72] in heart failure, and beta-carotene in patients with prior myocardial infarction [73] were associated with an increased mortality rate. Similarly, an RCT was necessary to establish the favorable effects of beta-blockers in reducing mortality in congestive heart failure, despite long-held beliefs that their negative inotropic action would be detrimental to these patients [74]. Well-conducted systematic reviews have equally contributed in improving the standards of healthcare [1]. Such examples include incorporating use of short course of oral steroids for community-acquired pneumonia [75] and establishing standards of care for early breast cancer [76]. Moreover, uptake of guidelines can have a major beneficial community effect, provided their development is supported by robust research evidence, as demonstrated by a decrease in asthma-related morbidity and mortality [77] and reductions in thromboembolic complications [78]. Of note, the Academy of Medical Royal Colleges in the United Kingdom has recently launched a booklet titled "Evidence based medicine matters", which contains 15 examples where EBM has benefited clinical practice in various medical specialties [79].

Evidence-Based Medicine Encourages the Development of Clinical Skills and Expertise

A common criticism of EBM is that it represents a "cookbook" in the sense that it regards clinical expertise mainly as a matter of collecting, analyzing and summarizing research done by others [80]. It has also been suggested that EBM, by encouraging blind adherence to guidelines, has shifted clinical decision making from the consultation room to the "professional association" [27].

Nevertheless, since the inception of EBM, its proponents have highlighted that external clinical evidence should not replace, but complement a physician's clinical intuition and judgement during the decision making process [13]. In fact, the original guidance series issued by the EBM Working Group underscore that a good understanding of the pathophysiological background of the disease in addition to clinical skills, such as careful history taking and physical examination, play a crucial part in the implementation of EBM [10]. Moreover, it is highlighted that teachers of EBM should be exceptional clinicians with a talent of precise observation, a gift for intuitive diagnosis and excellent judgment in making difficult management decisions [10]. Therefore, rather than diminishing the role of expertise and judicious clinical judgment, appropriate application of EBM values experiential thinking and encourages physicians to continuously improve or acquire new clinical skills. Even though some practitioners of EBM may also do research, it is important to remember that its practice is a method for providing care for patients and not a method for performing research [35].

Patients Are at the Core of Evidence-Based Medicine

Evidence-based medicine has also been accused that it disregards patients' unique knowledge and experience and ignores their needs and preferences [81]. Sweeney et al. suggest that EBM represents a doctor centered, rather than a patient centered, approach, claiming that it focuses on the clinician's interpretation of the evidence and diminishes the importance of human relationships and the patient's role in decision making [82].

Again, these claims are inconsistent with the true definition of EBM. The practice of EBM strongly emphasizes the importance of adjusting the evidence to patients' preferences and incorporating their personal values and perspective into decision making. Moreover, shared decision making, albeit originally developed as a separate concept, is now being recognized as an integral component of the third principle of EBM [83]. Without shared decision making, authentic EBM cannot occur, since it is only through evidence-informed deliberations that patients can construct informed preferences and subsequently incorporate the evidence, along with their values and their clinician's expertise, into their decision making [83]. As a result, in recent years a lot of research has focused on how to effectively implement shared decision making using decision aid tools. Interestingly, a recent Cochrane systematic review has identified 105 RCTs of shared decision making tools, assessing 50 different decisions and involving approximately 31,000 patients [64].

Implementation of Evidence-Based Medicine Is Practical and Not Time-Consuming

It is true that certain skills, such as being able to identify and critically appraise research evidence, are prerequisites for effective application of EBM. On this account, one could claim that EBM is intended only for those few who have the time and resources to develop these skills and implement them in their daily clinical practice. This argument, often cited as the "ivory tower" concept, suggests that most busy clinicians are not able keep pace with the rapid advances in healthcare research and are unwilling to invest additional time in acquiring EBM skills [35].

To overcome these time-related barriers and facilitate faster retrieval of high quality evidence, EBM makes use of systematic reviews and more importantly of sources of pre-appraised evidence [42], which can be quickly assessed at the point of care [84]. Even when searching for primary studies is deemed necessary, use of certain search strategy guidance [51] or certain applications, such as PubMed Clinical Queries [85], can help save considerable time. Finally, according to survey studies, most physicians have shown interest in acquiring EBM skills [35], which can be done at any stage of the clinical training, even during medical school. In fact, a cross-sectional study has shown that early introduction of EBM in pre-clinical years was favorable for students and enabled them to critically apprehend and appraise new research findings and medical innovations [86].

Evidence-Based Medicine Makes Effective Use of Different Types of Research

EBM has been criticized for placing great focus on RCTs, resulting in lack of applicability in individual patients, as well as being largely industry driven [69]. However, these claims do not do justice to EBM. Although RCTs are usually considered the "gold standard" for establishing the effects of an intervention, EBM recognizes that other study designs are more suitable for providing answers about diagnosis, prognosis or harms [35]. Moreover, from its early days, EBM has acknowledged the necessity for individualization of care. In particular, EBM has provided guidance on the credibility of subgroup analyses and the effect of baseline characteristics on treatment outcomes [87]. Additionally, it has championed N of 1 trials, which are conducted in individual patients in whom the benefits and harms of treatments are uncertain [88]. Finally, EBM has given great consideration to issues related to researchers' conflicts of interest and industry's influence on the publication of research findings [89].

Uptake of Evidence-Based Medicine Can Improve Healthcare-Related Outcomes

It is reasonable for critics of EBM to ask for actual evidence that practicing EBM can actually improve patient outcomes [90]. However, assessing the effectiveness of EBM as a whole concept is most likely impractical, as it is not clear how to define "non evidence-based" medical practice, while it is also questionable whether withholding access to evidence from a control arm would be ethical [35]. However, research has been done on evaluating various individual steps of the EBM process, mainly related to identification or application of evidence retrieved from literature searches, and implementation of shared decision making.

In a cross-sectional study, rapid answering strategies based on searching PubMed and Epistemonikos proved feasible to implement by internal medicine clinicians and provided appropriate guidance for clinical questions [91]. In another study, 33 internal medicine physicians were presented with research information from standardized literature searches, after they had committed to a specific diagnosis and treatment plan for 146 inpatients [92]. Physicians changed treatment for 23 (18%) patients, while quality of patient care, as judged by an independent panel, improved in 18 (78%) of these patients [92].

Moreover, a study comparing hospitals with online access to UpToDate with other acute care hospitals, found that hospitals with UpToDate access were associated with significantly lower mortality and complications rates and a shorter length of stay [93]. In a similar retrospective study, in addition to reduced mortality and shorter length of stay, hospitals that had adopted UpToDate demonstrated higher quality performance across various inpatient quality measures for four common medical conditions [94].

Furthermore, a systematic review of studies that evaluated shared decision making, concluded that patients reporting that they had participated in shared decision making, are likely to enjoy better affective-cognitive outcomes, such as improved satisfaction and decisional comfort [95]. Finally, according to a Cochrane systematic review on decision aids, patients exposed to decision aids had better knowledge about treatment options and outcomes, felt clearer about their values, and were more likely to actively engage in decision making, in comparison to usual care [64].

Current Challenges and Future Implications

Despite its numerous achievements and benefits, EBM is not devoid of barriers or limitations. Leaders and proponents of EBM have highlighted that EBM is an evolving concept, and cautioned against its inappropriate use [29, 96]. Recently, a report summarizing the current challenges of EBM has been published in The BMJ [96], while a relevant website, named EBM manifesto [97], has been developed with the intention to encourage working groups to identify, suggest and implement solutions for better evidence and healthcare. Based on these data, the key challenges of EBM at its current state are mainly related to improving the quality and applicability of research and facilitating its efficient uptake in clinical practice.

A Call for Improving the Applicability of Primary Research

As mentioned earlier, an important disadvantage of RCTs is their limited generalizability in real-world patients, given that they recruit selected patients who fulfil specific eligibility criteria and are studied under a highly controlled environment. As a result, there is an increasing call from the medical and academic community for trials that produce more transferable findings to the daily clinical practice [98]. On this account, pragmatic trials have been proposed as a viable alternative to RCTs. Such trials are conducted under usual conditions, have broad inclusive criteria and offer practitioners considerable freedom in deciding how to apply the intervention or comparators of interest [99]. Pragmatic trials aim to answer the clinically relevant question of "which of two (or more) treatments should we prefer" for our real-world patients, as opposed to traditional explanatory RCTs, which address "whether a difference exists between two treatments (one usually being a placebo) that are specified by strict definitions" [99]. Of note, specific tools related to both the design and critical appraisal of pragmatic trials have been developed [100, 101]. Notably, randomized registry trials are an innovative type of pragmatic trials that can further facilitate the incorporation or "real-world data" in primary research [102]. In a randomized registry trial, a clinical registry can be used to identify patients for enrolment, perform randomization, collect baseline variables, and detect end points. In comparison to traditional RCTs, they are inexpensive, less selective and enable fast enrolment and the possibility of very long-term follow-up [102].

A Need for More Patient-Oriented Research

Patient centered care may have acquired a prominent role in the healthcare agenda of various nations and medical associations, however considerable efforts are still required in order to determine what patients consider important and to ensure that their expectations are met by healthcare providers [31]. In addition to shifting the focus from clinically important outcomes to patient important outcomes [103], the field of patient-oriented care would be significantly enriched by qualitative research. Indeed, a lot of people in the EBM community acknowledge the utility of qualitative research in describing patients' experience and understanding their views [104]. Qualitative research can yield more valid information about subjective experiences, whereas a quantitative study might lose this depth and meaning [105]. In addition, information from qualitative studies may highlight important areas which require further quantitative assessment. Therefore, qualitative research should be viewed as complementary to quantitative research, and not as a type of study with lesser validity and robustness.

Moreover, despite the considerable progress that has occurred in the field of shared decision making during the last decade, current research has not yet established the link between shared decision making and patient behavioral or health outcomes [95]. Therefore, future studies should assess the impact of shared decision making across a continuum of outcomes and clinical settings and address the methodological challenges on how best to measure shared decision making [95]. Furthermore, it is unknown whether currently available decision aid tools can actually promote patient participation in making important healthcare decisions, other than merely presenting a summary of relevant research information [106]. On this account, future research should probably focus on designing more efficient and practical conversation aids that make intellectual and emotional sense to patients and encourage them to have meaningful conversations with their clinician [106].

Bridging the Gap Between Research and Clinical Practice

Engaging healthcare professionals in learning EBM and making it part of their clinical routine has always been one of the main challenges of EBM. To achieve a wider and more efficient uptake of EBM in daily clinical practice, physicians should be introduced to its principles at an early stage of their professional development, ideally during their medical training. Indeed, the need to develop a curriculum outlining the minimum standard requirements for training health professionals in EBM is now well recognized [107]. Other methods of teaching EBM to practice clinicians include morning reports, teaching conferences, and journal clubs [108]. However, EBM is best taught at the bedside, on the grounds that it is all about practicing medicine on actual patients at a real clinical setting and not about doing research. In addition, timely uptake and application of evidence-based knowledge requires, not only ready access to modern and high-quality information sources, but also efficient production and dissemination of both systematic reviews and practice guidelines [109]. In turn, this can be accomplished by creating experienced research teams focused in producing rigorous evidence summaries and in developing electronic platforms that facilitate rapid updating of the medical literature [1].

References

1. Djulbegovic B, Guyatt GH. Progress in evidence-based medicine: a quarter century on. Lancet. 2017;390(10092):415–23.
2. Bartholomew M. James Lind's treatise of the scurvy (1753). Postgrad Med J. 2002;78(925):695–6.
3. Eddy DM. Evidence-based medicine: a unified approach. Health Aff. 2005;24(1):9–17.
4. Greene JA, Podolsky SH. Reform, regulation, and pharmaceuticals–the Kefauver-Harris Amendments at 50. N Engl J Med. 2012;367(16):1481–3.
5. Cochrane AL. Archie Cochrane in his own words. Selections arranged from his 1972 introduction to "effectiveness and efficiency: random reflections on the health services" 1972. Control Clin Trials. 1989;10(4):428–33.
6. Eddy D. ACS report on the cancer-related health checkup. CA Cancer J Clin. 1980;30(4):193–240.
7. Sackett DL. Rules of evidence and clinical recommendations on the use of antithrombotic agents. Chest. 1986;89(2 Suppl):2S–3S.
8. Eddy DM. Practice policies: where do they come from? JAMA. 1990;263(9):1265, 9, 72 passim.
9. Guyatt GH. Evidence-based medicine. ACP J Club. 1991;114:A16.
10. Evidence-Based Medicine Working G. Evidence-based medicine. A new approach to teaching the practice of medicine. JAMA. 1992;268(17):2420–5.
11. Guyatt GH, Rennie D. Users' guides to the medical literature. JAMA. 1993;270(17):2096–7.
12. Dickersin K, Straus SE, Bero LA. Evidence based medicine: increasing, not dictating, choice. BMJ. 2007;334(Suppl 1):s10.
13. Sackett DL, Rosenberg WM, Gray JA, Haynes RB, Richardson WS. Evidence based medicine: what it is and what it isn't. 1996. Clin Orthop Relat Res. 2007;455:3–5.
14. Sackett DL, Strauss SE, Richardson WS, Rosenberg W, Haynes RB. Evidence-based medicine: how to practice and teach EBM. 2nd ed. Edinburgh: Churchill Livingstone; 2000.
15. Haynes RB, Devereaux PJ, Guyatt GH. Clinical expertise in the era of evidence-based medicine and patient choice. ACP J Club. 2002;136(2):A11–4.
16. McMaster University Health Sciences. Resources for evidence-based practice: About EBP. Available from: http://hsl.mcmaster.libguides.com/c.php?g=306765&p=2044668.
17. Guyatt GH, Sackett DL, Sinclair JC, Hayward R, Cook DJ, Cook RJ. Users' guides to the medical literature. IX. A method for grading health care recommendations. Evidence-Based Medicine Working Group. JAMA. 1995;274(22):1800–4.
18. Streptomycin treatment of pulmonary tuberculosis. Br Med J. 1948;2(4582):769–82.
19. Akobeng AK. Understanding randomised controlled trials. Arch Dis Child. 2005;90(8):840–4.
20. Murad MH, Asi N, Alsawas M, Alahdab F. New evidence pyramid. Evid Based Med. 2016;21(4):125–7.
21. Atkins D, Best D, Briss PA, Eccles M, Falck-Ytter Y, Flottorp S, et al. Grading quality of evidence and strength of recommendations. BMJ. 2004;328(7454):1490.
22. Akobeng AK. Understanding systematic reviews and meta-analysis. Arch Dis Child. 2005;90(8):845–8.
23. Price AI, Djulbegovic B, Biswas R, Chatterjee P. Evidence-based medicine meets person-centred care: a collaborative perspective on the relationship. J Eval Clin Pract. 2015;21(6):1047–51.
24. Guyatt GH, Haynes RB, Jaeschke RZ, Cook DJ, Green L, Naylor CD, et al. Users' Guides to the Medical Literature: XXV. Evidence-based medicine: principles for applying the Users' Guides to patient care. Evidence-Based Medicine Working Group. JAMA. 2000;284(10):1290–6.
25. Richardson WS, Doster LM. Comorbidity and multimorbidity need to be placed in the context of a framework of risk, responsiveness, and vulnerability. J Clin Epidemiol. 2014;67(3):244–6.
26. Richardson WS. The practice of evidence-based medicine involves the care of whole persons. J Clin Epidemiol. 2017;84:18–21.
27. Bensing J. Bridging the gap. The separate worlds of evidence-based medicine and patient-centered medicine. Patient Educ Couns. 2000;39(1):17–25.
28. Devereaux PJ, Anderson DR, Gardner MJ, Putnam W, Flowerdew GJ, Brownell BF, et al. Differences between perspectives of physicians and patients on anticoagulation in patients with atrial fibrillation: observational study. BMJ. 2001;323(7323):1218–22.
29. Montori VM, Guyatt GH. Progress in evidence-based medicine. JAMA. 2008;300(15):1814–6.
30. Stephenson BJ, Rowe BH, Haynes RB, Macharia WM, Leon G. The rational clinical examination. Is this patient taking the treatment as prescribed? JAMA. 1993;269(21):2779–81.
31. Epstein RM, Street RL Jr. The values and value of patient-centered care. Ann Fam Med. 2011;9(2):100–3.
32. Laine C, Davidoff F. Patient-centered medicine. A professional evolution. JAMA. 1996;275(2):152–6.
33. The NHS Constitution for England. Available from: https://www.gov.uk/government/publications/the-nhs-constitution-for-england/the-nhs-constitution-for-england.
34. Institute of Medicine (US) Committee on Quality of Health Care in America. Crossing the quality chasm: a new health system for the 21st century. Washington (DC): National Academies Press (US); 2001.
35. Straus SE, McAlister FA. Evidence-based medicine: a commentary on common criticisms. CMAJ. 2000;163(7):837–41.

36. McMaster University Health Sciences. Resources for evidence-based practice: forming questions. Available from: https://hslmcmaster.libguides.com/c.php?g=306765&p=2044787.
37. Akobeng AK. Principles of evidence based medicine. Arch Dis Child. 2005;90(8):837–40.
38. Richardson WS, Wilson MC, Nishikawa J, Hayward RS. The well-built clinical question: a key to evidence-based decisions. ACP J Club. 1995;123(3):A12–3.
39. Schardt C, Adams MB, Owens T, Keitz S, Fontelo P. Utilization of the PICO framework to improve searching PubMed for clinical questions. BMC Med Inform Decis Mak. 2007;7:16.
40. Villanueva EV, Burrows EA, Fennessy PA, Rajendran M, Anderson JN. Improving question formulation for use in evidence appraisal in a tertiary care setting: a randomised controlled trial [ISRCTN66375463]. BMC Med Inform Decis Mak. 2001;1:4.
41. Booth A, O'Rourke AJ, Ford NJ. Structuring the pre-search reference interview: a useful technique for handling clinical questions. Bull Med Libr Assoc. 2000;88(3):239–46.
42. DiCenso A, Bayley L, Haynes RB, ACP Journal Club. Editorial: Accessing preappraised evidence: fine-tuning the 5S model into a 6S model. Ann Intern Med. 2009;151(6):JC3–2–3.
43. Garg AX, Adhikari NK, McDonald H, Rosas-Arellano MP, Devereaux PJ, Beyene J, et al. Effects of computerized clinical decision support systems on practitioner performance and patient outcomes: a systematic review. JAMA. 2005;293(10):1223–38.
44. DynaMed. Available from: http://www.dynamed.com/home/.
45. UpToDate. Available from: https://www.uptodate.com/home.
46. BMJ Clinical Evidence. Available from: http://www.clinicalevidence.com/x/index.html.
47. BMJ Best Practice. Available from: http://bestpractice.bmj.com/info/.
48. CRD Database. Available from: https://www.crd.york.ac.uk/CRDWeb/Homepage.asp.
49. ACP Journal Club Archives. Available from: http://www.acpjc.org/.
50. Evidence-Based Medicine. Available from: http://ebm.bmj.com/.
51. Ho GJ, Liew SM, Ng CJ, Hisham Shunmugam R, Glasziou P. Development of a search strategy for an evidence based retrieval service. PLoS One. 2016;11(12):e0167170.
52. Trip. Available from: https://www.tripdatabase.com/.
53. Epistemonikos. Available from: https://www.epistemonikos.org/en/.
54. Slack MK, Draugalis JR. Establishing the internal and external validity of experimental studies. Am J Health Syst Pharm AJHP. 2001;58(22):2173–81; quiz 82–3.
55. Enhancing the QUAlity and Transparency of health Research (EQUATOR). Available from: http://www.equator-network.org/.
56. Schulz KF, Altman DG, Moher D, Group C. CONSORT 2010 statement: updated guidelines for reporting parallel group randomized trials. Ann Intern Med. 2010;152(11):726–32.
57. von Elm E, Altman DG, Egger M, Pocock SJ, Gotzsche PC, Vandenbroucke JP, et al. Strengthening the Reporting of Observational Studies in Epidemiology (STROBE) statement: guidelines for reporting observational studies. BMJ. 2007;335(7624):806–8.
58. Moher D, Liberati A, Tetzlaff J, Altman DG, Group P. Preferred reporting items for systematic reviews and meta-analyses: the PRISMA statement. PLoS Med. 2009;6(7):e1000097.
59. Chen Y, Yang K, Marusic A, Qaseem A, Meerpohl JJ, Flottorp S, et al. A reporting tool for practice guidelines in health care: the RIGHT statement. Ann Intern Med. 2017;166(2):128–32.
60. Critical Appraisal Skills Programme (CASP). Available from: http://www.casp-uk.net/casp-tools-checklists.
61. Charles C, Gafni A, Whelan T. Shared decision-making in the medical encounter: what does it mean? (or it takes at least two to tango). Soc Sci Med. 1997;44(5):681–92.
62. Stiggelbout AM, Van der Weijden T, De Wit MP, Frosch D, Legare F, Montori VM, et al. Shared decision making: really putting patients at the centre of healthcare. BMJ. 2012;344:e256.
63. Greenhalgh T, Howick J, Maskrey N, Evidence Based Medicine Renaissance G. Evidence based medicine: a movement in crisis? BMJ. 2014;348:g3725.
64. Stacey D, Legare F, Lewis K, Barry MJ, Bennett CL, Eden KB, et al. Decision aids for people facing health treatment or screening decisions. Cochrane Database Syst Rev. 2017;4:CD001431.
65. Elwyn G, Frosch D, Volandes AE, Edwards A, Montori VM. Investing in deliberation: a definition and classification of decision support interventions for people facing difficult health decisions. Med Decis Mak. 2010;30(6):701–11.
66. Kunneman M, Montori VM, Castaneda-Guarderas A, Hess EP. What is shared decision making? (and what it is not). Acad Emerg Med Off J Soc Acad Emerg Med. 2016;23(12):1320–4.
67. Evidence-Based Medicine Toolbox. Available from: https://ebm-tools.knowledgetranslation.net/self-evaluation.
68. Ivers N, Jamtvedt G, Flottorp S, Young JM, Odgaard-Jensen J, French SD, et al. Audit and feedback: effects on professional practice and healthcare outcomes. Cochrane Database Syst Rev. 2012;6:CD000259.
69. Fava GA. Evidence-based medicine was bound to fail: a report to Alvan Feinstein. J Clin Epidemiol. 2017;84:3–7.
70. Takala J, Ruokonen E, Webster NR, Nielsen MS, Zandstra DF, Vundelinckx G, et al. Increased mortality associated with growth hormone treatment in critically ill adults. N Engl J Med. 1999;341(11):785–92.

71. Hampton JR, van Veldhuisen DJ, Kleber FX, Cowley AJ, Ardia A, Block P, et al. Randomised study of effect of ibopamine on survival in patients with advanced severe heart failure. Second Prospective Randomised Study of Ibopamine on Mortality and Efficacy (PRIME II) Investigators. Lancet. 1997;349(9057):971–7.
72. Califf RM, Adams KF, McKenna WJ, Gheorghiade M, Uretsky BF, McNulty SE, et al. A randomized controlled trial of epoprostenol therapy for severe congestive heart failure: the Flolan International Randomized Survival Trial (FIRST). Am Heart J. 1997;134(1):44–54.
73. Rapola JM, Virtamo J, Ripatti S, Huttunen JK, Albanes D, Taylor PR, et al. Randomised trial of alpha-tocopherol and beta-carotene supplements on incidence of major coronary events in men with previous myocardial infarction. Lancet. 1997;349(9067):1715–20.
74. The Cardiac Insufficiency Bisoprolol Study II (CIBIS-II): a randomised trial. Lancet. 1999;353(9146):9–13.
75. Siemieniuk RA, Meade MO, Alonso-Coello P, Briel M, Evaniew N, Prasad M, et al. Corticosteroid therapy for patients hospitalized with community-acquired pneumonia: a systematic review and meta-analysis. Ann Intern Med. 2015;163(7):519–28.
76. Early Breast Cancer Trialists' Collaborative G, Peto R, Davies C, Godwin J, Gray R, Pan HC, et al. Comparisons between different polychemotherapy regimens for early breast cancer: meta-analyses of long-term outcome among 100,000 women in 123 randomised trials. Lancet. 2012;379(9814): 432–44.
77. Majeed A, Ferguson J, Field J. Prescribing of beta-2 agonists and inhaled steroids in England: trends between 1992 and 1998, and association with material deprivation, chronic illness and asthma mortality rates. J Public Health Med. 1999;21(4):395–400.
78. Lau BD, Haut ER. Practices to prevent venous thromboembolism: a brief review. BMJ Qual Saf. 2014;23(3):187–95.
79. Academy of Medical Royal Colleges, Sense About Science. Evidence based medicine matters. Available from: http://www.testingtreatments.org/wp-content/uploads/2016/11/Evidence-Based-Medicine-Matters.pdf.
80. Charlton BG, Miles A. The rise and fall of EBM. QJM. 1998;91(5):371–4.
81. Maynard A. Evidence-based medicine: an incomplete method for informing treatment choices. Lancet. 1997;349(9045):126–8.
82. Sweeney KG, MacAuley D, Gray DP. Personal significance: the third dimension. Lancet. 1998;351(9096):134–6.
83. Hoffmann TC, Montori VM, Del Mar C. The connection between evidence-based medicine and shared decision making. JAMA. 2014;312(13):1295–6.
84. Sackett DL, Straus SE. Finding and applying evidence during clinical rounds: the "evidence cart". JAMA. 1998;280(15):1336–8.
85. Corrao S, Colomba D, Arnone S, Argano C, Di Chiara T, Scaglione R, et al. Improving efficacy of PubMed clinical queries for retrieving scientifically strong studies on treatment. J Am Med Inform Assoc JAMIA. 2006;13(5):485–7.
86. Acharya Y, Raghavendra Rao MV, Arja S. Evidence-based medicine in pre-clinical years: a study of early introduction and usefulness. J Adv Med Educ Prof. 2017;5(3):95–100.
87. Bassler D, Busse JW, Karanicolas PJ, Guyatt GH. Evidence-based medicine targets the individual patient, part 2: guides and tools for individual decision-making. Evid Based Med. 2008;13(5):130–1.
88. Guyatt G, Sackett D, Taylor DW, Chong J, Roberts R, Pugsley S. Determining optimal therapy–randomized trials in individual patients. N Engl J Med. 1986;314(14):889–92.
89. Guyatt GH, Oxman AD, Montori V, Vist G, Kunz R, Brozek J, et al. GRADE guidelines: 5. Rating the quality of evidence–publication bias. J Clin Epidemiol. 2011;64(12):1277–82.
90. Miles A, Bentley P, Polychronis A, Grey J. Evidence-based medicine: why all the fuss? This is why. J Eval Clin Pract. 1997;3(2):83–6.
91. Izcovich A, Criniti JM, Popoff F, Ragusa MA, Gigler C, Gonzalez Malla C, et al. Answering medical questions at the point of care: a cross-sectional study comparing rapid decisions based on PubMed and Epistemonikos searches with evidence-based recommendations developed with the GRADE approach. BMJ Open. 2017;7(8):e016113.
92. Lucas BP, Evans AT, Reilly BM, Khodakov YV, Perumal K, Rohr LG, et al. The impact of evidence on physicians' inpatient treatment decisions. J Gen Intern Med. 2004;19(5 Pt 1):402–9.
93. Bonis PA, Pickens GT, Rind DM, Foster DA. Association of a clinical knowledge support system with improved patient safety, reduced complications and shorter length of stay among Medicare beneficiaries in acute care hospitals in the United States. Int J Med Inform. 2008;77(11): 745–53.
94. Isaac T, Zheng J, Jha A. Use of UpToDate and outcomes in US hospitals. J Hosp Med. 2012;7(2):85–90.
95. Shay LA, Lafata JE. Where is the evidence? A systematic review of shared decision making and patient outcomes. Med Decis Mak. 2015;35(1):114–31.
96. Heneghan C, Mahtani KR, Goldacre B, Godlee F, Macdonald H, Jarvies D. Evidence based medicine manifesto for better healthcare. BMJ. 2017;357:j2973.
97. Manifesto. Better evidence for better healthcare. Available from: http://evidencelive.org/manifesto/.
98. Sonnad SS, Mullins CD, Whicher D, Goldsack JC, Mohr PE, Tunis SR. Recommendations for the design of Phase 3 pharmaceutical trials that are more informative for patients, clinicians, and payers. Contemp Clin Trials. 2013;36(2):356–61.
99. Ford I, Norrie J. Pragmatic Trials. N Engl J Med. 2016;375(5):454–63.

100. Loudon K, Treweek S, Sullivan F, Donnan P, Thorpe KE, Zwarenstein M. The PRECIS-2 tool: designing trials that are fit for purpose. BMJ. 2015;350:h2147.
101. Zwarenstein M, Treweek S, Gagnier JJ, Altman DG, Tunis S, Haynes B, et al. Improving the reporting of pragmatic trials: an extension of the CONSORT statement. BMJ. 2008;337:a2390.
102. Li G, Sajobi TT, Menon BK, Korngut L, Lowerison M, James M, et al. Registry-based randomized controlled trials- what are the advantages, challenges, and areas for future research? J Clin Epidemiol. 2016;80:16–24.
103. Guyatt G, Montori V, Devereaux PJ, Schunemann H, Bhandari M. Patients at the center: in our practice, and in our use of language. ACP J Club. 2004;140(1):A11–2.
104. Greenhalgh T, Snow R, Ryan S, Rees S, Salisbury H. Six 'biases' against patients and carers in evidence-based medicine. BMC Med. 2015;13:200.
105. Kitzinger J. Qualitative research. Introducing focus groups. BMJ. 1995;311(7000):299–302.
106. Montori VM, Kunneman M, Brito JP. Shared decision making and improving health care: the answer is not in. JAMA. 2017;318(7):617–8.
107. Das K, Malick S, Khan KS. Tips for teaching evidence-based medicine in a clinical setting: lessons from adult learning theory. Part one. J R Soc Med. 2008;101(10):493–500.
108. Ismach RB. Teaching evidence-based medicine to medical students. Acad Emerg Med Off J Soc Acad Emerg Med. 2004;11(12):e6–10.
109. Schunemann HJ, Moja L. Reviews: rapid! rapid! rapid! … and systematic. Syst Rev. 2015;4:4.

Medical Biostatistics: Basic Concepts

2

Konstantinos I. Bougioukas
and Anna-Bettina Haidich

Introduction

When physicians begin to read the research literature in their chosen field, one of the first things they will discover is that knowledge of statistics is essential. This chapter provides an overview of essential statistical methods available to landmarks trials that investigate hypertension. It begins with an introduction to the types of variables and then demonstrates methods for summarizing, visualizing, and understanding data. The chapter continues with basic principles in the context of hypothesis testing and interpretation of effect sizes, confidence intervals and p-values. The authors also describe the process of selecting the appropriate statistical test in bivariable analysis (e.g., t-test, ANOVA, Kruskal-Wallis, chi-squared test) and outline basic regression models (multivariable analysis), with a special emphasis on survival analysis and Cox proportional hazards model. It also briefly covers topics such as intention-to-treat and per protocol analyses, interim analysis, subgroup and sensitivity analyses, sample size calculation and power of the study. The focus of the chapter is not on computational formulas, but on basic concepts and ideas with practical examples from published trials. At the end, the reader will have learned the essential principles and tools of biostatistics required for research in hypertension field.

Population, Sampling, Study Design and Randomization

In epidemiology and biostatistics, the term *population* is used for any collection of units, which are often people, but may be, for example, institutions, events, etc. about which the researcher wish to investigate particular properties and draw some conclusions [1].

The *sample* is a finite part or subset of the accessible population that participates in the study [1]. The gold standard for ensuring generalizability (external validity) is the *probability sampling*. These methods use a random process to guarantee that each unit of the population has the same probability of being chosen in the sample [2, 3].

Clinical trials can be classified in several ways, depending on their design. From most to least common in the healthcare literature [4], the major categories of randomized trials are summarized in Table 2.1.

The random procedure that is used by a trial design is called *randomization method*. The most usual randomization methods are simple randomization, block randomization and stratified randomization [11, 12]. A combination of these methods can also be used in trial designs, and other special methods do exist.

An example from the literature with these basic concepts is presented below:

K. I. Bougioukas · A.-B. Haidich (✉)
Department of Hygiene, Social-Preventive Medicine and Medical Statistics, Medical School, Aristotle University of Thessaloniki, Thessaloniki, Greece
e-mail: haidich@gapps.auth.gr

V. Papademetriou et al. (eds.), *Management of Hypertension*,
https://doi.org/10.1007/978-3-319-92946-0_2

Example: Treatment of Hypertension in Patients 80 Years of Age or Older-Hypertension in the Very Elderly Trial (HYVET) [13]

Population: Patients of 80 years of age or older with persistent hypertension (defined as a sustained systolic blood pressure of 160 mm Hg) living in Western and Eastern Europe, China, Australasia, and North Africa.

Sample (size): Entry of 4761 patients

Study design: 3845 patients; 1933 patients assigned to diuretic indapamide and 1912 patients to matching placebo alone (parallel groups).

Randomization method: Randomization was stratified according to age (80–89 years and 90 years or older) and sex; permuted blocks of 4 and 6 of any 10 patients were used to ensure roughly equal assignment to each of the two groups within large centers. (Stratified and blocked randomization).

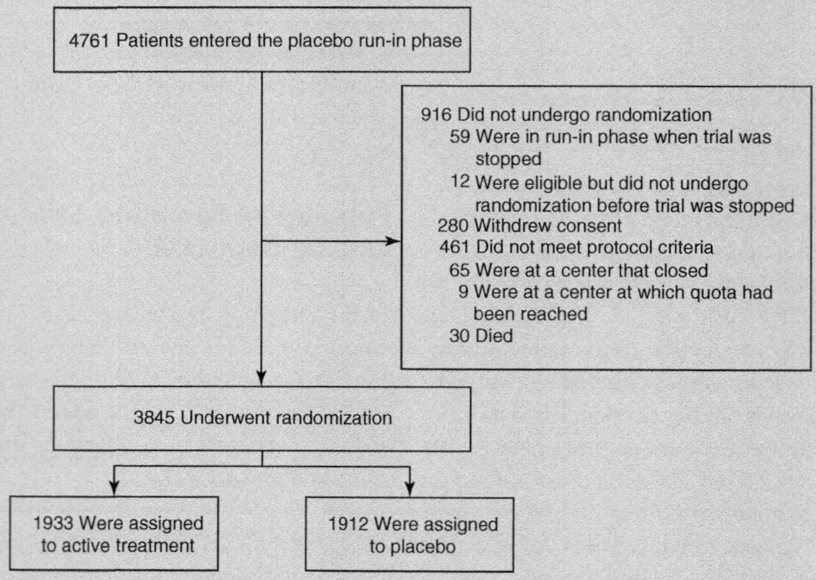

Table 2.1 Classification of randomized trials based on design

Study design (guidelines)	Defining characteristics	Example of trial
Parallel group (CONSORT 2010 [5])	Each participant is randomized to one of the intervention arms.	The Valsartan Antihypertensive Long-Term Use Evaluation (VALUE) Trial [6].
Crossover (under development[a])	Each participant is exposed to each intervention in a random sequence (all patients eventually get all treatments in varying order).	Spironolactone versus placebo, bisoprolol, and doxazosin to determine the optimal treatment for drug-resistant hypertension (PATHWAY-2): a randomized, double-blind, crossover trial [7].
Cluster (CONSORT extension 2012 [8])	Clusters of individuals (for example, clinics and schools) are randomly allocated to different study arms.	Patient education and provider decision support to control blood pressure in primary care: A cluster randomized trial [9].
Factorial (under development[a])	Participants are randomly assigned to individual interventions or a combination of interventions	Effect of blood pressure lowering and antihypertensive drug class on progression of hypertensive kidney disease: results from the AASK trial [10]. (3 × 2 factorial design)

[a]http://www.equator-network.org/library/reporting-guidelines-under-development/

Characteristics of the Subjects as Variables: Basic Types

In any particular trial, several characteristics (such as sex, age, ethnicity, smoking status, systolic blood pressure, or even an event like death from cardiovascular causes) are recorded for the participants of the study. In statistical terms these characteristics are called *variables* since they vary from subject to subject or from time to time [1]. Variables can take either categorical (qualitative data) or numerical (quantitative data) values (Fig. 2.1). The type of data is crucial for the decision regarding presentation (summary measures and graphs) and the techniques of data analysis that are employed [14, 15].

Categorical Variables

Variables are categorical when their data are placed into distinct groups with appropriate labels according to some qualitative characteristic or attribute, for instance place of birth, ethnic group, or type of drug [1, 16]. Categorical variables can be further divided into either nominal or ordinal variables. *Nominal* variables have two or more categories such as sex (male or female) or blood group (A, B, AB, or O) without natural ordering, while *ordinal* variables have an intrinsic order such as degree of pain (none, mild, moderate, or severe) [14, 15]. Note: A nominal variable like sex (male or female) or survival status (alive or dead) which can take only two possible categories is also called *binary* or *dichotomous* [14, 16].

Numerical Variables

Numerical variables take arithmetic values. They can be subdivided in discrete or continuous variables. *Discrete* variables can only take values of a countable set of numbers (which are usually the whole numbers 0, 1, 2, 3, etc.). Examples of discrete variables are the heart rate (beats/min), the number of visits to a GP in a year and the hospitalization days. In contrast, *continuous* variables have no limitation on the values that they can take. The baseline characteristics such as weight, height or blood pressure of the participants are examples of common continuous variables in a trial. However, the actual measurements are restricted by the accuracy of the method used for measuring the value [14, 15].

Moreover, categorization of numerical variables is also common in clinical research although there is a cost of loosing information [1]. For example, in the Systolic Blood Pressure Intervention Trial (SPRINT) [17] the continuous variable of systolic blood pressure was categorized into three categories (≤132 mm Hg, >132 mm Hg to <145 mm Hg, ≥145 mm Hg) and was presented in the table of baseline characteristics.

Variables from a Different Point of View

Information on a particular variable is usually collected for one of two reasons. The first is when the variable is an *outcome* of interest. An outcome variable is a characteristic which is believed to be affected by the values taken by other

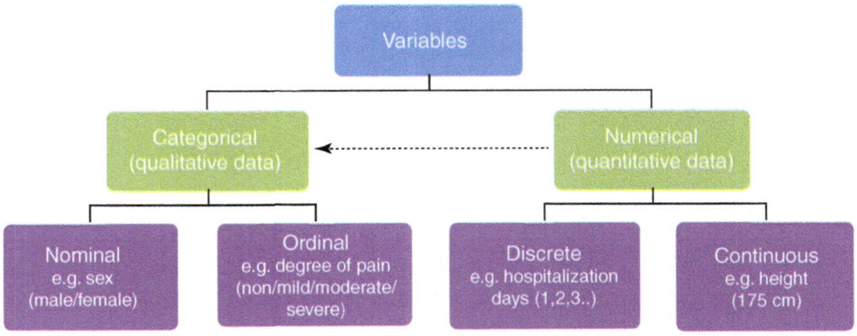

Fig. 2.1 Different types of variables. They can take either categorical (qualitative data) or numerical (quantitative data) values. The numerical variables can be converted into categorical variables. (Adapted from Aviva and Sabin [14])

variables [18]. It is also called a *response* or *dependent* variable. The outcomes measures can be defined as *primary* or *secondary endpoints* [19] based on the primary or secondary objectives of the trial, respectively. For example, in the main Hypertension in the Very Elderly Trial (HYVET) [13] that investigated the relative benefits and risks of antihypertensive treatment in patients 80 years of age or older, the primary endpoint was any stroke (fatal or nonfatal). Secondary endpoints included death from any cause, death from cardiovascular causes, death from cardiac causes, and death from stroke.

The second type of variable that the researcher would want to collect information on is an *explanatory* variable [18]. This is a factor that may influence the outcome or the association of the exposure and outcome (confounding factor). Such a variable partly explains the variability of the outcome. They are also called *independent* or *predictor* variables. In the HYVET study some of the explanatory variables were sex, age, baseline systolic blood pressure while seated, and previous cardiovascular disease.

Presenting Summaries of Variables

Summary Measures and Graphs for Categorical Variables

Categorical data are typically summarized by reporting the number (absolute frequencies) and the percentage (relative frequencies) of cases occurring into each category. The information from two categorical variables at once can be presented in a *two-way table* (*cross table* or *contingency table*), such as the one shown in Table 2.2 (one categorical variable is the race/ethnicity with five categories and the other is the treatment groups of the trial; data are from the Controlled Onset Verapamil Investigation of Cardiovascular End Points [CONVINCE] trial [20]) and this display of data is called a *frequency distribution* [21].

From this table we can see that in both treatment groups the majority of patients were white (COER verapamil group = 84.2%, Atenolol or Hydrochlorothiazide group = 84.5%). Another, important feature of this table is that the percentages within each treatment group (column percentages) add up to 100% (e.g., COER Verapamil group 84.2% + 6.9% + 1.2% + 7.3% + 0.4% = 100%). Moreover, this is a way to cross-check that the calculations have been performed correctly.

Table 2.2 Cross table of the race/ethnicity and the treatment group for the participants in CONVINCE trial

	Treatment No. (%) of participants	
Race/ ethnicity	COER Verapamil (n = 8179)	Atenolol or Hydrochlorothiazide (n = 8297)
White	6864 (84.2)	6981 (84.5)
Black	559 (6.9)	563 (6.8)
Asian	99 (1.2)	100 (1.2)
Hispanic	592 (7.3)	579 (7.0)
Other	36 (0.4)	41 (0.5)

Data are available in CONVINCE trial [20]
Abbreviation: COER controlled-onset extended-release

For categorical demographic variables, such as race/ethnicity, authors may well find that tables suffice for simple and concise recording of data. However, if the information in the table is sufficiently important, communicating it graphically may be a better choice [22]. For example, the reader of CONVINCE study [23] can immediately recognize from the presented side by side (or grouped) bar graph (Fig. 2.2) that for the primary end point, in each treatment group, more participants had primary events between 6 AM and noon than any other 6-h period.

Bar graphs are frequently used to present categorical variables. Another study that provides informative bar graphs is the Symplicity HTN-1 study [24]. This open-label study investigated the long term changes in blood pressure after renal denervation (RDN) in patients with treatment-resistant Hypertension. The proportion of patients with systolic blood pressure of 180 mm Hg or higher decreased over the duration of the study, from 30% at baseline to 5% at 36 months. The proportion who achieved target systolic blood pressure values of less than 140 mm Hg increased significantly at all time points (Fig. 2.3; stacked bar graph). At 1 month after RDN, 55 of 80 (69%) patients had reductions in systolic blood pressure of at least 10 mm Hg, which rose

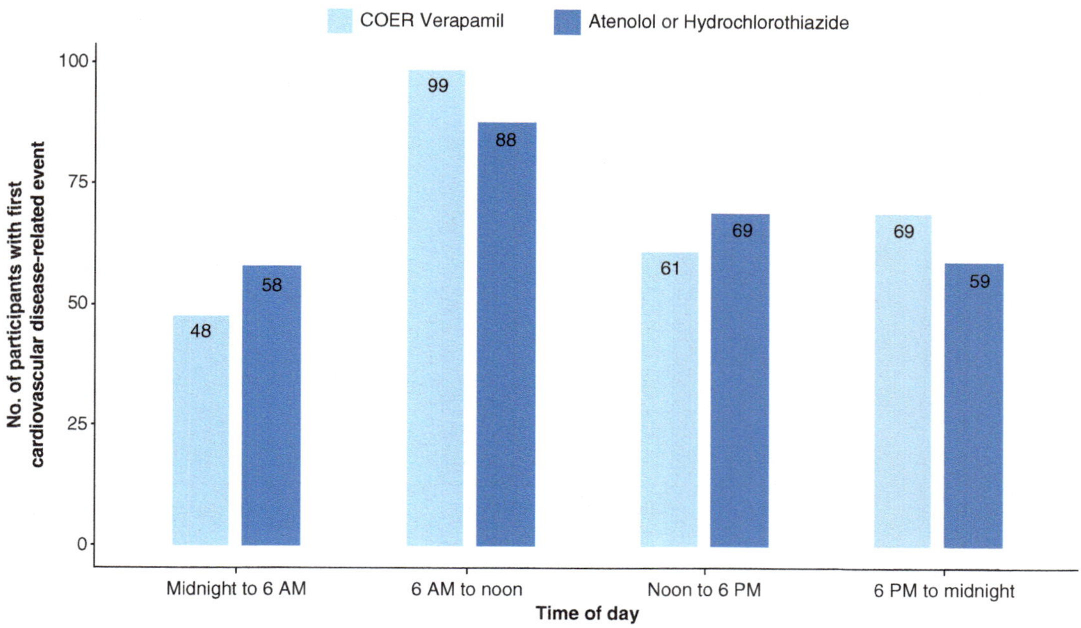

Fig. 2.2 Time of onset of first cardiovascular disease–related event was determined for 277 participants in the controlled onset extended-release (COER) verapamil group and 274 participants in the atenolol or hydrochlorothiazide group. (Grouped bar graph with frequencies; adapted from CONVINCE study [23])

Fig. 2.3 Distribution of changes in systolic blood pressure for all treated patients (stacked bar graph). (Adapted from Symplicity HTN-1 study [24])

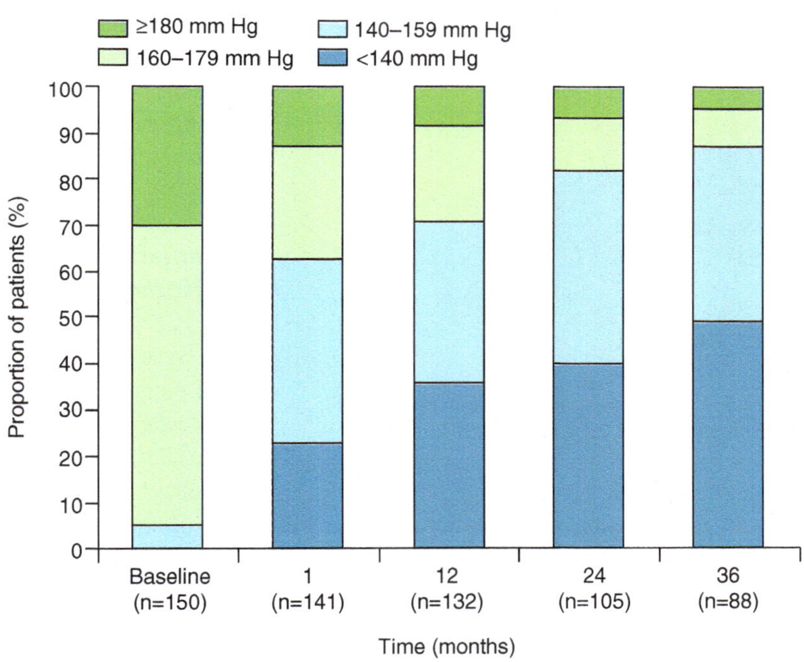

progressively to 82 of 88 (93%) at 36 months. Reductions of 20 mm Hg or more were seen in 68 of these 88 patients (77%) (Fig. 2.4; grouped bar graph with percentages).

A pie chart is another graph that can be used for the presentation of the categorical variables. The chart consists of a circle subdivided into sections, one for each category or group, so that the

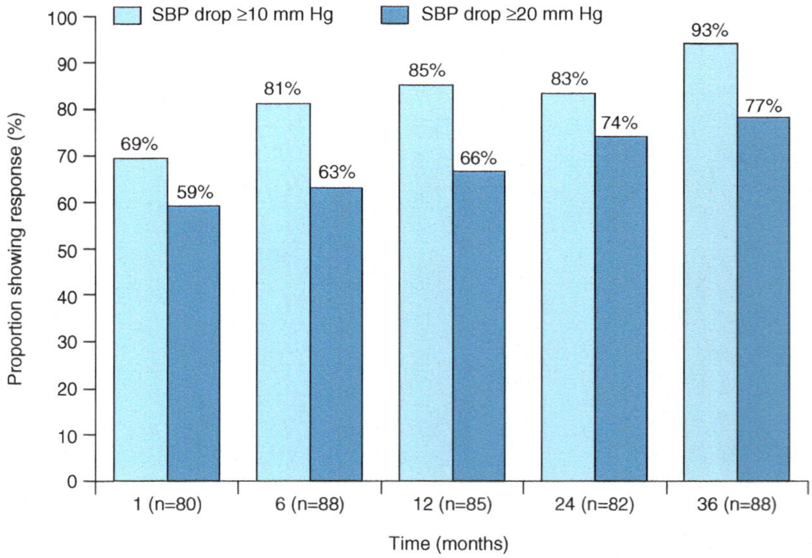

Fig. 2.4 Proportion of patients assessed to 36 months who showed treatment responses at different time points in the study (grouped bar graph with percentages). (Adapted from Symplicity HTN-1 study [24])

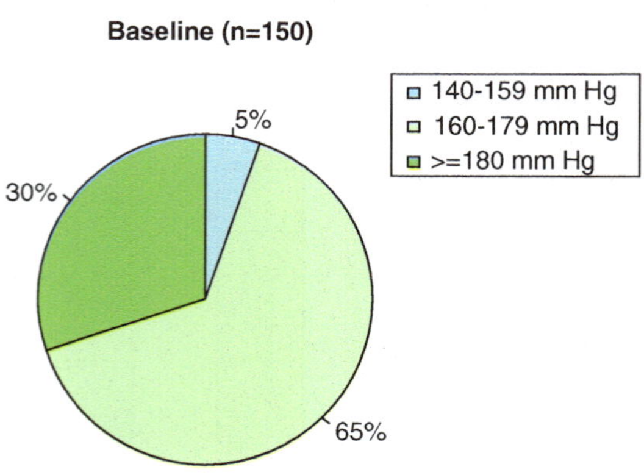

Fig. 2.5 Distribution of patients (n = 150) according to their blood pressure value at baseline

area of each section is proportional to the frequency in that category [14]. This type of chart is rarely used in scientific papers [25] because it requires too much space to present too little information, whereas there are better visualization alternatives such as bar charts. For example, the pie chart in Fig. 2.5 represents the distribution of patients (n = 150) according to their blood pressure value at baseline, that is the first stacked bar (baseline) of the Fig. 2.3. If the researcher had decided to present all the information of the graph, it would be needed multiple pie charts (five different pie graphs). However, multiple pie charts takes up a lot of the limited manuscript space and are difficult to analyze and interpret, especially when comparing adjacent pies [26, 27].

Summary Measures and Graphs for Numerical Variables

Two basic *summary measures* should be reported for a numerical variable. The first measure indicates where the center of the distribution of the values lies. This is an index of location (or central tendency) because it defines the center, or middle, of the sample data. The second measure describes the 'spread' of the observations, how widely the values are spread above and below the central value, and is called *variability* (or *dispersion*) of the distribution.

Measures of Location

There are three measures commonly used to describe the location or 'center' of the distribution of a numerical variable [28]:

1. *Arithmetic Mean*

The mean (or average), of a set of values is calculated by summing up all the values of observations and dividing by the total number of observations. The mathematical formula for n observations is

$$\overline{x} = \frac{x_1 + x_2 + x_3 + \ldots + x_{n-1} + x_n}{n} = \frac{1}{n}\sum_{i=1}^{n} x_i$$

where x_i is the ith observation of the sample. The capital Greek sigma Σ is a summation sign and is simply a short way of writing the quantity $x_1 + x_2 + x_3 + \ldots + x_{n-1} + x_n$.

The arithmetic mean is, in general, a natural measure of location and uses all the data values. However, it is influenced by extreme values, known as outliers or distorted by skewed data.

2. *The Median*

The median of a variable is the place that divides the data in half, once the data are ordered from smallest to largest. It is thought to be the "middle" value.

The sample median is:

- The $\left(\frac{n+1}{2}\right)$ th largest observation if n is odd
- The average of the $\left(\frac{n}{2}\right)$ th and $\left(\frac{n}{2}+1\right)$ th largest observations if n is even

The median can be more appropriate for distributions that are skewed. When the distribution is symmetrical, the median equals the mean.

3. *The Mode*

The mode is the most frequently occurring value among all the observations in a sample. There may be more than one mode if two values are equally frequent. The major disadvantage is that it ignores most of the information.

Measures of Variability

Several different measures can be used to describe the variability of a sample [28]. Two different variables can have the same arithmetic mean but can be made up of very different values.

1. *Range*

Perhaps the simplest measure is the range. It is defined as the difference between the largest and the smallest observations in a sample. The range is markedly influenced by extreme values.

2. *Variance*

The average of the squares of the deviations from the sample mean. The resulting measure of spread, denoted by s^2, is:

$$s^2 = \frac{\sum_{i=1}^{n}(x_i - \overline{x})^2}{n-1}$$

The units of the variance are the square of the units of the original observations. Variance is sensitive to outliers and it is inappropriate for skewed data.

3. *Standard deviation*

The standard deviation (SD) is defined as the square root of variance.

$$sd = \sqrt{s^2} = \sqrt{\frac{\sum_{i=1}^{n}(x_i - \overline{x})^2}{n-1}}$$

It is evaluated in the same units as the raw data. As the variance, it is sensitive to outliers and thus it is inappropriate for skewed data.

4. *Interquartile range (IQR)*

Range between percentiles (percentile is the value below which a given percentage of the data observations occur. e.g., the 25th percentile is the value below which 25% of the observations may lie) can also measure the variability of the sample. A common range used is the *interquartile range* (IQR), which is the range between the 25th and 75th percentile, thus the middle 50% (75%–25%) of the data is included between these two values. Again, data have to be ordered first from smallest to largest value. It is appropriate for skewed data.

Example
Suppose 11 baseline home systolic blood pressure records (mm Hg) in a trial with resistant hypertension:

134.9, 143.7, 151.0, 132.4, 150.2, 148.0, 148.7, 162.3, 131.5, 162.3, 137.8

Mean

$$\bar{x} = \frac{134.9+143.7+151.0+132.4+150.2+148.0+148.7+162.3+131.5+162.3+137.8}{11} =$$

$$\bar{x} = \frac{1602.8}{11} = 145.7\,\text{mm Hg}$$

Median
131.5, 132.4, 134.9, 137.8, 143.7, **148.0**, 148.7, 150.2, 151.0, 162.3, 162.3
Md = 148.0

Mode
134.9, 143.7, 151.0, 132.4, 150.2, 148.0, 148.7, **162.3**, 131.5, **162.3**, 137.8
Mo = 162.3 mm Hg

Range
Range = 162.3–131.5 = 30.8 mm Hg

Standard deviation (sd) and percentiles can be easily calculated with a statistical package such as R program:

Standard deviation (sd)
sd = 10.8 mm Hg

Interquartile range (IQR)
Percentiles

0%	**25%**	50%	**75%**	100%
131.5	**136.4**	148.0	**150.6**	162.3

Therefore
IQR = (150.6–136.4) = 14.2 mm Hg.

Histogram

The *histogram* is a graphical representation of the distribution of numerical data. They are typically used as tools for inspecting the distribution of numerical variables and get a "feel" for the data. A histogram gives information about [29]:

- How the data are distributed (Fig. 2.6): (a) left-skewed, (b) symmetric (e.g., normal distribution), (c) right-skewed.
- The amount of variability in the data
- Where the "center" of the data is (approximately) located

In an approximately normal distribution such as Fig. 2.6b, the mean (red line), the median (blue line) and the mode (green line) have very close values and the histogram is symmetric about the mean. Moreover, "nearly all" values (99.7%) of a normal distribution are within the interval ($\bar{x}$ − 3*sd*, $\bar{x}$ + 3*sd*).

Box Plot

A *box plot* chart is another graph that can be used for conveying location and variation information for continuous data, particularly for detecting changes between different groups of data before any formal analyses are performed. Figure 2.7 illustrates such a diagram that examines the yearly risk of recurrent lobar intracerebral hemorrhage (ICH) based on systolic blood pressure categories [30].

Box lower and upper margins indicate 25th (known as Q1; the value at which 25% of the data fall below) and 75th percentiles (known as Q3; the value at which 25% of the data fall

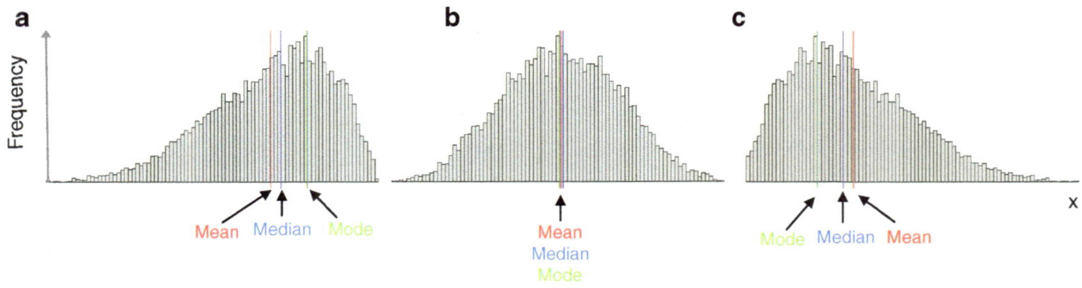

Fig. 2.6 Histograms of (**a**) a negative asymmetric distribution (left-skewed), (**b**) a normal (bell-shaped) distribution and (**c**) a positive asymmetric distribution (right-skewed)

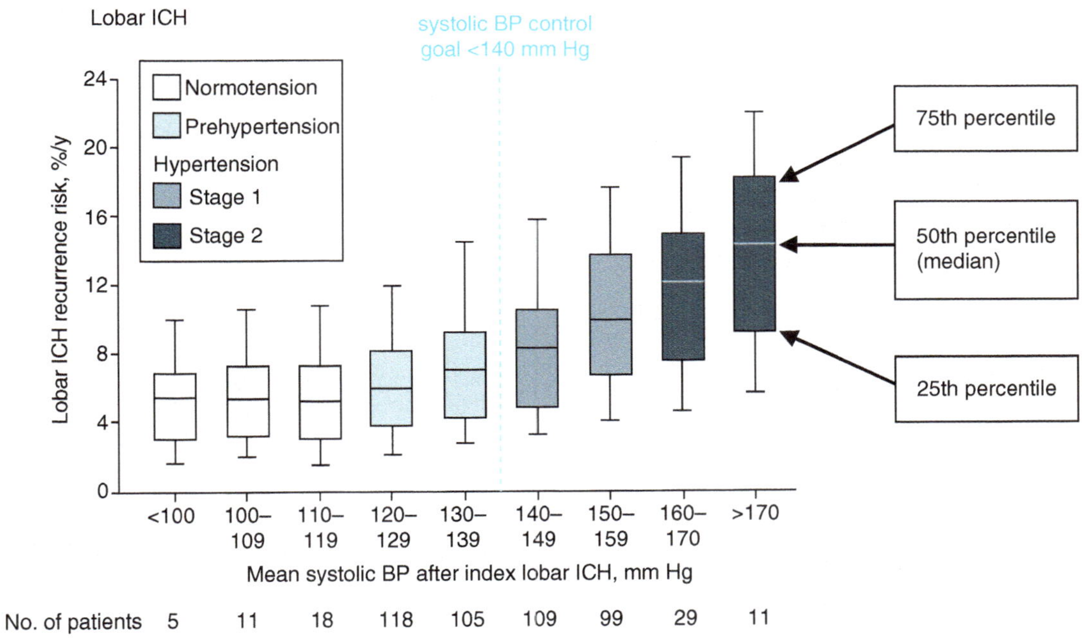

Fig. 2.7 Estimated yearly risk of recurrent lobar ICH (intracerebral hemorrhage) based on systolic BP (blood pressure) measurements during follow-up. (Adapted from Biffi et al. [30])

above) of yearly risk of recurrent lobar ICH, respectively; therefore, the boxes include the middle 50% of the observations. Horizontal lines in boxes indicate median values (50th percentile; Q2); error bars (or whiskers) indicate maximum and minimum estimated values in each distribution (Spear-style). Note: Tukey-style whiskers extend to a maximum of 1.5 × IQR beyond the box, while Altman-style whiskers can also be defined to span the 95% central range of the data [31].

A boxplot that is symmetric with the median line at approximately the center of the box and with symmetric whiskers suggests that the data may have come from a normal distribution.

In the statistical analysis methodology of a research paper, it should be indicated clearly how demographic data and clinical outcomes will be summarized. The following format is recommended [32]:

- Mean (standard deviation [sd]) for continuous or discrete variables with symmetric distributions.
- Median (first quartile [Q1], third quartile [Q3] or minimum [min], maximum [max]) for those with skewed distributions.
- Number (percentage) for categorical variables.

Examples from the literature:

"The Mean (SD), or median (interquartile range) values are quoted for the biometric and biochemical variables" (UKPDS 1998 [33]).

"We expressed continuous variables as means and standard deviations and qualitative variables as percentages" (Duran-Cantolla J. et al. [34]).

Other Popular Charts and Graphs for Numerical Data Used in Trials

Other commonly used graphs for presenting important numerical data are time charts (or line graphs), scatter plots and dynamite plots.

Time Chart (or Line Graph)

Typically a time chart has some unit of time on the horizontal axis (year, day, month, and so on) and a numerical variable on the vertical axis (usually systolic or diastolic blood pressure in mm Hg for trials with hypertension patients). At each time period, the amount is shown as a dot, and the dots connect to form the time chart [29]. Moreover, error bars can be added to each dot (Fig. 2.8).

Figure 2.8 shows that the two therapeutic strategies quickly resulted in different systolic blood-pressure levels. After the first year of therapy, the average systolic blood pressure at the 4-month protocol visits that both groups attended was 119.3 mm Hg in the intensive-therapy group and 133.5 mm Hg in the standard-therapy group, resulting in an average between-group difference of 14.2 mm Hg.

Scatter Plots

When two continuous variables are measured, the nature of the association between them can be explored graphically with a scatter plot [22]. Scatter plots are usually used prior to analyses to help assess the association of the variables to particular analytical procedures. Figure 2.9 is an example of a (grouped) scatter plot that investigates the association of office systolic blood pressure (SBP) and 24-h mean SBP in individual patients at baseline for sustained hypertension (red dots) and white-coat hypertension (blue dots) (European Lacidipine Study on Atherosclerosis [ELSA] trial that investigated white-coat hypertension [36]).

As shown in Fig. 2.9, in SH, 24-h mean SBP correlated with office SBP values (progressively lower values of one pressure were associated with progressively lower values of the other). In striking contrast, in WCH, 24-h mean SBP values were all in a narrow range, independently of the level of office SBP. In both SH and WCH patients, 24-h SBP was always lower than office SBP, the two values becoming progressively closer as SBP became less and the difference seems to disappear at about 130–120 mm Hg office SBP.

Dynamite Plots

Dynamite plots are bar plots where group means (usually mean changes from baseline blood pressure for studies examining hypertension) are represented by the tops of bars or columns and are very often presented in trials [37]. In this graph from ROX CONTROL HTN study [38] the reader can see that mean changes in office and 24 h ambulatory systolic blood pressure at 6 months were greater in the arteriovenous coupler group than in the control group (Fig. 2.10). Net mean differences were all in favour of the arteriovenous coupler group (office blood pressure −23.2 mm Hg systolic and −17.7 mm Hg diastolic, and ambulatory blood pressure −13.0 mm Hg systolic, and −13.4 mm Hg diastolic). However, the body of the bar has no logical interpretation and this

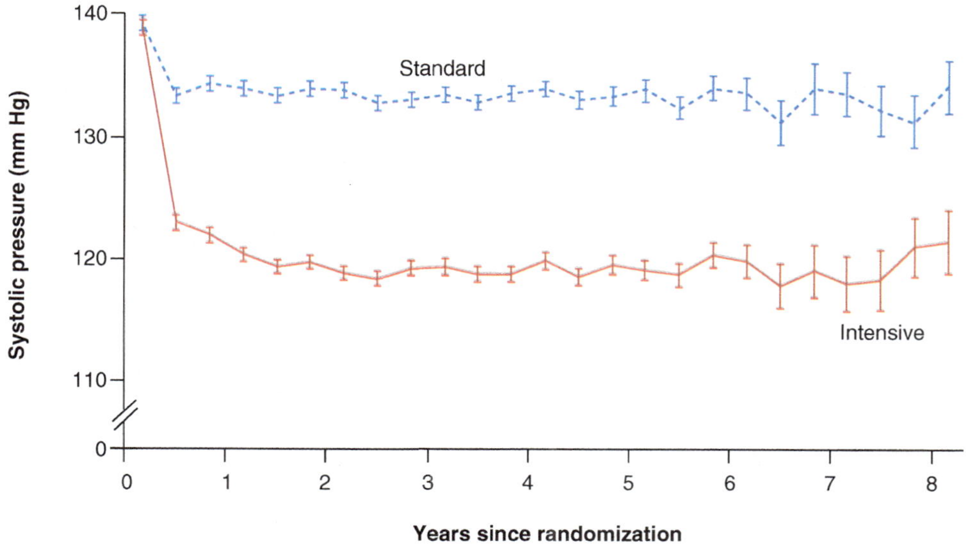

Mean no. of medications prescribed

	1	2	3	4	5	6	7	8
Intensive	3.2	3.4	3.4	3.5	3.5	3.5	3.4	3.4
Standard	1.9	2.1	2.1	2.2	2.2	2.3	2.3	2.3

No. of patients

	1	2	3	4	5	6	7	8
Intensive	2174	2071	1973	1792	1150	445	156	156
Standard	2208	2136	2077	1860	1241	504	203	201

Fig. 2.8 Mean systolic blood-pressure levels at each study visit with error bars. (Adapted from ACCORD [35])

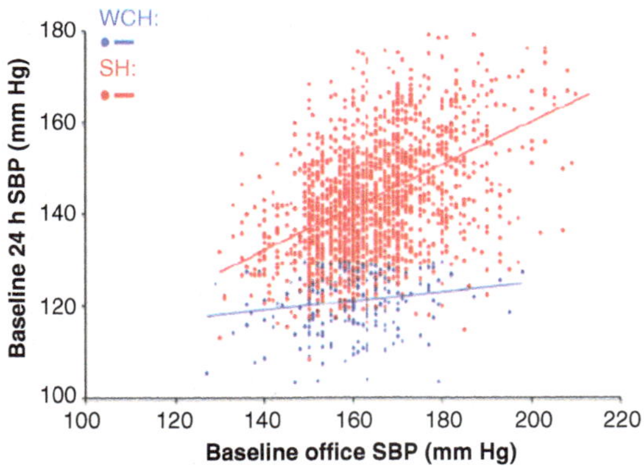

Fig. 2.9 Correlation between office systolic blood pressure (SBP) and 24-h mean SBP in individual patients at baseline. Data are shown separately for sustained hypertension (SH) and white-coat hypertension (WCH). (Adapted from Mancia et al. [36])

graph may not be appropriate for representing means [31]. Better alternative graphs are box plots or means plots (means presented by points with error bars).

Common Measures of Association

Measures of association such as risk ratio (RR) and odds ratio (OR) can be defined by constructing two-by-two contingency tables [39]. However, the most common measure that is reported in hypertension landmark trials is the hazard ratio (HR) that is derived from Cox models.

Risk Ratio

In a clinical trial to assess the impact of a new treatment on occurrence of an event, the risk ratio (RR) (or relative risk) could be calculated. For example in ALLHAT trial [40] for the heart failure outcome (Table 2.3) the risk ratio was reported comparing the Lisinopril treatment with Clorthalidone treatment (the hazard ratio could not be estimated because proportional hazards assumption was violated-see the section "Survival

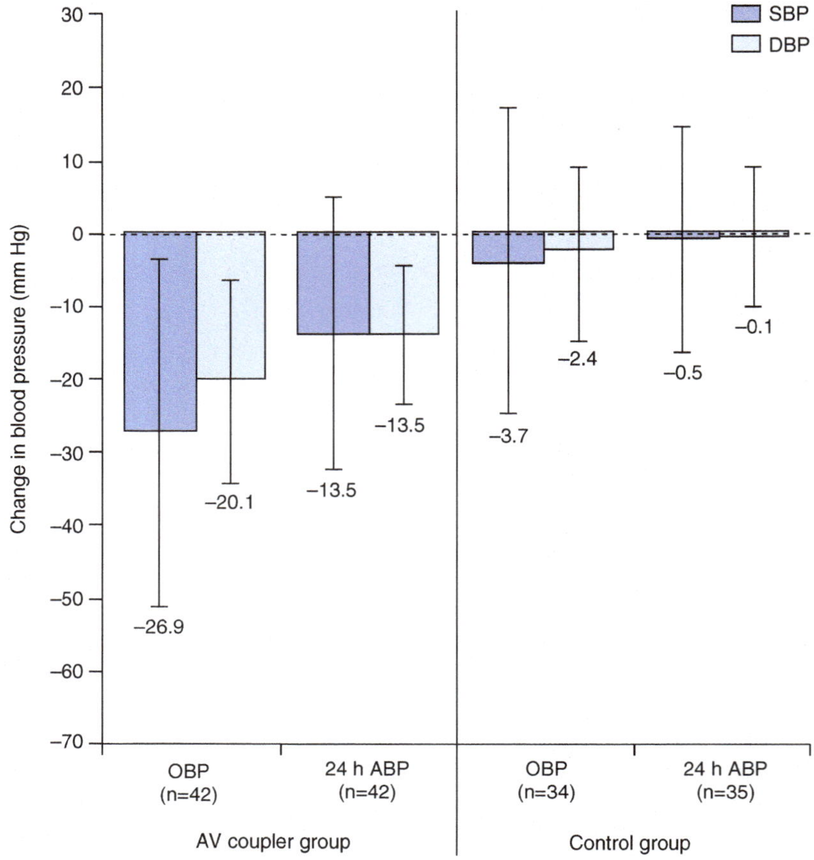

Fig. 2.10 Change from baseline in blood pressure at 6 months. Data are mean (SD). SBP systolic blood pressure, DBP diastolic blood pressure, OBP office blood pressure, ABP ambulatory blood pressure, AV arteriovenous. (Adapted from ROX CONTROL HTN study [38])

Table 2.3 Two-by-two contingency table for calculating risk ratio (data are available in ALLHAT trial [40])

		Outcome *Heart failure*		
		Yes	No	Total
Exposure	Treatment A: *Lisinopril*	a = 612	b = 6053	a + b = 6665
	Treatment B (control): *Chlorthalidone*	c = 870	d = 10491	c + d = 11361

Analysis and Cox Regression" p. 41). In this situation, the risk ratio is the ratio of the probability of occurrence of an event (risk) between two groups (e.g., treatment A vs treatment B; treatment B can be considered as control group):

$$Risk\ Ratio(RR) = \frac{risk\,in\,treatment A}{risk\,in\,treatment B(control)}$$

A risk ratio of 1 occurs when the risks are the same in the two groups and is equivalent to no association between the exposure to different treatments and the outcome. A risk ratio greater than 1 occurs when the risk of the outcome is higher among those exposed to the treatment A than among the treatment B. A risk ratio less than 1 occurs when the risk is lower among those exposed to treatment A, suggesting that the treatment A may be more protective than B when the outcome is negative e.g., heart failure. The further the risk ratio is from 1, the stronger the association between treatment and outcome. Note that a risk ratio is always a positive number (0, ∞).

The risk ratio in ALLHAT trial (Table 2.3) is calculated:

$$Risk\ in\ treatment\ A = \frac{a}{a+b} = \frac{612}{6665} = 0.0918$$

$$Risk\,in\,treatment\,B(control) = \frac{c}{c+d}$$

$$= \frac{870}{11361} = 0.0766$$

$$\textbf{Risk Ratio}: RR = \frac{\frac{a}{a+b}}{\frac{c}{c+d}} = \frac{\frac{612}{6665}}{\frac{870}{11361}} = \frac{0.0918}{0.0766} = 1.19$$

The risk of heart failure was 1.19 times higher in Lisinopril than in Clorthalidone group. In other words, the Lisinopril group had a 19% (1.19–1 = 0.19) higher risk for heart failure compared to Clorthalidone group.

Odds Ratio

The odds ratio can also be calculated from the Table 2.3. The odds ratio (OR) is the ratio of the odds of the outcome event in the treatment group compared to the control group:

$$Odds\ in\ treatment\ A = \frac{a}{b}$$

$$Odds\ in\ treatment\ B\ (control) = \frac{c}{d}$$

$$Odds\ Ratio(OR) = \frac{odds\,in\,treatment A}{odds\,in\,treatment\,B(control)}$$

OR = 1 Exposure does not affect odds of outcome (no association)
OR > 1 Exposure to treatment A associated with higher odds of outcome
OR < 1 Exposure to treatment A associated with lower odds of outcome

For ALLHAT trial example (Table 2.3) the odds ratio is calculated:

$$\textbf{Odds Ratio}: OR = \frac{\left(\frac{a}{b}\right)}{\left(\frac{c}{d}\right)} = \frac{a*d}{b*c} = \frac{612*10491}{6053*870} = 1.2$$

The odds of heart failure were 1.2 times higher in Lisinopril group than in Clorthalidone group. In other words, the odds of heart failure were 20% (1.2–1 = 0.2) higher in Lisinopril group. In this example the incidence of the heart failure was low and the OR is similar to RR.

Hazard Ratio

The majority of clinical trials record the length of time from study entry to a disease endpoint for a treatment and a control group. In this occasion, the hazard ratio is the most appropriate measure to be calculated and reported. Hazard ratio is a measure of relative risk over time in circumstances where we are interested not only in the total number of events, but in their timing as well. It is an estimate of the ratio of the hazard rate in the treated versus the control group. The Cox proportional hazards model (see the section "Survival Analysis and Cox Regression" p. 41) is usually used to calculate the hazard ratio, as it cannot be calculated directly from the crude numbers.

The hazard ratio is interpreted in a similar manner to the risk or odds ratio therefore values above one indicate a raised hazard, values below one indicate a decreased hazard and values equal to one indicate that there is no increased or decreased hazard of the endpoint. For example, in the SPRINT trial the hazard of heart failure was 38% (HR = 0.62; 0.62–1 = −0.38) lower in the intensive treatment than in standard treatment.

The hazard ratio is sometimes used interchangeably to mean a relative risk; however, this interpretation is not correct. The hazard ratio incorporates the change over time, whereas the relative risk can only be computed at single time points, generally at the end of the study.

Parameters and Statistics

Parameters are the summary description of the characteristics of the population (Fig. 2.11). For example the mean baseline home systolic blood pressure, μ_{SBP}, and its standard deviation, σ_{SBP}, in the population of patients assigned in the PATHWAY-2 study [7] were unknown parameters of interest. These unknown values were estimated from the sample data (n = 335) using the statistics $\bar{x}$ (sample mean) and *sd* (sample standard deviation) that equal to 147.6 mm Hg and 13.2 mm Hg, respectively. Therefore, *statistics* are measures of

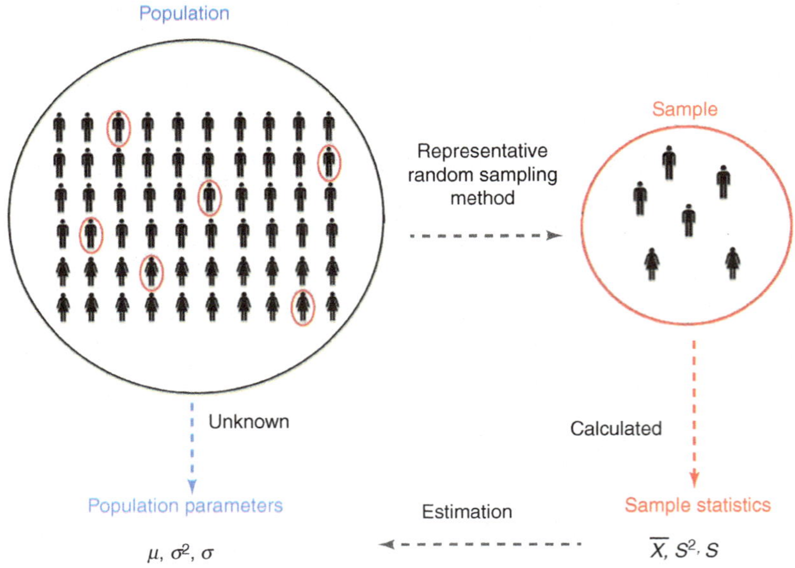

Fig. 2.11 Parameters are referred to the population while statistics are referred to the sample

numerical characteristics that describe the sample and can be considered as estimates of unknown population parameters. (Note: Greek letters refer to population attributes while their sample counterparts are Roman letters).

A **test statistic,** such as t statistic, is a quantity derived from the sample and is used in statistical hypothesis testing.

General Method for Hypothesis Testing (p-Value Approach)

In the statistical methods of the ACCORD BP trial [35] is reported that "the ACCORD BP trial was designed to have 94% power to detect a 20% reduction in the rate of the primary outcome for participants in the intensive therapy group, as compared with those in the standard-therapy group, assuming a two-sided alpha level of 0.05".

In another trial (UKPDS 38) [33] is referred that "in the text relative risks are quoted as risk reductions and significance tests were two sided. For aggregate end points 95% confidence intervals are quoted, whereas for single end points 99% confidence intervals are quoted to allow for potential type 1 errors."

The reader of the articles comes across with concepts such as power, type of errors, significance tests, confidence intervals, two-sided tests and alpha level of 0.05. The theory behind these elements is based on hypothesis testing. The basic steps of this theory is outlined below [14, 41]:

Basic Steps of Hypothesis Testing

Step-by-step hypothesis testing is following with more details:

Steps in hypothesis testing

1. From the research question, determine the appropriate null hypothesis, H_0, and the alternative, H_a.
2. Set the level of significance, α (usually 0.05).
3. Identify the appropriate test statistic and calculate the observed test statistic from the data.
4. Using the known distribution of the test statistic, calculate the p-value.

   Compare the *p*-value to significant level α. If *p*-value < α, reject the null hypothesis. If *p*-value ≥ α, do not reject the null hypothesis.
5. Interpret the results.

Step 1: State the Null and Alternative Hypotheses

The two types of hypotheses are the null and alternative. The null hypothesis (H_0) is a statement that indicates that no difference exists between conditions, groups, or variables while the alternative hypothesis (H_a) indicates a difference or association. The alternative hypothesis may be one-tailed or two-tailed, depending on the context of the research. One-tailed, hypothesis indicates a statistically significant change in a particular direction. For example, a treatment that is expected to show an improvement would be one-tailed. A two-tailed, hypothesis indicates a statistically significant change, but in no particular direction. For example, a researcher may compare two new conditions with no assumed difference between them. However, it is not known which condition would show the largest result.

Step 2: Set the Level of Significance Associated with the Null Hypothesis

When the researcher performs a particular statistical test, there is always a chance that the result is due to chance instead of any real difference. This means that the findings will lead to reject the null hypothesis when it is actually true. In this situation, a *type I error* is occurred. Therefore, statistical tests assume some level of uncertainty that it is called level of significance or alpha (the Greek letter α). The researcher chooses, before the data are collected, the level of significance (usually $\alpha = 0.05$) associated with the null hypothesis. In situations in which the clinical implications of incorrectly rejecting the null hypothesis are severe, it may require stronger evidence (more strict criteria) before rejecting the null hypothesis e.g., $\alpha = 0.01$ or $\alpha = 0.001$.

Step 3: Choose and Calculate the Appropriate Test Statistic Specific to H_0

The researcher should choose a particular type of test statistic based on characteristics of the data. For example, some tests are appropriate for comparing independent groups, while other tests are appropriate for dependent groups. Normal distribution of the data also plays an important role in choosing an appropriate test statistic.

Step 4: Compare the p-Value to Significant Level α. Reject or Not Reject the Null Hypothesis

The test statistic follows a known theoretical probability distribution. The value of the test statistic obtained from the sample is related to a known distribution to obtain the p-value, the area in both (or occasionally one) tails of the probability distribution. **The p-value is the probability of obtaining the observed results, or something more extreme, if the null hypothesis is true.** Most statistical packages provide the two-tailed p-value automatically. The smaller the p-value, the greater the evidence against the null hypothesis.

Conventionally, if p-value < 0.05, there is sufficient evidence to reject the null hypothesis, as there is only a small chance of the results occurring if the null hypothesis was true. In this occasion, the results are significant at the 5% level.

In contrast, if p-value ≥ 0.05, there is insufficient evidence to reject the null hypothesis and the results are not significant at the 5% level. This does not mean that the null hypothesis is true; but simply that there is not enough evidence to reject it.

Quoting a result only as significant at a certain cut-off level (e.g., stating only that $p < 0.05$) can be misleading. For example, H_0 would be rejected for $p = 0.049$ but not for $p = 0.051$. Therefore, it is recommended quoting the exact p-value obtained from the computer output. P-values less than 0.001 usually are reported as $p < 0.001$.

Step 5: Interpret the Results

Communicating results in a meaningful and comprehensible manner makes the research useful to others.

We present an example (e.g., chi-squared test) with the steps of hypothesis testing in Table 2.4.

In decision making, there are four possible scenarios that can happen regarding the truth in the population versus the results in the study sample, which are shown in Table 2.5:

Table 2.4 Practical procedures for hypothesis testing

Steps	Procedure	Example from ACCORD trial [35]
Step 1	State the null and alternative hypotheses.	H_0: There is no association between serious adverse events attributed to antihypertensive treatment and treatment strategy (adverse events and treatment strategy are independent). Ha (two-sided): There is an association between serious adverse events and treatment strategy (adverse events and treatment strategy are dependent).
Step 2	Set the level of significance associated with the null hypothesis.	Two-sided alpha level of $\alpha = 0.05$.
Step 3	Choose and calculate the appropriate test statistic specific to H_0.	Chi-squared test ($\chi^2 = 20.4$).
Step 4	Compare the p-value to the level of significance. Reject or not reject the null hypothesis.	The p-value < 0.001 is smaller than 0.05. Reject the null hypothesis.
Step 5	Interpret the results.	Adverse events and treatment strategy are dependent. As compared with the standard-therapy group, the intensive-therapy group had significantly higher rates of serious adverse events attributed to antihypertensive treatment.

Table 2.5 Type I and II errors in hypothesis testing

		In population the null hypothesis is	
		True (there is no difference)	False (there is difference)
Decision based on the sample	Not reject the null hypothesis	Correct decision: $1-\alpha$	Type II error: β (False negative)
	Reject the null hypothesis	Type I error: α (False positive)	Correct decision: $1-\beta$ (power of the study)

Errors in Hypothesis Testing

Types of error in hypothesis testing

Type I error: the null hypothesis is rejected while it is true; it is also called a false positive result. It is concluded that there is an effect when, in reality, there is none. The maximum chance (probability) of making a Type I error is denoted by α (alpha). This is the significance level of the test.

Type II error: we do not reject the null hypothesis when it is false, and conclude that there is no effect when one really exists; it is also called a false negative result. The chance of making a Type II error is denoted by β (beta); its compliment, (1 − β), is the power of the test. The ***power***, therefore, is the probability of rejecting the null hypothesis when it is false.

Hypothesis Testing and Confidence Interval (CI)

In medical statistics, a confidence interval (CI) is a type of interval estimate that shows the precision of an effect of interest. For example, a 95% confidence interval (95% CI) of the effect of interest (e.g., the difference in means) indicates that if the experiment was repeated many times under the same conditions (same sample sizes, same sampling method) on the same population and the 95% CIs of the effect (difference in means) were calculated, then 95% of these CIs would be expected to capture the true effect (that is the true parameter value) [1, 42]. In Fig. 2.12 the confidence intervals of the 100 randomly generated samples (sample size = 60) are presented. Each vertical bar is a confidence interval, centered on a sample mean (green point). The intervals all have the same length, but are centered on different sample means as a result of random sampling. The five red confidence intervals do not cover the true population mean (the horizontal red line $\mu = 2.25$). This is what we would expect using a 95% confidence level–approximately 95% of the intervals covering the population mean.

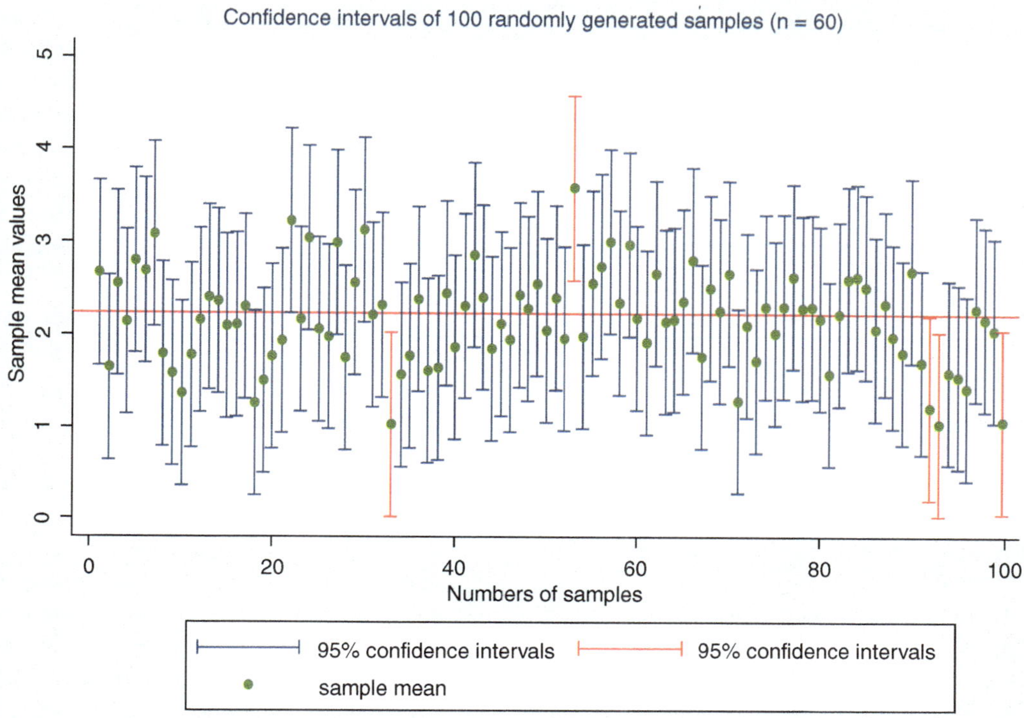

Fig. 2.12 The confidence intervals of the 100 randomly generated samples (sample size = 60). Ninety-five of them covering the population mean (the horizontal red line μ = 2.25). (Source: http://sites.nicholas.duke.edu/statsreview/ci/)

Confidence intervals and hypothesis tests are closely linked. The primary aim of a hypothesis test is to make a decision and provide an exact p-value. A confidence interval quantifies the effect of interest (e.g., the difference in means), and enables us to assess the clinical implications of the results. However, because it provides a range of plausible values for the true effect, it can also be used to make a decision although an exact p-value is not provided. If the confidence interval does not contain the null hypothesis value (e.g., the value zero when the effect of interest is the mean difference, or the value 1 for ratios, such as the risk or odds ratio), the p-value is less than the alpha level and the results are statistically significant ($p < \alpha$). If the confidence interval contains the null hypothesis value, the p-value is equal or larger than the alpha level and the results are not statistically significant ($p \geq \alpha$).

For example in ALLHAT [40], no significant difference (HR = 0.98; 95% CI: 0.90–1.07; p = 0.65) was observed between amlodipine and chlorthalidone for the primary outcome (fatal coronary heart disease or nonfatal myocardial infarction) as the confidence interval included the value 1 and $p = 0.65 > 0.05$.

Basic Statistical Tests

Principles for Choosing Statistical Test in Bivariable Analysis

Basic statistical tests can be categorized as parametric or non-parametric. A *parametric statistical test* makes assumptions about the parameters of the population distribution from which one's data are drawn. Examples of such tests are t-test and analysis of variance (ANOVA) test. *Non-parametric tests* (also called distribution-free tests) are the ones that make no such assumptions. Examples of non-parametric tests include the Mann-Whitney test and Kruskal-Wallis test [43]. If the sample size is large enough, the parametric tests usually have more statistical power than nonparametric tests counterparts.

We present the principles in guiding the choice of basic statistical tests in bivariable analysis with one dependent (numerical or categorical) variable and one categorical independent variable with levels-groups [44]. First of all, the researcher should answer what type of measurement is the dependent variable (numerical or categorical) and then how many groups are included in the independent variable. The next step is to inspect whether the groups of measurements are related (dependent groups) or not (independent groups). Measurements taken from the same participants at different time points (e.g., before-after studies, cross-over trials) must be analyzed using tests for paired data. The groups of measurements collected in these study designs are dependent.

In case of a numerical dependent variable (Table 2.6 and Fig. 2.13), the researcher further has to decide whether a parametric or a non-parametric test is more appropriate to be used. For example, if a continuous variable is approximately normally distributed in two independent groups (or the sample size per group is large enough), a two sample t-test can be conducted, else the corresponding non-parametric test, Mann-Whitney test, can be used (for highly skewed data or small sample sizes). There are various methods to check for normal distribution, e.g., plotting histograms or using one of the many "normality tests" (such as the Shapiro-Wilk test).

For examining the association between two categorical variables the tests presented in Table 2.7 are used. The flow chart for choosing each test is shown in Fig. 2.14.

Multiple Comparisons Problem

For comparison of three or more groups the researcher usually applies classical statistical tests such as analysis of variance (ANOVA) or Kruskal-Wallis test. For example in ANOVA the null hypothesis is that all means are equal while the alternative hypothesis is that there is at least

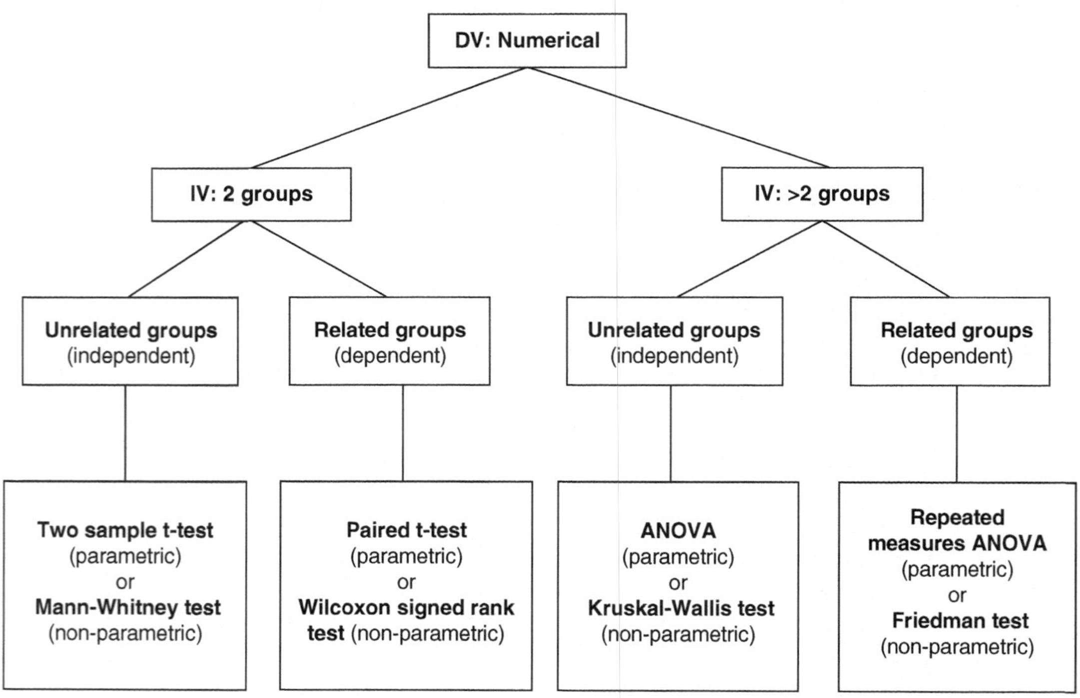

Fig. 2.13 Flow chart for choosing statistical when the dependent variable is numerical. DV Dependent variable, IV Independent variable

Table 2.6 Basic statistical tests in bivariable analysis with a numerical dependent variable

	Groups	Number of groups	Parametric statistical test	Description	Corresponding non-parametric statistical test	Description
Independent variable: categorical	Unrelated groups (independent)	2 groups	Two-sample t-test	Two sample t-test is used to compare the means of two independent samples. Each sample should follow an approximately normal distribution and the variances should be approximately equal. (The test can also be applied when each group has large number of observations). Example: Comparison of baseline systolic blood pressure in the intensive treatment group with the standard treatment group.	Mann-Whitney test	The Mann-Whitney is used to test the null hypothesis that two independent samples come from identical population distributions when the dependent variable is either ordinal or continuous.
		>2 groups	One-way analysis of variances (ANOVA)	One-way ANOVA is used to compare the means of several independent samples. Each sample has to follow an approximately normal distribution and the variances should be equal (homogeneity). (It can also be applied when each group has large number of observations). Example: Comparison of baseline systolic blood pressure in four race or ethnic groups (black, white, hispanic, and other) of patients at high risk for cardiovascular events.	Kruskal-Wallis test	The Kruskal-Wallis test is a rank-based non-parametric test that can be used to decide whether more than two population distributions are identical without assuming them to follow the normal distribution.
	Related groups (dependent)	2 groups (paired data)	Paired t-test	Paired t-test is used to assess whether the mean of the differences between two related measurements is significantly different from zero. Differences should follow approximately the normal distribution. (The test can also be applied when the number of patients is large). Example: Comparison of changes from baseline of 24-h mean systolic blood pressure at 12 and 24 months treatment in sustained hypertension patients.	Wilcoxon signed rank test	The Wilcoxon signed-rank test makes use of the sign and the magnitude of the rank of the differences between pairs of measurements.
		>2 groups (repeated measurements)	Repeated measurements ANOVA	Repeated measures analysis of variance (ANOVA) can be used when several measurements of the same dependent variable are taken at different time points. Assumptions: Normality of the residuals[a] by time point. Sphericity: variances of all possible difference scores are equal. (The test can also be applied for large number of measurements). Example: Comparison of changes from baseline of 24-h mean systolic blood pressure at 12, 24, 36 and 48 months treatment in sustained hypertension patients.	Friedman test	The Friedman test is used when the data arise from more than two related samples. It is based on ranks.

[a]residuals: the difference between the observed value and the estimated value of the quantity of interest

Table 2.7 Basic statistical tests in bivariable analysis with a categorical dependent variable

	Groups	Number of groups	Statistical test	Description
Independent variable: categorical	Unrelated groups (independent)	≥2 groups	Chi-squared test or Fisher's exact test (if there are expected frequencies less than 5)	Chi-squared test is used to determine whether there is a significant association between two categorical variables. It works well when the expected frequencies are large, otherwise Fisher's exact test can be applied. Example: Investigate the association between serious adverse events (yes/no) and treatment (Placebo, Spironolactone, Doxazosin or Bisoprolol).
	Related groups (dependent)	2 groups	McNemar's test or Exact binomial test (for small samples)	McNemar's test, for 2 × 2 tables, is used to assess whether there is a significant change in proportions over time for paired data or whether there is a significant difference in proportions between matched cases and controls. Alternatively, Exact binomial test can be used for small samples. Example: Investigate if the proportion of patients with systolic blood pressure > 130 mm Hg (yes/no) differs between the baseline and completion of the treatment (paired groups).
		>2 groups	Cochran's Q test	Cochran's *Q* test is used to determine if there are differences on a dichotomous dependent variable between three or more related groups. It is an extension to the McNemar's test. Example: Investigate if the proportion of patients with systolic blood pressure > 140 mm Hg (yes/no) differs between baseline, 6, 12 and 18 months treatment (four dependent groups of measurements).

one mean which is different from others. Rejecting the null hypothesis does not indicate which groups differ from the other groups. Consequently, researcher needs to examine patterns of differences among groups. However, this requires multiple comparisons of group means that lead to inflation of the Type I errors (the probability of falsely rejecting H_0) [45, 46]. For example, if there are g = 4 groups and pairwise comparisons are conducted with individual t tests at the significant level of 0.05 (5%) (individual error rate, IER), there are k = g(g–1)/2 = 12/2 = 6 possible pairwise comparisons (1 with 2, 1 with 3, 1 with 4, 2 with 3, 2 with 4 and 3 with 4). In this situation, the probability of at least one Type I error for the family of 6 tests (familywise error rate, FWER) is approximately FWER = $1 - (1 - \text{IER})^k = 1 - (1 - 0.05)^6 = 1 - (0.95)^6 = 0.265$ (26.5%).

Post-hoc Adjustment (Bonferroni Correction)

It is possible to use some form of post-hoc adjustments to take account of the number of tests performed. Many methods exist to manage the multiplicity problem [46, 47]. A commonly used approach is the Bonferroni correction which adjusts the statistical significance threshold by the number of tests [45]. For example, for a

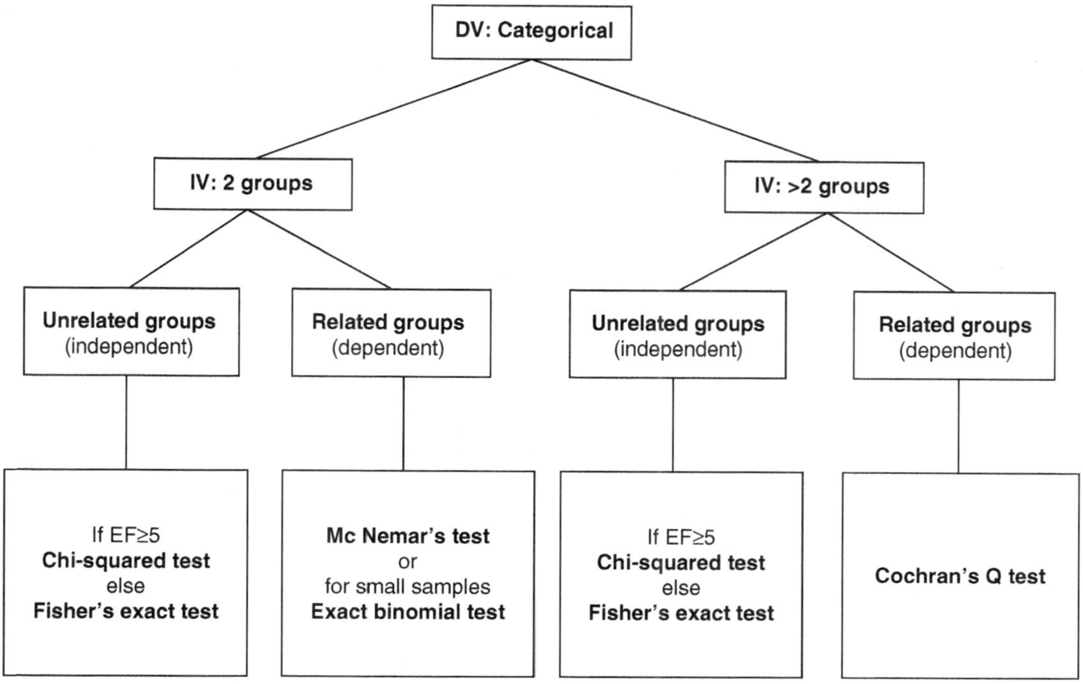

Fig. 2.14 Flow chart for choosing statistical when the dependent variable is categorical. DV Dependent variable, IV independent variable, EF expected frequencies

FWER fixed at 5%, the IER in a group of six tests is set at FWER/k = 0.05/6 = 0.008; therefore, an individual t-test must have a *p*-value less than 0.008 to be considered statistically significant. Even though the Bonferroni test controls the FWER, in many situations it may be too conservative and not have enough power to detect significant differences [46].

(Note: Equivalently, the researcher may multiply each individual p-value by the number of tests carried out in order to compute p_{adj}-values; any decisions about significance are then based on these adjusted p-values [14]. For example, if the researcher conducts six comparisons with t tests while keeping FWER = 0.05, each p-value of the t tests should be multiplied by 6 and then be compared with 0.05).

Basic Regression Models (Multivariable Analysis)

Clinical outcomes come in a variety of different types. Some are continuous, such as systolic blood pressure, and can be analyzed with linear regression. If the observed outcome is dichotomous/binary such as if a patient dies from a specific disease or not, logistic regression can be applied. However, if the information on the time to death is the observed outcome of interest, data are analyzed using statistical methods for survival analysis [48]. This statistical analysis uses the generic term "survival", although this method can be applied for any *time-to-event* outcome other than mortality. For example the outcome measured could be the time that the patient remains free of certain complications (*event-free survival-EFS)* or the time that the disease does not get worse (*progression free survival-PFS)*.

Regression analysis is used for explaining or modeling the association between a single variable *Y*, let's call this *response* variable (or just outcome), and one or *more explanatory* variables, $X1,\ldots, Xp$. When the number of parameters (p) is $p = 1$, it is called simple regression but when $p > 1$ it is called multiple regression. The most common models that are used in medical research are the linear, logistic and Cox regression models [28]. The characteristics of these models are outlined in Table 2.8. The survival analysis and

Table 2.8 Common regression models that are used in medical research

Type of outcome variable	Regression model	Measure of exposure effect	Basic assumptions	Description
Numerical	**Linear** $\mathbf{y = b_o + b_1x_1 + b_2x_2 + \ldots + b_px_p}$ The number of subjects per variable (SPV) should be at least 10.	Mean difference	1. Independence of the residuals 2. Linearity: associations between explanatory variables and response variable are linear 3. Homoscedacity 4. No multicollinearity 5. Normality of the residuals	Association between a numerical response variable and one or more (numerical or categorical) explanatory variables. Example: We would like to see if the treatment strategy adjusted for other covariates (age, sex, weight and smoking status) has an effect on 24-h mean systolic blood pressure (SBP) in sustained hypertension patients.
Dichotomous	**Logistic** $\mathbf{logit(P) = b_o + b_1x_1 + b_2x_2 + \ldots + b_px_p}$ 10 outcome events per variable (EPV) with the least common event determining the maximum number of independent variables. For example, in a study of 170 participants, assume that 100 patients achieved the goal of home systolic blood pressure of <135 mm Hg and 70 patients did not achieve it after antihypertensive treatment. Therefore at most, seven independent variables can be included (since 70 is the smallest outcome).	Odds ratio (OR)	1. Linearity of independent continuous variables with the log odds of the model 2. No multicollinearity	Association between a dichotomous response variable and one or more (numerical or categorical) explanatory variables. Example: We would like to see if the treatment strategy adjusted for other prespecified baseline covariates (sex, age, height, weight, smoking history, and the baseline value of home systolic blood pressure) has an effect on achieving a home systolic blood pressure of <135 mm Hg.
Time to a binary event	**Cox (proportional hazards)** $\mathbf{ln(h(t)) = ln(ho(t)) + b_1x_1 + b_2x_2 + \ldots + b_px_p}$ 10 outcome events per variable (EPV)	Hazard ratio (HR)	1. Linearity of independent continuous variables with the ln (hazard) 2. No multicollinearity 3. The hazard ratios are assumed to be constant over time (proportionality assumption).	Association between time to a binary event (death, failure, relapse) and one or more (numerical or categorical) explanatory variables. Example: We would like to see if the antihypertensive treatment strategy adjusted for other covariates (body size, age, sex, diabetes, and previous history of cardiovascular events, stroke, or chronic kidney disease) has an effect on time to cardiovascular death for hypertension high risk patients.

Residuals: the difference between the observed value and the estimated value of the quantity of interest interest; logit(P): ln(P) = ln(P/1−P) where P is the probability for the event to occur and ln is the natural logarithm
Homoscedacity: constant variance of the residuals
Multicollinearity: can occur in the regression model if two or more explanatory variables are significantly related to each other

Cox regression is presented more analytically in the following sections because these statistical approaches are used in the majority of the landmark trials that examine hypertension.

Survival Analysis and Cox Regression

In analyzing survival or time-to-event data, there are several important quantities of interest to define.

Event Definition

A clearly defined event is crucial for the presentation of survival data. Examples of potential events are: (1) death from any cause, (2) disease progression, (3) diagnosis with a specific disease, or (4) recovery (e.g., return to work) [49].

Start Time

Another crucial component of any survival analysis is the start time or time zero. This is the time point that is most important in relation to the time at which the event under study occurs. In a clinical trial this is typically the time of randomization and ensures comparability of the treatment arms. Because the time variable used in plots and analyses is the time since time zero, it also defines all the times at which surviving subjects are assumed to be comparable [50].

Censoring

The distinguishing feature of survival data is that at the end of the follow-up period, the event will probably not have occurred for all participants in the study (Fig. 2.15) (only participants 1, 5, and 7 experienced the event). This can be because the participant is lost to follow-up (e.g., has moved away) (participant 6) or is withdrawn (participant 3), or because the end of the study observation period is reached without the subject having an event (participants 2 and 4). For these participants, survival time is said to be right-censored. Although these may seem to be cases of missing data as the time-to-event is not actually observed, these subjects are highly valuable as the observation that they went a certain amount of time without experiencing an event is itself informative. One of the most important properties of survival methods is their ability to handle such censored observations which are ignored by methods such as a Mann-Whitney test (non-parametric test because time-to-event data are usually skewed)

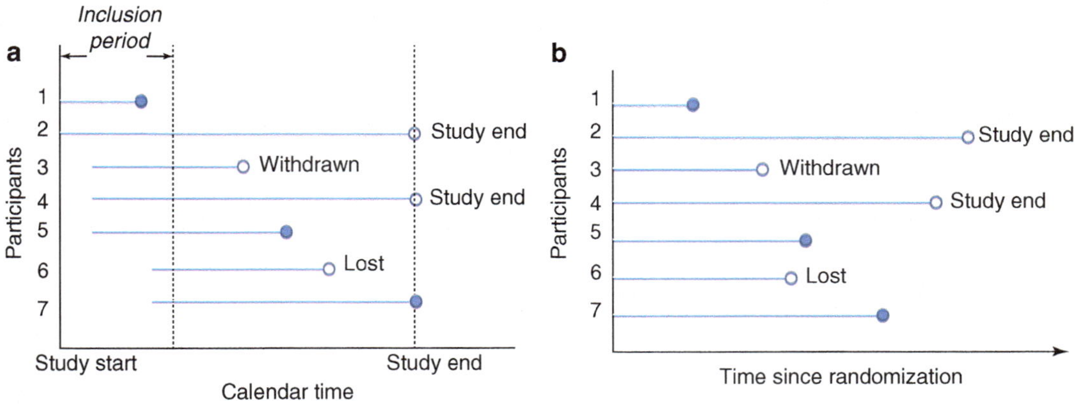

Fig. 2.15 Diagram (**a**) shows participants profiles in calendar time. The participants may enter the study at different times during the inclusion period. Diagram (**b**) ignores the different starting times and convert calendar time into survival time. Solid blue circles indicate participants who had the event while white circles indicate those who had censored data

for comparing survival times of two independent groups.

Survival analysis takes into account censored data and, therefore, utilizes the information available from a clinical trial more fully [18, 49, 51].

Survival Function

One of the most important quantities is the *survival function*, denoted by S(*t*), which provides the probability of surviving beyond a specific point in time (denoted *t*) [52]. As *t* gets larger, the probability of an event increases and therefore *S*(*t*) decreases. Plotting a graph of probability against time produces a *survival curve*, which is a useful component in the analysis of such data (Fig. 2.16). Since *S*(*t*) is a probability, it is always between zero and one for all values of *t*, $0 \leq S(t) \leq 1$. When $t = 0$, $S(0) = 1$, indicating that all patients are event-free at the start of study and theoretically, if the study period increased without limit, everyone will experience the event, so the survivor curve must eventually fall to zero. In practice, when using actual data, we usually obtain graphs that are step functions. Cumulative survival drops with every experienced event, whereas it remains unchanged with every censored observation (indicated by the red plus signs). Moreover, because the study period is never infinite in length, it is possible that not everyone studied gets the event. Thus, *S*(t) may not go all the way down to zero at the end of the study [49].

Hazard Function

Hazard is defined as the immediate risk of event occurrence. The hazard function *h(t)* gives the instantaneous potential per unit time for the event to occur, given that the individual has survived up to time t. Note that, in contrast to the survivor function, which focuses on not failing, the hazard function focuses on failing, that is, on the event occurring. It is always non-negative and has no upper bound [49].

Regardless of which function S(t) or h(t) one prefers, there is a clearly defined relationship between the two. In fact, if one knows the form of S(t), one can derive the corresponding h(t), and vice versa.

Kaplan-Meier Approach and Log-Rank Test

In comparing the survival distributions of two or more groups (for example, new therapy vs standard of care), Kaplan-Meier estimation and the log-rank test are the basic statistical methods of analyses.

Kaplan-Meier approach is usually presented in placing curves for different treatment groups on the same graph that allows the reader to graph-

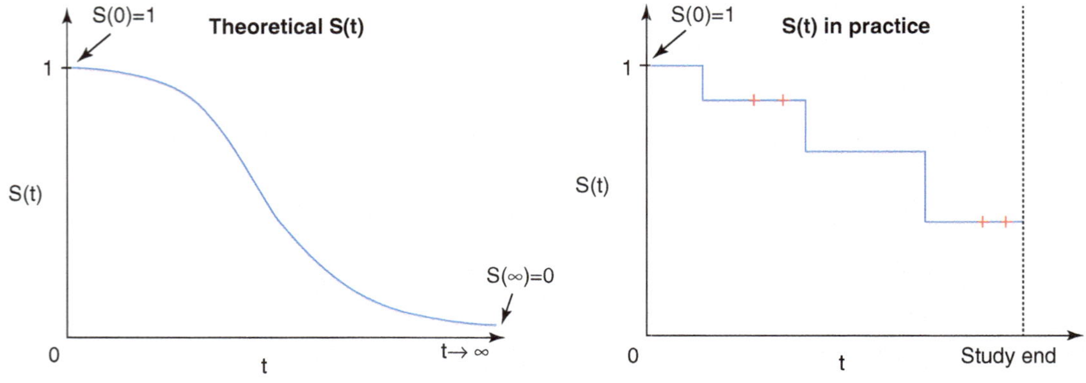

Fig. 2.16 The theoretical survival curve (on the left) and the step chart for the S(t) that is produced in practice (on the right)

ically review any treatment differences. This can be done in one of two ways [53]:

Kaplan-Meier Survival Plots

A Kaplan-Meier survival (K-M) plot presents an estimate (Kaplan-Meier estimator) of the probability of surviving beyond each time (vertical axis) versus time (horizontal axis). The curves in a K-M plot decrease with time from 1 (or 100%), displaying the proportion of patients that have survived (or remain event-free) (Fig. 2.17).

Samples of survival times are frequently highly skewed, therefore, the median is generally a better measure of central location than the mean. This value (the point at which half the patients have experienced the event) can be estimated for each curve by proceeding horizontally from the 0.5 point on the Y-axis until the survivor curve is reached and then proceeding vertically downward until the X-axis is crossed at the median survival time. For example in Fig. 2.17 the median overall survival (OS) time for metastatic colorectal cancer patients treated with bevacizumab-containing therapy was estimated to be 19.9 months in patients with hypertension (HTN) and 12.3 months in normotensive patients [54]. (Note: each patient's HTN status was determined 3 months after date of initiation of bevacizumab-containing therapy and from that time point was calculated the OS time).

Figure 2.18 depicts event free Kaplan-Meier curves for the participants in the SPRINT trial in a paper that conducted subgroup analysis [55]. It shows that the proportion of event free acute decompensated heart failure (ADHF) for the treatment group consistently lies above that for the placebo group; this difference indicates that the intensive treatment has better prognosis than the standard treatment at all time points of follow-up. Notice, however, that the two survival functions are somewhat closer together in the six months of follow-up, but thereafter they are quite spread apart. This widening gap suggests that the treatment is more effective later during follow-up than at the start. However, the estimated median event free time was not reached either for the

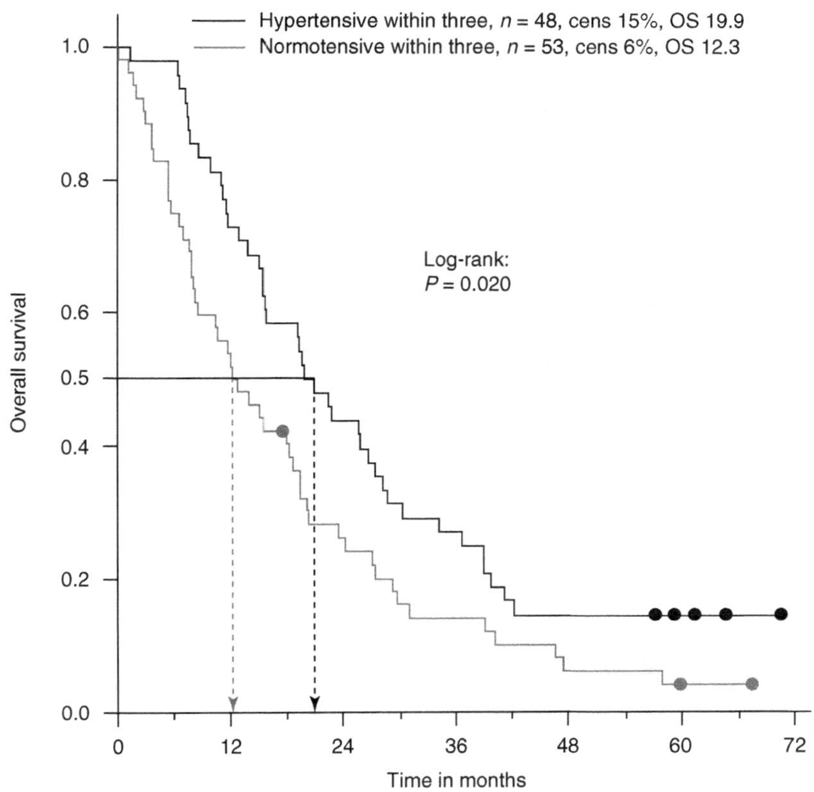

Fig. 2.17 Kaplan Meier survival curves of overall survival (OS) for metastatic colorectal cancer patients with hypertension and no hypertension treated with bevacizumab-containing therapy. The median overall survival time is calculated (on-study date: after 3 months of the initiation of bevacizumab-containing therapy) for each group. (Adapted from Österlund et al. [54])

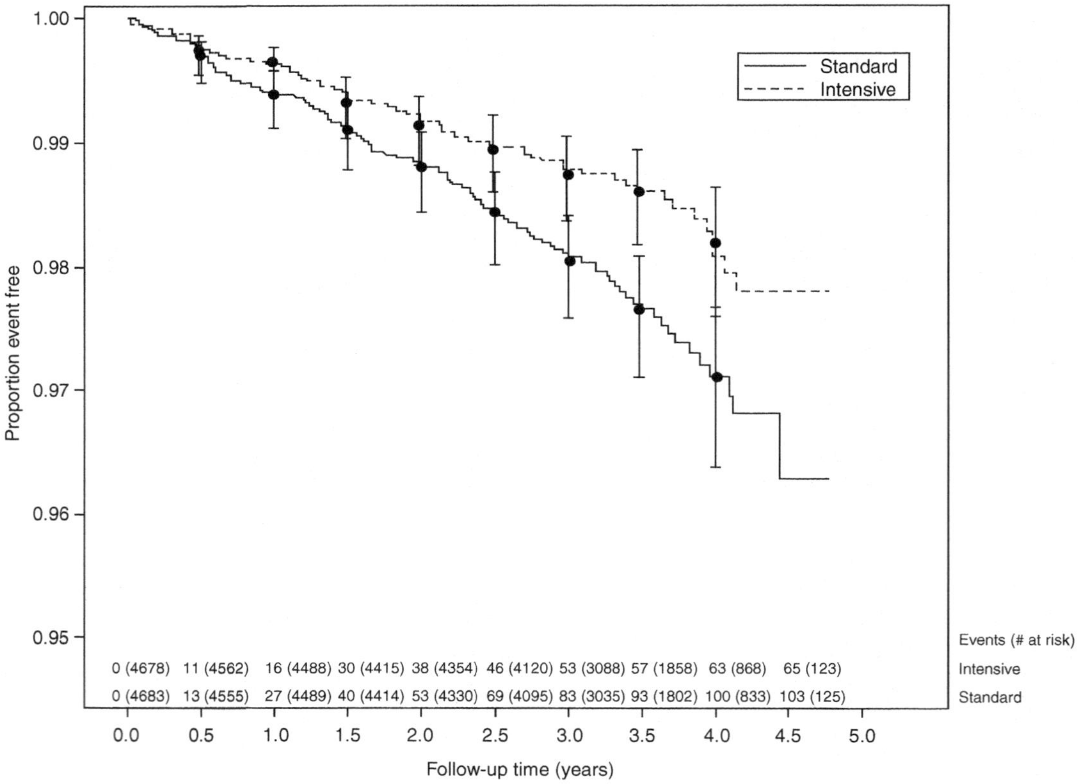

Fig. 2.18 Kaplan–Meier curves for the SPRINT (Systolic Blood Pressure Reduction Intervention Trial [55]) acute decompensated heart failure outcome by treatment group. Vertical bars indicate 95% confidence intervals. Number at risk and number of events is shown every 6 months

intensive treatment or for the standard treatment. (Note: for this reason, studies sometimes report the estimated time point at which a lower percentile (e.g., 25th) of the study population has the event [50]).

The 95% confidence intervals of the event free survival curves are shown with vertical bars in Fig. 2.18. In practice, there are usually patients who are lost to follow-up or event free at the end of follow-up, and confidence intervals are often wide at the tail of the curves due to lower number of patients, making meaningful interpretations difficult [56].

Cumulative Incidence Plots

Cumulative incidence plots are an alternative to Kaplan-Meier survival curve plots and are used very often in clinical trials. This plot shows the cumulative probability that the event of interest has occurred over the course of the observation period. The increase in event rates is shown starting from 0 (or 0%) subjects at time zero with an increasing curve over time [18, 53]. An informative example is shown in Fig. 2.19 obtained from the PREDIMED trial [57] that compares three different groups (Mediterranean Diet with extra-virgin olive oil (EVOO), Mediterranean Diet with Nuts and Control Diet). Actually, it presents the same plot in two different vertical scales. The y-axis of the nested plot, in the right side of the graph, is limited to the maximum estimated incidence (without using the full range 0–1 for the y-axis) in order to provide more detail [50, 53].

If two survival curves (or cumulative incidence plots) cross at any point, such as Med diet,

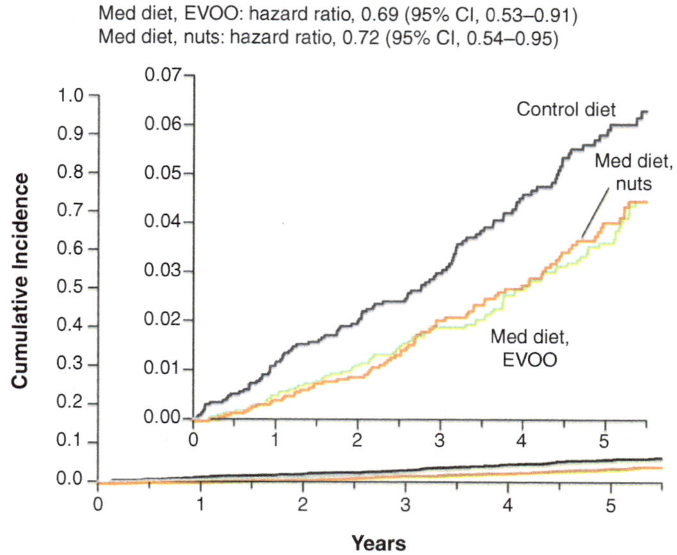

No. at Risk						
Control diet	2450	2268	2020	1583	1268	946
Med diet, EVOO	2543	2486	2320	1987	1687	1310
Med diet, nuts	2454	2343	2093	1657	1389	1031

Fig. 2.19 The plot shows the incidence of the primary end point (a composite of acute myocardial infarction, stroke, and death from cardiovascular causes) for the three groups of the study (Mediterranean Diet with extra-virgin olive oil (EVOO), Mediterranean Diet with Nuts and Control Diet) [57]. EVOO extra-virgin olive oil, Med Mediterranean

nuts and Med diet, EVOO (see the nested scaled graph in the right side of the Fig. 2.19) this might suggest that the hazard ratio between the two groups has reversed and the proportionality assumption (an assumption that is required in Cox analysis) has been violated.

Log-Rank Test

While a Kaplan-Meier plot elegantly represents differences between various groups' survival curves over time, it gives little indication of their statistical significance. The most common method of comparing independent groups of survival times is the log-rank test. This test, however, does not account for confounding variables, such as differences in patient demographics (e.g., age, sex) between groups [58].

Cox Regression Model

If an investigator is interested in quantifying or investigating the effects of known covariates (e.g., age, or race) or predictor variables (e.g., blood pressure), regression models are utilized. A rule of thumb is that Cox models should have a minimum of 10 outcome events per predictor variable.

Compared to the Kaplan–Meier method where only categorical variables can be used to predict the event, with the Cox regression analysis a combination of categorical and/or continuous variables can be used to predict survival. In addition, Cox regression models can also manage censored data.

Among the available survival regression models, the Cox proportional hazards model developed by Sir David Cox is the most commonly used and it is given by the following equation:

$$\ln\left(h(t)\right) = \ln\left(h_0(t)\right) + \beta_1 X_1 + \beta_2 X_2 + \ldots + \beta_p X_p$$

or

$$h(t) = h_0(t) \cdot e^{\left(\beta_1 X_1 + \beta_2 X_2 + \ldots + \beta_p X_p\right)}$$

where h(t) is the hazard at time t, $h_0(t)$ is an arbitrary baseline hazard (in which we are not interested),

$x_1, \ldots, x_p$ are explanatory variables in the model and $\beta_1, \ldots, \beta_p$ are the corresponding coefficients. The exponential values of the coefficients, $e^{\beta i}$, are the estimated **hazard ratios (HR)**. The hazard ratio is assumed to be constant over time in this model (i.e. the hazards for the groups to be compared are assumed to be *proportional*). It is important to check this assumption either by using graphical methods (e.g., Schoenfeld residuals plot) or specific statistical techniques (e.g., interaction between time and treatment) [48, 49, 59]. For example in ALLHAT trial [40] it is reported that "The Cox proportional hazards regression model assumption was examined by using log-log plots and testing a treatment×time (time-dependent) interaction term."

The Cox regression model was used in the sub-analysis of the ACCOMPLISH randomised controlled trial [60] as well. The Fig. 2.20 shows the hazard ratios for different endpoints comparing two treatments groups (benazepril and amlodipine vs benazepril and hydrochlorothiazide) within each of the three BMI categories. In the obese group, the primary or secondary endpoints did not differ between treatment arms ($p > 0.05$). However, in the overweight category, the hazard of primary endpoint was 24% (HR = 0.76; 0.76–1 = −0.24) lower in patients assigned to benazepril and amlodipine than to benazepril and hydrochlorothiazide, adjusted for all the other covariates (age, sex, diabetes, and previous history of cardiovascular events, stroke, or chronic kidney disease) in the model. The 95% confidence interval (0.59–0.94) does not include one, which indicates that the result is significant. As expected, the corresponding p-value = 0.037 is less than 0.05.

Differences between treatment arms were greatest in the normal weight category. Hazard rates for both the composite primary endpoint and total myocardial infarction were lower in patients assigned to benazepril and amlodipine than to benazepril and hydrochlorothiazide ($p < 0.05$).

Intention to Treat Analysis and Per Protocol Analysis

Intention-to-treat (ITT) analysis is a comparison of the treatment groups that includes all subjects as originally allocated after randomization, regardless of whether they completed the trial or even received the treatment after randomization [1, 61]. It serves to protect from biases in RCTs

	Benazepril and amlodipine	Benazepril and hydrochlorothiazide	Hazard ratio (95% CI)	p value
Obese				
Primary endpoint	142/2887 (5%)	152/2822 (5%)	0.89 (0.71–1.12)	0.3189
Cardiovascular death	48/2887 (2%)	47/2822 (2%)	0.97 (0.65–1.45)	0.8844
Total myocardial infarction	67/2887 (2%)	66/2822 (2%)	0.97 (0.68–1.36)	0.8426
Total stroke	52/2887 (2%)	51/2887 (2%)	0.99 (0.67–1.46)	0.9541
Overweight				
Primary endpoint	103/2059 (5%)	137/2098 (7%)	0.76 (0.59–0.94)	0.0369
Cardiovascular death	38/2059 (2%)	53/2098 (3%)	0.73 (0.48–1.11)	0.1372
Total myocardial infarction	44/2059 (2%)	65/2098 (3%)	0.69 (0.47–1.00)	0.0522
Total stroke	43/2059 (2%)	54/2098 (3%)	0.81 (0.54–1.21)	0.2953
Normal				
Primary endpoint	43/791 (5%)	75/825 (9%)	0.57 (0.39–0.84)	0.0037
Cardiovascular death	21/791 (3%)	34/825 (4%)	0.62 (0.36–1.07)	0.0853
Total myocardial infarction	14/791 (2%)	28/825 (3%)	0.50 (0.26–0.96)	0.0364
Total stroke	17/791 (2%)	28/825 (3%)	0.60 (0.33–1.11)	0.1025

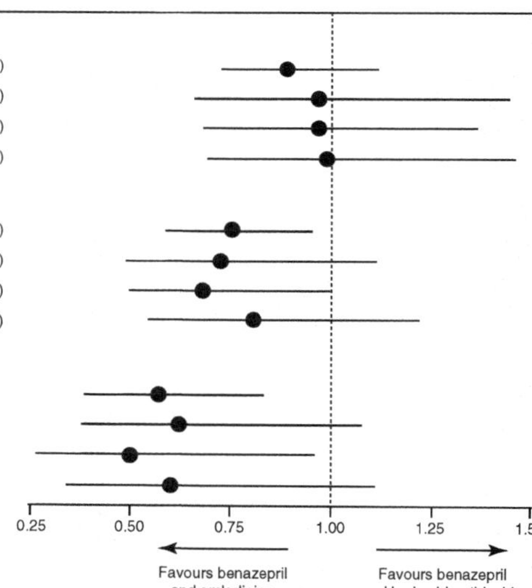

Fig. 2.20 Comparison of hazard rates within obese, overweight, and normal weight categories. Hazard ratio was calculated by Cox regression and adjusted for age, sex, diabetes, and previous history of cardiovascular events, stroke, or chronic kidney disease. BMI: body-mass index. (Adapted from Weber et al. [60])

associated with noncompliance and missing outcomes [62–64]. This method is recommended in superiority trials and assumes that if the subjects are randomized adequately then noncompliant subjects will be balanced across all the treatment groups [18].

Per-protocol analysis is a comparison of treatment groups that includes only those participants who completed the treatment originally allocated (fulfill the protocol in the terms of the eligibility, interventions, and outcome assessment) [64]. By focusing only on the fully compliant subjects, one can determine the maximal efficacy of a treatment [18]. If done alone, this analysis leads to bias.

In noninferiority trials, both intention to treat and per-protocol analyses are recommended; both approaches should support noninferiority [64].

Interim Analysis

Many trials recruit participants over a long period of time. Interim analyses of randomized controlled trials involve early looks at the data, usually by an independent data monitoring committee to protect the welfare of subjects [18, 65]. In practice, this can be done by stopping enrollment/treatment as soon as a drug is determined to be harmful (e.g., a large number of serious adverse events in one of the treatment groups), highly beneficial (e.g., large effect size suggests superiority of one treatment over the other and clinical equipoise no longer exists) or have negligible chance of demonstrating efficacy if fully enrolled, given results to date (that is, stopping for futility) [5, 66]. For example ACCOMPLISH [67] and SPRINT [17, 55] trials were stopped early at the recommendation of the data and safety monitoring board because the observed difference between the treatment groups exceeded the boundary of the pre-specified stopping rule.

However, performing multiple statistical examinations of accumulating data without appropriate correction can lead to erroneous results and interpretations. If the accumulated data from a trial are examined at five interim analyses that use a p-value of 0.05, the overall false positive rate is nearer to 19% than to the nominal 5% [5]. Adjustment for multiple analyses in interim analysis can be conducted using group sequential methods. The approaches described by Pocock [68, 69], O'Brien & Fleming [70] and Lan and DeMets [71] are popular implementations of group sequential testing for clinical trials. For example, ACCORD trial [35] quoted that "during the trial, an independent data and safety monitoring committee appointed by the NHLBI monitored the primary outcome (11 times) and total rate of death (7 times) with the use of O'Brien–Fleming boundaries determined by the Lan–DeMets approach. For these two outcomes, P values were adjusted to account for the number, timing, and results of interim analyses".

Subgroup and Sensitivity Analyses

Subgroup Analysis

Patients recruited in a major trial (such as SPRINT trial [17]) are not a homogeneous bunch: demographics (e.g., age, gender, race), their medical history (e.g., previous chronic kidney disease or previous cardiovascular disease), and other baseline characteristics (e.g., systolic blood pressure) may vary. Hence, it is reasonable to undertake subgroup analyses to inspect whether the overall result of the trial appears to apply to all eligible patients, or whether there is evidence that real treatment effects depend on certain baseline features [18, 72].

Subgroup analyses for the SPRINT trial [17] are shown in Fig. 2.21. This kind of figure, called a forest plot [72], is the usual way of documenting the estimated treatment effect within each subgroup (an HR in this case) together with its 95% CI. It shows that the effects of the intervention on the rate of the primary outcome was consistent across the six pre-specified subgroups, all being in the direction of superiority for intensive treatment compared with standard treatment. For reference, the results for all patients, with their inevitably tighter CIs, are shown at the top of Fig. 2.21.

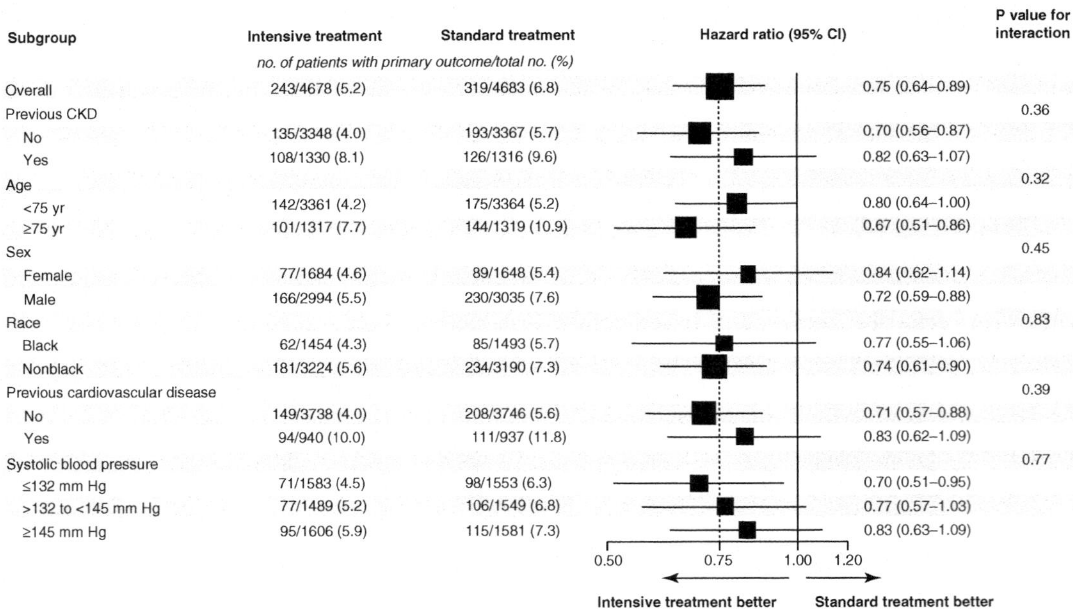

Fig. 2.21 Forest plot of primary outcome according to subgroups. The dashed vertical line represents the hazard ratio for the overall study population. The box sizes are proportional to the precision of the estimates (with larger boxes indicating a greater degree of precision [larger studies]). CKD Chronic kidney disease. (Adapted from SPRINT trial [17])

Scanning across subgroups, one can see that estimated HRs vary by chance and CIs are wider for smaller subgroups which have tinier squared bolb. Some CIs overlap the line of unity, indicating that the subgroup p-value does not reach 5% significance level; this will inevitably happen, especially in smaller subgroups, and is not helpful in interpreting subgroup findings [72]. For example for the subgroup analysis of sex (female/male) in the SPRINT trial, the effect in females was not statistical significant (95%CI: 0.62 to 1.14, $p > 0.05$) but in males (95%CI: 0.59 to 0.88, $p < 0.05$) it was. Comparing p-values for separate analyses of the treatment effect in each group can be misleading [73].

Instead, a statistical test of interaction should accompany each subgroup display as shown in Fig. 2.21. This interaction test examines the extent to which the observed difference in HRs across subgroups may be attributed to chance variation. However, the greater the number of statistical test for interaction performed, the greater the probability of a false-positive finding caused by chance alone (the overall Type I error rate for all subgroup analyses is inflated), so the p-values for interaction test should be adjusted [74]. The SPRINT trial reported that "Interactions between treatment effect and prespecified subgroups were assessed with a likelihood-ratio test for the interaction with the use of Hommel-adjusted p-values" (Hommel adjustment method is a modification of Bonferroni correction [75]). In conclusion, for the SPRINT trial there were no significant interactions between treatment and subgroup with respect to the primary outcome.

Sensitivity Analysis

Sensitivity analysis is an approach to inspect the impact, effect or influence of key assumptions or variations—such as different methods of analysis, different cut-offs or definitions of outcomes, protocol deviations, different missing data management and manipulation of outliers—on the final interpretations and overall conclusions of a study. In other words, it is a technique to assess the robustness of the findings based on primary analyses of data in clinical trials [76].

For example for the longitudinal analysis of systolic blood pressure in ACCORD trial [35], a sensitivity analysis was presented that compared Maximum Likelihood Repeated Measures Analysis (ML) under the assumption that the missing data were missing at random (MAR) with analysis of observed data under the assumption that the missing values were missing completed at random (MCAR).

Sample Size Calculation and Power

The sample size of a randomized controlled trial (RCT) is the number of subjects needed to detect a clinically relevant treatment effect. Usually, the number of participants in a trial is restricted because of scientific and ethical reasons. However, if the sample size is too small, one may not be able to detect an important existing effect (low power), whereas samples that are unduly large may waste time, research resources, money, and raise ethical considerations. It is therefore important to plan carefully and optimize the sample size of a clinical trial [5, 77].

Elements of the sample size calculation are [5, 18, 77, 78]:

1. The estimated outcomes in each group (which implies the clinically important target difference between the intervention groups, e.g., minimum expected difference of means, $\mu_1 - \mu_2$, or proportions, $p_1 - p_2$)
2. The significance level alpha and whether a one-tailed or two-tailed statistical analysis is planned, usually 5%
3. The desired statistical power ($1 - \beta$), usually 80% or 90%
4. The estimated measurement variability (e.g., standard deviation) for continuous outcomes
5. The study design (parallel or crossover, etc.)
6. The expected dropout rate of subjects during the study
7. Adjustments for interim or/and subgroup analyses

The power of the study is a measure of how likely it is that the hypothesis test will produce a statistically significant result, for a population effect of a given magnitude, if an effect truly exists. For example, a study power of 80% means that if the study were to be repeated many times, a statistically significant result would be obtained 8 times out of 10, if there truly is an effect of the specified size.

The power needed is usually decided before the start of the study for calculating the sample size. However, it is also possible to work backwards, to estimate the power of a study given a fixed sample size. For example, there may be circumstances where the number of participants who are available or affordable (due to cost or time constraints) is limited. The power of a clinical trial is increased when the level of alpha, the expected difference, or the sample size are increased [79].

Authors should indicate how the sample size was estimated. They should identify the primary endpoint on which the calculation was based, all the elements used in the computation, and report the resulting target sample size [5]. This information is usually provided in statistical methods of the research paper. For example, in PATHWAY-2 trial [7] is reported that "the sample size was estimated to be 294 patients, based on detecting a difference of 3 mm Hg (SD 12) in home systolic blood pressure between each of the experimental drugs and the placebo treatment, with 90% power using a single sample *t* test at the 0.003 significance level (this was chosen in order that the 0.01 level could be adjusted for three planned comparisons)".

Nowadays, the sample size calculation can be conducted with specialized tools such as G*Power or software environment R (Fig. 2.22).

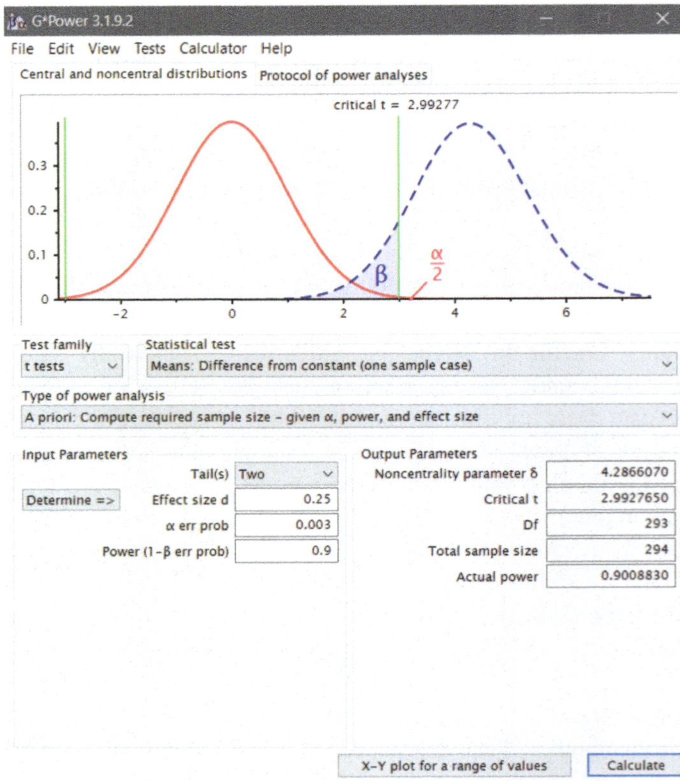

Fig. 2.22 The sample size calculation can be conducted with specialized tools such as G*Power or R programming language

R programming language

```
library(pwr)

pwr.t.test(d=0.25,n=NULL,power=0.9, sig.level=0.003,type="one.sample",alternative="two.sided")


     One-sample t test power calculation

          n = 293.3132
          d = 0.25
  sig.level = 0.003
      power = 0.9
alternative = two.sided
```

where $d = \frac{|\mu_1 - \mu_2|}{\sigma}$ is the standardized difference or effect size.

References

1. Everitt BS. Medical statistics from A to Z. Cambridge, UK: Cambridge University Press; 2006.
2. Peters TJ, Eachus JI. Achieving equal probability of selection under various random sampling strategies. Paediatr Perinat Epidemiol England. 1995;9:219–24.
3. Martinez-Mesa J, Gonzalez-Chica DA, Duquia RP, Bonamigo RR, Bastos JL. Sampling: how to select participants in my research study? An Bras Dermatol Brazil. 2016;91:326–30.
4. Hopewell S, Dutton S, Yu L-M, Chan A-W, Altman DG. The quality of reports of randomised trials in 2000 and 2006: comparative study of articles indexed in PubMed. BMJ [Internet]. 2010;340. Available from: http://www.bmj.com/content/340/bmj.c723.abstract.
5. Moher D, Hopewell S, Schulz KF, Montori V, Gotzsche PC, Devereaux PJ, et al. CONSORT 2010 explanation and elaboration: updated guidelines for reporting parallel group randomised trials. Int J Surg England. 2012;10:28–55.
6. Julius S, Weber MA, Kjeldsen SE, McInnes GT, Zanchetti A, Brunner HR, et al. The Valsartan

Antihypertensive Long-Term Use Evaluation (VALUE) trial. Hypertension [Internet]. 2006;48:385–391. Available from: http://hyper.ahajournals.org/content/48/3/385.abstract.
7. Williams B, MacDonald TM, Morant S, Webb DJ, Sever P, McInnes G, et al. Spironolactone versus placebo, bisoprolol, and doxazosin to determine the optimal treatment for drug-resistant hypertension (PATHWAY-2): a randomised, double-blind, crossover trial. Lancet [Internet]. Elsevier; 2017;386:2059–68. Available from: https://doi.org/10.1016/S0140-6736(15)00257-3.
8. Campbell MK, Piaggio G, Elbourne DR, Altman DG. Consort 2010 statement: extension to cluster randomised trials. BMJ. England. 2012;345:e5661.
9. Bosworth HB, Olsen MK, Dudley T, Orr M, Goldstein MK, Datta SK, et al. Patient education and provider decision support to control blood pressure in primary care: a cluster randomized trial. Am Heart J United States. 2009;157:450–6.
10. Wright JTJ, Bakris G, Greene T, Agodoa LY, Appel LJ, Charleston J, et al. Effect of blood pressure lowering and antihypertensive drug class on progression of hypertensive kidney disease: results from the AASK trial. JAMA. United States. 2002;288:2421–31.
11. Vickers AJ. How to randomize. J Soc Integr Oncol Canada. 2006;4:194–8.
12. Suresh KP. An overview of randomization techniques: an unbiased assessment of outcome in clinical research. J Hum Reprod Sci [Internet]. India: Medknow Publications Pvt Ltd; 2011;4:8–11. Available from: http://www.ncbi.nlm.nih.gov/pmc/articles/PMC3136079/.
13. Beckett NS, Peters R, Fletcher AE, Staessen JA, Liu L, Dumitrascu D, et al. Treatment of hypertension in patients 80 years of age or older. N Engl J Med [Internet]. Massachusetts Medical Society; 2008;358:1887–98. Available from: https://doi.org/10.1056/NEJMoa0801369.
14. Aviva P, Caroline S. Medical statistics at a glance. 3rd ed. Oxford, UK: Wiley Blackwell; 2009.
15. Thomas E. An introduction to medical statistics for health care professionals: describing and presenting data. Musculoskeletal Care England. 2004;2:218–28.
16. Kirkwood BR, Sterne JAC. Essential medical statistics. 2nd ed. Hoboken: Wiley-Blackwell; 2003.
17. SPRINT Research Group. A randomized trial of intensive versus standard blood-pressure control. N Engl J Med [Internet]. Massachusetts Medical Society; 2015;373:2103–16. Available from: https://doi.org/10.1056/NEJMoa1511939.
18. Wang D, Bakhai A. Clinical trials: a practical guide to design, analysis, and reporting. London: Remedica; 2006.
19. Paul S. Clinical endpoint. Encycl Biopharm Stat. 3rd ed. [Internet]. CRC Press; 2012. p. 273–5. Available from: https://doi.org/10.1201/b14674-43.
20. Black HR, Elliott WJ, Grandits G, Grambsch P, Lucente T, White WB, Neaton JD, Grimm Jr. RH, Hansson L, Lacourcière Y, Muller J. Principal results of the controlled onset verapamil investigation of cardiovascular end points (CONVINCE) trial. JAMA [Internet]. 2003;289:2073–82. Available from: https://doi.org/10.1001/jama.289.16.2073.
21. Duquia RP, Bastos JL, Bonamigo RR, González-Chica DA, Martínez-Mesa J. Presenting data in tables and charts. An Bras Dermatol [Internet]. Sociedade Brasileira de Dermatologia; 2014;89:280–5. Available from: http://www.ncbi.nlm.nih.gov/pmc/articles/PMC4008059/.
22. Rice K, Lumley T. Graphics and statistics for cardiology: comparing categorical and continuous variables. Heart. England. 2016;102:349–55.
23. Black HR, Elliott WJ, Grandits G, Grambsch P, Lucente T, White WB, et al. Principal results of the controlled onset verapamil investigation of cardiovascular end points (CONVINCE) trial. JAMA. United States. 2003;289:2073–82.
24. Krum H, Schlaich MP, Sobotka PA, Böhm M, Mahfoud F, Rocha-Singh K, et al. Percutaneous renal denervation in patients with treatment-resistant hypertension: final 3-year report of the Symplicity HTN-1 study. Lancet [Internet]. Elsevier; 2017;383:622–9. Available from: https://doi.org/10.1016/S0140-6736(13)62192-3.
25. Annesley TM. Bars and pies make better desserts than figures. Clin Chem United States. 2010;56:1394–400.
26. Hink JK, Eustace JK, Wogalter MS. Do grables enable the extraction of quantitative information better than pure graphs or tables? Int J Ind Ergon [Internet]. 1998;22:439–47. Available from: http://www.sciencedirect.com/science/article/pii/S0169814197000176.
27. Kozak M, Hartley J, Wnuk A, Tartanus M. Multiple pie charts: unreadable, inefficient, and overused. J Sch Publ [Internet]. University of Toronto Press; 2015;46:282–9. Available from: https://doi.org/10.3138/jsp.46.3.05.
28. Rosner B. Fundamentals of biostatistics. Boston: Cengage Learning; 2010.
29. Rumsey DJ. Statistics for dummies. Hoboken: Wiley; 2011.
30. Biffi A, CD A, TK B, et al. Association between blood pressure control and risk of recurrent intracerebral hemorrhage. JAMA [Internet]. 2015;314:904–12. Available from: https://doi.org/10.1001/jama.2015.10082.
31. Nuzzo RL. The box plots alternative for visualizing quantitative data. PM&R [Internet]. 2016;8:268–72. Available from: http://www.sciencedirect.com/science/article/pii/S1934148216000678.
32. Thabane L, Akhtar-Danesh N. Guidelines for reporting descriptive statistics in health research. Nurse Res England. 2008;15:72–81.
33. Tight blood pressure control and risk of macrovascular and microvascular complications in type 2 diabetes: UKPDS 38. BMJ [Internet]. 1998;317:703–713. Available from: http://www.bmj.com/content/317/7160/703.abstract.
34. Duran-Cantolla J, Aizpuru F, Montserrat JM, Ballester E, Teran-Santos J, Aguirregomoscorta JI, et al. Continuous positive airway pressure as treatment for systemic hypertension in people with obstructive sleep apnoea: randomised controlled trial. BMJ. England. 2010;341:c5991.

35. Effects of intensive blood-pressure control in type 2 diabetes mellitus. N Engl J Med [Internet]. Massachusetts Medical Society; 2010;362:1575–85. Available from: https://doi.org/10.1056/NEJMoa1001286.
36. Mancia G, Facchetti R, Parati G, Zanchetti A. Effect of long-term antihypertensive treatment on white-coat hypertension. Hypertens (Dallas, Tex 1979) United States. 2014;64:1388–98.
37. Logan M. Biostatistical design and analysis using R: a practical guide. Chichester: Wiley; 2011.
38. Lobo MD, Sobotka PA, Stanton A, Cockcroft JR, Sulke N, Dolan E, et al. Central arteriovenous anastomosis for the treatment of patients with uncontrolled hypertension (the ROX CONTROL HTN study): a randomised controlled trial. Lancet (London, England) England. 2015;385:1634–41.
39. Kirkwood BR, Sterne JAC. Essential medical statistics. Hoboken: Wiley; 2010.
40. Major outcomes in high-risk hypertensive patients randomized to angiotensin-converting enzyme inhibitor or calcium channel blocker vs diuretic: The Antihypertensive and Lipid-Lowering Treatment to Prevent Heart Attack Trial (ALLHAT). JAMA United States. 2002;288:2981–97.
41. Chernick MR, Friis RH. Introductory biostatistics for the health sciences: modern applications including bootstrap. Hoboken: Wiley; 2003.
42. Dunn OJ, Clark VA. Basic statistics: a primer for the biomedical sciences. Hoboken: Wiley; 2009.
43. Sedgwick P. A comparison of parametric and non-parametric statistical tests. BMJ. England. 2015;350:h2053.
44. du Prel J-B, Rohrig B, Hommel G, Blettner M. Choosing statistical tests: part 12 of a series on evaluation of scientific publications. Dtsch Arztebl Int Germany. 2010;107:343–8.
45. Cao J, Zhang S. Multiple comparison procedures. JAMA. United States. 2014;312:543–4.
46. Kim H-Y. Statistical notes for clinical researchers: post-hoc multiple comparisons. Restor Dent Endod Korea (South). 2015;40:172–6.
47. Write PS. Adjusted P-values for simultaneous inference. Biometrics. 1992;43:1005–13.
48. George B, Seals S, Aban I. Survival analysis and regression models. J Nucl Cardiol [Internet]. 2014;21:686–94. Available from: http://www.ncbi.nlm.nih.gov/pmc/articles/PMC4111957/.
49. Kleinbaum D, Klein M. Survival analysis: a self-learning text (Statistics for Biology and Health) [Internet]. Springer; 2005. Available from: citeulike-article-id:3504416.
50. May S, McKnight B. Graphics and statistics for cardiology: survival analysis. Heart England. 2017;103:335–40.
51. Altman DG. Practical statistics for medical research. 1st ed. London/New York: Chapman and Hall; 1991.
52. Selvin S. Survival analysis for epidemiologic and medical research [Internet]. Pract Guid Biostat Epidemiol. Cambridge: Cambridge University Press; 2008. Available from: https://www.cambridge.org/core/books/survival-analysis-for-epidemiologic-and-medical-research/021027404E37FCD99D5A9176D9EAB051.
53. Jager KJ, van Dijk PC, Zoccali C, Dekker FW. The analysis of survival data: the Kaplan-Meier method. Kidney Int United States. 2008;74:560–5.
54. Österlund P, Soveri L-M, Isoniemi H, Poussa T, Alanko T, Bono P. Hypertension and overall survival in metastatic colorectal cancer patients treated with bevacizumab-containing chemotherapy. Br J Cancer [Internet]. Nature Publishing Group; 2011;104:599–604. Available from: http://www.ncbi.nlm.nih.gov/pmc/articles/PMC3049598/.
55. Upadhya B, Rocco M, Lewis CE, Oparil S, Lovato LC, Cushman WC, et al. Effect of intensive blood pressure treatment on heart failure events in the systolic blood pressure reduction intervention trial. Circ Heart Fail United States. 2017;10:e003613.
56. Clark TG, Bradburn MJ, Love SB, Altman DG. Survival analysis part I: basic concepts and first analyses. Br J Cancer England. 2003;89:232–8.
57. Estruch R, Ros E, Salas-Salvado J, Covas M-I, Corella D, Aros F, et al. Primary Prevention of Cardiovascular Disease with a Mediterranean Diet Supplemented with Extra-Virgin Olive Oil or Nuts. N Engl J Med [Internet]. 2018;378(25):e34. Available from: https://doi.org/10.1056/NEJMoa1800389.
58. Tolles J, Lewis RJ. Time-to-event analysis. JAMA. United States. 2016;315:1046–7.
59. Bradburn MJ, Clark TG, Love SB, Altman DG. Survival analysis Part III: multivariate data analysis – choosing a model and assessing its adequacy and fit. Br J Cancer [Internet]. Nature Publishing Group; 2003;89:605–11. Available from: http://www.ncbi.nlm.nih.gov/pmc/articles/PMC2376927/.
60. Weber MA, Jamerson K, Bakris GL, Weir MR, Zappe D, Zhang Y, et al. Effects of body size and hypertension treatments on cardiovascular event rates: subanalysis of the ACCOMPLISH randomised controlled trial. Lancet [Internet]. Elsevier; 2017;381:537–45. Available from: https://doi.org/10.1016/S0140-6736(12)61343-9.
61. Newell DJ. Intention-to-treat analysis: implications for quantitative and qualitative research. Int J Epidemiol England. 1992;21:837–41.
62. Moher D, Hopewell S, Schulz KF. CONSORT 2010 explanation and elaboration: updated guidelines for reporting parallel group randomised trials. BMJ [Internet]. 2010;340. Available from: https://doi.org/10.1136/bmj.c869.
63. Lewis JA, Machin D. Intention to treat--who should use ITT? Br J Cancer England. 1993;68:647–50.
64. Shah PB. Intention-to-treat and per-protocol analysis. C Can Med Assoc J [Internet]. Canadian Medical Association; 2011;183:696. Available from: http://www.ncbi.nlm.nih.gov/pmc/articles/PMC3071397/.
65. Friedman LM, Furberg CD, DeMets DL. Fundamentals of clinical trials. New York: Springer; 2010.
66. Spieth PM, Kubasch AS, Penzlin AI, Illigens BM-W, Barlinn K, Siepmann T. Randomized controlled tri-

als – a matter of design. Neuropsychiatr Dis Treat New Zealand. 2016;12:1341–9.
67. Jamerson K, Weber MA, Bakris GL, Dahlöf B, Pitt B, Shi V, et al. Benazepril plus amlodipine or hydrochlorothiazide for hypertension in high-risk patients. N Engl J Med [Internet]. Massachusetts Medical Society; 2008;359:2417–28. Available from: https://doi.org/10.1056/NEJMoa0806182.
68. POCOCK SJ. Group sequential methods in the design and analysis of clinical trials. Biometrika [Internet]. 1977;64:191–9. Available from: https://doi.org/10.1093/biomet/64.2.191.
69. Pocock SJ. Interim analyses for randomized clinical trials: the group sequential approach. Biometrics [Internet]. [Wiley, International Biometric Society]; 1982;38:153–62. Available from: http://www.jstor.org/stable/2530298.
70. O'Brien PC, Fleming TR. A multiple testing procedure for clinical trials. Biometrics [Internet]. [Wiley, International Biometric Society]; 1979;35:549–56. Available from: http://www.jstor.org/stable/2530245.
71. Gordon Lan KK, Demets DL. Discrete sequential boundaries for clinical trials. Biometrika [Internet]. 1983;70:659–63. Available from: https://doi.org/10.1093/biomet/70.3.659.
72. Pocock SJ, McMurray JJV, Collier TJ. Statistical controversies in reporting of clinical trials: part 2 of a 4-part series on statistics for clinical trials. J Am Coll Cardiol United States. 2015;66:2648–62.
73. Matthews JN, Altman DG. Statistics notes. Interaction 2: compare effect sizes not P values. BMJ England. 1996;313:808.
74. Lagakos SW. The challenge of subgroup analyses--reporting without distorting. N Engl J Med United States. 2006;354:1667–9.
75. Hommel G. A stagewise rejective multiple test procedure based on a modified Bonferroni test. Biometrika [Internet]. 1988;75:383–6. Available from: https://doi.org/10.1093/biomet/75.2.383.
76. Thabane L, Mbuagbaw L, Zhang S, Samaan Z, Marcucci M, Ye C, et al. A tutorial on sensitivity analyses in clinical trials: the what, why, when and how. BMC Med Res Methodol England. 2013;13:92.
77. Noordzij M, Tripepi G, Dekker FW, Zoccali C, Tanck MW, Jager KJ. Sample size calculations: basic principles and common pitfalls. Nephrol Dial Transplant England. 2010;25:1388–93.
78. Eng J. Sample size estimation: how many individuals should be studied? Radiology United States. 2003;227:309–13.
79. Krzywinski M, Altman N. Points of significance: Power and sample size. Nat Meth [Internet]. Nature Publishing Group, a division of Macmillan Publishers Limited. All Rights Reserved.; 2013;10:1139–40. Available from: https://doi.org/10.1038/nmeth.2738.

Part II

Major Trials in Hypertension Research and Their Application in Clinical Practice

Arterial Hypertension and Cardiovascular Risk

3

Renata Cifkova

Hypertension as a Cardiovascular Risk Factor

In a comparative risk assessment of 67 risk factors and risk factor clusters in 21 regions, hypertension ranked first for global disease burden [1]. It is the most prevalent cardiovascular disorder affecting 20–50% of the adult population worldwide. At the same time, hypertension has been identified as a risk factor for coronary heart disease, stroke, peripheral arterial disease, heart and renal failure in both men and women in a large number of epidemiological studies [2–5]. Hypertension has also been shown to increase the risk of atrial fibrillation [6]. There is also evidence from observational studies that blood pressure (BP) correlates inversely with cognitive function and that hypertension is associated with an increased incidence of dementia [7, 8].

In the year 2001, the worldwide burden of disease attributable to high systolic BP (≥115 mmHg) was 54% for stroke, and 47% for ischemic heart disease [9]. About half of this burden was experienced by individuals with hypertension, the other part in those with a lesser degree of high BP. More than 80% of the attributable burden of the disease was found in low- and middle-income regions.

A meta-analysis of individual data of one million adults from 61 prospective observational studies found a continuous graded independent relationship with the risk of stroke and coronary events [10]. Coronary heart disease (CHD) and stroke mortality increases progressively and linearly from BP levels as low as 115 mmHg systolic and 75 mmHg diastolic upward (Figs. 3.1 and 3.2). The increased risks are seen in all age groups from 40 to 89 years of age. For every 20 mmHg systolic or 10 mmHg diastolic BP increase, there is a doubling of mortality from CHD and stroke.

The current text is an extension and update of the following chapter:
Cífková R. Assessment of Total Cardiovascular Risk in Hypertension: The Role of Subclinical Organ Damage. In: Berbari AE, Mancia G (eds). Special Issues in Hypertension. Springer Milan Heidelberg New York Dordrecht London, pp. 199–212. ISBN 978–88–470-2600-1.

R. Cifkova (✉)
Center for Cardiovascular Prevention, Charles University in Prague, First Faculty of Medicine and Thomayer Hospital, Prague, Czech Republic

Department of Medicine II – Cardiology and Angiology, Charles University in Prague, First Faculty of Medicine and General University Hospital, Prague, Czech Republic
e-mail: renata.cifkova@ftn.cz

V. Papademetriou et al. (eds.), *Management of Hypertension*,
https://doi.org/10.1007/978-3-319-92946-0_3

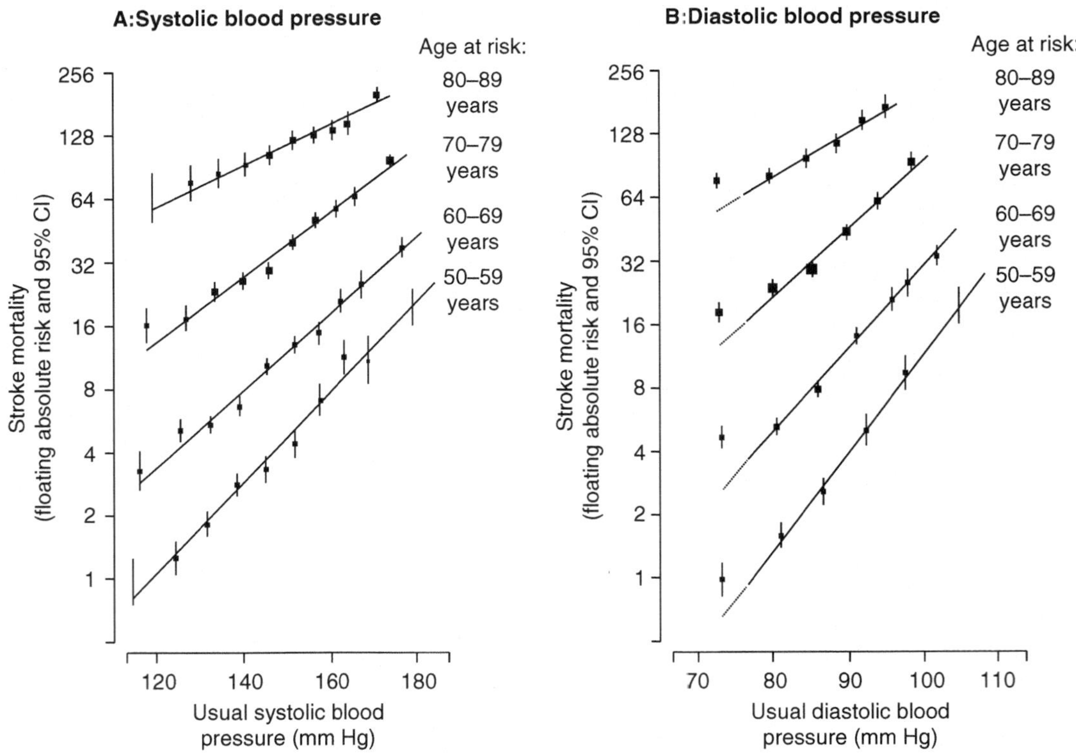

Fig. 3.1 Stroke mortality rate in each decade of age plotted for the usual systolic (*left*) and diastolic (*right*) blood pressure at the start of that decade. Data from one million adults in 61 prospective studies. (Adapted from Ref. [10])

Assessment of Total Cardiovascular Risk in Hypertension

Introduction

Historically, hypertension guidelines long focused on BP values as the only or main variables determining therapeutic interventions. Although this approach was maintained in the 2003 Joint National Committee (JNC) 7 guidelines [11] and was found cost effective [12], the ESH-ESC guidelines have since 2003 [13–15] emphasized that management of hypertension should be related to quantification of total cardiovascular (CV) risk. Finally, this approach was also adopted by the most recent US hypertension guidelines [16]. The rationale for this approach is that only a small proportion of the hypertensive population has an elevation of BP alone with the great majority exhibiting additional CV risk factors [17–21], with a relationship between the severity of BP elevation and that of alterations in glucose and lipid metabolism [22]. When elevated BP and metabolic risk factors are concomitantly present, they potentiate each other risk [17, 23, 24]. Thresholds and goals for antihypertensive treatment as well as treatment strategies for concomitant risk factors may differ based on total CV risk. Therefore, estimation of total CV risk is essential for guiding patient management.

The use of total CV risk estimation may also improve physicians´ behavior in drug prescription and patient adherence [25, 26]; however, there are some reports showing no impact on provider behaviors [27] and inadequate use in routine clinical practice [28, 29].

How to Assess Total CV Risk

A number of complex and computerized methods have been developed for estimating total CV risk,

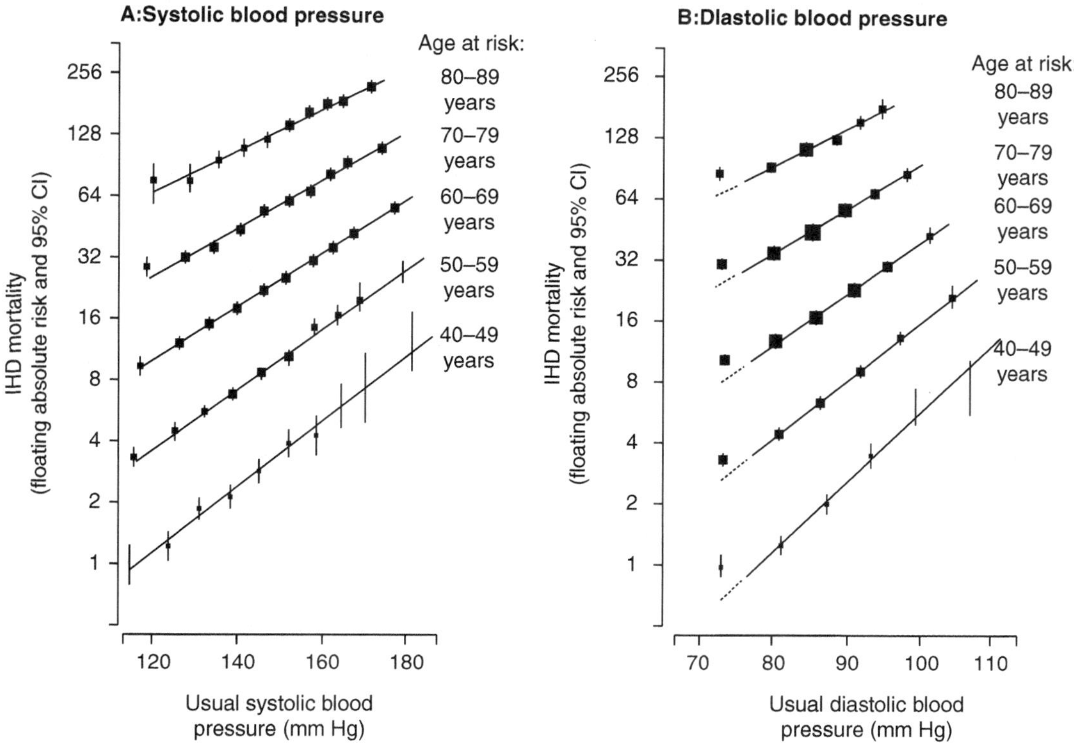

Fig. 3.2 Ischemic heart disease (IHD) mortality rate in each decade of age plotted for the usual systolic (*left*) and diastolic (*right*) blood pressure at the start of that decade. Data from one million adults in 61 prospective studies. (Adapted from Ref. [10])

i.e., the likelihood of experiencing a CV event, usually within the next 10 years. Many risk stratification systems are based on the Framingham study [30], estimating the 10-year risk for both fatal and non-fatal CHD by systolic BP and presence of other risk factors. The easy and rapid calculation of the Framingham risk score using published tables (National Cholesterol Education Program, NCEP) [31] may assist the physician and patient in demonstrating the benefits of treatment.

The Framingham risk stratification has been shown to be reasonably applicable to some European populations [32] but requiring recalibration in other populations [33, 34] due to geographic differences in the incidence of coronary and stroke events.

The latest US hypertension guidelines [16] recommend use of the ACC/AHA Pooled Cohort Equation (http://tools.acc.org/ASCVD-Risk-Estimator/) to estimate the 10-year risk of atherosclerotic CVD (ASCVD) to establish the BP threshold for treatment [35].

Given the need for a European model based on a large database, the SCORE (Systemic Coronary Risk Evaluation) project [36] was used to develop SCORE charts for high- and low-risk countries in Europe estimating the risk of dying from CV (not just coronary) disease over 10 years, and allowing calibration of the charts for individual countries provided that national mortality statistics and estimates of the prevalence of major CV risk factors are available. The SCORE model has also been used in the HeartScore, the official European Society of Cardiology management tool for implementation of CVD prevention in clinical practice (www.escardio.org).

The main disadvantage associated with an intervention threshold based on relatively short-term absolute risk is that younger adults (particularly women), while having more than one risk factor, are unlikely to reach treatment thresholds despite being at high risk relative to their peers. By contrast, most elderly men (e.g., those aged 65) will often reach treatment thresholds whilst being at very little increased risk relative to their peers. This situation results in most resources being concentrated on the oldest subjects whose potential lifespan, despite intervention, is relatively limited, while young subjects at high relative risk remain untreated despite, in the absence of intervention, a predicted significant shortening of their otherwise much longer potential lifespan [37, 38].

Use of the SCORE chart for estimating total CV risk in hypertension should be considered a minimal requirement taking into account the fact that total CV risk can be underestimated [39].

On the basis of these considerations, the 2013 ESH-ESC guidelines [15] suggest total CV risk be stratified as shown in Table 3.1. The terms *low (<1%)*, *moderate (<1 and <5%)*, *high (≥5 and <10%)*, and *very high (≥10%) risk* refer to the 10-year risk of CV mortality as defined by the 2012 ESC prevention guidelines [40]. The factors on which this stratification is based are listed in Table 3.2. They include risk factors, asymptomatic organ damage, diabetes mellitus, and established CV or renal disease.

Table 3.1 Stratification of total CV risk

Other risk factors, asymptomatic organ damage or disease	Blood pressure (mmHg)			
	High normal SBP 130–139 or DBP 85–89	Grade 1 HT SBP 140–159 or DBP 90–99	Grade 2 HT SBP 160–179 or DBP 100–109	Grade 3 HT SBP ≥180 or DBP ≥110
No other RF		Low risk	Moderate risk	High risk
1–2 RF	Low risk	Moderate risk	Moderate to high risk	High risk
≥3 RF	Low to Moderate risk	Moderate to high risk	High risk	High risk
OD, CKD stage 3 or diabetes	Moderate to high risk	High risk	High risk	High to very high risk
Symptomatic CVD, CKD stage ≥4 or diabetes with OD/RFs	Very high risk	Very high risk	Very high risk	Very high risk

BP = blood pressure; CKD = chronic kidney disease; CV = cardiovascular; CVD = cardiovascular disease; DBP = diastolic blood pressure; HT = hypertension; OD = organ damage; RF = risk factor; SBP = systolic blood pressure.

Table 3.2 Factors—other than office BP—influencing prognosis; used for stratification of total CV risk

Risk factors
Male sex
Age (men ≥55 years; women ≥65 years)
Smoking
Dyslipidemia
total cholesterol >4.9 mmol/l (190 mg/dl), and/or;
LDL-cholesterol >3.0 mmol/l (115 mg/dl), and/or;
HDL-cholesterol: men <1.0 mmol/l (40 mg/dl), women <1.2 mmol/l (46 mg/dl), and/or
triglycerides >1.7 mmol/l (150 mg/dl)
Fasting plasma glucose 5.6–6.9 mmol/l (102–125 mg/dl)
Abnormal glucose tolerance test
Obesity (BMI ≥ 30 kg/m^2)
Abdominal obesity (waist circumference: men ≥102 cm, women ≥88 cm in Caucasians)
Family history of premature CV disease (men aged <55 years; women aged <65 years)

Table 3.2 (continued)

Asymptomatic organ damage
Pulse pressure (in the elderly) ≥ 60 mmHg
Left ventricular hypertrophy
electrocardiogram:
Sokolow-Lyon index >3.5 mV; RaVL >1.1 mV; Cornell voltage duration product
> 244 mV×ms; or
echocardiogram:
LVM index[a]: men >115 g/m^2; women >95 g/m^2
Carotid wall thickening (IMT > 0.9 mm) or plaque
Carotid-femoral pulse wave velocity > 10 m/s
Ankle-brachial index <0.9
CKD with eGFR 30–60 ml/min/1.73 m^2
Microalbuminuria 30–300 mg/24 h or albumin-creatinine ratio 30–300 mg/g; 3.4–34 mg/mmol preferentially in morning spot urine
Diabetes mellitus
Fasting plasma glucose ≥7.0 mmol/l (126 mg/dl) on 2 repeated measurements, and/or
HbA_{1c} > 7% (53 mmol/mol), and/or
Post-load plasma glucose >11.0 mmol/l (198 mg/dl)
Established CV or renal disease
Cerebrovascular disease:
ischemic stroke;
cerebral hemorrhage;
transient ischemic attack
CHD:
myocardial infarction;
angina;
coronary revascularization with PCI or CABG;
heart failure
Heart failure, including heart failure with preserved EF
Symptomatic lower extremities PAD
CKD with eGFR <30 ml/min/1.73 m^2; proteinuria (> 300 mg/24 h)
Advanced retinopathy:
hemorrhages or exudates;
papilledema

Adopted from [15]

BMI body mass index, *CABG* coronary artery bypass grafting, *CHD* coronary heart disease, *CKD* chronic kidney disease, *CV* cardiovascular, *EF* ejection fraction, *eGFR* estimated glomerular filtration rate, *HbA_{1c}* glycated hemoglobin, *HDL-C* high-density lipoprotein cholesterol, *IMT* intima-media thickness, *LDL-C* low-density lipoprotein cholesterol, *LVM* left ventricular mass, *PCI* percutaneous coronary intervention, *PWV* pulse wave velocity

[a]Risk maximal for concentric LVH: increased LVM index with a wall thickness to radius ratio of 0.42

Searching for Subclinical (Asymptomatic) Organ Damage

Given the importance of subclinical organ damage as an intermediate stage in the continuum of vascular disease and as a determinant of overall CV risk, signs of organ involvement in hypertensive individuals should be sought for carefully using appropriate techniques.

The presence of any of the four following markers, i.e., increased urinary albumin excretion (UAE), increased pulse wave velocity (PWV), left ventricular hypertrophy (LVH), and carotid plaques predicts CV mortality independently of SCORE stratification [41–43]. This is an argument favoring routine use of organ damage assessment, particularly in specialized centers or clinics. The risk increases with the number of damaged organs [41].

Heart

Electrocardiography

Electrocardiography (EKG) is part of routine assessment of hypertensive individuals in order to detect LVH, pattern of "strain", ischemia, and arrhythmias. Its sensitivity in detecting LVH is low, nonetheless hypertrophy detected by Sokolow-Lyons index, modified Sokolow-Lyons index (largest S wave plus largest R wave >3.5 mV) or by Cornell voltage QRS duration is an independent predictor of CV events [44]. In a prospective survey including 7495 American adults, a new indicator of LVH, the Novacode estimate of left ventricular mass index (LVMI) (based on both voltage and strain pattern criteria), has been reported to be significantly related to 10-year CV mortality [45]. A further analysis from the LIFE trial has shown that hypertensive patients with EKG LVH or left bundle branch block are at increased risk of CV mortality and hospitalization for heart failure [46]. A prospective study by Verdecchia et al. [47] documented that R-wave voltage in aVL is closely associated with left ventricular mass (LVM) and predictive of CV events when hypertension is not accompanied by EKG LVH. The prevalence of EKG LVH increases the severity of hypertension [48].

Electrocardiography seems to be valuable at least in patients over 55 years of age [49, 50]. Electrocardiographic ST-T abnormalities are often present in conjunction with EKG LVH. Adding EKG repolarization changes to EKG voltage and QRS duration may improve the detection of LVH [51]. It can also be used to detect LV strain indicating higher risk [44, 49]. In the LIFE study, new development of EKG strain was a strong predictor of adverse outcome in the setting of EKG LVH regression [52].

Longer QRS duration is an independent predictor of sudden cardiac death and heart failure in patients with hypertension [52, 53].

Electrocardiography and/or 24-h Holter EKG monitoring play a crucial role in detecting atrial fibrillation, an independent predictor of adverse outcomes such as stroke, heart failure, and CV mortality in hypertensive patients [54]. There is growing evidence that new-onset atrial fibrillation should be considered target organ damage [55].

Echocardiography (Two-Dimensional Transthoracic)

Standard two-dimensional transthoracic echocardiography (2TTE) is more sensitive than electrocardiography in diagnosing LVH [56] and predicting CV and renal risk [57]; it may also be more helpful in risk stratification [58].

There are also some technical limitations such as inter-observer variability, low-quality imaging in obese individuals and in patients with obstructive lung disease. Although the relation between LVMI and CV risk is continuous, thresholds of 115 g/m^2 for men and 95 g/m^2 for women are widely used for conservative estimates of LVH [59]. Concentric hypertrophy (wall-to-radius ratio $\geq$0.42 with an increased LVM), eccentric hypertrophy (increased LVM and wall-to-radius ratio <0.42), and concentric remodeling (wall-to-radius ratio $\geq$0.42 with normal LVM) all predict an increased incidence of CVD but concentric hypertrophy has consistently been shown to be associated with the highest risk [60–62].

In addition, echocardiography is a tool for assessing left ventricular systolic and diastolic function; ejection fraction as well as midwall fractional shortening have been proposed as possible additional predictors of CV events. Alterations of diastolic function (i.e., alterations of LV relaxation and filling) are frequent in hypertensives, and particularly in the elderly [63]. Hypertension-induced diastolic dysfunction is associated with concentric geometry and can induce symptoms/signs of heart failure, even when ejection fraction (EF) is still normal (heart failure with preserved ejection fraction) [64]. Diastolic dysfunction is associated with increased risk of atrial fibrillation [65], heart failure [66], and increased total mortality [67]. Filing abnormalities can be quantified by Doppler transmitral inflow pattern and predict heart failure and all-cause mortality [66, 68].

Finally, echocardiography provides information on the size of the left atrium; left atrial enlargement is associated with a higher risk of atrial fibrillation, CVD, and death [69–72].

Table 3.3 Definitions of LVH, concentric geometry, left ventricular chamber, systolic/diastolic function, and LA dilation

Parameter	Measure	Cutoff point
LVH	LV mass/height^2 (g/m^2)	Men >50 Women >47
LVH	LV mass/BSA (g/m^2)	Men >115 Women >95
LV concentric geometry	RWT	≥ 0.43
LV chamber size	LV end-diastolic diameter/height (cm/m)	Men >3.3 Women >3.4
Systolic function	LV ejection fraction (%)	>55
Diastolic function	Septal e´ velocity (cm/s) Lateral e´ velocity (cm/s)	<8 <10
LV filling pressures	E/e´ (averaged) ratio	≥13
LA size (Simpson)	LA volume/BSA (ml/m^2)	≥34
LA size (elliptical)	LA volume/height^2 (ml/m^2)	Men >17.7 Women >16.7

BSA body surface area, *LA* left atrial, *LV* left ventricular, *LVH* left ventricular hypertrophy, *RWT* relative wall thickness

Normal ranges and cutoff values of parameters to be included in the echocardiographic report are listed in Table 3.3.

Subclinical systolic dysfunction can be assessed using speckle-tracking echocardiography to quantify longitudinal contractile function (longitudinal strain).

Other Cardiac Imaging Techniques

Three-dimensional echocardiography (3DE) is a more reliable method for quantitative analysis, and for LVM in particular. There is limited evidence for 3DE reference values and prognostic validation [73].

Cardiac magnetic resonance imaging is the gold standard for cardiac anatomical and functional quantification; it has the same limitations as 3DE and is more expensive. Cardiac magnetic resonance imaging should be used when 2D-TTE or 3DE is unavailable and LV geometry is important for the decision to treat.

Blood Vessels

Carotid Arteries

Ultrasound examination of the carotid arteries with measurement of intima-media thickness (IMT) or the presence of plaques have been shown to predict stroke and myocardial infarction [74, 75]. The relationship between carotid IMT and CV events is a continuous one but, for the common carotid arteries, an IMT > 0.9 mm is considered abnormal [76]. Ultrasound scans limited to the common carotid arteries (an infrequent site of atherosclerosis) are likely to measure vascular hypertrophy only whereas assessment of atherosclerosis also requires scanning of the bifurcations and/or internal carotids where plaques are more frequent [77–79]. Further analysis from ELSA [80] has shown baseline carotid IMT (both at carotid bifurcations and at the level of the common carotid artery) predicts CV events independent of BP (clinic and ambulatory). This suggests that both atherosclerosis (reflected by the IMT at bifurcations) and vascular hypertrophy (reflected by the common carotid IMT) exert an adverse prognostic effect in addition to that of high BP.

Quantitative B-mode ultrasound of carotid arteries requires training and methodological standardization for IMT measurement. Lack of standardization regarding the definition and measurement of IMT were responsible for high variability and low intra-individual reproducibility. A meta-analysis failed to show any added value of IMT compared with the Framingham risk score in predicting future CVD even in the intermediate risk group [81]. Thus, the 2016 European guidelines on CVD prevention in clinical practice do not recommend systematic use of carotid IMT to improve risk assessment [82].

Presence of a plaque can be identified by an IMT > 1.3 mm or 1.5 mm, or by a focal increase in thickness of 0.5 mm or 50% of the surrounding IMT value [77–79]. There is evidence that, in untreated hypertensive individuals without target organ damage by routinely performed tests, these alterations are common and thus carotid ultrasound examination may often detect vascular damage and make risk stratification more precise [39]. An adverse prognostic significance of carotid plaques (hazard ratio 2.3) has also been reported in a sample of Copenhagen county residents free of overt CVD, followed for about 13 years [83].

Carotid plaque has a stronger predictive value for both stroke and myocardial infarction, higher than that of IMT and independent of traditional CV risk factors. The presence of a carotid plaque automatically reclassifies patients from intermediate to high risk [76]; however, routine carotid ultrasound imaging is not recommended unless there is a clinical indication (bruit, previous TIA or stroke).

Ankle-Brachial Index

A low ankle-brachial index (ABI, <0.9) signals peripheral arterial disease and, in general, advanced atherosclerosis [84, 85] whereas carotid IMT measurements are able to detect earlier changes. A reduced ABI (< 0.9) relates to further development of angina, myocardial infarction, congestive heart failure, need for coronary artery bypass surgery, stroke, carotid and peripheral vascular surgery [86–89] and, in patients with multi-vessel coronary disease, it confers additional risk [90].

Pulse Wave Velocity

Large artery stiffening has been identified as the most important pathophysiological determinant of isolated systolic hypertension and age-related pulse pressure increase [91]. Measurement of carotid-femoral pulse wave velocity (PWV) provides a comprehensive non-invasive assessment of arterial stiffness [92]. Carotid-femoral PWV is currently considered the gold standard for large artery stiffening, a measure shown to have an independent predictive value for all-cause mortality and CV morbidity, coronary events and strokes in patients with uncomplicated essential hypertension [93–97]. Reference values for PWV are available from 16,867 subjects enrolled in 13 different centers in eight European countries [98]. A PWV > 10 m/s is considered a conservative estimate of an abnormal value in middle-aged hypertensive patients [99]. The additive predictive value of PWV beyond traditional risk scoring systems (including SCORE and the Framingham Risk Score) has been shown by the Copenhagen county population [83].

Indirect indices of aortic stiffness and wave reflection such as central blood pressure and augmentation index have been confirmed as independent predictors of CV events in two studies [100, 101]. In one of these studies, only central systolic blood pressure consistently and independently predicted CV mortality after adjustment for various CV risk factors including LVM and carotid IMT [101]. In the Conduit Artery Function Evaluation (CAFE) study, a substudy of ASCOT, central pulse pressure was significantly associated with a post-hoc defined composite outcome of fatal CV events/procedures and development of renal impairment [102]. The BP GUIDE study [103] showed that management of hypertension guided by central aortic blood pressure (compared with best practice care) was associated with less use of medication to achieve BP control.

In conclusion, PWV may be useful in refining risk stratification in selected patients but is not yet recommended for routine practice.

Kidney

The diagnosis of induced renal damage is based on the finding of a reduced renal function and/or the detection of elevated urinary albumin excretion [104]. Renal function is represented mainly by glomerular filtration rate (GFR) depending on the number and function of nephrons, and decreasing with age after the third decade (progressive loss of 1% per year).

Renal function is currently classified based on the estimated glomerular filtration rate (eGFR) calculated using various formulas of which the 2009 CKD EPI formula seems to be the most reliable for a wide range of patients [105]. Values of eGFR <60 ml/min/1.73 m^2 indicate chronic kidney disease (CKD) stage 3 whilst values <30 and <15 ml/min/1.73 m^2 indicate CKD stages 4 and 5 (kidney failure), respectively [106] (Table 3.4).

A reduction in GFR and an increase in CV risk are also reflected in increased serum cystatin C [107].

While elevated serum creatinine or low eGFR (or creatinine clearance) indicate reduced glomerular filtration, an increase in urinary albumin or protein excretion reflects derangement in the glomerular filtration barrier. Urinary albumin excretion (UAR) has been shown to predict the development of overt diabetic nephropathy in both type 1 and 2 diabetics [108] while the presence of overt proteinuria generally indicates the presence of established renal parenchymal damage [109]. Urinary albumin excretion, even below the current threshold values, has been shown to predict CV events in both diabetic and non-diabetic hypertensive patients [110, 111]. There is a continuous relationship between CV and non-CV mortality and urinary protein excretion [112, 113]. Albuminuria can be measured from spot urine samples, preferably early morning urine (24-h or night urine samples are discouraged due to the inaccuracy of urine collection) by indexing the urinary albumin concentration to the urinary creatinine concentration [106].

Progressive reduction in eGFR and increased albuminuria indicate progressive loss of renal function towards end-stage renal disease and are

Table 3.4 Prognosis of CKD by GFR and albuminuria category

Prognosis of CKD by GFR and albuminuria categories: KDIGO 2012				Persistent albuminuria categories description and range		
				A1	A2	A3
				Normal to mildly increased	Moderately increased	Severely increased
				<30 mg/g <3mg/mmol	30-300 mg/g 3-30 mg/mmol	>300 mg/g >30mg/mmol
GFR categories (ml/min/ 1.73 m^2) Description and range	G1	Normal or high	≥90			
	G2	Mildly decreased	60–89			
	G3a	Mildly to moderately decreased	45–59			
	G3b	Moderately to severely decreased	30–44			
	G4	Severely decreased	15–29			
	G5	Kidney failure	<15			

Green: low risk (if no other markers of kidney disease, no CKD); Yellow: moderately increased risk;
Orange: high risk; Red, very high risk.
CKD= chronic kidney disease; GFR = glomerular filtration rate

both independent predictors of increased CV risk in diabetic and non-diabetic kidney disease [114]. The presence of both increased albuminuria and reduced eGFR is associated with a greater risk of renal and CV complications (Table 3.4).

Hyperuricemia is frequently seen in untreated hypertensives (particularly in pre-eclampsia) and has also been shown to correlate with reduced renal blood flow and the presence of nephrosclerosis [115].

Serum creatinine, eGFR, and urinalysis including measurement of albumin-to-creatinine ratio are considered routine laboratory tests to be performed in all hypertensive patients and repeated at least annually.

Retinal Vessels

Most hypertensive patients usually present early in the process of their disease, and hemorrhages and exudates (grade 3) and papilledema (grade 4) are observed very rarely but are highly reproducible and always associated with an increased risk of CV events [116, 117]. On the other hand, grade 1 (focal or general arteriolar narrowing) and 2 (arteriovenous nipping) retinal changes are reported much more frequently than other subclinical organ damage with documented clinical significance (LVH, carotid plaques, and albuminuria), but the prognostic significance of these mild retinal changes has been questioned [118–121] and their reproducibility is limited. These changes appear to be largely non-specific except for young patients, in whom a deviation from an entirely normal retina should raise concern. More selective methods for objective assessment of the eye fundus have been developed, e.g., digitalized retinal photographs, which showed that retinal arteriolar and venular narrowing may precede the development of hypertension [122, 123].

Brain

Hypertension is associated with an increased risk of ischemic and hemorrhagic stroke, and vascular brain injury (VBI) [124]. Brain imaging in hypertension may be used to detect VBI considered a sign of cerebral small vessel disease (SVD) and an important mediator of the relationship between hypertension and brain aging. Cerebral SVD is associated with cognitive, psychiatric, and physical disabilities contributing to the risk of stroke, cognitive dysfunction, and dementia [125–127]. The following signs of VBI can be recognized on brain imaging: white matter hyperintensity, cerebral microbleeds, recent small subcortical infarcts, lacunes, dilated perivascular space, and atrophy [128].

Several studies have shown that VBI detected using magnetic resonance imaging (MRI) is quite common in the general population [125, 129], with prevalence increasing with age and hypertension. The availability and cost considerations do not allow widespread use of MRI in the evaluation of elderly patients but silent brain infarcts should be sought in all hypertensives with neural disturbance and, particularly, memory loss. Cognitive tests should be used in the clinical assessment of elderly hypertensives [130].

Prognostic Value of Treatment-Induced and Multiorgan Subclinical Organ Damage

Treatment-induced changes in organ damage affect the incidence of CV events, hence organ damage should be assessed also during treatment [131] because LVH regression and reduction of urinary protein excretion indicate treatment-induced CV protection [131, 132]. There is also some evidence that treatment-induced changes in eGFR predict CV events [133–139].

On the other hand, two meta-analyses did not show any predictive value of treatment-induced reduction in carotid IMT for CV events [140, 141]. There is no or limited evidence for the predictive power of treatment-induced changes in PWV and ABI.

Whenever possible, search for subclinical organ damage should be made simultaneously in various organs because multiorgan subclinical organ damage is associated with a worse prognosis.

A population-based study from Denmark showed that subclinical organ damage predicted CV death independently of SCORE and use of the combination of SCORE and subclinical organ damage may improve risk prediction, particularly in subjects with moderate CV risk, by assessing urinary albumin excretion and pulse wave velocity [41].

Regression of target organ damage may not be achieved even under satisfactory BP control. Some changes may be irreversible because they are too advanced. Blood pressure-lowering treatment can also prevent development of target organ damage [142]. If target organ damage develops during antihypertensive treatment, it may be associated with an increased risk [143].

In conclusion, it is important to assess target organ damage on treatment; if there is target organ damage at baseline, its evaluation should be repeated at least once during the first year of effective BP control. If there is no target organ damage at baseline, the re-assessment may be postponed.

References

1. Lim SS, et al. A comparative risk assessment of burden of disease and injury attributable to 67 risk factors and risk factor clusters in 21 regions, 1990–2010: a systematic analysis for the global burden of disease study 2010. Lancet. 2012;380(9859):2224–60. https://doi.org/10.1016/S0140-6736(12)61766-8.
2. MacMahon S, Peto R, Cutler J, et al. Blood pressure, stroke, and coronary heart disease. Part 1. Prolonged differences in blood pressure: prospective observational studies corrected for the regression dilution bias. Lancet. 1990;335(8692):765–74.
3. Kannel WB. Blood pressure as a cardiovascular risk factor: prevention and treatment. JAMA. 1996;275:1571–6.
4. Assmann G, Schulte H. The prospective cardiovascular Munster (PROCAM) study: prevalence of hyperlipidemia in persons with hypertension and/or diabetes mellitus and the relationship to coronary heart disease. Am Heart J. 1988;116(6 Pt 2):1713–24.
5. Walker WG, Neaton JD, Cutler JA, Neuwirth R, Cohen JD. Renal function change in hypertensive members of the multiple risk factor intervention trial. Racial and treatment effects. The MRFIT research group. JAMA. 1992;268:3085–91.
6. Lloyd-Jones DM, Wang TJ, Leip EP, Larson MG, Levy D, Vasan RS, D'Agostino RB, Massaro JM, Beiser A, Wolf PA, Benjamin EJ. Lifetime risk for development of atrial fibrillation: the Framingham heart study. Circulation. 2004;110:1042–6. Epub 2004 Aug 16.
7. Skoog I, Lernfelt B, Landahl S, et al. 15-year longitudinal study of blood pressure and dementia. Lancet. 1996;347(9009):1141–5.
8. Hajjar I, Goldstein FC, Martin GS, Quyyumi AA. Roles of arterial stiffness and blood pressure in hypertension-associated cognitive decline in healthy adults. Hypertension. 2016;67:171–5. https://doi.org/10.1161/HYPERTENSIONAHA.115.06277. Epub 2015 Nov 2.
9. Lawes CM, Vander Hoorn S, Rodgers A, International Society of Hypertension. Global burden of blood-pressure-related disease, 2001. Lancet. 2008;371(9623):1513–8. https://doi.org/10.1016/S0140-6736(08)60655-8.
10. Lewington S, Clarke R, Qizilbash N, Peto R, Collins R, Prospective Studies Collaboration. Age-specific relevance of usual blood pressure to vascular mortality: a meta-analysis of individual data for one million adults in 61 prospective studies. Lancet. 2002;360(9349):1903–13.
11. Chobanian AV, Bakris GL, Black HR, Cushman WC, Green LA, Izzo L Jr, Jones DW, Materson BJ, Oparil S, Wright JT Jr, Roccella EJ, National Heart, Lung, Blood Institute; National High Blood Pressure Education Program Coordinating Committee. Seventh report of the joint National Committee on prevention, detection, evaluation, and treatment of high blood pressure. Hypertension. 2003;42:1206–52.
12. Rubinstein A, Colantonio L, Bardach A, Caporale J, Martí SG, Kopitowski K, Alcaraz A, Gibbons L, Augustovski F, Pichón-Rivière A. Estimation of the burden of cardiovascular disease attributable to modifiable risk factors and cost-effectiveness analysis of preventative interventions to reduce this burden in Argentina. BMC Public Health. 2010;10:627. https://doi.org/10.1186/1471-2458-10-627.
13. Guidelines Committee. 2003 European Society of Hypertension-European Society of Cardiology guidelines for the management of arterial hypertension. J Hypertens. 2003;21:1011–53.
14. Mancia G, De Backer G, Dominiczak A, Cifkova R, Fagard R, Germano G, Grassi G, Heagerty AM, Kjeldsen SE, Laurent S, Narkiewicz K, Ruilope L, Rynkiewicz A, Schmieder RE, Boudier HA, Zanchetti A, Vahanian A, Camm J, De Caterina R, Dean V, Dickstein K, Filippatos G, Funck-Brentano C, Hellemans I, Kristensen SD, McGregor K, Sechtem U, Silber S, Tendera M, Widimsky P, Zamorano JL, Erdine S, Kiowski W, Agabiti-Rosei E, Ambrosioni E, Lindholm LH, Viigimaa M, Adamopoulos S, Agabiti-Rosei E, Ambrosioni E, Bertomeu V, Clement D, Erdine S, Farsang C, Gaita D, Lip G, Mallion JM, Manolis AJ, Nilsson

PM, O'Brien E, Ponikowski P, Redon J, Ruschitzka F, Tamargo J, van Zwieten P, Waeber B, Williams B, Management of Arterial Hypertension of the European Society of Hypertension; European Society of Cardiology. 2007 Guidelines for the Management of Arterial Hypertension: The Task Force for the Management of Arterial Hypertension of the European Society of Hypertension (ESH) and of the European Society of Cardiology (ESC). J Hypertens. 2007;25:1105–87. No abstract available. Erratum in: J Hypertens 2007;25(8):1749.
15. Mancia G, Fagard R, Narkiewicz K, Redón J, Zanchetti A, Böhm M, Christiaens T, Cifkova R, De Backer G, Dominiczak A, Galderisi M, Grobbee DE, Jaarsma T, Kirchhof P, Kjeldsen SE, Laurent S, Manolis AJ, Nilsson PM, Ruilope LM, Schmieder RE, Sirnes PA, Sleight P, Viigimaa M, Waeber B, Zannad F, Task Force Members. 2013 ESH/ESC Guidelines for the management of arterial hypertension: the Task Force for the management of arterial hypertension of the European Society of Hypertension (ESH) and of the European Society of Cardiology (ESC). J Hypertens. 2013;31:1281–357. https://doi.org/10.1097/01.hjh.0000431740.32696.cc. No abstract available.
16. Whelton PK, Carey RM, Aronow WS, Casey DE Jr, Collins KJ, Dennison Himmelfarb C, DePalma SM, Gidding S, Jamerson KA, Jones DW, MacLaughlin EJ, Muntner P, Ovbiagele B, Smith SC Jr, Spencer CC, Stafford RS, Taler SJ, Thomas RJ, Williams KA Sr, Williamson JD, Wright JT Jr. 2017 ACC/AHA/AAPA/ABC/ACPM/AGS/APhA/ASH/ASPC/NMA/PCNA guideline for the prevention, detection, evaluation, and management of high blood pressure in adults: a report of the American College of Cardiology/American Heart Association Task Force on Clinical Practice Guidelines. Hypertension. 2018;71:1269–324. https://doi.org/10.1161/HYP.0000000000000065. pii: HYP.0000000000000065. [Epub ahead of print].
17. Kannel WB. Risk stratification in hypertension: new insights from the Framingham Study. Am J Hypertens. 2000;13(Suppl 1):S3–S10.
18. Thomas F, Rudnichi A, Bacri AM, Bean K, Guize L, Benetos A. Cardiovascular mortality in hypertensive men according to presence of associated risk factors. Hypertension. 2001;37:1256–61.
19. Wei M, Mitchell BD, Haffner SM, Stern MP. Effects of cigarette smoking, diabetes, high cholesterol, and hypertension on all-cause mortality and cardiovascular disease mortality in Mexican Americans. The San Antonio Heart Study. Am J Epidemiol. 1996;144:1058–65.
20. Assmann G, Schulte H. The Prospective Cardiovascular Münster (PROCAM) study: prevalence of hyperlipidemia in persons with hypertension and/or diabetes mellitus and the relationship to coronary heart disease. Am Heart J. 1988;116(6 Pt 2):1713–24.
21. Mancia G, Parati G, Borghi C, Ghironzi G, Andriani E, Marinelli L, Valentini M, Tessari F, Ambrosioni E, SMOOTH Investigators. Hypertension prevalence, awareness, control and association with metabolic abnormalities in the San Marino population: the SMOOTH study. Hypertension. 2006;24:837–43.
22. Mancia G, Facchetti R, Bombelli M, Polo Friz H, Grassi G, Giannattasio C, Sega R. Relationship of office, home, and ambulatory blood pressure to blood glucose and lipid variables in the PAMELA population. Hypertension. 2005;45:1072–7.
23. Asia Pacific Cohort Studies Collaboration. Joint effects of systolic blood pressure and serum cholesterol on cardiovascular disease in the Asia Pacific region. Circulation. 2005;112:3384–90.
24. Multiple Risk Factor Intervention Trial Research Group. Relationship between baseline risk factors coronary heart disease total mortality in the Multiple Risk Factor Intervention Trial. Mult Risk Factor Interv Trial Res Group Prev Med. 1986;15:254–73.
25. Viera AJ, Sheridan SL. Global risk of coronary heart disease: assessment and application. Am Fam Physician. 2010;82:265–74.
26. Brett T, Arnold-Reed D, Phan C, Cadden F, Walker W, Manea-Walley W, Mora N, Young J, Bulsara M. The Fremantle Primary Prevention Study: a multicentre randomised trial of absolute cardiovascular risk reduction. Br J Gen Pract. 2012;62:e22–8. https://doi.org/10.3399/bjgp12X616337.
27. Vagholkar S, Zwar N, Jayasinghe UW, Denney-Wilson E, Patel A, Campbell T, Harris MF. Influence of cardiovascular absolute risk assessment on prescribing of antihypertensive and lipid-lowering medications: a cluster randomized controlled trial. Am Heart J. 2014;167:28–35. https://doi.org/10.1016/j.ahj.2013.10.002. Epub 2013 Oct 17
28. Frikke-Schmidt R, Tybjærg-Hansen A, Schnohr P, Jensen GB, Nordestgaard BG. Common clinical practice versus new PRIM score in predicting coronary heart disease risk. Atherosclerosis. 2010;213:532–8. https://doi.org/10.1016/j.atherosclerosis.2010.07.028. Epub 2010 Jul 27
29. Shillinglaw B, Viera AJ, Edwards T, Simpson R, Sheridan SL. Use of global coronary heart disease risk assessment in practice: a cross-sectional survey of a sample of U.S. physicians. BMC Health Serv Res. 2012;12:20. https://doi.org/10.1186/1472-6963-12-20.
30. Anderson KM, Wilson PW, Odell PM, Kannel WB. An updated coronary risk profile. A statement for health professionals. Circulation. 1991;83:356–62.
31. National Cholesterol Education Program. (NCEP) expert panel on detection, evaluation, and treatment of high blood cholesterol in adults (adult treatment panel III). Third report of the National Cholesterol Education Program (NCEP) expert panel on detection, evaluation, and treatment of high blood choles-

terol in adults (adult treatment panel III) final report. Circulation. 2002;106:3143–421.
32. Haq IU, Ramsay LE, Yeo WW, Jackson PR, Wallis EJ. Is the Framingham risk function valid for northern European populations? A comparison of methods for estimating absolute coronary risk in high risk men. Heart. 1999;81:40–6.
33. Menotti A, Puddu PE, Lanti M. Comparison of the Framingham risk function-based coronary chart with risk function from an Italian population study. Eur Heart J. 2000;21:365–70.
34. Hense HW, Schulte H, Löwel H, Assmann G, Keil U. Framingham risk function overestimates risk of coronary heart disease in men and women from Germany–results from the MONICA Augsburg and the PROCAM cohorts. Eur Heart J. 2003;24:937–45.
35. Goff DC Jr, Lloyd-Jones DM, Bennett G, Coady S, D'Agostino RB, Gibbons R, Greenland P, Lackland DT, Levy D, O'Donnell CJ, Robinson JG, Schwartz JS, Shero ST, Smith SC Jr, Sorlie P, Stone NJ, Wilson PW, Jordan HS, Nevo L, Wnek J, Anderson JL, Halperin JL, Albert NM, Bozkurt B, Brindis RG, Curtis LH, DeMets D, Hochman JS, Kovacs RJ, Ohman EM, Pressler SJ, Sellke FW, Shen WK, Smith SC Jr, Tomaselli GF, American College of Cardiology/American Heart Association Task Force on Practice Guidelines. 2013 ACC/AHA guideline on the assessment of cardiovascular risk: a report of the American College of Cardiology/American Heart Association Task Force on Practice Guidelines. Circulation. 2014;129(25 Suppl 2):S49–73. https://doi.org/10.1161/01.cir.0000437741.48606.98. Epub 2013 Nov 12.
36. Conroy RM, Pyörälä K, Fitzgerald AP, Sans S, Menotti A, De Backer G, De Bacquer D, Ducimetière P, Jousilahti P, Keil U, Njølstad I, Oganov RG, Thomsen T, Tunstall-Pedoe H, Tverdal A, Wedel H, Whincup P, Wilhelmsen L, Graham IM, SCORE Project Group. Estimation of ten-year risk of fatal cardiovascular disease in Europe: the SCORE project. Eur Heart J. 2003;24:987–1003.
37. Simpson FO. Guidelines for antihypertensive therapy: problems with a strategy based on absolute cardiovascular risk. J Hypertens. 1996;14:683–9.
38. Zanchetti A. Antihypertensive therapy: how to evaluate the benefits. Am J Cardiol. 1997;79:3–8. discussion 47–8
39. Cuspidi C, Ambrosioni E, Mancia G, Pessina AC, Trimarco B, Zanchetti A, APROS Investigators. Role of echocardiography and carotid ultrasonography in stratifying risk in patients with essential hypertension: the Assessment of Prognostic Risk Observational Survey. J Hypertens. 2002;20:1307–14.
40. Perk J, De Backer G, Gohlke H, Graham I, Reiner Z, Verschuren M, Albus C, Benlian P, Boysen G, Cifkova R, Deaton C, Ebrahim S, Fisher M, Germano G, Hobbs R, Hoes A, Karadeniz S, Mezzani A, Prescott E, Ryden L, Scherer M, Syvänne M, Scholte op Reimer WJ, Vrints C, Wood D, Zamorano JL, Zannad F, European Association for Cardiovascular Prevention & Rehabilitation (EACPR); ESC Committee for Practice Guidelines (CPG). European guidelines on cardiovascular disease prevention in clinical practice (version 2012). The fifth joint task force of the European Society of Cardiology and Other Societies on cardiovascular disease prevention in clinical practice (constituted by representatives of nine societies and by invited experts). Eur Heart J. 2012;33:1635–701. https://doi.org/10.1093/eurheartj/ehs092. Epub 2012 May 3.
41. Sehestedt T, Jeppesen J, Hansen TW, Wachtell K, Ibsen H, Torp-Pedersen C, et al. Risk prediction is improved by adding markers of subclinical organ damage to SCORE. Eur Heart J. 2010;31:883–91.
42. Sehestedt T, Jeppesen J, Hansen TW, Rasmussen S, Wachtell K, Ibsen H, et al. Thresholds for pulse wave velocity, urine albumin creatinine ratio and left ventricular mass index using SCORE, Framingham and ESH/ESC risk charts. J Hypertens. 2012;30:1928–36.
43. Volpe M, Battistoni A, Tocci G, Agabiti Rosei E, Catapano AL, Coppo R, et al. Cardiovascular risk assessment beyond systemic coronary risk estimation: a role for organ damage markers. J Hypertens. 2012;30:1056–64.
44. Levy D, Salomon M, D'Agostino RB, Belanger AJ, Kannel WB. Prognostic implications of baseline electrocardiographic features and their serial changes in subjects with left ventricular hypertrophy. Circulation. 1994;90:1786–93.
45. Havranek EP, Froshaug DB, Emserman CD, Hanratty R, Krantz MJ, Masoudi FA, Dickinson LM, Steiner JF. Left ventricular hypertrophy and cardiovascular mortality by race and ethnicity. Am J Med. 2008;121:870–5.
46. Li Z, Dahlöf B, Okin PM, Kjeldsen SE, Wachtell K, Ibsen H, Nieminen MS, Jern S, Devereux RB. Left bundle branch block and cardiovascular morbidity and mortality in hypertensive patients with left ventricular hypertrophy: the Losartan Intervention for Endpoint Reduction in Hypertension study. J Hypertens. 2008;26:1244–9.
47. Verdecchia P, Angeli F, Cavallini C, Mazzotta G, Repaci S, Pede S, Borgioni C, Gentile G, Reboldi G. The voltage of R wave in lead aVL improves risk stratification in hypertensive patients without ECG left ventricular hypertrophy. J Hypertens. 2009;27:1697–704.
48. Bacharova L, Schocken D, Estes EH, Strauss D. The role of ECG in the diagnosis of left ventricular hypertrophy. Curr Cardiol Rev. 2014;10:257–61.
49. Okin PM, Devereux RB, Jern S, Kjeldsen SE, Julius S, Nieminen MS, et al. Regression of electrocardiographic left ventricular hypertrophy during antihypertensive treatment and the prediction of major cardiovascular events. JAMA. 2004;292:2343–9.
50. Fagard RH, Staessen JA, Thijs L, Celis H, Birkenhager WH, Bulpitt CJ, et al. Prognostic significance of electrocardiographic voltages and their

serial changes in elderly with systolic hypertension. Hypertension. 2004;44:459–64.
51. Hancock EW, Deal BJ, Mirvis DM, et al. AHA/ACCF/HRS recommendations for the standardization and interpretation of the electrocardiogram: part V: electrocardiogram changes associated with cardiac chamber hypertrophy: a scientific statement from the America Heart Association Electrocardiography and Arrhythmias Committee, Council on Clinical Cardiology; the American College of Cardiology Foundation; and the Heart Rhythm Society. Endorsed by the International Society for Computerized Electrocardiology. J Am Coll Cardiol. 2009;53:992–1002.
52. Okin PM, Oikarinen L, Viitasalo M, Toivonen L, Kjeldsen SE, Nieminen MS, et al. Prognostic value of changes in the electrocardiographic strain pattern during antihypertensive treatment: the Losartan Intervention for End-Point Reduction in Hypertension Study (LIFE). Circulation. 2009;119:1883–91.
53. Morin DP, Oikarinen L, Viitasalo M, et al. QRS duration predicts sudden cardiac death in hypertensive patients undergoing intensive medical therapy: the LIFE study. Eur Heart J. 2009;30:2908–14.
54. Wachtell K, Hornestam B, Lehto M, et al. Cardiovascular morbidity and mortality in hypertensive patients with a history of atrial fibrillation: the Losartan Intervention for End Point Reduction in Hypertension (LIFE) study. J Am Coll Cardiol. 2005;45:705–11.
55. Chrispin J, Jain A, Soliman EZ, et al. Association of electrocardiographic and imaging surrogates of left ventricular hypertrophy with incident atrial fibrillation: MESA (Multi-Ethnic Study of Atherosclerosis). J Am Coll Cardiol. 2014;63:2007–13.
56. Reichek N, Devereux RB. Left ventricular hypertrophy: relationship of anatomic, echocardiographic and electrocardiographic findings. Circulation. 1981;63:1391–8.
57. Levy D, Garrison RJ, Savage DD, Kannel WB, Castelli WP. Prognostic implications of echocardiographically determined left ventricular mass in the Framingham Heart Study. N Engl J Med. 1990;322:1561–6.
58. Tsioufis C, Kokkinos P, Macmanus C, Thomopoulos C, Faselis C, Doumas M, et al. Left ventricular hypertrophy as a determinant of renal outcome in patients with high cardiovascular risk. J Hypertens. 2010;28:2299–308.
59. Lang RM, Bierig M, Devereux RB, Flachskampf FA, Foster E, Pellikka PA, et al. Recommendations for chamber quantification. Eur J Echocardiogr. 2006;7:79–108.
60. Koren MJ, Devereux RB, Casale PN, Savage DD, Laragh JH. Relation of left ventricular mass and geometry to morbidity and mortality in uncomplicated essential hypertension. Ann Intern Med. 1991;114:345–52.
61. Verdecchia P, Schillaci G, Borgioni C, Ciucci A, Battistelli M, Bartoccini C, et al. Adverse prognostic significance of concentric remodeling of the left ventricle in hypertensive patients with normal left ventricular mass. J Am Coll Cardiol. 1995;25:871–8.
62. Muiesan ML, Salvetti M, Monteduro C, Bonzi B, Paini A, Viola S, et al. Left ventricular concentric geometry during treatment adversely affects cardiovascular prognosis in hypertensive patients. Hypertension. 2004;43:731–8.
63. Zanchetti A, Cuspidi C, Comarella L, Rosei EA, Ambrosioni E, Chiariello M, Leonetti G, Mancia G, Pessina AC, Salvetti A, Trimarco B, Volpe M, Grassivaro N, Vargiu G. Left ventricular diastolic dysfunction in elderly hypertensives: results of the APROS-diadys study. J Hypertens. 2007;25:2158–67.
64. Hogg K, Swedberg K, McMurray J. Heart failure with preserved left ventricular systolic function: epidemiology, clinical characteristics and prognosis. J Am Coll Cardiol. 2004;43:317–27.
65. Tsang TS, Barnes ME, Gersh BJ, Bailey KR, Seward JB. Risks for atrial fibrillation and congestive heart failure in patients ≥ 65 years of age with abnormal left ventricular diastolic relaxation. Am J Cardiol. 2004;93:54–8.
66. Aurigemma GP, Gottdiener JS, Shemanski L, Gardin J, Kitzman D. Predictive value of systolic and diastolic function for incident congestive heart failure in the elderly: the cardiovascular health study. J Am Coll Cardiol. 2001;37:1042–8.
67. Redfield MM, Jacobsen SJ, Burnett JC Jr, Mahoney DW, Bailey KR, Rodeheffer RJ. Burden of systolic and diastolic ventricular dysfunction in the community: appreciating the scope of the heart failure epidemic. JAMA. 2003;289:194–202.
68. Bella JN, Palmieri V, Roman MJ, Liu JE, Welty TK, Lee ET, et al. Mitral ratio of peak early to late diastolic filling velocity as a predictor of mortality in middle-aged and elderly adults: the Strong Heart Study. Circulation. 2002;105:1928–33.
69. Laukkanen JA, Kurl S, Eränen J, Huttunen M, Salonen JT. Left atrium size and the risk of cardiovascular death in middle-aged men. Arch Intern Med. 2005;165:1788–93.
70. Verdecchia P, Reboldi G, Gattobigio R, Bentivoglio M, Borgioni C, Angeli F, Carluccio E, Sardone MG, Porcellati C. Atrial fibrillation in hypertension: predictors and outcome. Hypertension. 2003;41:218–23.
71. Kizer JR, Bella JN, Palmieri V, Liu JE, Best LG, Lee ET, Roman MJ, Devereux RB. Left atrial diameter as an independent predictor of first clinical cardiovascular events in middle-aged and elderly adults: the Strong Heart Study (SHS). Am Heart J. 2006;151:412–8.
72. Abhayaratna WP, Seward JB, Appleton CP, Douglas PS, Oh JK, Tajik AJ, Tsang TS. Left atrial size physi-

ologic determinants and clinical applications. J Am Coll Cardiol. 2006;47:2357–63.
73. Takeuchi M, Nishikage T, Mor-Avi V, Sugeng L, Weinert L, Nakai H, Salgo IS, Gerard O, Lang RM. Measurement of left ventricular mass by real-time three-dimensional echocardiography: validation against magnetic resonance and comparison with two-dimensional and m-mode measurements. J Am Soc Echocardiogr. 2008;21:1001–5.
74. Bots ML, Hoes AW, Koudstaal PJ, Hofman A, Grobbee DE. Common carotid intima-media thickness and risk of stroke and myocardial infarction: the Rotterdam Study. Circulation. 1997;96:1432–7.
75. Hodis HN, Mack WJ, Labree L, Selzer RH, Liu CR, Liu CH, Azen SP. The role of carotid arterial intima-media thickness in predicting clinical coronary events. Ann Intern Med. 1998;128:262–9.
76. Vlachopoulos C, Xaplanteris P, Aboyans V, Brodmann M, Cifkova R, Cosentino F, De Carlo M, Gallino A, Landmesser U, Laurent S, Lekakis J, Mikhailidis DP, Naka KK, Protogerou AD, Rizzoni D, Schmidt-Trucksass A, Van Bortel L, Weber T, Yamashina A, Zimlichman R, Boutouyrie P, Cockcroft J, O'Rourke M, Park JB, Schillaci G, Sillesen H, Townsend RR. The role of vascular biomarkers for primary and secondary prevention. A position paper from the European Society of Cardiology Working Group on peripheral circulation: endorsed by the Association for Research into Arterial Structure and Physiology (ARTERY) Society. Atherosclerosis. 2015;241:507–32.
77. Zanchetti A, Bond MG, Hennig M, Neiss A, Mancia G, Dal Palù C, Hansson L, Magnani B, Rahn KH, Reid JL, Rodicio J, Safar M, Eckes L, Rizzini P, European Lacidipine Study on Atherosclerosis investigators. Calcium antagonist lacidipine slows down progression of asymptomatic carotid atherosclerosis: principal results of the European Lacidipine Study on Atherosclerosis (ELSA), a randomized, double-blind, long-term trial. Circulation. 2002;106:2422–7.
78. Zanchetti A, Bond MG, Hennig M, Tang R, Hollweck R, Mancia G, Eckes L, Micheli D, ELSA Investigators. Absolute and relative changes in carotid intima-media thickness and atherosclerotic plaques during long-term antihypertensive treatment: further results of the European Lacidipine Study on Atherosclerosis (ELSA). J Hypertens. 2004;22:1201–12.
79. Zanchetti A, Rosei EA, Dal Palù C, Leonetti G, Magnani B, Pessina A. The Verapamil in Hypertension and Atherosclerosis Study (VHAS): results of long-term randomized treatment with either verapamil or chlorthalidone on carotid intima-media thickness. J Hypertens. 1998;16:1667–76.
80. Zanchetti A, Hennig M, Hollweck R, Bond G, Tang R, Cuspidi C, Parati G, Facchetti R, Mancia G. Baseline values but not treatment-induced changes in carotid intima-media thickness predict incident cardiovascular events in treated hypertensive patients: findings in the European Lacidipine Study on Atherosclerosis (ELSA). Circulation. 2009;120:1084–90.
81. Den Ruijter HM, Peters SA, Anderson TJ, Britton AR, Dekker JM, Eijkemans MJ, Engstrom G, Evans GW, de Graaf J, Grobbee DE, Hedblad B, Hofman A, Holewijn S, Ikeda A, Kavousi M, Kitagawa K, Kitamura A, Koffijberg H, Lonn EM, Lorenz MW, Mathiesen EB, Nijpels G, Okazaki S, O'Leary DH, Polak JF, Price JF, Robertson C, Rembold CM, Rosvall M, Rundek T, Salonen JT, Sitzer M, Stehouwer CD, Witteman JC, Moons KG, Bots ML. Common carotid intima-media thickness measurements in cardiovascular risk prediction: a meta-analysis. JAMA. 2012;308:796–803.
82. Piepoli MF, Hoes AW, Agewall S, Albus C, Brotons C, Catapano AL, Cooney MT, Corra U, Cosyns B, Deaton C, Graham I, Hall MS, Hobbs FD, Lochen ML, Lollgen H, Marques-Vidal P, Perk J, Prescott E, Redon J, Richter DJ, Sattar N, Smulders Y, Tiberi M, van der Worp HB, van Dis I, Verschuren WM. 2016 European guidelines on cardiovascular disease prevention in clinical practice: The Sixth Joint Task Force of the European Society of Cardiology and Other Societies on Cardiovascular Disease Prevention in Clinical Practice (constituted by representatives of 10 societies and by invited experts). Developed with the special contribution of the European Association for Cardiovascular Prevention & Rehabilitation (EACPR). Eur Heart J. 2016;37:2315–81.
83. Sehestedt T, Jeppesen J, Hansen TW, Rasmussen S, Wachtell K, Ibsen H, Torp-Pedersen C, Olsen MH. Which markers of subclinical organ damage to measure in individuals with high normal blood pressure? J Hypertens. 2009;27:1165–71.
84. Criqui MH, Langer RD, Fronek A, Feigelson HS, Klauber MR, McCann TJ, Browner D. Mortality over a period of 10 years in patients with peripheral arterial disease. N Engl J Med. 1992;326:381–6.
85. Fowkes FG, Murray GD, Newman AB, Lee RJ. Ankle brachial index combined with Framingham Risk Score to predict cardiovascular events and mortality: a meta-analysis. JAMA. 2008;300:197–208.
86. Hiatt WR. Medical treatment of peripheral arterial disease and claudication. N Engl J Med. 2001;344:1608–21.
87. Vogt MT, Cauley JA, Newman AB, Kuller LH, Hulley SB. Decreased ankle/arm blood pressure index and mortality in elderly women. JAMA. 1993;270:465–9.
88. McKenna M, Wolfson S, Kuller L. The ratio of ankle and arm arterial pressure as an independent predictor of mortality. Atherosclerosis. 1991;87:119–28.
89. Vogt MT, McKenna M, Anderson SJ, Wolfson SK, Kuller LH. The relationship between ankle-arm index and mortality in older men and women. J Am Geriatr Soc. 1993;41:523–30.
90. Burek KA, Sutton-Tyrrell K, Brooks MM, Naydeck B, Keller N, Sellers MA, Roubin G, Jandová R,

Rihal CS. Prognostic importance of lower extremity arterial disease in patients undergoing coronary revascularization in the Bypass Angioplasty Revascularization Investigation (BARI). J Am Coll Cardiol. 1999;34:716–21.
91. Safar ME, Levy BI, Struijker-Boudier H. Current perspectives on arterial stiffness and pulse pressure in hypertension and cardiovascular diseases. Circulation. 2003;107:2864–9.
92. Laurent S, Cockcroft J, Van Bortel L, Boutouyrie P, Giannattasio C, Hayoz D, Pannier B, Vlachopoulos C, Wilkinson I, Struijker-Boudier H, European Network for Non-invasive Investigation of Large Arteries. Expert consensus document on arterial stiffness: methodological issues and clinical applications. Eur Heart J. 2006;27:2588–605.
93. Willum-Hansen T, Staessen JA, Torp-Pedersen C, Rasmussen S, Thijs L, Ibsen H, Jeppesen J. Prognostic value of aortic pulse wave velocity as index of arterial stiffness in the general population. Circulation. 2006;113:664–70.
94. Laurent S, Boutouyrie P, Asmar R, Gautier I, Laloux B, Guize L, Ducimetiere P, Benetos A. Aortic stiffness is an independent predictor of all-cause and cardiovascular mortality in hypertensive patients. Hypertension. 2001;37:1236–41.
95. Laurent S, Katsahian S, Fassot C, Tropeano AI, Gautier I, Laloux B, Boutouyrie P. Aortic stiffness is an independent predictor of fatal stroke in essential hypertension. Stroke. 2003;34:1203–6.
96. Boutouyrie P, Tropeano AI, Asmar R, Gautier I, Benetos A, Lacolley P, Laurent S. Aortic stiffness is an independent predictor of primary coronary events in hypertensive patients: a longitudinal study. Hypertension. 2002;39:10–5.
97. Ben-Shlomo Y, Spears M, Boustred C, et al. Aortic pulse wave velocity improves cardiovascular event prediction: an individual participant meta-analysis of prospective observational data from 17,635 subjects. J Am Coll Cardiol. 2014;63:636–46.
98. Reference Values for Arterial Stiffness' Collaboration. Determinants of pulse wave velocity in healthy people and in the presence of cardiovascular risk factors: 'establishing normal and reference values'. Eur Heart J. 2010;31:2338–50.
99. Van Bortel LM, Laurent S, Boutouyrie P, Chowienczyk P, Cruickshank JK, De Backer T, Filipovsky J, Huybrechts S, Mattace-Raso FU, Protogerou AD, Schillaci G, Segers P, Vermeersch S, Weber T, Artery Society, European Society of Hypertension Working Group on Vascular Structure and Function, European Network for Noninvasive Investigation of Large Arteries. Expert consensus document on the measurement of aortic stiffness in daily practice using carotid-femoral pulse wave velocity. J Hypertens. 2012;30:445–8.
100. Jankowski P, Kawecka-Jaszcz K, Czarnecka D, Brzozowska-Kiszka M, Styczkiewicz K, Loster M, Kloch-Badełek M, Wiliński J, Curyło AM, Dudek D, Aortic Blood Pressure and Survival Study Group. Pulsatile but not steady component of blood pressure predicts cardiovascular events in coronary patients. Hypertension. 2008;51:848–55.
101. Wang KL, Cheng HM, Chuang SY, Spurgeon HA, Ting CT, Lakatta EG, Yin FC, Chou P, Chen CH. Central or peripheral systolic or pulse pressure: which best relates to target organs and future mortality? J Hypertens. 2009;27:461–7.
102. Williams B, Lacy PS, Thom SM, Cruickshank K, Stanton A, Collier D, Hughes AD, Thurston H, O'Rourke M, CAFE Investigators; Anglo-Scandinavian Cardiac Outcomes Trial Investigators; CAFE Steering Committee and Writing Committee. Differential impact of blood pressure-lowering drugs on central aortic pressure and clinical outcomes: principal results of the Conduit Artery Function Evaluation (CAFE) study. Circulation. 2006;113:1213–25.
103. Sharman JE, Marwick TH, Gilroy D, Otahal P, Abhayaratna WP, Stowasser M, Value of Central Blood Pressure for GUIDing ManagEment of Hypertension Study Investigators. Randomized trial of guiding hypertension management using central aortic blood pressure compared with best practice care: principal findings of the BP GUIDE study. Hypertension. 2013;62:1138–45.
104. Stevens LA, Coresh J, Greene T, Levey AS. Assessing kidney function--measured and estimated glomerular filtration rate. N Engl J Med. 2006;354:2473–83.
105. Levey AS, Stevens LA, Schmid CH, Zhang YL, Castro AF 3rd, Feldman HI, Kusek JW, Eggers P, Van Lente F, Greene T, Coresh J, CKD EPI. A new equation to estimate glomerular filtration rate. Ann Intern Med. 2009;150:604–12.
106. Kidney Disease: Improving Global Outcomes (KDIGO) CKD Work Group. KDIGO 2012 clinical practice guideline for the evaluation and management of chronic kidney disease. Kidney Int Suppl. 2013;3:1–150.
107. Shlipak MG, Katz R, Sarnak MJ, Fried LF, Newman AB, Stehman-Breen C, Seliger SL, Kestenbaum B, Psaty B, Tracy RP, Siscovick DS. Cystatin C and prognosis for cardiovascular and kidney outcomes in elderly persons without chronic kidney disease. Ann Intern Med. 2006;145:237–46.
108. Parving HH. Initiation and progression of diabetic nephropathy. N Engl J Med. 1996;335:1682–3.
109. Ruilope LM, Rodicio JL. Clinical relevance of proteinuria and microalbuminuria. Curr Opin Nephrol Hypertens. 1993;2:962–7.
110. Redon J, Williams B. Microalbuminuria in essential hypertension: redefining the threshold. J Hypertens. 2002;20:353–5.
111. Arnlöv J, Evans JC, Meigs JB, Wang TJ, Fox CS, Levy D, Benjamin EJ, D'Agostino RB, Vasan RS. Low-grade albuminuria and incidence of cardiovascular disease events in nonhypertensive and nondiabetic individuals: the Framingham Heart Study. Circulation. 2005;112:969–75.

112. Hillege HL, Fidler V, Diercks GF, van Gilst WH, de Zeeuw D, van Veldhuisen DJ, Gans RO, Janssen WM, Grobbee DE, de Jong PE, Prevention of Renal and Vascular End Stage Disease (PREVEND) Study Group. Urinary albumin excretion predicts cardiovascular and noncardiovascular mortality in general population. Circulation. 2002;106:1777–82.
113. National Kidney Foundation. Executive summary. Am J Kid Dis. 2004;43(Suppl 1):S16–33.
114. Gerstein HC, Mann JF, Yi Q, Zinman B, Dinneen SF, Hoogwerf B, Halle JP, Young J, Rashkow A, Joyce C, Nawaz S, Yusuf S, Study Investigators HOPE. Albuminuria and risk of cardiovascular events, death, and heart failure in diabetic and non-diabetic individuals. JAMA. 2001;286:421–6.
115. Mallat SG, Al Kattar S, Tanios BY, Jurjus A. Hyperuricemia, hypertension, and chronic kidney disease: an emerging association. Curr Hypertens Rep. 2016;18:74.
116. Wong TY, Klein R, Sharrett AR, Duncan BB, Couper DJ, Tielsch JM, Klein BE, Hubbard LD. Retinal arteriolar narrowing and risk of coronary heart disease in men and women. The Atherosclerosis Risk in Communities Study. JAMA. 2002;287:1153–9.
117. Wong TY, Klein R, Couper DJ, Cooper LS, Shahar E, Hubbard LD, Wofford MR, Sharrett AR. Retinal microvascular abnormalities and incident stroke: the Atherosclerosis Risk in Communities Study. Lancet. 2001;358(9288):1134–40.
118. Cuspidi C, Macca G, Salerno M, Michev L, Fusi V, Severgnini B, Corti C, Meani S, Magrini F, Zanchetti A. Evaluation of target organ damage in arterial hypertension: which role for qualitative funduscopic examination? Ital Heart J. 2001;2:702–6.
119. Dimmitt SB, West JN, Eames SM, Gibson JM, Gosling P, Littler WA. Usefulness of ophthalmoscopy in mild to moderate hypertension. Lancet. 1989;20(8647):1103–6.
120. Fuchs FD, Maestri MK, Bredemeier M, Cardozo SE, Moreira FC, Wainstein MV, Moreira WD, Moreira LB. Study of the usefulness of optic fundi examination of patients with hypertension in a clinical setting. J Hum Hypertens. 1995;9:547–51.
121. Sairenchi T, Iso H, Yamagishi K, Irie F, Okubo Y, Gunji J, Muto T, Ota H. Mild retinopathy is a risk factor for cardiovascular mortality in Japanese with and without hypertension: the Ibaraki Prefectural Health Study. Circulation. 2011;124:2502–11.
122. Antonios TF, Singer DR, Markandu ND, Mortimer PS, MacGregor GA. Rarefaction of skin capillaries in borderline essential hypertension suggests an early structural abnormality. Hypertension. 1999;34(4 Pt 1):655–8.
123. Noon JP, Walker BR, Webb DJ, Shore AC, Holton DW, Edwards HV, Watt GC. Impaired microvascular dilatation and capillary rarefaction in young adults with a predisposition to high blood pressure. J Clin Invest. 1997;99:1873–9.
124. Henskens LH, van Oostenbrugge RJ, Kroon AA, Hofman PA, Lodder J, de Leeuw PW. Detection of silent cerebrovascular disease refines risk stratification of hypertensive patients. J Hypertens. 2009;27:846–53.
125. Longstreth WT Jr, Manolio TA, Arnold A, Burke GL, Bryan N, Jungreis CA, Enright PL, O'Leary D, Fried L. Clinical correlates of white matter findings on cranial magnetic resonance imaging of 3301 elderly people. The Cardiovascular Health Study. Stroke. 1996;27:1274–82.
126. Prins ND, van Dijk EJ, den Heijer T, Vermeer SE, Koudstaal PJ, Oudkerk M, Hofman A, Breteler MM. Cerebral white matter lesions and the risk of dementia. Arch Neurol. 2004;61:1531–4.
127. Vermeer SE, Hollander M, van Dijk EJ, Hofman A, Koudstaal PJ, Breteler MM, Rotterdam Scan Study. Silent brain infarcts and white matter lesions increase stroke risk in the general population: the Rotterdam Scan Study. Stroke. 2003;34:1126–9.
128. Wardlaw JM, Smith EE, Biessels GJ, Cordonnier C, Fazekas F, Frayne R, Lindley RI, O'Brien JT, Barkhof F, Benavente OR, Black SE, Brayne C, Breteler M, Chabriat H, Decarli C, de Leeuw FE, Doubal F, Duering M, Fox NC, Greenberg S, Hachinski V, Kilimann I, Mok V, Oostenbrugge R, Pantoni L, Speck O, Stephan BC, Teipel S, Viswanathan A, Werring D, Chen C, Smith C, van Buchem M, Norrving B, Gorelick PB, Dichgans M. Neuroimaging standards for research into small vessel disease and its contribution to ageing and neurodegeneration. Lancet Neurol. 2013;12(8):822–38.
129. Vermeer SE, Koudstaal PJ, Oudkerk M, Hofman A, Breteler MM. Prevalence and risk factors of silent brain infarcts in the population-based Rotterdam Scan Study. Stroke. 2002;33:21–5.
130. Tsoi KK, Chan JY, Hirai HW, Wong SY, Kwok TC. Cognitive tests to detect dementia: a systematic review and meta-analysis. JAMA Intern Med. 2015;175:1450–8.
131. Devereux RB, Wachtell K, Gerdts E, Boman K, Nieminen MS, Papademetriou V, Rokkedal J, Harris K, Aurup P, Dahlof B. Prognostic significance of left ventricular mass change during treatment of hypertension. JAMA. 2004;292:2350–6.
132. Ibsen H, Olsen MH, Wachtell K, Borch-Johnsen K, Lindholm LH, Mogensen CE, Dahlöf B, Devereux RB, de Faire U, Fyhrquist F, Julius S, Kjeldsen SE, Lederballe-Pedersen O, Nieminen MS, Omvik P, Oparil S, Wan Y. Reduction in albuminuria translates to reduction in cardiovascular events in hypertensive patients: losartan intervention for endpoint reduction in hypertension study. Hypertension. 2005;45:198–202.
133. Inker LA, Levey AS, Pandya K, Stoycheff N, Okparavero A, Greene T, et al. Early change in proteinuria as a surrogate end point for kidney disease progression: an individual patient meta-analysis. Am J Kidney Dis. 2014;64:74–85.
134. Bakris GL, Sarafidis PA, Weir MR, Dahlöf B, Pitt B, Jamerson K, Velazquez EJ, Staikos-Byrne L, Kelly RY, Shi V, Chiang YT, Weber MA, ACCOMPLISH

Trial Investigators. Renal outcomes with different fixed-dose combination therapies in patients with hypertension at high risk for cardiovascular events (ACCOMPLISH): a prespecified secondary analysis of a randomised controlled trial. Lancet. 2010;375(9721):1173–81. https://doi.org/10.1016/S0140-6736(09)62100-0. Epub 2010 Feb 18.

135. Haller H, Ito S, Izzo JL Jr, Januszewicz A, Katayama S, Menne J, Mimran A, Rabelink TJ, Ritz E, Ruilope LM, Rump LC, Viberti G, ROADMAP Trial Investigators. Olmesartan for the delay or prevention of microalbuminuria in type 2 diabetes. N Engl J Med. 2011;364(10):907–17. https://doi.org/10.1056/NEJMoa1007994.

136. Holtkamp FA, de Zeeuw D, de Graeff PA, Laverman GD, Berl T, Remuzzi G, Packham D, Lewis JB, Parving HH, Lambers Heerspink HJ. Albuminuria and blood pressure, independent targets for cardioprotective therapy in patients with diabetes and nephropathy: a post hoc analysis of the combined RENAAL and IDNT trials. Eur Heart J. 2011;32:1493–9. https://doi.org/10.1093/eurheartj/ehr017. Epub 2011 Mar 18.

137. Drawz PE, Rosenberg ME. Slowing progression of chronic kidney disease. Kidney Int Suppl. 2013;3:372–6.

138. de Galan BE, Perkovic V, Ninomiya T, Pillai A, Patel A, Cass A, Neal B, Poulter N, Harrap S, Mogensen CE, Cooper M, Marre M, Williams B, Hamet P, Mancia G, Woodward M, Glasziou P, Grobbee DE, MacMahon S, Chalmers J, ADVANCE Collaborative Group. Lowering blood pressure reduces renal events in type 2 diabetes. J Am Soc Nephrol. 2009;20:883–92. https://doi.org/10.1681/ASN.2008070667. Epub 2009 Feb 18.

139. Ninomiya T, Perkovic V, de Galan BE, Zoungas S, Pillai A, Jardine M, Patel A, Cass A, Neal B, Poulter N, Mogensen CE, Cooper M, Marre M, Williams B, Hamet P, Mancia G, Woodward M, MacMahon S, Chalmers J, ADVANCE Collaborative Group. Albuminuria and kidney function independently predict cardiovascular and renal outcomes in diabetes. J Am Soc Nephrol. 2009;20:1813–21. https://doi.org/10.1681/ASN.2008121270. Epub 2009 May 14

140. Costanzo P, Perrone-Filardi P, Vassallo E, Paolillo S, Cesarano P, Brevetti G, et al. Does carotid intima-media thickness regression predict reduction of cardiovascular events? A meta-analysis of 41 randomized trials. J Am Coll Cardiol. 2010;56:2006–20.

141. Wang JG, Staessen JA, Li Y, Van Bortel LM, Nawrot T, Fagard R, et al. Carotid intima-media thickness and antihypertensive treatment: a meta-analysis of randomized controlled trials. Stroke. 2006;37:1933–40.

142. Verdecchia P1, Sleight P, Mancia G, Fagard R, Trimarco B, Schmieder RE, Kim JH, Jennings G, Jansky P, Chen JH, Liu L, Gao P, Probstfield J, Teo K, Yusuf S, ONTARGET/TRANSCEND Investigators. Effects of telmisartan, ramipril, and their combination on left ventricular hypertrophy in individuals at high vascular risk in the Ongoing Telmisartan Alone and in Combination with Ramipril Global End Point Trial and the Telmisartan Randomized Assessment Study in ACE Intolerant Subjects with Cardiovascular Disease. Circulation. 2009;120:1380–9. https://doi.org/10.1161/CIRCULATIONAHA.109.865774. Epub 2009 Sep 21.

143. Izzo R, Losi MA, Stabile E, Lonnebakken MT, Canciello G, Esposito G, et al. Development of left ventricular hypertrophy in treated hypertensive outpatients: the Campania salute network. Hypertension. 2017;69:136–42.

The VA Co-operative Studies; The First RCTs in Cardiovascular Disease – A Tribute to Edward D. Freis

4

Vasilios Papademetriou, Michael Doumas, Costas Tsioufis, Kyriakos Dimitriadis, and Charles Faselis

Introduction

The relationship between elevated blood pressure and premature death was first demonstrated from data collected by insurance companies in the 1920s [1], and the association continued to be strengthened by data from the same source accumulated over the next 3 decades. The beneficial effects of blood pressure reduction however, remained controversial till the mid 1950s because of the luck of effective therapies and the fear of harming vital organs and actually increasing cardiovascular events with lower pressures [2]. Thus therapeutic nihilism prevailed for a long time.

The advent of effective and well tolerated antihypertensive therapies offered an attractive choice for the reduction of elevated blood pressure, which rapidly replaced prior difficult and not well tolerated therapeutic strategies, such as Kempner's rice diet, splachnicectomy, and adrenalectomy [3]. Although antihypertensive drugs were widely accepted for the management of malignant hypertension – a devastating condition with very high morbidity and mortality – the place of antihypertensive therapy in severe hypertension and especially in mild to moderate hypertension remained uncertain for a long time [3].

The two landmark VA Co-operative studies [4, 5], designed and spearheaded by Edward Freis (Fig. 4.1) were the first multicenter, prospective, placebo-controlled, double-blind, randomized trial ever conducted in the cardiovascular field. In the words of Edward Freis: "the VA studies established a model for future trials" [6]. Ed Freis solved many problems and had change many minds in order to be successful in conducting those trials, but as many pioneers he was persistent and determined. These studies changed the history of cardiovascular medicine. Needless to say that history is written by people who have bright ideas and are determined to overcome all obstacles.

This chapter presents the findings of the VA Co-operative studies in both patients with severe hypertension and patients with mild-moderate hypertension, describes the unfriendly environment of the times and summarizes the influence of the VA studies in cardiovascular medicine, medical research and daily practice. Finally this

V. Papademetriou (✉)
Georgetown University and VA Medical Center, Washington, DC, USA
e-mail: vpapademetriou@va.gov

M. Doumas · C. Faselis
VA Medical Center and George Washington University, Washington, DC, USA

C. Tsioufis
VA Medical Center and Georgetown University, Washington, DC, USA

1st Academic Department of Cardiology, Athens, Greece

K. Dimitriadis
1st Academic Department of Cardiology, Athens, Greece

V. Papademetriou et al. (eds.), *Management of Hypertension*,
https://doi.org/10.1007/978-3-319-92946-0_4

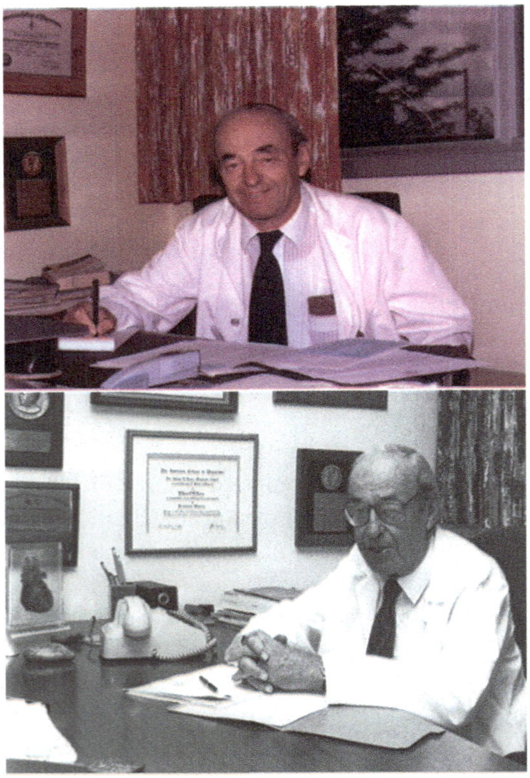

Fig. 4.1 Edward D. Freis at his office at the VA Medical Center, Washington, DC. (On the top, younger age; on the bottom, older age)

chapter pays a tribute to Ed Freis, the man, the physician and the pioneer of cardiovascular clinical trials.

The VA Co-operative Studies

The idea for landmark VA Co-operative studies started in the early 1960s when Ed Freis formed the VA co-op study group, aiming to test his idea that lowering elevated blood pressure will result in fewer cardiovascular events, the opposite of what his opponents supported. At that time many believed that high BPs were needed to perfused organs with diseased arteries and lowering BPs would be detrimental. The studies included male Veterans with average diastolic blood pressure between 90 and 129 mmHg not on any antihypertensive medication [4, 5]. Patients were excluded from the study if they had: (a) malignant hypertension, (b) very severe target organ damage (cardiac, cerebrovascular, optic, renal), (c) surgically curable hypertension, (d) malignancy, (e) history of cerebral or subarachnoid hemorrhage, dissecting aneurism, and treatment-resistant congestive heart failure, (f) been unwilling or unable to attend the study, and (g) been uncooperative or judged unreliable (alcohol abuse, vagrants, poorly motivated). Patients with prior myocardial infarction or ischemic stroke were allowed to participate in the study. A vigorous pre-randomization work-up and a meticulous post-randomization follow-up plan were applied and will be later described in detail. Patients were randomized to receive either triple antihypertensive therapy (100 mg HCTZ, 0.2 mg reserpine, and 150 mg hydralazine) or placebo. Drug doses were down-titrated in case of severe adverse effects or hypotensive episodes. A total of 523 patients were found eligible and entered the study from April 1964. Of those, 143 patients had average baseline diastolic blood pressure between 115 and 129 mmHg, while 380 patients had average baseline diastolic blood pressure between 90 and 114 mmHg. The first study for patients with severe hypertension (average diastolic blood pressure: 115–129 mmHg), was terminated prematurely in May 1967 due to substantial benefits of active therapy and ended as scheduled in October 1969 for patients with less severe hypertension (average diastolic blood pressure: 90–114 mmHg). The findings of the study will be presented separately for the two blood pressure categories.

Patients with Severe Hypertension (DBP: 115–129 mmHg)

A total of 143 middle-aged (mean age: 51 years; range 30–73 years) Caucasian and African American male Veterans were included in this study [4]. The cardiovascular risk of study participants at baseline was very high: quite severe target organ damage, prior cardiovascular thrombotic event (8%), enlarged heart at roentgenogram (42%), electrocardiographic left ventricular hypertrophy (32%), cardiac symptoms (30%), diabetes mellitus (9%), and dyslipidemia (mean total cholesterol: 250 mg/dl). The average baseline blood pressure was 185.6/121.2 mmHg in the active treatment group and 186.8/121.0 mmHg in the placebo group. There were no significant differences between the two groups in any baseline demographic or clinical parameter.

The average blood pressure reduction at the end of the study was 43 mmHg for systolic and 29.7 mmHg for diastolic blood pressure. In particular, diastolic blood pressure was significantly decreased with active therapy from 121.2 mmHg at baseline to 91.5 mmHg at the end of the study. Blood pressure reduction was observed from the beginning of the study (diastolic blood pressure: 93.1 mmHg at 4 months) and remained stable between 90 and 92 mmHg in average throughout the study. Of note, blood pressure dropped significantly (by 10–80 mmHg for systolic and by 5–60 mmHg for diastolic) in the vast majority (>90%) of study participants in the active therapy group, with most patients experiencing impressive blood pressure reductions of 28–60 mmHg for systolic and 12–44 mmHg for diastolic blood pressure. In contrast, diastolic blood pressure remained practically unaffected by placebo (from 121.0 mmHg at baseline to 119.7 mmHg at study end).

Overall, 27 events occurred in the placebo group compared with only two events in the actively treated group (Table 4.1), and the difference was highly statistically significant ($p < 0.0001$). The overall dropout rate was small (8.4%) and equally divided between the two groups. Even if all patients who dropped out in the active therapy group had an event and all patients who dropped out in the placebo group were free of an event, the difference in outcomes remained statistically significant ($p < 0.001$). There were 7 cardiovascular events (myocardial infarction: 2, congestive heart failure: 3, stroke/TIA: 3), 6 with placebo and 1 with active therapy. Moreover, there were 21 terminating events with placebo, including 4 deaths (sudden death, dissecting aortic aneurysm, ruptured abdominal aneurysm), progression to malignant hypertension, cerebrovascular and subarachnoid hemorrhage, treatment resistant congestive heart failure, and severe blood pressure elevation (office diastolic blood pressure > 140 mmHg and in-hospital diastolic blood pressure > 130 mmHg). In contrast, only 1 event occurred with active therapy, consisting of hyperglycemia, hypokalemia, and depression).

Standard doses of antihypertensive therapy (100 mg HCTZ, 0.2 mg reserpine, and 150 mg hydralazine) were administered in 45/73 patients on active therapy, while the doses were reduced to the rest due to either hypotension or side effects (headache, weakness, depression, hyperglycemia).

Table 4.1 Morbid and fatal events in the VA Co-operative study in patients with severe hypertension (Diastolic blood pressure: 115–129 mmHg; modified from Ref. [4])

	Placebo n = 70	Therapy n = 73
Accelerated hypertension	12	0
Stroke	4	1
Coronary event	2	0
CHF	2	0
Renal damage	2	0
Deaths	4	0

Patients with Less Severe Hypertension (DBP: 90–114 mmHg)

In total, 380 patients with average baseline blood pressure between 90 and 114 mmHg were included in the study, with 186 assigned to triple antihypertensive therapy and 194 assigned to placebo [5]. Most patients were middle-aged, for a median age of 49.2 years in the control group and 48.1 years in the placebo group. Most participants were Caucasians, but a significant portion was African-Americans (active therapy: 41%, control: 42%). Office baseline blood pressure was in average 162.1/103.8 mmHg in the active therapy group and 165.1/104.7 mmHg in the control group. Study participants in both the active therapy and control group had moderate target organ damage, enlarged heart at x-ray (29% and 22%, respectively), electrocardiographic left ventricular hypertrophy (16% in both groups), and dyslipidemia (total cholesterol: 245.0 and

250.1, respectively). There were no significant differences between the two groups in any demographic or clinical parameter at baseline.

Both systolic and diastolic blood pressure fell significantly with active therapy and promptly within the first 4 months of therapy, while remaining practically unaltered with placebo. In particular, systolic blood pressure dropped by 27.2 mmHg in average with active therapy and increased by 4.2 mmHg in average with placebo. Likewise, diastolic blood pressure fell by 17.4 mmHg in average with active therapy and increased by 1.2 mmHg with placebo. A large variation in individual responses was observed, with many patients experiencing systolic blood pressure reductions of 10–50 mmHg, while the corresponding diastolic blood pressure reductions were mainly 5–30 mmHg.

Overall, 98 events occurred throughout the study follow-up period. Participants in the control group experienced 76 events while participants assigned to active therapy experienced 22 events. Severe blood pressure elevation (diastolic blood pressure >124 mmHg on 3 visits and persisting >3 months) occurred in 20 patients assigned to placebo and these patients were not included for analysis, leaving 56 events in the control group. The efficacy of intervention was defined as the difference in complications (%) between control and active therapy groups divided by the complications (%) in the control group. The overall efficacy of active therapy was 70% and when the 20 patients with progression to severe hypertension were excluded, the efficacy remained substantial (59%). The efficacy of intervention was 73% when the terminating morbid events were considered, i.e. cardiovascular deaths, class A events (dissecting aneurysm, subarachnoid hemorrhage, malignant hypertension, uncontrolled heart failure), and treatment failures.

There were 19 deaths in the control group compared with 8 deaths in the active therapy group (Table 4.2). In the control group, 5 deaths were due to hemorrhagic events (cerebrovascular, subarachnoid, dissecting aneurysm), 6 due to thrombotic events (myocardial infarction, stroke), and 8 sudden deaths. In the active therapy group, there were no deaths due to hemorrhagic events; there were 4 sudden deaths and 4 due to thrombotic events (myocardial infarction, stroke). The benefits of active therapy were even more impressive in nonfatal events. There were 16 events in the placebo group (stroke, malignant hypertension, uncontrolled congestive heart failure, and hemorrhagic events) compared with only one nonfatal event (hypotension) in the active therapy group. The benefits were highly apparent in the prevention of heart failure, cerebrovascular and renal events but not in the prevention of coronary events. Life-table analysis revealed that the benefits of active therapy appeared early in the study and were maintained and even enhanced throughout the 5-year follow-up period.

Table 4.2 Morbid and fatal events in the VA Co-operative study in patients with mild to moderate hypertension (Diastolic blood pressure: 90–114 mmHg; modified from Ref. [5])

	Placebo n = 194	Therapy n = 186
Accelerated hypertension	4	0
Stroke	20	5
Total coronary event	13	11
Fatal coronary event	11	6
Congestive heart failure	11	0
Renal damage	3	0
Deaths	19	8

Subgroup analysis was also performed according to age, race, and baseline blood pressure levels. According to age, the majority of events were observed in participants older than 50 years, both in the active therapy and the control group. Of major clinical importance, the benefits of active therapy were similar both in the older (>50 years) and younger (<50 years) participants (efficacy: 59% and 55%, respectively). According to race, there were no differences in morbid events between Caucasian and African American participants. Likewise, the benefits of active therapy were essentially the same in the two racial groups (efficacy: 59% and 54%, respectively). Very important information was extracted from the subgroup analysis according to baseline blood pressure levels. Morbid events were significantly higher in patients with higher baseline blood pressure levels: 42.7% vs 15.3% for patients with baseline systolic blood pressure over vs under 165 mmHg, and 31.8% vs 25% for patients with baseline diastolic blood pressure over vs under 105 mmHg in the placebo group. The benefits of antihypertensive therapy were greater in patients with higher baseline blood pressure levels. In particular, efficacy was 64% vs 40% in patients with systolic blood pressure over vs under 165 mmHg, while the corresponding percentages were even more impressive (75% vs 35%) in patients with diastolic blood pressure over or under 105 mmHg.

Regarding safety, dose adjustments were frequently required due to hypotensive or other symptoms. Reserpine or HCTZ (or their matching placebos) were withdrawn in 29 participants. Reserpine (or its matching placebo) was withdrawn in 12 participants due to depressive symptoms; however, only 7 of these patients were actually receiving reserpine, while the rest 5 participants were on matching placebo. Likewise, peptic ulcer was experienced by 10 patients, 6 on active therapy and 4 on placebo. Side effects of active therapy included sleepiness, nasal stuffiness, gout, hypotension-induced seizures, and abnormal glucose tolerance tests in 6 patients.

Prevailing Unfriendly Environment Prior to the VA Co-operative Studies

> *Now what is done to this poor fellow in an effort to bring his blood pressure down? Because of an ill-founded idea that protein is responsible for hypertension in kidney disease, he is denied meat and eggs, especially red meat which for some reason is looked upon with particular dread. Then, his diet is rendered even more unpalatable by the withdrawal of salt. One would sympathize with this half-starved fellow except that he probably would not be able to eat anyway, his teeth having been removed on the theory that focal infection has something to do with hypertension. Even before this he had sacrificed his tonsils and had had his sinuses punctured because of the same theory. In case some food was consumed, the slight colonic residue was washed out by numerous colonic irrigations, especially during the period when the theory of auto-intoxication was enjoying a wave of popularity. To add to his unhappiness, he may be told to stop work and exercise. Of course, he is denied alcohol and tobacco, as well as coffee and tea, and now to cap the climax of his difficulties, the unfortunate person with hypertension seems about to fall into the clutches of the neurosurgeon, who is prepared to separate him from his sympathetic nervous system. The only thing I can add would be that the surgeon is now also prepared to remove the adrenals.* Edward Weiss, The New York Academy Bulletin, 1953

The psychic element of blood pressure elevation was greatly appreciated at that time. Characteristically, one study evaluated the effect of patient reassurance in the management of benign hypertensive disease in 31 outpatients (9 of them were previously hospitalized) [7]. The authors fabricated an 'electron gun' with no physiologic action and informed the patients that this device is highly effective in hypertensive patients, offering dramatic blood pressure reductions. It was found that 'electron gun' was associated with substantial blood pressure reduction in 15 out of 31 study participants, and the average reduction in responders was 36 mmHg for systolic and 27 mmHg for diastolic blood pressure. Of note, blood pressure was even controlled (diastolic blood pressure <90 mmHg) in 8 of the 15 responders to this 'fake-device' therapy. Similar results were obtained among hospitalized patients (39/28 mmHg drop in 6 out of 9 patients). In addition, subjective symptoms (headache, fatigue, dizziness, nervousness, and chest pain) were significantly improved among all study participants, permitting previously partially incapacitated patients to resume normal activities. Of note blood pressure reduction was transient and blood pressure returned to prior levels within 8 weeks after the termination of 'electron-gun' use [7].

In the 1960's four different approaches struggled to prevail for the management of patients with arterial hypertension: (a) a dietary approach, with Walter Kempner at Duke University as leading figure, (b) splachnicectomy that started in the 1920's with Adson, Peet, and Page, and was represented by Reginald Smithwick at Boston University as the leading figure of that time, (c) drug therapy, with many excellent physicians around the globe leading the field, such as Robert Wilkins and Edward Freis in the United States of America, Horace Smirk in New Zealand, and

Colin Dollery in United Kingdom, and (d) a nihilistic approach, with Willian Goldring, Herbert Chasis, and George Perrera as leading figures.

Walter Kempner introduced a low-calorie diet that consisted mainly of rice and fruits, which was mainly low in sodium (<30 mmol/day), fat, and protein. Kempner's diet was associated with a reduction in body weight and blood pressure [8], but was very difficult to adhere, and caused ketosis. The enthusiasm over Kempner's diet has gradually subsided over the years. In the words of Arthur Fishberg: "*Apparently the only essential feature of the rice diet is sodium restriction and the rest is what you might call window dressing*", George Perrera from Columbia University adds: "*The only virtue in the rice diet rests in its low sodium content*", Edward Weiss writes: "*When people have their attention focused too much on a weird diet, the harm that is done to them by obsession is often worse than what is produced by the disease*", and Herbert Chasis from NY University College finishes: "*Our experience with the rice diet was disappointing … We observed no great falls in blood pressure … We concluded we would not advice the rice diet*" [9]. But even salt restriction was not considered very helpful by many physicians. George Perrera stated characteristically: "*Salt restriction forms only a small part of what we can do for the hypertensive subject; when carried to excess it places undue emphasis on a feature of limited value; and it must always be remembered that diets can do harm*".

The recognition of sympathetic nervous system importance in blood pressure regulation generated the hypothesis that the surgical destruction of sympathetic nerves will effectively lower blood pressure. Surgical sympathectomy was an extensive operation, included the resection of sympathetic nerves of the abdominal organs for maximum efficacy, and was thus called splachnicectomy [10]. Sympathectomy was found to be very effective in the management of malignant hypertension, lowering the blood pressure and attenuating or even reversing organ damage in about half of patients suffering from this mortal condition. Sympathectomy required prolonged hospitalization and recovery, and was associated with devastating adverse effects [11, 12]. The enthusiasm over sympathectomy waned over the years as well. In the words of Arthur Fishberg: "*The proportion of patients with essential hypertension in whom sympathectomy is indicated seems to be extremely small … The indications in general are hypertension in an individual below the age of fifty, who is definitely deteriorating despite every non-surgical therapeutic measure and in whom there are no arteriosclerotic complications … Sympathectomy is indicated in only a few very sick hypertensives*", and Herbert Chasis adds: "*Sympathectomy and adrenalectomy are desperate maneuvers in desperately ill patients, with the family and the physician eventually becoming desperate … The interest in sympathectomy is on the wane*", while he mentions the controversy on indications: "*It is the opinion of some that the best kind of patients to operate on is the one with early labile essential hypertension. On the other hand, there are other physicians who don't advice sympathectomy until the prognosis is extremely poor*" [9]. The concept of modulating the sympathetic nervous system recently revived with renal sympathetic denervation [13–16]. The intervention is minimally invasive and requires the ablation of renal sympathetic nerves that travel at the adventitia of renal arteries. Renal sympathetic denervation was found very effective in the management of resistant hypertension and several conditions associated with sympathetic overdrive [17–30]. The first large randomized, sham-controlled study however failed to uncover significant greater blood pressure reductions compared to placebo, raising concerns about the efficacy of this interventional approach [31–33]. Recently however, the interest on renal sympathetic denervation came back following the positive results of the intervention in patients with elevated blood pressure who were not taking antihypertensive drugs [34].

Therapeutic nihilism describes an extended skepticism and a negative attitude over drug use and prescription for the management of diseased individuals. The roots of therapeutic nihilism go way back to Aristotle who said that most of the patients die through the medicines of physicians, and shaped by Maimonides (a famous Egyptian physician of the twelfth century) who wrote: "*Most physicians are greatly in error in that they think that medication strengthens the health: it weakens and perverts it*". Such a critical approach was adopted by Sir William Osler, the leading figure of modern medicine, who lived in Baltimore and practiced in John Hopkins University, and recognized only a dozen of drugs for being of therapeutic benefit, being a major advocate against the wide use of medications for patient management. The therapeutic nihilism expressed by Osler at the beginning of the twentieth century (partly justified by the limited knowledge about drugs at that time) was characterized by his reserve and aversion to prescription of drugs, and greatly influenced therapeutic strategies until the '70s.

In 1953, a questionnaire was sent to 15 top experts in antihypertensive drugs worldwide, including Edward Freis. Among those 15 experts, 14 answered that antihypertensive therapy should not be used in benign essential hypertension, termed as 'mild hypertension', 'labile hypertension', symptomless hypertension' benign with no vascular sequelae', and 'diastolic blood pressure less than 120 mmHg' [to 39]. Prof. Edward Freis also added that "*the satisfactory agent has not been found and the drugs now available are stop-gaps*". It has to be kept in mind however, that at that time the only available antihypertensive agents included hexamethonium, ergot and veratrum viride derivatives, and hydrazinophthalazine. Prof. Arthur Fishberg, Director of Medicine at Beth Israel Hospital stated characteristically: "*… (Hexamethonium) may do some terrible things to the patient. He may be much worse in spite of reduction in blood pressure. You cannot be too careful with the drug, I myself have had one fatality in a patient treated with hexamethonium who really had had only very minimal symptoms of coronary insufficiency*" [9].

George Perrera evaluated the role of antihypertensive drugs on mortality in patients with essential hypertension (excluding patients with accelerated hypertension and overt cardiovascular disease) [35]. The study included 29 middle-aged patients for a 7-year follow-up period, while an equally numbered group matched for age, sex, race, baseline blood pressure, clinical and laboratory parameters, was formed retrospectively as control group. The blood pressure of treated patients was maintained below 160/104 mmHg, while the blood pressure of control patients remained over 200/120 mmHg. In total, death occurred in 16/29 patients on antihypertensive therapy and in 16/29 control patients, for an average survival period of 42 and 45 months, respectively. It was thus suggested by Perrera in 1960: "*… the burden of proof, that drugs which lower the arterial pressure will prolong the lives of patients with primary hypertension who do not have the accelerated form of disease, must rest with those who make such claims*" [35].

The Influence of the VA Studies

The findings of the VA studies have not been adopted and implemented in everyday life practice right away. It took many years and intense efforts by many physicians to overcome the therapeutic nihilism and the concerns about treating patients with mild and moderate hypertension.

The findings of a large epidemiological study among industrial employees in metropolitan Chicago uncover the remaining skepticism of practicing physicians to treat mild hypertension despite the impressive findings of the VA studies. Among almost 23,000 employees in Chicago, 75.3% had undetected or untreated hypertension [36]. Of great interest, this study assessed whether the publication of the VA studies in 1967 and 1970 had a measurable impact on community practice and patterns of care for patients with arterial hypertension. Surprisingly, the proportion of patients receiving antihypertensive therapy among the whole study population and among those with identified hypertension was consistently lower in 1971 than in 1967 for all age, sex, and race subgroups [36]. These findings highlight the time delay in the adoption of the VA findings in real life practice.

This is also better reflected in the findings of the Hypertension Detection and Follow-up Program (HDFP) trial. HDFP was a large, community-based, randomized, controlled trial sponsored by the National Heart, Lung, and Blood Institute with more than $60 million, a huge amount of money in the '70s. The study included almost 11,000 patients with essential hypertension, mostly (71%) in its mild form (diastolic blood pressure: 90–104 mmHg). Patients were assigned either to intensive therapy or usual therapy in the community [37]. The study revealed a 17% survival benefit in the intensively treated group. In contrast however to the findings of the VA studies, the survival benefits were greater in patients with mild hypertension than in patients with more severe hypertension. This can be attributed to the fact that the community physicians were less likely to treat mild hypertension and thus the differences between intensive and usual treatment were maximized, while community physicians were more likely to treat severe hypertension and thus the differences between intensive and usual care were minimized.

Despite the aforementioned time delay in the adoption and implementation of the VA findings in real life practice, the intense efforts of Edward Freis and other advocates of drug therapy have finally prevailed. First, the findings of the HDFP trial strengthened the belief that antihypertensive therapy is beneficial even in patients with slightly elevated blood pressure. The VA and HDFP findings led the NHLBI to advise physicians accustomed to treating mild hypertension with benign neglect to reconsider their practice and prescribe antihypertensive drugs. Many studies thereafter verified the findings of the VA Co-operative studies leading to the generalization of treating all stages of hypertension nowadays [38–45].

The Legacy of Edward Freis

Edward Freis is considered among the most prominent scientists in the field of arterial hypertension and cardiovascular disease [46]. His major contribution was the conduction of the VA Co-operative studies that were the first randomized, controlled studies in the cardiovascular field and demonstrated for the first time the substantial benefits of antihypertensive therapy in all stages of essential hypertension [4, 5, 47]. Although the findings of the first VA Co-operative study in patients with severe hypertension were well accepted by the scientific community, this was not the case with the second VA Co-operative study in patients with less severe hypertension. Freis tried very hard to advertise the findings of the VA mild-to-moderate hypertension study in order to maximize attention and change the behavior of practicing physicians. However, this was really tough. A relevant press release attracted very little attention by the media, an Associated Press dispatch was buried in the inside papers of only a few newspapers, and the most powerful weapon – television – actually ignored the study apart from a brief comment by Walter Cronkite [48]. Only the Lasker Award recognition in 1971 boosted some publicity, which however might have subsided as well if one defining event has not had happened: Mrs. Lasker approached Elliot Richardson - whose father had hypertension and died from stroke – with reprints of the VA studies and convinced him as Head of the High Blood Pressure Education Program to design and run a media campaign about hypertension that aimed primarily at the public. The idea was also embraced by Theodore Cooper, who was the Director of the National Heart, Lung and Blood Institute, and was carried out with great success, attracting wide attention in the treatment of mild hypertension by both patients and physicians.

Another major contribution of Edward Freis was his research on the hemodynamic effects of the first antihypertensive drugs that became available in the fifties [49–54]. Of major clinical importance was his work on thiazide diuretics, a class of drugs that revolutionized antihypertensive therapy. Fries was among the very first to study their efficacy and believe that diuretics is the cornerstone of antihypertensive therapy [55–57]. Edward Freis remained a strong advocate of thiazide diuretics for the rest of his life and defended their use with solid arguments during the times of severe accusations about toxicity and reduced efficacy compared to newer antihypertensive drugs.

Edward Fries was also convinced that antihypertensive therapy was more effective when being aggressive. In the light of the recently published SPRINT trial [58–62], it seems worth mentioning to say what Edward Freis was doing for his personal health: he himself was suffering from hypertension and was taking antihypertensive drugs with aggressive blood pressure goals. It is characteristic that at the age of 91 he maintained his blood pressure as low as 110–125/60–70 mmHg without experiencing any feeling of weakness or any episodes of fainting [6].

Edward Freis: Prior Work

Edward Freis joined Robert Wilkins (chief of Cardiology at Boston University) as a research fellow at the end of World War II in 1945. His first assignment was to evaluate the hemodynamic effects of novel antihypertensive drugs, and the first such agent to study was pentaquine. Pentaquine was a drug for malaria that resulted in orthostatic hypotension and was tested in patients with malignant hypertension. It was found that pentaquine use was associated with blood pressure reduction and some reversal of malignant hypertension in some patients [63], but the drug was later withdrawn due to a lot of adverse effects.

The period between 1945 and 1955 was full of new developments in the field of antihypertensive therapy. A variety of new agents was developed and needed to be tested for efficacy and safety in patients with essential hypertension. Freis and Wilkins were among the first to study several new drugs: rauwolfia serpentina, veratrum alkaloid, ganglionic blockers, and hydralazine [64, 65]. Very soon they were convinced that, despite the variety of adverse effects, the blood pressure can be effectively lowered in the majority of patients with the new drugs, especially when drugs with different mechanisms of action were combined.

Freis moved to Georgetown University, Washington, DC and started working at the Veterans Administration Medical Center at the US Capital city. He continued to assess the hemodynamic effects of the new antihypertensive agents and was excited by the discovery of a new class, thiazide diuretics. Freis, a lover of sport cars and fast driving, entered the rally of testing diuretics in patients with essential hypertension along with many other famous researchers, including his prior mentor Robert Wilkins. The competition was so hard that both Freis and Wilkins published in 1957 the effects of chlorothiazide in hypertensive patients almost at the same time in local journal (for rapid publication): Freis at the Medical Annals of the District of Columbia and Wilkins at the Boston Medical Quarterly [66, 67]. However, Freis was the first to present the blood pressure lowering capacity of thiazides, either alone or in combination with other antihypertensive agents, at the American Heart Association Annual Meeting in fall 1957. Wilkins was immediately recognized with the much esteemed Lasker Award in 1958, while Freis received the Lasker Award in 1971 after the publication of the two seminal VA studies.

Multi-centric Studies

Until the conduction of the landmark VA trials, both observational and clinical studies originated from only one clinic and reflected the opinions and habits of the Head of the Department. Therefore, available information about the natural history of hypertension and its complications, and the effects of intervention was scarce, fragmented, and many times controversial due to the small number of participants in each study and the infinite variety of approaches. Edward Freis decided to conduct a multicenter study to overcome these obstacles, inspired by the multi-clinic studies of anti-tuberculosis therapy. He quickly realized that a multicenter clinical trial was feasible in the extended and friendly VA environment. He then took advantage of his reputation as a pioneer in the field of hypertension to form a team of physicians in many VA centers across the East Coast that could conduct a multicenter, long-term, controlled clinical trial. He respected the physicians conducting the antihypertensive VA studies so much that he did not present the data in any Congress before the publication of the

VA studies in order not to be solely recognized and take the credit for himself alone.

The organization of a multicenter trial was not an easy task and it took more than 5 years to organize it. He first contacted other teams at a meeting of the Chiefs of the VA Medical Services in 1956 with two ideas: to assess the relative efficacy of antihypertensive drugs and to evaluate the long-term effects of antihypertensive therapy on cardiovascular morbidity and mortality. There were too many obstacles to overcome: an unfriendly environment, ethical and financial issues. The strong objections about the efficacy and safety of antihypertensive therapy expressed primarily by Goldring and Chasis have dominated the field and greatly influenced practicing physicians at that time. Moreover, ethical considerations about the use of a placebo arm in an antihypertensive drug trial were expressed primarily by Horace Smirk who was a strong advocate of drug therapy. Finally, financial resources were significantly limited. The finalization of the study protocol was done in 1962 during a meeting of the American Federation of Clinical Research. However, since the resources were not enough to rent a room, the meeting was held at the lobby of the Seaview Hotel in Atlantic City. At last, 27 physicians agreed to join Edward Freis for the conduction of the VA studies, including Edward Frohlich who then became himself an emblematic figure in hypertension research.

Exclusion of White-Coat Hypertension

To unveil the real effects of antihypertensive therapy, study participants had to have 'real' hypertension and not white coat hypertension. In order to exclude or at least minimize the white coat effect, a rigorous screening and pre-randomization protocol has been implemented for the first time. Patients with essential hypertension that seemed to be eligible for the study were initially hospitalized for 1 week. Male patients with diastolic blood pressure between 90 and 129 mmHg from the fourth till the sixth day of hospitalization without antihypertensive therapy and fulfilling inclusion/exclusion criteria were considered potentially eligible for the study and entered a pre-randomization trial period. This period lasted 2–4 months with several blood pressure recordings at the outpatient clinic. Patients were excluded from study participation if the average diastolic blood pressure during this period was below 90 mmHg.

This extended, multi-month, double-phase screening and pre-randomization period, both in the hospital and at the outpatient clinic, is greatly different than the one who is almost always used in current clinical trials. The VA-method not only included patients with 'real' hypertension avoiding the inclusion of patients with white coat hypertension with the best possible way at that time (ambulatory blood pressure measurement was not available), but also 'educated' patients for the participation in a clinical trial. It is thus not surprising that placebo was not associated with significant blood pressure reduction during the whole course of the VA Co-operative studies. This has to be compared with recent trials, where placebo results in substantial blood pressure reduction and might mask the real effects of intervention, as recently observed in the Symplicity-3 trial [31–33].

Adherence to Therapy

Compliance was checked by pill counts, as performed in clinical trials nowadays. However, in order to ensure the best possible compliance, another brilliant method was used. Riboflavin was incorporated in placebo tablets; riboflavin is a substance that results in yellow urine fluorescence when ultraviolet lighting is used.

A urine specimen was obtained and tested for yellow fluorescence at each visit during the 2–4 months pre-randomization period. In addition, patients returned all medication bottles and pills were counted at each visit. Patients were considered as adherent to therapy if they have received >90% of the estimated pills. Two consequent successive visits without any violation (unjustified loss of a visit, >90% of dispensed drugs, yellow fluorescence of urine specimen) were required for study participation.

Another method to limit poor adherence was the exclusion of patients with dubious reliability or seemingly poor motivation. Therefore, patients with alcohol abuse and vagrants were not included in the study.

The aforementioned adherence criteria were very strict. Consequently, almost half of eligible patients did not qualify for the study because they failed to pass the adherence tests.

Biostatistics

Statistics were not much appreciated and thus applied in medical research at that time. Edward Fries first heard about the utility of statistics from Dr. Martini (a European expert in Clinical trials) during a trip in Europe for the attention of the European Meeting of Cardiology in Bonn. He then realized the importance of biostatics by reading the work of Fisher and Hill. The VA Central Office had a Department of Biostatistics, which consisted by only one statistician: Jack Williams. The biostatistics department was not only poorly powered but also poorly used. When Freis contacted Williams he realized that he was the only one interested to use biostatistics in a clinical trial and thus took his full attention. The unfortunate death of Williams led to his replacement by Lawrence Shaw, a very experienced biostatistician who was supported by R. Tewksbury. When Shaw joined the team of antihypertensive drug trials he was actively involved not only in the analysis of data but also in the design of the studies. Shaw immediately realized that too many questions were trying to be answered in only one study: the effects of antihypertensive therapy on mortality and morbidity and the comparative efficacy and safety of each one of antihypertensive drugs available at that time along with their long-term effects on morbidity and mortality. It was thanks to his critical approach and his objections about the feasibility and the validity of such a study that the objectives were separated. Therefore, the landmark VA studies evaluated only one question: whether antihypertensive therapy is associated with a reduction in cardiovascular events, while the other objectives were addressed in different trials [51, 52]. It was the first time in cardiovascular medicine that a biostatistician was not used an aid for data analysis but was actively involved in the design of the study, paving the way for the modern use of biostatistics in clinical trials.

Premature Termination

The VA-severe hypertension study (baseline diastolic blood pressure: 115–129 mmHg) was the first clinical trial that was prematurely terminated. The study was initiated in April 1964 and rumors about excessive mortality were first heard at the end of the first year; however, study investigators did not meet immediately based solely on rumors. By the time that study investigators were gathered for an emergency safety meeting, it was realized that 29 morbid events have occurred, and the difference in events between the two groups was huge: 27 events in the placebo group with 4 of them being fatal compared with only 2 events in the control group. The study was prematurely terminated unanimously and the study investigators expressed their regret for not recognizing the difference between the two groups earlier and subsequently terminate the study earlier. In their own words: "the events occurred so rapidly they caught us by surprise". Such a difference was not observed in the VA mild-to-moderate hypertension study and thus it was continued for 2 more years.

Summary and Conclusions

The landmark VA Co-operative studies establish in an undisputable way that treatment of treatment of mild to moderate or severe hypertension reduces cardiovascular events and cardiovascular mortality. Furthermore treatment of hypertension prevents the development of accelerated hypertension and progression to malignant hypertension, a form of hypertension with high mortality.

The VA studies address diastolic blood pressure as the target of therapy, simply because at the time it was not recognized that systolic was as or more important than diastolic blood pressure. When asked Dr. Fries why he chose diastolic blood pressure as the target he declared that it was easier to measure and more stable. Of note his VA study on mild to moderate hypertension demonstrated benefit by reducing diastolic blood pressure to around 100 mmHg. Since the early 70s when the paper was published [5], it took many subsequent studies that included 100 s of thousands of patients to prove the point that reducing diastolic to from 100 mmHg to <90 mmHg is beneficial.

Yet the results that Edward D Freis produced from these two landmark studies still hold water. The % reduction of cardiovascular events remained unchanged through the years: about 42% reduction in stroke and 16% reduction in MIs for every 5–6 mmHg diastolic blood pressure reduction. His work ignited cardiovascular research in a major way and made cardiology the leading specialty for medical research.

Furthermore, ED Freis contributed to the widespread efforts to treat hypertension by establishing the "Hypertension Diagnosis and Treatment Clinics" that help improve the control rates of hypertension up to 80% in our days.

All in all, Ed Freis deserves a lot of the credit not only from proving to the word that treating hypertension is beneficial, but also for his contribution for improvement of awareness and control of hypertension through the years.

In remembrance of his dedication and contribution we dedicate this chapter to Edward D. Freis, the man, the teacher, the healer, the scientist, the researcher.

References

1. Hunter ARO. Mortality study of impaired lives. Actuarial Soc. 1923;24:453–6.
2. Perera GA. Hypertensive vascular disease: description and natural history. J Chronic Dis. 1955;1:33–42.
3. Doumas M, Papademetriou V, Douma S, et al. Benefits from treatment and control of patients with resistant hypertension. Int J Hypertens. 2010;2011:318549.
4. Veterans Administration Cooperative Study Group on Antihypertensive Agents. Effects of treatment on morbidity in hypertension. Results in patients with diastolic blood pressure averaging 115 through 129 mm Hg. JAMA. 1967;202:1028–34.
5. Veterans Administration Cooperative Study Group on Antihypertensive Agents. Effects of treatment on morbidity in hypertension. II. Results in patients with diastolic blood pressure averaging 90 through 114 mm Hg. JAMA. 1970;213:1143–52.
6. Freis E. Hypertension treatment: contributions and comments on challenges. J Clin Hypertens. 2004;6:45–6.
7. Goldring W, Chasis H, Schreiner GE, Smith HW. Reassurance in the management of benign hypertensive disease. Circulation. 1956;14:260–4.
8. Kempner W. Treatment of hypertensive vascular disease with rice diet. Am J Med. 1948;4:545–77.
9. Goldring W, Chasis H, Fishberg AM, et al. Hypertensive vascular disease; transcription of a panel meeting on therapeutics. Bull N Y Acad Med. 1954;30:376–98.
10. Adson AW, McCraig W, Brown GE. Surgery in its relation to hypertension. Surg Gynecol Obstet. 1936;62:314–31.
11. Peet MM. Hypertension and its surgical treatment by supradiaphragmatic splanchnicectomy. Am J Surg. 1948;LXXV:48–68.
12. Papademetriou V, Doumas M, Tsioufis C. Renal sympathetic denervation for the treatment of difficult to control or resistant hypertension. Int J Hypertens. 2011;2011:196518.
13. Krum H, Schlaich M, Whitbourn R, et al. Catheter-based renal sympathetic denervation for resistant hypertension: a multicentre safety and proof-of-principle cohort study. Lancet. 2009;373:1275–81.
14. Doumas M, Douma S. Interventional management of resistant hypertension. Lancet. 2009;373:1228–30.
15. Symplicity HTN-2 Investigators, Esler MD, Krum H, Sobotka PA, Schlaich MP, Schmieder RE, Bohm M. Renal sympathetic denervation in patients with treatment-resistant hypertension (the Symplicity HTN-2 trial): a randomised controlled trial. Lancet. 2010;376:1903–9.
16. Doumas M, Douma S. Renal sympathetic denervation: the jury is still out. Lancet. 2010;376:1878–80.
17. Tsioufis C, Dimitriadis K, Kordalis A, et al. Renal denervation therapy: can it contribute to better blood pressure control in hypertension? Curr Vasc Pharmacol. 2017;16:66–9. https://doi.org/10.2174/15701611156661704226151649.
18. Tsioufis C, Dimitriadis K, Thomopoulos C, et al. Renal and Cardiac Effects of Renal Sympathetic Denervation and Carotid Baroreceptor Stimulation. Curr Vasc Pharmacol. 2014;12:55–62.
19. Faselis C, Doumas M, Kokkinos P, Tsioufis C, Papademetriou V. The role of renal nerve ablation for the management of resistant hypertension and other disease conditions: benefits and concerns. Curr Vasc Pharmacol. 2014;12:38–46.

20. Raman VK, Tsioufis C, Doumas M, Papademetriou V. Renal denervation therapy for drug-resistant hypertension: does it still work? Curr Treat Options Cardiovasc Med. 2017;19:39.
21. Papademetriou V, Doumas M, Anyfanti P, Faselis C, Kokkinos P, Tsioufis C. Renal nerve ablation for hypertensive patients with chronic kidney disease. Curr Vasc Pharmacol. 2014;12:47–54.
22. Doumas M, Faselis C, Papademetriou V. Renal sympathetic denervation in hypertension. Curr Opin Nephrol Hypertens. 2011;20:647–53.
23. Doumas M, Athyros V, Karagiannis A. Transcatheter renal sympathetic denervation: chasing a chimera or a matter of technological improvements. Cardiology. 2015;131:186–8.
24. Doumas M, Lazaridis A, Papademetriou V. Renal nerve ablation for resistant hypertension: the dust has not yet settled. J Clin Hypertens. 2014;16:399–400.
25. Doumas M, Anyfanti P, Bakris G. Should ambulatory blood pressure monitoring be mandatory for future studies in resistant hypertension: a perspective. J Hypertens. 2012;30:874–6.
26. Doumas M, Faselis C, Kokkinos P, Tsioufis C, Papademetriou V. Clinical studies of renal nerve ablation. Unanswered questions for its efficacy and safety. Curr Clin Pharmacol. 2013;8:212–6.
27. Petidis K, Anyfanti P, Doumas M. Renal sympathetic denervation: renal function concerns. Hypertension. 2011;58:e19.
28. Worthley SG, Tsioufis CP, Worthley MI, et al. Safety and efficacy of a multi-electrode renal sympathetic denervation system in resistant hypertension. Eur Heart J. 2013;34:2132–40.
29. Papademetriou V, Doumas M, Tsioufis C. Renal sympathetic denervation: hibernation or resurrection? Cardiology. 2016;135:87–97.
30. Papademetriou V, Rashidi AA, Tsioufis C, Doumas M. Renal nerve ablation for resistant hypertension: how did we get here, present status and future directions. Circulation. 2014;129:1440–51.
31. Bhatt DL, Kandzari DE, O'Neill WW, Symplicity HTN-3 Investigators, et al. A controlled trial of renal denervation for resistant hypertension. N Engl J Med. 2014;370:1393–401.
32. Papademetriou V, Tsioufis C, Doumas M. Renal denervation and Symplicity HTN-3: "Dubium sapientiae initium" (doubt is the beginning of wisdom). Circ Res. 2014;115:211–4.
33. Tsioufis C. Hypertension: is the sham-procedure 'toxic' for renal denervation? Nat Rev Nephrol. 2014;10:186–7.
34. Townsend RR, Mahfoud F, Kandzari DE, et al. Catheter-based renal denervation in patients with uncontrolled hypertension in the absence of antihypertensive medications (SPYRAL HTN-OFF MED): a randomized, sham-controlled, proof-of-concept trial. Lancet. 2017;390:2160–70. https://doi.org/10.1016/S0140-6736(17)32281-X.
35. Perera GA. Antihypertensive drug versus symptomatic treatment in primary hypertension: effect on survival. J Am Med Assoc. 1960;173:11–3.
36. Schoenberger JA, Stamler J, Shekelle RB, Shekelle S. Current status of hypertension control in an industrial population. JAMA. 1972;222:559–62.
37. Hypertension Detection and Follow-Up Program Cooperative Group. Five-year findings of the Hypertension Detection and Follow-Up Program: I. Reduction in mortality of persons with high blood pressure, including mild hypertension. JAMA. 1979;242:2562–71.
38. Management Committee of the Australian National Blood Pressure Study. The Australian therapeutic trial in mild hypertension. Lancet. 1980;1:1261–7.
39. Medical Research Council Working Party. MRC trial of treatment of mild hypertension: principal results. BMJ. 1985;291:97–104.
40. SHEP Cooperative Research Group. Prevention of stroke by antihypertensive treatment in older persons with isolated systolic hypertension: final results of the Systolic Hypertension in the Elderly Program (SHEP). JAMA. 1991;265:3255–64.
41. Hansson L, Zanchetti A, Carruthers SG, Dahlof B, Elmfeldt D, Julius S, Menard J, Rahn KH, Wedel H, Westerling S. Effects of intensive blood-pressure lowering and low-dose aspirin in patients with hypertension: principal results of the Hypertension Optimal Treatment (HOT) randomised trial. HOT Study Group. Lancet. 1998;351:1755–62.
42. Lewington S, Clarke R, Qizilbash N, Peto R, Collins R, Prospective Studies Collaboration. Age-specific relevance of usual blood pressure to vascular mortality: a meta-analysis of individual data for one million adults in 61 prospective studies. Lancet. 2002;360:1903–13.
43. Mancia G, Fagard R, Narkiewicz K, Redón J, Zanchetti A, Böhm M, Task Force Members, et al. 2013 ESH/ESC Guidelines for the management of arterial hypertension: the Task Force for the management of arterial hypertension of the European Society of Hypertension (ESH) and of the European Society of Cardiology (ESC). J Hypertens. 2013;31:1281–357.
44. James PA, Oparil S, Carter BL, et al. 2014 evidence-based guideline for the management of high blood pressure in adults: report from the panel members appointed to the Eighth Joint National Committee (JNC 8). JAMA. 2014;311:507–20.
45. Leung AA, Nerenberg K, Daskalopoulou SS, McBrien K, Zarnke KB, Dasgupta K, CHEP Guidelines Task Force, et al. Hypertension Canada's 2016 Canadian hypertension education program guidelines for blood pressure measurement, diagnosis, assessment of risk, prevention, and treatment of hypertension. Can J Cardiol. 2016;32:569–88.
46. Moser M. Salute to the icons of hypertension. J Clin Hypertens. 2004;6:8–9.
47. Freis ED. The Veterans Administration cooperative study on antihypertensive agents. Implications for stroke prevention. Stroke. 1974;5:76–7.
48. Freis ED. Reminiscences of the Veterans Administration Trial of the treatment of hypertension. Hypertension. 1990;16:472–5.

49. Veterans Administration Cooperative Study on Antihypertensive Agents. A double blind control study of antihypertensive agents: I. Comparative effectiveness of reserpine, reserpine and hydralazine, and three ganglionic blocking agents, chlorisondamine, mecamylamine, and pentolinium tartrate. Arch Intern Med. 1960;106:81–96.
50. Veterans Administration Cooperative Study on Antihypertensive Agents. Double blind control study of antihypertensive agents: II. Further report on the comparative effectiveness of reserpine, reserpine and hydralazine, and three ganglionic blocking agents, chlorisondamine, mecamylamine, and pentolinium tartrate. Arch Intern Med. 1962;110:126–33.
51. Freis ED, Stanton JR. A clinical evaluation of veratrum viride in the treatment of essential hypertension. Am Heart J. 1948;36:723–38.
52. Freis ED, Stanton JR. The hemodynamic effects of hypotensive drugs in man; dihydroergocomine. J Clin Invest. 1949;28:1387–402.
53. Finnerty FA, Fries ED. Experimental and clinical evaluation in man of hexamethonium (C6), a new ganglionic blocking agent. Circulation. 1950;2:828–36.
54. Freis ED, Rose JC, Higgins TF, et al. The hemodynamic effects of hypotensive drugs in man. IV. 1-Hydralazinophthalazine. Circulation. 1953;8:199–204.
55. Freis ED, Wanko A, Wilson IM, Parrish AE. Treatment of essential hypertension with chlorothiazide (diuril); its use alone and combined with other antihypertensive agents. J Am Med Assoc. 1958;166:137–40.
56. Freis ED, Wanko A, Wilson IM, Parrish AE. Chlorothiazide in hypertensive and normotensive patients. Ann N Y Acad Sci. 1958;71:450–5.
57. Frohlich ED, Schnaper HW, Wilson IM, Freis ED. Hemodynamic alterations in hypertensive patients due to chlorothiazide. N Engl J Med. 1960;262:1261–3.
58. The SPRINT Research Group. A randomized trial of intensive versus standard blood pressure control. N Engl J Med. 2015;373:2103–16.
59. SPRINT Research Group. Effects of intensive systolic blood pressure control on kidney and cardiovascular outcomes in persons without kidney disease: a secondary analysis of a randomized trial. Ann Intern Med. 2017;167:375–83. https://doi.org/10.7326/M16-2966.
60. SPRINT Research Group. Effect of intensive blood pressure treatment on patient-reported outcomes. N Engl J Med. 2017;377:733–44.
61. SPRINT Research Group. Effect of intensive versus standard blood pressure treatment according to baseline prediabetes status: a post hoc analysis of a randomized trial. Diabetes Care. 2017;40:1401–8. https://doi.org/10.2337/dc17-0885.
62. Stergiou GS, Doumas M, Kollias A, Papademetriou V. Important practice lessons from the SPRINT study beyond the blood pressure goal: all well known and now confirmed. J Am Soc Hypertens. 2016;10:613–7.
63. Freis ED, Wilkins RW. The effects of pentaquine in patients with hypertension. Proc Soc Exp Biol Med. 1947;64:455–8.
64. Wilkins RW. New drug therapies in arterial hypertension. Ann Intern Med. 1952;37:1144–55.
65. Wilkins RW, Judson WE. The use of Rauwolfia serpentina in hypertensive patients. N Engl J Med. 1953;248:48–53.
66. Freis ED, Wilson IM. Potentiating effect of chlorothiazide (Diuril) in combination with antihypertensive agents: preliminary report. Med Ann Dist Columbia. 1957;26:468–71.
67. Hollander W, Wilkins RW. Chlorothiazide: a new type of drug for the treatment of arterial hypertension. BMQ. 1957;8:69–75.

The Role of Dietary Modifications in Controlling Blood Pressure

5

K. Dimitriadis, C. Filippou, and C. Tsioufis

Introduction

Body weight increase is closely related to blood pressure (BP) levels augmentation in almost a linear fashion [1], augmenting overall cardiovascular risk [2]. More specifically in the Framingham Heart Study, data regarding 45.000 subjects during a follow-up of 44 years showed that overweight and obese men had a 48% and 123% higher risk of developing hypertension compared to normal weight individuals. In the same manner, overweight and obese women compered to normal weight ones had a 70% and 175% higher risk for developing hypertension [3].

The important INTERSALT study performed in 10.074 adults 20–59 years old in 32 countries worldwide showed that an intake of more than 2.3 gr/day is linked with increased BP by 6 mmHg and diastolic by 2.5 mmHg [4]. In another cross-sectional work including more than 100,000 subjects from 18 countries it was found that for an increase of consumption of salt by 1 gr/day the systolic BP augments by 2.6 mmHg and diastolic BP by 1.8 mmHg [5]. Thus, the higher the intake of salt the higher by 25% the probability of being hypertensive as shown in a prospective study of 4500 normotensives [6, 7].

There is an inverse correlation between consumption of potassium and hypertension [6, 7]. In the NHANES study 1gr/day higher potassium was associated with lower systolic BP by 1.2 mmHg [8], while in another population the higher quartile of sodium/potassium ratio (7.9–9.7) had more increased systolic and diastolic BP by 8 mmHg and 7 mmHg, respectively compared to those in the lower quartile of sodium/potassium ratio (2.1–2.3) [9]. In this sense low consumption of potassium leads to hypertension [7] and more specifically this risk augments by 20% in the subjects with less than 2600 mg urine excretion for males and less than 2200 mg for females [10].

Although moderate alcohol intake compared to full abstinence is associated with higher HDL cholesterol levels and decreased risk for cardiovascular events, the correlation with BP is positive leading to higher hemodynamic load [11]. For each 10 gr of alcohol BP rises for approximately 11 mmHg and the latter is reversed after 2–4 weeks when no or minimal consumption is present [12]. In a randomized clinical study of 44 treated hypertensive men moderate compared to low alcohol consumption was linked to higher BP by 5 mmHg for systolic and 3 mmHg for the diastolic component [13]. Additionally a 45% increased risk for the development of hypertension is observed in normotensives who consumed more than 1 drink for more than 5 days per week compared to no alcohol [14].

K. Dimitriadis (✉) · C. Filippou · C. Tsioufis
Clinical Dietician-Nutritionist. First Cardiology Clinic, Hippokration Hospital, University of Athens, Athens, Greece

V. Papademetriou et al. (eds.), *Management of Hypertension*,
https://doi.org/10.1007/978-3-319-92946-0_5

Dietary Interventions for BP Lowering

Lifestyle changes are the pillars for both prevention and management of hypertension [15, 16]. In the PREMIER study, that was a randomized clinical study in 810 subjects >25 years old with systolic BP ranging 120–159 mmHg and diastolic BP 80–95 mmHg, on no antihypertensive medication, it was shown that after 6 months the behavioral intervention alone or with the adoption of the DASH diet lowered systolic BP by 3.7 mmHg and 4.3 mmHg, while diastolic BP was decreased by 1.7 mmHg and 2.6 mmHg respectively. The 18 months results concluded that the combination of the DASH diet with behavioral alterations compared to the latter alone are linked to 23% less possibilities for hypertension [17].

The current guidelines suggest for subjects with high normal BP to prevent the development of hypertension and for the hypertensive individuals with ow cardiovascular risk and no target organ damage to base their management on lifestyle/dietary interventions, whereas in those who drug therapy is initiated it should be always accompanied by non-pharmacological management [18]. In the innovative American guidelines for hypertension, subjects of low cardiovascular risk with hypertension grade1 should follow a healthy lifestyle without any medication taken [19]. The proposed in the guidelines dietary interventions are weight loss, decrease in sodium intake, increase in potassium consumption, reduction of alcohol and the adoption of a healthy dietary pattern like the DASH or the Mediterranean diet [18, 19].

Weight Loss and BP Control

Losing excess weight is directly related to BP levels reduction 38, 39, 40. In a meta-analysis of 25 randomized trials a weight loss of 5.1 kgr reduces systolic and diastolic BP by 4.4 mmHg and 3.6 mmHg respectively. The higher the decrease in weight the higher is the reduction of BP with 1 mmHg corresponding to the loss of approximately 1 kgr [20]. TOHP study was one of the largest randomized studies for the investigation of the effects of weight reduction on BP levels. In the weight reduction group with intense education the lost weight after 6 months was 4.4 kgr, in 18 months 2 kgr and after 3 years only 0.2 kgr, underscoring the difficulty in maintaining the positive results.

[21]. Compared to the control group in the abovementioned timepoints of the study systolic/diastolic BP was lowered by 3.7/2.7 mmHg, 1.8/1.3 mmHg and 1.3/0.9 mmHg [22]. After 7 years there was no difference in body weight but the risk of developing hypertension was 77% less in the intervention group [23].

The short-term effects of weight reduction on BP are rather beneficial, however there is a problem with the long-term results since 50% of subjects gain their initial weight before any intervention after a mean period of 3 years and this causes an increase in BP 45–47. In patients with morbid obesity drugs and bariatric surgery are therapeutic solutions although the impact on BP remain controversial [24, 25].

Sodium and BP Control

The reduction of salt to 2.300 mg per day is one of the most important dietary interventions for maintaining normal BP [18, 26, 27]. There are many randomized well-designed studies showing the beneficial effects of reducing dietary salt [7, 28–38]. In a recent meta-analysis reduction of salt intake from 4.500 mg to 1.500 mg per day decreases systolic BP by 1 mmHg, with no effects on diastolic BP in normotensives, whereas in hypertensive individuals the same salt restriction results in lower systolic/diastolic BP by 5.5/2.9 mmHg [39]. In these lines data from the TOHP study reveal that restriction of sodium was lower than 1.150 mg per day for the 6 months of follow-up and 920 mg per day for 3 years compared to controls leading to lower BP [22]. In treated hypertensives the TONE study investigated the effects of weight reduction and sodium restriction <1.8 gr/day on BP levels. The combination of salt and weight decrease was accompanied by attenuated systolic BP of 5.3 mmHg and diastolic of 3.4 mmHg compared to controls [40]. Regarding cross-sectional studies excretion of sodium in the urine is closely associated with both the BP levels as well as the hypertension risk [41]. The INTERMAP study showed that in 4.680 adults 40–59 years showed that in China and Japan the sodium/potassium ratio was higher (6.0–6.8) in China and compared to Great Britain and America (2.2–3.1) and BP levels were higher in the Eastern compared to Western countries [42].

One of the most important trials on the way salt affects BP is the double-blind randomized trial of modest salt restriction in older people by Cappucio F et al., published more than 2 decades ago [43]. This crossover trial was conducted to examine the effect on BP of a modest reduction in salt intake from 10 g to 5 g per day in both hypertensive and normotensive individuals. The study was conducted in 47 older adults, aged 60 years or more, with systolic BP <210 mmHg and diastolic BP <115 mmHg on no drugs. For 2 weeks participants were told to reduce their salt intake to about 5 g (80 mmoles sodium) daily. Participants achieved this reduction by not adding salt at the table or in cooking, and by avoiding foods that contain large amounts of salt. After the 2 weeks of reduced sodium intake, participants were allocated in random order to take 12 Slow Sodium tablets daily (10 mmoles sodium per tablet) or 12 Slow Sodium matching placebo tablets daily. After 1 month, measurements were repeated, and participants crossed over to the opposite treatment for a further month. It should be noted that energy restriction was not suggested and an average reduction in sodium intake of 80 mmol/day (about 5 g salt) was associated with a reduction in both systolic BP and diastolic BP of 7.2 mmHg and 3.2 mmHg, respectively. There was no significant difference in the BP fall between 18 normotensives and 29 hypertensive participants (8.2/3.97 mmHg vs 6.6/2.7 mmHg) [43].

Based on the abovementioned results one could suggest that the fall of BP in this study is similar to that in the controlled-outcome trials of drug therapy in older hypertensive people for example with the use of thiazide diuretics. Additionally, a modest reduction in sodium intake is feasible and can be achieved over a long period, provided salt is not added to food or in cooking, and highly salted processed foods are avoided.

Two of the most recent meta-analyses of randomized, controlled clinical trials that have been performed in adults investigating the magnitude of the effect of salt reduction on BP found that the salt restriction has significant beneficial effects. Specifically, Graudal et al. found that a mean reduction of salt intake from 11.5 g to 3.8 g per day reduces significantly systolic BP by 5.5 mmHg and diastolic BP by 2.9 mmHg in people with hypertension, while in people without hypertension has very little or no effect [39]. He FJ et al. found that a mean reduction of salt intake of 4.4 g per day in people with hypertension reduces significantly systolic BP by 5.4 mmHg and diastolic BP by 2.8 mmHg. In normotensive individuals the same reduction of salt intake reduces significantly systolic BP by 2.4 mmHg and diastolic BP by 1.0 mmHg [26].

Potassium and BP Control

The augmented intake of potassium up to 3.500–5.000 mg per day through diet and not by supplements remains a recommendation for better BP levels, unless the subject has chronic kidney disease or taking drugs that reduce the excretion of sodium [2] [44]. Up to now there are several randomized studies on the above [45]. A meta-analysis showed that an intake of 3.500–4.700 mg potassium per day reduces systolic BP by 7.1 mmHg and diastolic BP by 4,0 mmHg, whereas there is no effect in normotensives [46]. Consistently, cross-sectional data suggest that potassium excretion in the urine is related to the BP levels and the risk of developing hypertension in the future [47]. The INTERSALT study showed that intake of more thatn 600 mg of potassium per day is linked to lower BP by 1 mmHg [48].

Dietary Patterns and BP Control

The real impact of diet on BP is not only due to the ingredients but also due to the patterns of diet that one follows. The diet patterns are mostly important clinically since they reflect better the dietary habits of each individuals and the interactions between foods consumed and other lifestyle parameters [49]. In this sense the effect of the totality of nutrients intake on the overall cardiovascular health as well as BP can be investigated through the study of the dietary patterns [50].

DASH Diet and BP

The DASH diet is associated with BP reduction 74 and is characterized by high consumption of fruits, vegetables and milk products with low fat content accompanied by low consumption of red meat. It is a diet rich in potassium, calcium, magnesium, proteins and fibers with low fat and cholesterol [51].

There are numerous randomized trials on the BP lowering impact of DASH diet in hypertension [51–71]. The historic study by Appel LJ et al., was a randomized, controlled-feeding clinical trial was conducted in order to test the effects on BP of three different diets: the control diet, the fruits-and-vegetables diet and the "combination" diet, which was rich in fruits, vegetables, and low-fat dairy products, now named the "DASH" diet [51]. The study was conducted in 459 adults with SBP <160 mmHg and DBP 80–95 mmHg. The assigned diets were prepared and given to the participants for 8 weeks. Sodium intake was kept constant at 3000 mg per day and it was the same among all three diets and body weight was maintained at constant levels. Among all subjects, the DASH diet reduced significantly systolic BP and diastolic BP by 5.5 and 3.0 mmHg, respectively, compared to the control diet and by 2.7 and 1.9 mmHg, respectively, compared to the fruits-and-vegetables diet. The results were more profound among the subjects with hypertension compared to the subjects without hypertension [51]. Specifically, among the 133 subjects with hypertension the DASH diet reduced significantly systolic BP and diastolic BP by 11.47 mmHg and 5.5 mmHg, respectively, more compared to the control diet and by 4.17 mmHg and 2.6 mmHg, respectively, more compared to the fruits-and-vegetables diet. Furthermore, among the 326 subjects without hypertension the DASH diet reduced significantly systolic BP and DBP by 3.57 mmHg and 2.1 mmHg, respectively, more compared to the control diet and by 2.77 mmHg and 1.8 mmHg, respectively, more compared to the fruits-and-vegetables diet. Given the findings of this pioneer studies one could comment that the gradient of BP reduction across diets indicates that some aspects of the fruits-and-vegetables diet reduced BP and that additional aspects of the combination (DASH) diet reduced it further. Known diet-related determinants of BP (sodium intake, body weight, and alcohol) could not be responsible for the reductions in BP, because changes in these potential confounders were small and similar for all the diets. Finally, regarding the composition of the diets compared the control and the fruits-and-vegetables diets contained more oils, table fats, salad dressings, and red meats and were higher in saturated fat, total fat, and cholesterol than was the DASH diet. The fruits-and-vegetables and the DASH diets contained relatively more servings of fruits, juices, vegetables, and nuts/seeds, and were higher in magnesium, potassium, and fiber than was the control diet [51]. Both the fruits-and-vegetables and DASH diets were low in sweets and sugar-containing drinks. The DASH diet contained a greater variety of fruits, and its high calcium content was obtained by increasing low-fat dairy products. It is worthy to note that the effect of an individual nutrient on BP levels may be too small to be detected. However, when several nutrients with small BP lowering effects are consumed together, the cumulative effect may be sufficient for detection. Also, people do not eat isolated nutrients, but they consume meals consisting of a variety of foods with complex combinations of nutrients. Thus, the approach of assessing whole dietary patterns, instead of assessing single nutrients or food items is considered more accurate [51]. However, the DASH clinical trial was not designed to identify the effective and ineffective components of this particular diet.

In a subgroup analysis of the DASH trial, the effect on the 24-h ambulatory hemodynamic load was tested and it was revealed that this dietary pattern reduces systolic/diastolic BP by 4.5/2.7 mmHg more than the control group. In the hypertensive setting compared to the normotensives the drop of BP was higher in the intervention arm [52]. More specifically, 24-h systolic/diastolic BP was more attenuated by 10.1/5/5 mmHg compared to the controls, whereas in normotensives DASH diet was accompanied by a lower 24-h systolic/diastolic BP by 2.3/1.6 mmHg [52].

The randomized cross-over DASH-Sodium study had the aim to investigate the impact of DAH on BP with the parallel restriction of sodium intake [53]. The study population were adults with baseline systolic BP 120–159 mmHg and diastolic BP 80–95 mmHg in whom the following interventions took place: control diet, DASH diet with three levels of sodium consumption: low, medium and high [53]. All meals were cooked and served in the participant for a period of 30 days and the energy intake was calculated foe each person in order to maintain stable weight. The results showed that the DASH diet with low sodium reduced BP by 3/1.6 mmHg compared to the DASH diet of high sodium. Additionally, the low sodium DASH diet was characterized by lower systolic/diastolic BP by 8.9/4.5 mmHg compared to the high sodium control diet [53].

When weight reduction is achieved while on DASH diet the BP lowering is enhanced [72, 73]. The ENCORE study was a randomized control trial in individuals with systolic BP of 130–159 mmHg and diastolic BP of 85–99 mmHg in whom the effect of DASH diet with or without weight loss on BP was investigated during a follow-up of 4 months. There were no directions regarding salt consumption and frequent dietary education and counseling took place. The DASH diet was related with lower BP by 7.7/3.6 mmHg compared to the control group, while when DASH was combined with weight loss the BP drop was more pronounced by 12.5/5.9 mmHg compared to controls at the end of the follow-up [62].

The cross-sectional data suggest that adoption of the DASH diet is linked with lower risk of hypertension and BP levels [74]. The difference in office BP between the higher and the lower quartile of compliance to the DASH pattern is 7.5 and 5.1 mmHg for men and women respectively, while the 24-h ambulatory data show a difference of 6.3 and 5.4 mmHg for men and women respectively [75].

In accordance to the previous, prospective works found that DASH diet is related with lower risk of future development of hypertension [76]. More specifically, in 2.751 normotensive subjects the upper quartile of compliance to the diet was associated with 15$ attenuated risk compared to the lower compliance quartile after a follow-up of 11 years [77].

In a recent meta-analysis of randomized trials for the BP effect of DASH diet it was shown that it leads to a lowering of systolic/diastolic BP of 4.9/2.6 mmHg [71]. Two other meta-analyses by Saneei et al. and Siervo et al. found that the DASH diet reduces significantly SBP by 6.7/5.2 mmHg and DBP by 3.5/2.6 mmHg, respectively [78, 79].

Mediterranean Diet and BP

The Mediterranean diet is based on the high consumption of lipids derived from extra virgin (cold pressed) olive oil, vegetables including leafy green vegetables, fruits, cereals, nuts and pulses/legumes, moderate intakes of fish and other meat, dairy products and red wine, and low intakes of eggs and sweets [80, 81]. It is associated with lower BP and this is supported by randomized trials [82–93].

Focusing on the PREDIMED study that is the largest in this setting, it was conducted in 772 adults with high cardiovascular risk and comparisons were made between the Mediterranean diet with olive oil versus the same diet with nuts without any energy restriction for 3 months [86]. There were no advise given for salt restriction or physical activity.

The results showed that the diet with nuts reduced systolic BP more by 7.1/2.6 mmHg compared to the low-fat group with no change in body weight in both arms [86].

In a subgroup analysis of 235 subjects of the PREDIMED study there was ambulatory 24-h BP monitoring after the intervention. In accordance to the office BP changes the 24-h systolic/diastolic BP was reduced more in the arm with the nuts intake [92]. In the same study there was no difference in the systolic BP after 4 years but the diastolic BP was lower in the nuts arm [94]. Importantly, subjects in the Mediterranean diet had less risk of developing hypertension compared to the control group after a 4 years follow-up [95].

A more recent randomized, parallel-group, controlled clinical trial was conducted in order to assess the effects on cardiovascular outcomes of two Mediterranean diets (MeDiets), one supplemented with extra-virgin olive oil and the other supplemented with mixed nuts, compared to a low-fat diet (control diet) [96]. The study was conducted in 7447 adults with type 2 diabetes or ≥3 cardiovascular risk factors. The participants of the two MeDiets groups, depending on the group assignment, were given for free either extra-virgin olive oil (1 L per week) or sachets of nuts (30 g per day: 15 g walnuts, 7.5 g hazelnuts and 7.5 g almonds) [96]. Participants in the two MeDiets groups received education to follow the MeDiet and consume the supplemental foods at the baseline and thereafter, once every 3 months in individual and group sessions, while those in the control group were given advice to reduce dietary fat. During the first 3 years of the trial they were given a leaflet explaining the low-fat diet on a yearly basis, but thereafter they were invited to individual and group sessions with the same frequency and intensity as those in the MeDiets groups [96]. Sodium intake was not restricted and energy restriction was not suggested, nor increase of physical activity was promoted. The primary end-point was a composite of myocardial infarction, stroke, and death from cardiovascular causes [96]. Additionally, secondary end-points were stroke, myocardial infarction, death from cardiovascular causes, and death from any cause. Participants were followed for a median of 4.8 years (interquartile range, 2.8–5.8). The multivariable-adjusted hazard ratios were 0.70 (0.54–0.92), p = 0.01 for the MeDiet supplemented with extra-virgin olive oil and 0.72 (0.54–0.96), p = 0.03 for the MeDiet supplemented with nuts, as compared to the low-fat diet with respect to the primary end-point [96]. Regarding components of the primary end-point, only the comparisons of stroke risk reached statistical significance: 0.67 (0.46–0.98), p = 0.04 for the MeDiet supplemented with extra-virgin olive oil and 0.54 (0.35–0.84), p = 0.006 for the MeDiet supplemented with nuts, as compared to the low-fat diet. During the 4-year follow-up participants allocated to the two MeDiets groups had significantly lower DBP than the participants in the low-fat diet group: −1.53 mmHg for the MeDiet supplemented with extra-virgin olive oil, and −0.65 mmHg for the MeDiet supplemented with nuts versus the low-fat diet. No between-group differences in changes of SBP were seen [96].

Based on these results among high-risk persons who were initially free of cardiovascular disease, an energy-unrestricted MeDiet supplemented with extra-virgin olive oil or nuts reduced the incidence of major cardiovascular events, for a relative risk reduction of approximately 30%. The findings support the benefits of the MeDiet for cardiovascular risk reduction. Perhaps there is a synergy among the nutrient-rich foods included in the MeDiet that fosters favorable changes in intermediate pathways of cardiometabolic risk, such as blood lipids, insulin sensitivity, resistance to oxidation, inflammation, and vasoreactivity. It should be noted that although the control group's diet was meant to be low fat, the participants did not achieve this, possibly due to the relatively low level of dietary education and personalized counseling at the start of the study. Their inability to reach the <30% fat target could also reflect the difficulty patients have, in general, in decreasing fat content in their diet, which may mean the diet they maintained was a more realistic comparison. Therefore, the major between-group difference involved the supplemental items and consequently, the differences in outcomes observed between the MeDiets groups and the low-fat diet group might be attributed to the supplemental foods provided. The interventions in all three groups were intended to improve the overall dietary pattern. The good quality of the diet in the control group may have impaired the ability to find large between-group differences in BP changes. Thus, if there was a "true" control group (for example, with a typical Western dietary pattern, or with no intervention at all) the between-group differences both in stroke and BP would have been greater. Concerning BP, significant reductions were apparent in both SBP and DBP for all three groups during follow-up, but a greater reduction in DBP was found in the two MeDiets groups versus the low-fat diet group. This could partly explain the benefit of the MeDiets on clinical disease end-points, especially the reduction in incidence of stroke, a cardiovascular event clearly related to high BP. However, other mechanisms apart from BP also need to be considered.

The PREDIMED clinical trial fits well into the paradigm of focusing on dietary patterns instead of isolated foods or nutrients. Overall patterns better represent dietary practices found in free-living populations and provide useful epidemiological information with a high potential for acceptability, palatability, and future compliance.

The Mediterranean diet is characterized by a high consumption of total fat, mainly from olive oil and nuts, whole-grain cereals, legumes, fruits, and vegetables. It also includes moderate to high intake of fish, moderate intake of dairy products, poultry, and wine, consumed with meals along with low intake of red/ processed meats, and sweets. Consequently, the Mediterranean diet is rich in anti-oxidant and anti-inflammatory nutrients, fiber, ω-3 and mono-unsaturated fat and low in saturated fat and dietary cholesterol. Extra-virgin olive oil is an excellent source of mono-unsaturated fat. It also contains significant amounts of phenolic anti-oxidants and other phytochemicals (tocopherols, polyphenols). Nuts are rich in mono-unsaturated fat (mostly oleic acid), whereas walnuts are high in poly-unsaturated fatty acids (linoleic and a-linolenic acids). Nuts are also good sources of arginine, potassium, vitamin E and other bioactive compounds. This may help explain their beneficial health effects. From a public health perspective, a behavioral intervention coupled with an easy (free) access to representative healthy foods is a realistic test of the effectiveness to be attained with official policies and health promotion activities. The PREDIMED trial attempts to obtain relevant information for public health use, because the nutritional intervention is undertaken in free-living persons who receive information, motivation, support, and empowerment to modify their food habits in a real-life context, i.e. they continue to buy their foods and cook their meals. Such an intervention provides a real-life scenario that may be easily applied to public health policies.

Meta-analyses

Two meta-analyses of randomized, controlled clinical trials have been performed in adults investigating the magnitude of the effect of the MeDiet on blood pressure. Both found that the MeDiet has significant beneficial effects on SBP and DBP. Specifically, Ndanuko et al. and Nissensohn et al. found that the MeDiet reduces significantly SBP by 3.0/1.4 mmHg and DBP by 1.9/0.7 mmHg, respectively [71, 79].

Conclusions

Diet interventions are important in the overall reduction of cardiovascular risk and particular in the development and clinical impact of the hypertensive phenotype. The use of dietary consultation by means of promoting reduction of salt, maintenance of healthy weight and adoption of certain dietary patterns constitute the pillars of lifestyle management in hypertension. The DASH and the Mediterranean diet have proved their favorable effect on BP levels rendering them current health choices for the modern societies. Implementing such interventions in a large scale is an important and urgent clinically meaningful task nowadays in order to reduce hypertension and cardiovascular disease burden.

References

1. Jordan J, Yumuk V, Schlaich M, Nilsson PM, Zahorska-Markiewicz B, Grassi G, Schmieder RE, Engeli S, Finer N. Joint statement of the European Association for the Study of Obesity and the European Society of Hypertension: obesity and difficult to treat arterial hypertension. J Hypertens. 2012;30(6):1047–55.
2. Leggio M, Lombardi M, Caldarone E, Severi P, D'Emidio S, Armeni M, Bravi V, Bendini MG, Mazza A. The relationship between obesity and hypertension: an updated comprehensive overview on vicious twins. Hypertens Res. 2017;40(12):947–63.
3. Wilson PW, D'Agostino RB, Sullivan L, Parise H, Kannel WB. Overweight and obesity as determinants of cardiovascular risk: the Framingham experience. Arch Intern Med. 2002;162(16):1867–72.
4. Elliott P, Stamler J, Nichols R, Dyer AR, Stamler R, Kesteloot H, Marmot M. Intersalt revisited: further analyses of 24 hour sodium excretion and blood pressure within and across populations. Intersalt Cooperative Research Group. BMJ (Clinical research ed). 1996;312(7041):1249–53.
5. Mente A, O'Donnell MJ, Rangarajan S, McQueen MJ, Poirier P, Wielgosz A, Morrison H, Li W, Wang X, Di C, et al. Association of urinary sodium and potassium excretion with blood pressure. N Engl J Med. 2014;371(7):601–11.
6. Adrogue HJ, Madias NE. The impact of sodium and potassium on hypertension risk. Semin Nephrol. 2014;34(3):257–72.
7. Takase H, Sugiura T, Kimura G, Ohte N, Dohi Y. Dietary sodium consumption predicts future blood pressure and incident hypertension in the Japanese Normotensive General Population. J Am Heart Assoc. 2015;4(8):e001959.
8. Zhang Z, Cogswell ME, Gillespie C, Fang J, Loustalot F, Dai S, Carriquiry AL, Kuklina EV, Hong Y, Merritt R, et al. Association between usual sodium and potassium intake and blood pressure and hypertension among U.S. adults: NHANES 2005–2010. PloS one. 2013;8(10):e75289.
9. Rodrigues SL, Baldo MP, Machado RC, Forechi L, Molina Mdel C, Mill JG. High potassium intake blunts the effect of elevated sodium intake on blood pressure levels. J Am Soc Hypertens (JASH). 2014;8(4):232–8.
10. Kieneker LM, Gansevoort RT, Mukamal KJ, de Boer RA, Navis G, Bakker SJ, Joosten MM. Urinary potassium excretion and risk of developing hypertension: the prevention of renal and vascular end-stage disease study. Hypertension (Dallas, Tex : 1979). 2014;64(4):769–76.
11. Klatsky AL. Alcohol and cardiovascular mortality: common sense and scientific truth. J Am Coll Cardiol. 2010;55(13):1336–8.
12. Puddey IB, Beilin LJ. Alcohol is bad for blood pressure. Clin Exp Pharmacol Physiol. 2006;33(9):847–52.
13. Puddey IB, Beilin LJ, Vandongen R. Regular alcohol use raises blood pressure in treated hypertensive subjects. A randomised controlled trial. Lancet (London, England). 1987;1(8534):647–51.
14. Nunez-Cordoba JM, Martinez-Gonzalez MA, Bes-Rastrollo M, Toledo E, Beunza JJ, Alonso A. Alcohol consumption and the incidence of hypertension in a Mediterranean cohort: the SUN study. Rev Esp Cardiol. 2009;62(6):633–41.
15. Frisoli TM, Schmieder RE, Grodzicki T, Messerli FH. Beyond salt: lifestyle modifications and blood pressure. Eur Heart J. 2011;32(24):3081–7.
16. The treatment of mild hypertension study. A randomized, placebo-controlled trial of a nutritional-hygienic regimen along with various drug monotherapies. The Treatment of Mild Hypertension Research Group. Arch Intern Med. 1991;151(7):1413–23.
17. Elmer PJ, Obarzanek E, Vollmer WM, Simons-Morton D, Stevens VJ, Young DR, Lin PH, Champagne C, Harsha DW, Svetkey LP, et al. Effects of comprehensive lifestyle modification on diet, weight, physical fitness, and blood pressure control: 18-month results of a randomized trial. Ann Intern Med. 2006;144(7):485–95.
18. Mancia G, Fagard R, Narkiewicz K, Redon J, Zanchetti A, Bohm M, Christiaens T, Cifkova R, De Backer G, Dominiczak A, Redon J, Tsioufis C, Bueno H, et al. 2013 ESH/ESC guidelines for the management of arterial hypertension: the task force for the management of arterial hypertension of the European Society of Hypertension (ESH) and of the European Society of Cardiology (ESC). J Hypertens. 2013;31(7):1281–357.
19. Whelton PK, Carey RM, Aronow WS, Casey DE Jr, Collins KJ, Dennison Himmelfarb C, Depalma SM, Gidding S, Jamerson KA, Jones DW, et al. ACC/AHA/AAPA/ABC/ACPM/AGS/APhA/ ASH/ASPC/NMA/PCNA guideline for the prevention, detection, evaluation, and Management of High Blood Pressure in adults: a report of the American College of Cardiology/American Heart Association Task Force on Clinical Practice Guidelines. J Am Coll Cardiol. 2018;71(19):2199–269.
20. Neter JE, Stam BE, Kok FJ, Grobbee DE, Geleijnse JM. Influence of weight reduction on blood pressure: a meta-analysis of randomized controlled trials. Hypertension (Dallas, Tex : 1979). 2003;42(5):878–84.
21. Stevens VJ, Obarzanek E, Cook NR, Lee IM, Appel LJ, Smith West D, Milas NC, Mattfeldt-Beman M, Belden L, Bragg C, et al. Long-term weight loss and changes in blood pressure: results of the Trials of Hypertension Prevention, phase II. Ann Intern Med. 2001;134(1):1–11.
22. Effects of weight loss and sodium reduction intervention on blood pressure and hypertension incidence in overweight people with high-normal blood pressure. The Trials of Hypertension Prevention,

phase II. The Trials of Hypertension Prevention Collaborative Research Group. Arch Intern Med. 1997;157(6):657–67.
23. He J, Whelton PK, Appel LJ, Charleston J, Klag MJ. Long-term effects of weight loss and dietary sodium reduction on incidence of hypertension. Hypertension (Dallas, Tex : 1979). 2000;35(2):544–9.
24. Straznicky N, Grassi G, Esler M, Lambert G, Dixon J, Lambert E, Jordan J, Schlaich M. European Society of Hypertension Working Group on Obesity Antihypertensive effects of weight loss: myth or reality? J Hypertens. 2010;28(4):637–43.
25. Ryan DH. The pharmacological and surgical management of adults with obesity. J Fam Pract. 2014;63(7 Suppl):S21–6.
26. He FJ, Li J, Macgregor GA. Effect of longer term modest salt reduction on blood pressure: Cochrane systematic review and meta-analysis of randomised trials. BMJ (Clinical research ed). 2013;346:f1325.
27. Aburto NJ, Ziolkovska A, Hooper L, Elliott P, Cappuccio FP, Meerpohl JJ. Effect of lower sodium intake on health: systematic review and meta-analyses. BMJ (Clinical research ed). 2013;346:f1326.
28. MacGregor GA, Markandu ND, Sagnella GA, Singer DR, Cappuccio FP. Double-blind study of three sodium intakes and long-term effects of sodium restriction in essential hypertension. Lancet (London, England). 1989;2(8674):1244–7.
29. Benetos A, Xiao YY, Cuche JL, Hannaert P, Safar M. Arterial effects of salt restriction in hypertensive patients. A 9-week, randomized, double-blind, crossover study. J Hypertens. 1992;10(4):355–60.
30. Fotherby MD, Potter JF. Effects of moderate sodium restriction on clinic and twenty-four-hour ambulatory blood pressure in elderly hypertensive subjects. J Hypertens. 1993;11(6):657–63.
31. Cappuccio FP, Markandu ND, Carney C, Sagnella GA, MacGregor GA. Double-blind randomised trial of modest salt restriction in older people. Lancet (London, England). 1997;350(9081):850–4.
32. Gates PE, Tanaka H, Hiatt WR, Seals DR. Dietary sodium restriction rapidly improves large elastic artery compliance in older adults with systolic hypertension. Hypertension (Dallas, Tex : 1979). 2004;44(1):35–41.
33. Melander O, von Wowern F, Frandsen E, Burri P, Willsteen G, Aurell M, Hulthen UL. Moderate salt restriction effectively lowers blood pressure and degree of salt sensitivity is related to baseline concentration of renin and N-terminal atrial natriuretic peptide in plasma. J Hypertens. 2007;25(3):619–27.
34. Kojuri J, Rahimi R. Effect of "no added salt diet" on blood pressure control and 24 hour urinary sodium excretion in mild to moderate hypertension. BMC Cardiovasc Disord. 2007;7:34.
35. Dickinson KM, Keogh JB, Clifton PM. Effects of a low-salt diet on flow-mediated dilatation in humans. Am J Clin Nutr. 2009;89(2):485–90.
36. He FJ, Marciniak M, Visagie E, Markandu ND, Anand V, Dalton RN, MacGregor GA. Effect of modest salt reduction on blood pressure, urinary albumin, and pulse wave velocity in white, black, and Asian mild hypertensives. Hypertension (Dallas, Tex : 1979). 2009;54(3):482–8.
37. He J, Gu D, Chen J, Jaquish CE, Rao DC, Hixson JE, Chen JC, Duan X, Huang JF, Chen CS, et al. Gender difference in blood pressure responses to dietary sodium intervention in the GenSalt study. J Hypertens. 2009;27(1):48–54.
38. Liu F, Chen P, Li D, Yang X, Huang J, Gu D. Ambulatory blood pressure and blood pressure load responses to low sodium intervention in Han Chinese population. Clin Exp Hypertens. 2015;37(7):551–6.
39. Graudal NA, Hubeck-Graudal T, Jurgens G. Effects of low sodium diet versus high sodium diet on blood pressure, renin, aldosterone, catecholamines, cholesterol, and triglyceride. Cochrane Database Syst Rev. 2017;4:Cd004022.
40. Whelton PK, Appel LJ, Espeland MA, Applegate WB, Ettinger WH Jr, Kostis JB, Kumanyika S, Lacy CR, Johnson KC, Folmar S, et al. Sodium reduction and weight loss in the treatment of hypertension in older persons: a randomized controlled trial of nonpharmacologic interventions in the elderly (TONE). TONE Collaborative Research Group. JAMA. 1998;279(11):839–46.
41. Stamler J. The INTERSALT Study: background, methods, findings, and implications. Am J Clin Nutr. 1997;65(2 Suppl):626s–42s.
42. Zhou BF, Stamler J, Dennis B, Moag-Stahlberg A, Okuda N, Robertson C, Zhao L, Chan Q, Elliott P. Nutrient intakes of middle-aged men and women in China, Japan, United Kingdom, and United States in the late 1990s: the INTERMAP study. J Hum Hypertens. 2003;17(9):623–30.
43. Cappucio FP, Markandu ND, Carney C, Sagnella GA, MacGregor GA. Double-blind randomized trial of modest salt restriction in older people. Lancet. 1997;350:850–4.
44. Koliaki C, Katsilambros N. Dietary sodium, potassium, and alcohol: key players in the pathophysiology, prevention, and treatment of human hypertension. Nutr Rev. 2013;71(6):402–11.
45. Geleijnse JM, Kok FJ, Grobbee DE. Blood pressure response to changes in sodium and potassium intake: a metaregression analysis of randomised trials. J Hum Hypertens. 2003;17(7):471–80.
46. Aburto NJ, Hanson S, Gutierrez H, Hooper L, Elliott P, Cappuccio FP. Effect of increased potassium intake on cardiovascular risk factors and disease: systematic review and meta-analyses. BMJ (Clinical research ed). 2013;346:f1378.
47. Whelton PK, He J. Health effects of sodium and potassium in humans. Curr Opin Lipidol. 2014;25(1):75–9.
48. Dyer AR, Elliott P, Shipley M. Urinary electrolyte excretion in 24 hours and blood pressure in the INTERSALT Study. II. Estimates of electrolyte-blood pressure associations corrected for regression dilution bias. The INTERSALT Cooperative Research Group. Am J Epidemiol. 1994;139(9):940–51.

49. Tapsell LC, Neale EP, Satija A, Hu FB. Foods, nutrients, and dietary patterns: interconnections and implications for dietary guidelines. Adv Nutr (Bethesda, Md). 2016;7(3):445–54.
50. Jacobs DR Jr, Steffen LM. Nutrients, foods, and dietary patterns as exposures in research: a framework for food synergy. Am J Clin Nutr. 2003;78(3 Suppl):508s–13s.
51. Appel LJ, Moore TJ, Obarzanek E, Vollmer WM, Svetkey LP, Sacks FM, Bray GA, Vogt TM, Cutler JA, Windhauser MM, et al. A clinical trial of the effects of dietary patterns on blood pressure. DASH Collaborative Research Group. N Engl J Med. 1997;336(16):1117–24.
52. Moore TJ, Vollmer WM, Appel LJ, Sacks FM, Svetkey LP, Vogt TM, Conlin PR, Simons-Morton DG, Carter-Edwards L, Harsha DW. Effect of dietary patterns on ambulatory blood pressure : results from the Dietary Approaches to Stop Hypertension (DASH) Trial. DASH Collaborative Research Group. Hypertension (Dallas, Tex : 1979). 1999;34(3):472–7.
53. Sacks FM, Svetkey LP, Vollmer WM, Appel LJ, Bray GA, Harsha D, Obarzanek E, Conlin PR, Miller ER 3rd, Simons-Morton DG, et al. Effects on blood pressure of reduced dietary sodium and the Dietary Approaches to Stop Hypertension (DASH) diet. DASH-Sodium Collaborative Research Group. N Engl J Med. 2001;344(1):3–10.
54. Lopes HF, Martin KL, Nashar K, Morrow JD, Goodfriend TL, Egan BM. DASH diet lowers blood pressure and lipid-induced oxidative stress in obesity. Hypertension (Dallas, Tex : 1979). 2003;41(3):422–30.
55. Nowson CA, Worsley A, Margerison C, Jorna MK, Frame AG, Torres SJ, Godfrey SJ. Blood pressure response to dietary modifications in free-living individuals. J Nutr. 2004;134(9):2322–9.
56. Appel LJ, Sacks FM, Carey VJ, Obarzanek E, Swain JF, Miller ER 3rd, Conlin PR, Erlinger TP, Rosner BA, Laranjo NM, et al. Effects of protein, monounsaturated fat, and carbohydrate intake on blood pressure and serum lipids: results of the OmniHeart randomized trial. JAMA. 2005;294(19):2455–64.
57. Marquez-Celedonio FG, Texon-Fernandez O, Chavez-Negrete A, Hernandez-Lopez S, Marin-Rendon S, Berlin-Lascurain S. Clinical effect of lifestyle modification on cardiovascular risk in prehypertensives: PREHIPER I study. Rev Esp Cardiol. 2009;62(1):86–90.
58. Nowson CA, Wattanapenpaiboon N, Pachett A. Low-sodium Dietary Approaches to Stop Hypertension-type diet including lean red meat lowers blood pressure in postmenopausal women. Nutr Res (New York, NY). 2009;29(1):8–18.
59. Al-Solaiman Y, Jesri A, Mountford WK, Lackland DT, Zhao Y, Egan BM. DASH lowers blood pressure in obese hypertensives beyond potassium, magnesium and fibre. J Hum Hypertens. 2010;24(4):237–46.
60. Malloy-McFall J, Barkley JE, Gordon KL, Burzminski N, Glickman EL. Effect of the DASH diet on pre- and stage 1 hypertensive individuals in a free-living environment. Nutr Metab Insights. 2010;3:15–23.
61. Harnden KE, Frayn KN, Hodson L. Dietary Approaches to Stop Hypertension (DASH) diet: applicability and acceptability to a UK population. J Hum Nutr Diet. 2010;23(1):3–10.
62. Blumenthal JA, Babyak MA, Hinderliter A, Watkins LL, Craighead L, Lin PH, Caccia C, Johnson J, Waugh R, Sherwood A. Effects of the DASH diet alone and in combination with exercise and weight loss on blood pressure and cardiovascular biomarkers in men and women with high blood pressure: the ENCORE study. Arch Intern Med. 2010;170(2):126–35.
63. Lin PH, Allen JD, Li YJ, Yu M, Lien LF, Svetkey LP. Blood pressure-lowering mechanisms of the DASH dietary pattern. J Nutr Metab. 2012;2012:472396.
64. Whitt-Glover MC, Hunter JC, Foy CG, Quandt SA, Vitolins MZ, Leng I, Hornbuckle LM, Sanya KA, Bertoni AG. Translating the Dietary Approaches to Stop Hypertension (DASH) diet for use in underresourced, urban African American communities, 2010. Prev Chronic Dis. 2013;10:120088.
65. Lima ST, da Silva Nalin de Souza B, Franca AK, Salgado Filho N, Sichieri R. Dietary approach to hypertension based on low glycaemic index and principles of DASH (Dietary Approaches to Stop Hypertension): a randomised trial in a primary care service. Br J Nutr. 2013;110(8):1472–9.
66. Wong MC, Wang HH, Kwan MW, Fong BC, Chan WM, Zhang DX, Li ST, Yan BP, Coats AJ, Griffiths SM. Dietary counselling has no effect on cardiovascular risk factors among Chinese Grade 1 hypertensive patients: a randomized controlled trial. Eur Heart J. 2015;36(38):2598–607.
67. Jenkins DJ, Jones PJ, Frohlich J, Lamarche B, Ireland C, Nishi SK, Srichaikul K, Galange P, Pellini C, Faulkner D, et al. The effect of a dietary portfolio compared to a DASH-type diet on blood pressure. Nutr Metab Cardiovasc Dis: NMCD. 2015;25(12):1132–9.
68. Sayer RD, Wright AJ, Chen N, Campbell WW. Dietary Approaches to Stop Hypertension diet retains effectiveness to reduce blood pressure when lean pork is substituted for chicken and fish as the predominant source of protein. Am J Clin Nutr. 2015;102(2):302–8.
69. Chiu S, Bergeron N, Williams PT, Bray GA, Sutherland B, Krauss RM. Comparison of the DASH (Dietary Approaches to Stop Hypertension) diet and a higher-fat DASH diet on blood pressure and lipids and lipoproteins: a randomized controlled trial. Am J Clin Nutr. 2016;103(2):341–7.
70. Kawamura A, Kajiya K, Kishi H, Inagaki J, Mitarai M, Oda H, Umemoto S, Kobayashi S. Effects of the DASH-JUMP dietary intervention in Japanese participants with high-normal blood pressure and stage 1 hypertension: an open-label single-arm trial. Hypertens Res. 2016;39(11):777–85.
71. Naseem S, Ghazanfar H, Assad S, Ghazanfar A. Role of sodium-restricted dietary approaches to control blood pressure in Pakistani hypertensive population. JPMA J Pak Med Assoc. 2016;66(7):837–42.

72. Azadbakht L, Mirmiran P, Esmaillzadeh A, Azizi T, Azizi F. Beneficial effects of a Dietary Approaches to Stop Hypertension eating plan on features of the metabolic syndrome. Diabetes Care. 2005;28(12):2823–31.
73. Kucharska A, Gajewska D, Kiedrowski M, Sinska B, Juszczyk G, Czerw A, Augustynowicz A, Bobinski K, Deptala A, Niegowska J. The impact of individualized nutritional therapy according to DASH diet on blood pressure, body mass and selected biochemical parameters in overweight/obese patients with primary arterial hypertension: a prospective randomized study. Kardiol Pol. 2017;76(1):158–65.
74. Wang HH, Wong MC, Mok RY, Kwan MW, Chan WM, Fan CK, Lee CL, Griffiths SM. Factors associated with grade 1 hypertension: implications for hypertension care based on the Dietary Approaches to Stop Hypertension (DASH) in primary care settings. BMC Fam Pract. 2015;16:26.
75. Harrington JM, Fitzgerald AP, Kearney PM, McCarthy VJ, Madden J, Browne G, Dolan E, Perry IJ. DASH diet score and distribution of blood pressure in middle-aged men and women. Am J Hypertens. 2013;26(11):1311–20.
76. Schulze MB, Hoffmann K, Kroke A, Boeing H. Risk of hypertension among women in the EPIC-Potsdam Study: comparison of relative risk estimates for exploratory and hypothesis-oriented dietary patterns. Am J Epidemiol. 2003;158(4):365–73.
77. Bai G, Zhang J, Zhao C, Wang Y, Qi Y, Zhang B. Adherence to a healthy lifestyle and a DASH-style diet and risk of hypertension in Chinese individuals. Hypertens Res. 2017;40(2):196–202.
78. Saneei P, Salehi-Abargouei A, Esmaillzadeh A, Azadbakht L. Influence of Dietary Approaches to Stop Hypertension (DASH) diet on blood pressure: a systematic review and meta-analysis on randomized controlled trials. Nutr Metab Cardiovasc Dis: NMCD. 2014;24(12):1253–61.
79. Siervo M, Lara J, Chowdhury S, Ashor A, Oggioni C, Mathers JC. Effects of the Dietary Approach to Stop Hypertension (DASH) diet on cardiovascular risk factors: a systematic review and meta-analysis. Br J Nutr. 2015;113(1):1–15.
80. Bach-Faig A, Berry EM, Lairon D, Reguant J, Trichopoulou A, Dernini S, Medina FX, Battino M, Belahsen R, Miranda G, et al. Mediterranean diet pyramid today. Science and cultural updates. Public Health Nutr. 2011;14(12a):2274–84.
81. Salas-Salvado J, Garcia-Arellano A, Estruch R, Marquez-Sandoval F, Corella D, Fiol M, Gomez-Gracia E, Vinoles E, Aros F, Herrera C, et al. Components of the Mediterranean-type food pattern and serum inflammatory markers among patients at high risk for cardiovascular disease. Eur J Clin Nutr. 2008;62(5):651–9.
82. Strazzullo P, Ferro-Luzzi A, Siani A, Scaccini C, Sette S, Catasta G, Mancini M. Changing the Mediterranean diet: effects on blood pressure. J Hypertens. 1986;4(4):407–12.
83. Esposito K, Marfella R, Ciotola M, Di Palo C, Giugliano F, Giugliano G, D'Armiento M, D'Andrea F, Giugliano D. Effect of a mediterranean-style diet on endothelial dysfunction and markers of vascular inflammation in the metabolic syndrome: a randomized trial. JAMA. 2004;292(12):1440–6.
84. Ros E, Nunez I, Perez-Heras A, Serra M, Gilabert R, Casals E, Deulofeu R. A walnut diet improves endothelial function in hypercholesterolemic subjects: a randomized crossover trial. Circulation. 2004;109(13):1609–14.
85. Vincent-Baudry S, Defoort C, Gerber M, Bernard MC, Verger P, Helal O, Portugal H, Planells R, Grolier P, Amiot-Carlin MJ, et al. The Medi-RIVAGE study: reduction of cardiovascular disease risk factors after a 3-mo intervention with a Mediterranean-type diet or a low-fat diet. Am J Clin Nutr. 2005;82(5):964–71.
86. Estruch R, Martinez-Gonzalez MA, Corella D, Salas-Salvado J, Ruiz-Gutierrez V, Covas MI, Fiol M, Gomez-Gracia E, Lopez-Sabater MC, Vinyoles E, et al. Effects of a Mediterranean-style diet on cardiovascular risk factors: a randomized trial. Ann Intern Med. 2006;145(1):1–11.
87. Rallidis LS, Lekakis J, Kolomvotsou A, Zampelas A, Vamvakou G, Efstathiou S, Dimitriadis G, Raptis SA, Kremastinos DT. Close adherence to a Mediterranean diet improves endothelial function in subjects with abdominal obesity. Am J Clin Nutr. 2009;90(2):263–8.
88. Athyros VG, Kakafika AI, Papageorgiou AA, Tziomalos K, Peletidou A, Vosikis C, Karagiannis A, Mikhailidis DP. Effect of a plant stanol ester-containing spread, placebo spread, or Mediterranean diet on estimated cardiovascular risk and lipid, inflammatory and haemostatic factors. Nutr Metab Cardiovasc Dis: NMCD. 2011;21(3):213–21.
89. Jones JL, Fernandez ML, McIntosh MS, Najm W, Calle MC, Kalynych C, Vukich C, Barona J, Ackermann D, Kim JE, et al. A Mediterranean-style low-glycemic-load diet improves variables of metabolic syndrome in women, and addition of a phytochemical-rich medical food enhances benefits on lipoprotein metabolism. J Clin Lipidol. 2011;5(3):188–96.
90. Damasceno NR, Perez-Heras A, Serra M, Cofan M, Sala-Vila A, Salas-Salvado J, Ros E. Crossover study of diets enriched with virgin olive oil, walnuts or almonds. Effects on lipids and other cardiovascular risk markers. Nutr Metab Cardiovasc Dis: NMCD. 2011;21(Suppl 1):S14–20.
91. Katsarou AL, Vryonis MM, Protogerou AD, Alexopoulos EC, Achimastos A, Papadogiannis D, Chrousos GP, Darviri C. Stress management and dietary counseling in hypertensive patients: a pilot study of additional effect. Prim Health Care Res Dev. 2014;15(1):38–45.
92. Domenech M, Roman P, Lapetra J, Garcia de la Corte FJ, Sala-Vila A, de la Torre R, Corella D, Salas-Salvado J, Ruiz-Gutierrez V, Lamuela-Raventos RM, et al. Mediterranean diet reduces 24-hour ambulatory blood pressure, blood glucose, and lipids: one-year random-

ized, clinical trial. Hypertension (Dallas, Tex : 1979). 2014;64(1):69–76.
93. Davis CR, Hodgson JM, Woodman R, Bryan J, Wilson C, Murphy KJ. A Mediterranean diet lowers blood pressure and improves endothelial function: results from the MedLey randomized intervention trial. Am J Clin Nutr. 2017;105(6):1305–13.
94. Toledo E, Hu FB, Estruch R, Buil-Cosiales P, Corella D, Salas-Salvado J, Covas MI, Aros F, Gomez-Gracia E, Fiol M, et al. Effect of the Mediterranean diet on blood pressure in the PREDIMED trial: results from a randomized controlled trial. BMC Med. 2013;11:207.
95. Estruch R. PREDIMED Study Investigators: primary prevention of cardiovascular disease with a Mediterranean diet. N Engl J Med. 2013; 368(14):1279–90.
96. Estruch R, Ros E, Salas-Salvadó J, Covas MI, Corella D, Arós F, et al. Primary prevention of cardiovascular disease with a Mediterranean diet. N Engl J Med. 2013;368(14):1279–90.

Hypertension Management in the Elderly

6

Samar A. Nasser and Keith C. Ferdinand

Introduction

Approximately 85.7 million American adults have hypertension, and the age-adjusted prevalence among United States (U.S.) adults ≥20 years of age is estimated to be 34.0% in the National Health and Nutrition Examination Survey (NHANES) 2011–2014 [1]. In 2011–2014, the prevalence of hypertension was 11.6% among those 20–39 years of age, 37.3% among those 40–59 years of age, and 67.2% among those ≥ 60 years of age [1]. During the same timeframe, the prevalence of hypertension was 67.2% among U.S. adults ≥ 60 years of age and only 54.0% had controlled blood pressure (BP). According to NHANES 2005–2010, 76.5% of U.S. adults ≥ 80 years of age had hypertension, representing an increase from 69.2% in 1988–1994 [2]. In elderly Americans, hypertension is the most important risk factor for cardiovascular disease (CVD), with estimates that 69% of patients with an incident myocardial infarction, 77% with incident stroke, and 74% with incident heart failure have antecedent hypertension [3]. Moreover, hypertension is a major risk factor for incident diabetes mellitus, atrial fibrillation, and chronic kidney disease ([3]).

The prevalence of hypertension continues to rise in the U.S. with population growth, population aging, and persistent adverse behavioral risk factors, including high sodium and low potassium dietary patterns, physical inactivity, and increasing obesity. With advancing age, there is a gender transition from the younger (< 45 years) where hypertension affects more men than women, to the older population (> 65 years) where hypertension affects more women than men [4] (Fig. 6.1). In addition to more prevalent hypertension in older women than men, BP control is more difficult to achieve in women than men [3]. Among patients 80 years of age with hypertension, only 23% of women (versus 38% of men) had BP < 140/90 mm Hg ([5]). Furthermore, older adults visiting their physicians for antihypertensive pharmacotherapy versus younger adults were significantly more likely to include three or more hypertensive medications. A total of 62% of all visits included the provision, prescription, or continuation of one or more hypertensive medications. In 2013, 82% of visits to office-based physicians by adults with hypertension were made by those who had additional chronic conditions [6].

Evidence-based guidelines provide inconsistent recommendations regarding the optimal systolic blood pressure (SBP) treatment targets in the elderly

S. A. Nasser
Department of Clinical Research & Leadership, School of Medicine and Health Sciences, The George Washington University, Washington, DC, USA
e-mail: snasser@gwu.edu

K. C. Ferdinand (✉)
Tulane Heart and Vascular Institute, Tulane University School of Medicine, New Orleans, LA, USA
e-mail: kferdina@tulane.edu

V. Papademetriou et al. (eds.), *Management of Hypertension*,
https://doi.org/10.1007/978-3-319-92946-0_6

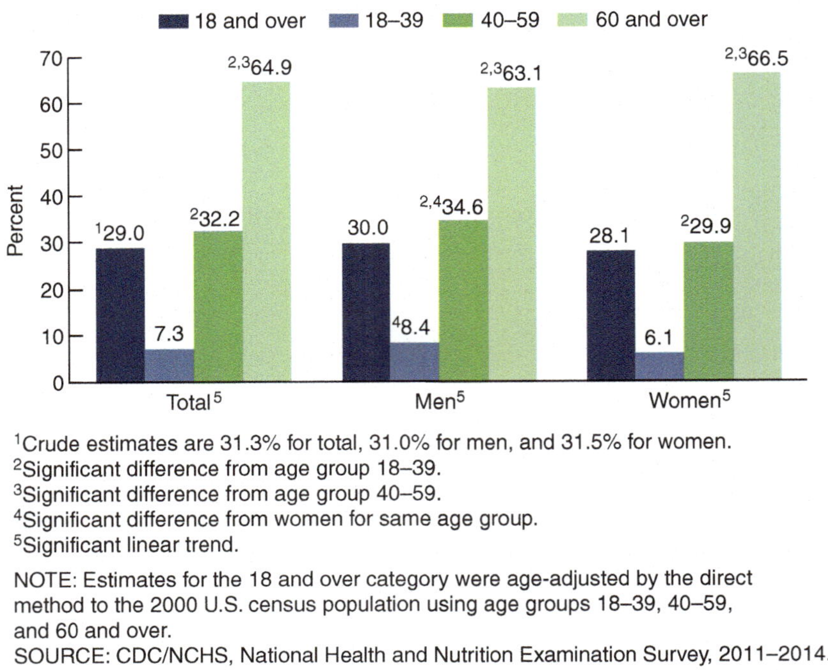

Fig. 6.1 Prevalence of hypertension among adults aged 18 and over, by sex and age: United States, 2011–2014 [1]Crude estimates are 31.3% for total, 31.0% for men, and 31.5% for women. [2]Significant difference from age group 18–39. [3]Significant difference from age group 40–59. [4]Significant difference from women for same age group. [5]Significant linear trend. NOTE: Estimates for the 18 and over category were age-adjusted by the direct method to the 2000 U.S. census population using age groups 18–39, 40–59, and 60 and over. (Source: CDC/NCHS, National Health and Nutrition Examination Survey, 2011–2014. Yoon et al. [45])

populations. Historically, in the period before the landmark Systolic Hypertension in the Elderly Program (SHEP) trial in 1991, elevated BP in this population (specifically systolic hypertension alone) had been somewhat controversial. Indeed, prior to landmark trials, hypertension was considered to be a normal compensatory phenomenon. For example in 1937, President Franklin Delano Roosevelt, who had a BP reading of 162/98 mm Hg at the age of 54 did not receive treatment to reduce his BP from his personal physician, as this was consistent with medical knowledge and opinion at that time [7]. Subsequently, significant cardiovascular benefits were demonstrated in the elderly in multiple studies.

Pathophysiologic Considerations in Elderly Patients

Specific considerations must be taken into account when treating hypertension in the elderly population. Blood pressure represents the confluence of cardiac and vascular properties such as arterial stiffness, endothelial dysfunction, increased cardiac output, high peripheral vascular resistance and extracellular/intravascular volume. Blood pressure is a function of blood flow and vascular resistance. In clinical practice, pressure refers to a pulsatile phenomenon defined in terms of SBP and diastolic blood pressure (DBP), representing the extremes of the BP oscillation around a mean BP value. These are quantitative measures of BP; however, BP and flow fluctuate during the cardiac cycle [3]. Systolic blood pressure increases with age until the eighth or ninth decade of life, in contrast to DBP, which rises only until middle age and then either levels off or slightly decreases.

As blood vessels become stiff due to age-related processes, and/or other co-morbidities, such as hypertension, hyperlipidemia, diabetes mellitus, and peripheral vascular diseases, SBP rises. The wider the pulse pressure, the smaller the ratio of DBP to SBP lowering with antihypertensive therapy, which is consistent with well-known hemodynamic principles. Indeed, DBP rises with increased peripheral arterial resistance but falls with increased stiffness of the large conduit arteries. Therefore, antihypertensive therapy will maximize the decrease in SBP and minimize the reduction in DBP in direct proportion to the age-related stiffening of large arteries [8].

Notably, elderly patients are prone to having isolated systolic hypertension (ISH)—SBP ≥ 140 mm Hg; DBP < 90 mm Hg. Isolated systolic hypertension is characterized by reduced vascular compliance, often combined with increased peripheral resistance and is a result of increased arterial stiffness from arteriosclerosis or impairment of nitric oxide–mediated vasodilation [9, 10]. The prevalence of ISH is very significant in elderly patients with hypertension demonstrated in more than 65% of hypertensive patients aged ≥ 60 years and more than 90% of those aged > 70 years [11].

Additionally, salt sensitivity is more frequently observed in older than in younger subjects [12] resulting in a higher SBP and higher pulse pressure when more salt is consumed by elderly individuals. Finally, elderly persons are at increased risk for orthostatic hypotension, which is present in up to 20 percent of patients older than 65 years [13] and can lead to increased risk for syncope, falls, and injuries.

Appropriate Determination of the Diagnosis of Hypertension

According to a recent Food and Drug Administration (FDA) Consumer Update, BP evaluations should be done in a clinic or a medical office, by using BP cuffs of various sizes to ensure the reading is accurate. There is no such thing as a "standard" cuff to fit a "standard" arm, thus the BP kiosks at various drug stores, pharmacies, or grocery stores may be inaccurate [14]. The most common error in BP measurement is use of an improperly sized cuff. The bladder length recommended by the American Heart Association is 80% of the patient's arm circumference, and the ideal width is at least 40% [15].

The Million Hearts Campaign is a national initiative of the Department of Health and Human Services whose goal is to prevent one million heart attacks and strokes by 2017 [16]. This collaborative effort involves multiple government agencies and nongovernmental collaborators. The initiative is co-led by the Centers for Disease Control and the Centers for Medicare and Medicaid Services within the Department of Health and Human Services. One of the Million Hearts main areas of focus is improving medication adherence through knowledge dissemination, stakeholder activation, creation of incentives, measuring and reporting, improving population health, and research. The Million Hearts Campaign supports self-monitoring BP particularly in certain types of patients, including the elderly, people with diabetes or chronic kidney disease, pregnant women, and those with suspected or confirmed white coat hypertension [17]. Clinicians should encourage patients to take any home BP monitor they use to their provider's office to measure its accuracy against a comparable device before the readings are accepted. The Canadian Hypertension Education Program Guidelines developed a technique for assessing automated office blood pressure (AOBP) to ensure accuracy (Table 6.1).

Table 6.1 Recommended technique for automated office blood pressure (AOBP)

1. Measurements should be taken with a validated sphygmomanometer known to be accurate.
2. Choose a cuff with an appropriate bladder size matched to the size of the arm. Select the cuff size as recommended by its manufacturer.
3. Place the cuff so that the lower edge is 3 cm above the elbow crease and the bladder is centered over the brachial artery. There is no rest period needed before measurement. The arm should be bare and supported with the BP cuff at heart level, as a lower position will result in an erroneously higher SBP and DBP. There should be no talking, and patients' legs should not be crossed.
4. When using automated office oscillometric devices, the patient should be seated in a quiet room (no specified period of rest). With the device set to take measures at 1- or 2-minute intervals. The first measurement is taken by a health professional to verify cuff position and validity of the measurement. The patient is left alone after the first measurement while the device automatically takes subsequent readings.
5. Record the average BP as displayed on the electronic device as well as the arm used and whether the patient was supine, sitting or standing. Record the heart rate.

Adapted from the Canadian hypertension education program guidelines
Ref.: Leung et al. [18]

For the elderly population, multiple BP readings should be done prior to diagnosing hypertension. Once hypertension is diagnosed, prescription initiation and intensification should proceed as, start low and go slow, and routinely monitor both seated and standing BP as orthostatic hypotension is more prevalent in the elderly population. If the patient has significant orthostasis, then the standing BP should take precedence.

Evolution of Clinical Trial Evidence

Based mainly on observational data, controversy lies in the J-shaped relation (J-curve) between the risk of myocardial infarction and treated BP which led to the suggestion that a reduction of pressure induced by drugs might cause *and* prevent myocardial ischemia [19], especially in the elderly population. Theoretically speaking, there is likely a turning point of BP below which the risk of cardiovascular events increases, as BP is essential for the perfusion of all organs. Overall, there have been conflicting views on the treatment of hypertension in very old patients as some studies suggested that BP and death were inversely related. Presently, the J-curve issue remains unresolved, however several randomized studies have attempted to address this controversy. Given that the J-curve demonstrated a link between DBP and coronary events, McEvoy and colleagues studied 11,565 adults in an observational trial from the Atherosclerosis Risk In Communities (ARIC) cohort, to evaluate the independent association of DBP with myocardial damage and with coronary heart disease (CHD), stroke, or death over 21 years. There was a trend toward higher risk of progression of subclinical myocardial damage and incident CHD among those with DBP < 60 and SBP ≥ 140 mm Hg [20]. Thus, suggesting that low DBP levels, particularly < 60 mm Hg, might harm the myocardium and are associated with subsequent CHD. However, this phenomenon appears to be most likely in clinical settings where SBP is ≥ 120 mm Hg and pulse pressure is higher.

Published in 1989, the European Working Party on High Blood Pressure in the Elderly (EWPHE) trial comprised 840 men and women over 60 years old, with a SBP in the range of 160–239 mm Hg and a diastolic pressure in the range 90–119 mm Hg, who were randomized to receive active treatment (hydrochlorothiazide with triamterene) or matching placebo. A significant BP difference of 20/8 mm Hg was obtained between the groups and maintained during 5 years of follow-up. The EWPHE trial demonstrated that active treatment was associated with a 27% reduction in cardiovascular mortality ($p = 0.037$), a 60% reduction in fatal myocardial infarctions ($p = 0.043$), a 52% reduction in strokes ($p = 0.026$), and a significant reduction in the incidence of severe congestive heart failure [21]. In a follow-up paper, Staessen and colleagues evaluated mortality and other possible correlates of mortality in the EWPHE patients, who were grouped in thirds of the distribution of treated blood pressure. The EWPHE trial demonstrated a U-shaped relation with treated systolic pressure and an inverse association with treated diastolic pressure. The U curve between mortality and diastolic pressure in patients taking placebo indicates that the increased mortality in the lower thirds of the actively treated patients may not be drug induced; however, it could be secondary to deterioration in general health, as suggested by the decreases in body weight and hemoglobin concentration ([22]).

The Swedish Trial in Old Patients with Hypertension (STOP-Hypertension) was a multicenter, randomized, double-blind study of 1,627 patients (mean age 76; mean BP 195/102 mm Hg) on antihypertensive treatment (atenolol, hydrochlorothiazide plus amiloride, metoprolol, or pindolol) compared to placebo.At study completion, the average BP reduction was 20/8 mm Hg in the actively treated group compared to placebo. The mean follow-up was 2.5 years [23].Compared with placebo, active treatment significantly reduced the number of primary endpoints (94 vs 58; p = 0.0031) and stroke morbidity and mortality (53 vs 29; p = 0.0081), as well as a significantly reduced number of deaths in the active treatment group (63 vs 36; p = 0.0079). These benefits were noticeable up to age 84 years, and STOP-Hypertension concluded that the elderly aged 70–84 conferred significant and clinically relevant reductions in cardiovascular morbidity and mortality as well as in total mortality in both men and women.

In 1991, the SHEP trial was the first randomized controlled trial to demonstrate the benefits of treating ISH in those with an average age of 72 years and an average SBP at entry of 170 with a mean diastolic of 77 mm Hg, randomized to either diuretic therapy (chlorthalidone plus atenolol or reserpine, if needed) or placebo. Out of 4,736 total and after an average of 4.5 years, the average BP at study end was 155/72 and 143/65 mm Hg, control and actively treated, respectively. The SHEP trial revealed a 37% reduction in nonfatal strokes, 32% decrease in cardiovascular events, 33% decrease in nonfatal myocardial infarctions, and a 55% reduction in heart failure in the treated versus placebo group ([24]). In support of the SHEP trial, the Medical Research Council trial of treatment of hypertension in older adults demonstrated that active treatment led to a significant reduction in cardiovascular events in men and women aged 65–74 with sustained mild to moderate hypertension [25]. Additionally, the Systolic Hypertension in Europe (Syst-Eur) revealed benefits of antihypertensive treatment (nitrendipine with enalapril and hydrochlorothiazide, if needed) that were similar to those trials in older patients with combined systolic and diastolic hypertension [26].

By 2008, nevertheless, there still was no solid evidence that antihypertensive drug treatment in the very elderly (≥ 80 years) was either safe or effective. Thus, the Hypertension in the Very Elderly Trial (HYVET) was the first randomized trial to demonstrate benefits of treating hypertension in 3,845 very elderly from Australia, China, Europe, and Tunisia [27]. Overall, the results demonstrated clear benefits in those patients 80 years or older whose SBP was > 160 mm Hg with active treatment (indapamide with or without perindopril) as compared to placebo. The BP in the active treatment group was 15/6.1 mm Hg lower than the placebo group, revealing a 30% reduction in the rate of fatal and non-fatal stroke (95% CI −1–51, $p = 0.06$), 39% reduction in rate of death from stroke (95% CI 1–62, $p = 0.05$), 21% reduction in rate of death from any causes (95% CI 4–35, $p = 0.02$), 23% reduction in the rate of death from cardiovascular causes (95% CI −1–40, $p = 0.06$), and a 64% reduction in the rate of heart failure (95% CI 42–78, $p < 0.001$).

Accordingly, Cardio-Sis (CARDIO vascolari del Controllodella Pressione Arteriosa SI Stolica) trial of 1,111 participants without diabetes with a mean age of 67 years compared a SBP of ≤ 130 mm Hg to the standard < 140 mm Hg SBP (open label therapywith combinations of furosemide, ramipril, telmisartan, amlodipine, bisoprolol, and transdermal clonidine; combinations of ramipril and of telmisartan with hydrochlorothiazide were also available). The primary (electrocardiographic left ventricular hypertrophy)and secondary end points (composite of cardiovascular events) 2 years post-randomization, were less frequent in the tightthan in the standard control group in patients with and without established CVD at initiation. Therefore, the advantage of a "tightly controlled group" as compared to a standard control group had a significantly lower incidence of new left ventricular hypertrophy, atrial fibrillation, and need for coronary revascularization [28], without any paradoxical rise in the risk of events at low levels of achieved BP during follow-up.

Recent Guidelines Endorsing Higher Systolic BP Goals in Elderly

A 2014 evidence-based guideline for the management of high BP in adults consisted of a report from the members appointed to the Eighth Joint National Committee Panel (JNC-8P). This nomenclature accurately reflects the *Journal of American Medical Association (JAMA)* publication from the JNC-8P and avoids the perception that the federal government and any of the 39 professional organizations that reviewed and endorsed the Seventh Report of the Joint National Committee on Prevention, Evaluation, and Treatment of High Blood Pressure (JNC-7) were responsible for conclusions. The JNC-8P members based their recommendations upon strict adherence of evidence-based medicine, consensus, and expert opinion, and their extensive review process recommended for those ≥ 60 years of age, a SBP ≥ 150 mm Hg threshold for initiating antihypertensive drug treatment and a treatment goal SBP of < 150 mm Hg [29].

The persistent controversy lies in the generalized recommendation for the higher threshold in the elderly hypertensive patients, as the higher SBP threshold is especially threatening to African Americans and women who are disproportionately affected with hypertension in this age demographic [30]. Furthermore, as most Americans ≥ 60 years of age with hypertension are women, women will be differentially affected by the recommendation to raise the SBP threshold for initiating treatment (to 150 mm Hg) and to raise the treatment target (<150 mm Hg) for people ≥ 60 years of age. Unfortunately, the JNC-8P 2014 recommendations offer no recognition that the elderly hypertensive population is primarily female, that older women generally have poorly controlled hypertension, and that approximately 40% of those with poor BP control are African American women, who have the highest risks for stroke, heart failure, and chronic renal disease.

In addition, according to new evidence-based guidelines jointly developed by the American College of Physicians (ACP) and the American Academy of Family Physicians (AAFP) in 2017, they collaboratively recommend that physicians initiate treatment in adults aged 60 years old and older with persistent SBP at or above 150 mm Hg to achieve a target SBP of less than 150 mm Hg in order to reduce the risk of mortality, stroke, and cardiac events (Grade: strong recommendation, high-quality evidence). The second recommendation is that clinicians consider initiating or intensifying pharmacologic treatment in adults aged 60 years or older with a history of stroke or transient ischemic attack to achieve a target SBP of less than 140 mm Hg to reduce the risk for recurrent stroke (Grade: weak recommendation, moderate-quality evidence). The final recommendation is that clinicians should consider initiating or intensifying pharmacologic treatment in some adults aged 60 years or older at high cardiovascular risk, based on individualized assessment, to achieve a target SBP of less than 140 mm Hg to reduce the risk for stroke or cardiac events (Grade: weak recommendation, low-quality evidence). These clinical recommendations regarding the benefits and harms of higher versus lower BP targets for hypertension in adults 60 years and older were developed for utilization by all clinicians caring for adults 60 years and older with hypertension [31]. Adapted from the Million Hearts® website, Table 6.2 provides practical approaches to effective provider-patient communication to control hypertensive patients.

Given that the JNC-8P recommendations were challenged by several in the cardiology community over the elevated hypertension treatment threshold, and in recognition of significant new clinical trial evidence in hypertension, the 2017 American College of Cardiology/American Heart Association/American Academy of Physician Assistants/Association of Black Cardiologists/American College of Preventative Medicine/American Geriatrics Society/American Pharmacists Association/American Society of Hypertension/American Society for Preventative Cardiology/National Medical Association/Preventive Cardiovascular Nurses Association Guideline for the Prevention, Detection, Evaluation and Management of High Blood Pressure in Adults is currently in development and will serve as an update to the 2003 JNC-7 that was the final hypertension guideline headed by the National Heart, Lung, and Blood Institute (NHLBI). The 2003 JNC-7 was the final and most recent hypertension management guideline to be endorsed by the ACC/AHA, however the JNC-8P was not endorsed by these organizations.

Impact OF SPRINT and Future Guidelines for Blood Pressure Control in Elderly

According to the landmark clinical trial sponsored by the National Institutes of Health, the Systolic Blood Pressure Intervention Trial (SPRINT) was a randomized trial of 9,361 community-dwelling adults (mean age 68 years) that evaluated whether lowering SBP to a target

Table 6.2 Practical approaches to effective provider-patient communication to control high blood pressure

Explain the roles of each member of the health care team.
Ask, "What is most important for you to accomplish during your visit today?" The answer helps set the agenda.
Review blood pressure goal against current reading(s).
Have an open conversation about goals, achievements, confidence, and barriers. Consider asking these questions to get a discussion going: What have you been doing since our last visit to control your blood pressure? What concerns you the most about your high blood pressure? What specifically would you like to work on to manage your high blood pressure? How confident are you that you could do [behavior] to help control your blood pressure? What might get in the way or keep you from being successful? What do you think would make it easier to control your high blood pressure?
Help set small, achievable goals based on patients' answers. For example, if the patient is working to improve diet, establish a goal to swap out favorite food items for lower sodium versions. Small changes can gradually lead to more heart-healthy meals, cooked at home.
Use the "Ask-Tell-Ask" technique to address actions for each behavioral goal: Ask permission to provide information on a specific topic. For example, for medication adherence, you might say, "There are several things I want to tell you about your new medication. Is that okay?" Tell the patient what they need to know (e.g., when they should take the medication, expected side effects, importance of taking it as directed). Use simple words and diagrams or pictures. Ask the patient to repeat back the information in their own words.
Consider asking these questions to get a discussion going: What have you been doing since our last visit to control your blood pressure? What concerns you the most about your high blood pressure? What specifically would you like to work on to manage your high blood pressure? How confident are you that you could do [behavior] to help control your blood pressure? What might get in the way or keep you from being successful? What do you think would make it easier to control your high blood pressure?

Adapted from: Million Hearts® is a national initiative to prevent one million heart attacks and strokes by 2017. It is led by the Centers for Disease Control and Prevention and the Centers for Medicare & Medicaid Services, two agencies of the Department of Health and Human Services. https://millionhearts.hhs.gov/files/TipSheet_HCP_Checklist.pdf

< 120 versus < 140 mm Hg reduced major cardiovascular (CV) events (i.e., myocardial infarction, acute coronary syndrome, stroke, acute heart failure and CV mortality) [32]. Of the 9,361 participants, 2,636 (28.2%) were aged 75 years and older, 3,332 (35.6%) were women, 5,399 (57.7%) were non-Hispanic white, 2,947 (31.5%) were black, and 984 (10.6%) were Hispanic. Cardiovascular disease was present in 1,877 persons (20.1%), and the Framingham 10-year CVD risk score was 15% and higher in 5,737 persons (61.3%). SPRINT was terminated early at 3.26 years due to overwhelming evidence of benefit. The SPRINT trial provided critical information on the efficacy and safety of lowering the SBP to < 120 mm Hg in elderly hypertensive adults. The primary outcome, myocardial infarction, acute coronary syndrome, stroke, congestive heart failure, or cardiovascular death, was significantly lowered in the intensive BP management arm compared with the routine management arm (5.2% vs. 6.8%, hazard ratio [HR] 0.75, 95% confidence interval [CI] 0.64–0.89; $p < 0.0001$). Thus, SPRINT demonstrated that a treatment goal for SBP of less than 120 mm Hg reduced incident CVD by 33% (from 3.85% to 2.59% per year) and totalmortality by 32% (from 2.63% to 1.78% per year) [32]. Overall, SPRINT demonstrated that intensive compared to standard SBP targets resulted in lower composite CVD outcomes and all-cause mortality in adults ≥ 75 years of age [33], however SPRINT was not a specific drug class study.

Consistent with the SPRINT cohort, the subgroup of participants aged ≥ 75 years also demonstrated impressive reductions in CVD events and total mortality with intensive as compared with standard therapy. The resultssupport and enhance the major SPRINT study findings in community-dwelling persons aged 75 years or older, demonstrating that a treatment goal for SBP of less than 120 mm Hg reduced incident CVD by 33% (from 3.85% to 2.59% per year) and total mortality by 32% (from 2.63% to 1.78% per year) ([33]). On the other hand, although elderly women are the predominant population with ISH, only 36% of the landmark SPRINT cohort were women and 28% of the entire SPRINT cohort were aged 75 years (the upper limit was age 80 years) [30].

Of note, the BP in SPRINT was measured using automated oscillometric blood pressure versus using manual (auscultatory) blood pressure, which was the technique used in other trials and which is more commonly used in routine practice than AOBP. Thus, the reported SPRINT SBP may be higher than usual clinic measurements.

Additionally, in SPRINT, diastolic pressures were greater than 70 mm Hg at baseline, and remained above 65 mm Hg during the course of the trial, even with intensive treatment. Given the concern for many older adults with isolated systolic hypertension experiencing low diastolic pressure (i.e., less than 60–65 mmHg), especially with coronary artery disease, aggressive lowering of the systolic pressure, may exacerbate myocardial ischemia and increase risk. Although there were increased adverse events with intensive BP lowering in SPRINT, such as syncope (2.3% versus 1.7%) and hyponatremia (3.8% versus 2.1%), the rates of orthostatic hypotension and falls resulting in hospitalization were similar between the groups.

From 2011 to 2017, according to the hypertension guidelines from the American College of Cardiology Foundation/American Heart Association 2011 expert consensus document on hypertension in the elderly developed in collaboration with the American Academy of Neurology, the American Geriatrics Society, the American Society for Preventive Cardiology, the American Society of Hypertension, the American Society of Nephrology, the Association of Black Cardiologists, and the European Society of Hypertension collectively recommended that the BP goals be lowered to less than 140/90 mm Hg in older persons younger than 80 years and to 140–145/<90 mm Hg, if tolerated in adults aged 80 years and older [3]. In addition, the Canadian 2016 hypertension guidelines recommend that high-risk adults aged 50 years and older with a SBP of 130 mmHg or higher obtained by an AOBP measurement should have a target SBP goal of 120 mmHg or lower [34].

The recent 2016 Canadian Hypertension Education Program (CHEP) Guidelines recommend intensive BP reduction in high risk patients, including, clinical or subclinical CVD or chronic kidney disease (nondiabetic nephropathy, proteinuria <1 g/d, estimated glomerular filtration rate 20–59 mL/min/1.73 m^2) or estimated 10-year global cardiovascular risk ≥15% or age ≥ 75 years [18]. However, even CHEP maintains in the very elderly (age ≥ 80 years), the SBP target is <150 mm Hg. Nevertheless, for high-risk patients, intensive management to a target SBP 120 mm Hg should be guided by AOBP measurements, not usual clinic measurements. Finally, patients should be prepared for more clinical encounters, monitoring, and medication usage, as individuals who received intensive treatment in SPRINT were followed monthly until target BP levels were achieved. On average, SPRINT participants were prescribed 2.7 antihypertensive agents, compared with 1.8 agents in the standard control group. Therefore, although SBP targets <120 mm Hg are beneficial in certain cases, intensive treatment also incurs greater health care utilization and potential treatment risks and should be closely monitored.

Sub-Studies from SPRINT: Prediabetes, Chronic Kidney Disease, Cognition

Given the strength of the rigorously conducted randomized controlled SPRINT study design with adjudicated outcomes in a large, racially diverse population allowed for large subgroups of those with prediabetes and those with fasting normoglycemia at baseline. Recent sub-group analysis in SPRINT revealed lower risk in outcomes in those with prediabetes [35]. Accordingly, the beneficial effects of intensive SBP treatment on CVD events and all-cause mortality continued to patients with prediabetes and were similar among those with prediabetes and fasting normoglycemia.

Among SPRINT patients with chronic kidney disease (CKD) and hypertension without diabetes, a target SBP of 120 mm Hg compared to 140 mm Hg reduced rates of major CV events and all-cause death without evidence of effect modifications by CKD or deleterious effect on the main kidney outcome. Thus, demonstrating the best available evidence to date in favor of intensive SBP reduction as a means to improve survival in patients with CKD and hypertension who are burdened with very high mortality rate [36].

Overall, data demonstrate that antihypertensive drug therapy either significantly or insignificantly reduces the incidence of dementia or of cognitive impairment [37–39] despite the short follow-up of the double-blind antihypertensive drug versus placebo trials on the incidence of dementia and cognitive impairment. The SPRINT study suggests that target SBP levels of lower than 140 mm Hg and possibly 120 mm Hg or lower extend to cognitive outcomes as well. According to Hajjar et al. [40], patients 70 years of age or older who receive hypertension treatment, a SPRINT SBP level of 120 mm Hg or lower was not associated with worsening cognitive outcome and may be superior to the JNC-8P target for cognition. Thus, the findings suggest that a lower SBP target for African American patients specifically is linked to greater cognitive benefit.

Best Antihypertensive Agents in the Elderly

Adoption of healthy lifestyles is critical to prevent high BP and isthe bedrock of BP management and control. According to the JNC 7, major lifestyle modifications shown to lower BP include weight reduction in those individuals who are overweight or obese, adoption of Dietary Approaches to Stop Hypertension (DASH) eating plan, dietary sodium reduction, physical activity, moderation of alcohol consumption, and smoking cessation, if applicable. The initiation of any antihypertensive agent dose should start low, and be up-titrated slowly while reducing BP gradually. Given the increased risk for hypotension and orthostatic hypotension, a single antihypertensive agent should be initiated at a time with careful monitoring of blood pressure. A strategy of initiating two drugs at low doses when the baseline BP is > 20 mm Hg above goal may be used cautiously, taking care to avoid overaggressive BP lowering especially given the frailty of the population.

Based upon evidence-based guidelines performed in patients aged ≥ 60 years, the antihypertensive treatment to be implemented in older hypertensive subjects are the same drug classes that are recommended for younger patients (i.e., diuretics, angiotensin receptor antagonist (ARB's), angiotensin-converting enzyme inhibitors (ACE-I), and calcium channel blockers, with an extension to β-blockers in the European Society of Cardiology (ESC)/European Society of Hypertension (ESH)guidelines) [3, 41]. The choice of the specific antihypertensive agentin the treatment of elderly persons with hypertension depends on efficacy, tolerability, presence of specific comorbidities and cost [3]. Angiotensin converting enzyme inhibitionor ARB is a reasonable initial approach, especially if there is concurrent CVD, diabetes, proteinuria, chronic kidney disease, or heart failure. According to the ESC/ESH guideline, a calcium antagonist or diuretic in elderly patients with ISH is recommended [42]. Consistent with ESC/ESH guidelines, the Antihypertensive and Lipid-Lowering Treatment to Prevent Heart Attack Trial (ALLHAT) data, also suggested that low-dose daily diuretic (chlorthalidone) is the most effective agent in this population [43]. On the other hand, hyponatremia is a valid consideration in elderly patients as many patients' free water intake is reduced. After 1 year of treatment, 7.2% of the participants randomized to chorthalidone-treatment had a serum potassium < 3.5 mmol/L compared with 1% of the participants randomized to placebo after 1 year. However, with addition of an ACEI/ARB and/or aldosterone antagonist, the hypokalemia can be ameliorated.

In the Scandinavian population, the Anglo-Scandinavian Cardiac Outcomes Trial-Blood

Pressure Lowering Arm (ASCOT-BPLA), data revealed a significant overall mortality benefit in subjects aged >60 years when using a combination of calcium channel blocker (amlopdipine) and ACEI (perindopril) when compared to a beta-blocker (atenolol) and thiazide (bendr oflumethia zide (BFZ) regimen [44]. Therefore, a long-acting dihydropyridine calcium channel blocker as the initial agent for the elderly is a safe option, with the addition of an ACEI/ARB or low-dose thiazide diuretic to the calcium channel blocker, if needed. Table 6.3 provides a comparison of recommended target BP goals recommended by the 2011–2017 Hypertension Guidelines in the elderly.

Conclusion

Age is a powerful risk factor for hypertension complications, however the treatment of hypertension in the elderly is complex. The current recommendation of less than 140/90 mm Hg has been associated with dramatic reductions in HTN complications with BP reduction. Multiple trials have shown more appropriate treatment of hypertension in the elderly is safe and will decrease stroke, heart failure, myocardial infarction and all-cause mortality. There is sufficient evidence of benefit and limited risk of harm if BP targets of less than 140/90 mm Hg are recommended for

Table 6.3 Blood pressure treatment goals recommended by the 2011–2017 hypertension guidelines

1. The BP should be lowered to less than 140/90 mm Hg in older persons younger than 80 years and to 140–145/<90 mm Hg, if tolerated in adults aged 80 years and older [ACCF/AHA 2011 expert consensus].
2. The BP should be lowered in older adults younger than 80 years to less than 140/90 mm Hg. In adults older than 80 years, the SBP should be lowered to between 140 and 150 mm Hg provided they are in good physical and mental conditions [ESH/ESC guidelines, 2013].
3. The BP should be lowered in adults aged 60 years or older to less than 150/90 mm Hg if they do not have diabetes mellitus or CKD and to less than 140/90 mm Hg if they have diabetes mellitus or CKD [JNC 8 Panel Members, 2014].
4. The BP should be lowered in adults aged 60 years and older to less than 140/90 mm Hg [47].
5. The BP should be lowered to less than 140/90 mm Hg in adults aged 60 to 79 years and to less than 150/90 mm Hg in adults aged 80 years and older [48].
6. The BP should be lowered to less than 140/90 mm Hg in adults aged 60 to 79 years and to less than 150/90 mm Hg in adults aged 80 years and older [Canadian Hypertension Education Program, 2013].
7. The BP should be lowered to less than 140/90 mm Hg in adults aged 60 to 79 years and to less than 150/90 mm Hg in adults aged 80 years and older [A statement by the American Society of Hypertension and the International Society of Hypertension, 2014].
8. The BP should be lowered to less than 140/90 mm Hg in patients with coronary artery disease and with an acute coronary syndrome if they are aged 80 years and younger but to less than 150 mm Hg if they are older than 80 years of age. Consideration can be given to reduce the blood pressure to less than 130/80 mm Hg. Caution is advised in reducing a DBP to less than 60 mm Hg in persons with diabetes mellitus or in persons older than 60 years of age [AHA/ACC/ASH scientific statement, 2015].
9. High-risk adults aged 50 years and older with a SBP of 130 mmHg or higher obtained by an automated office blood pressure measurement should have a target systolic blood pressure goal of 120 mm Hg or lower. High-risk patients for treatment with intensive blood pressure management include those with clinical or subclinical cardiovascular disease or CKD or an estimated 10-year global cardiovascular risk of 15% and higher or an age of 75 years and higher [Canadian Hypertension Education Program (CHEP), 2016].
10. Selected high cardiovascular risk persons should have a SBP goal of less than 120 mm Hg to improve cardiovascular outcomes. Close monitoring should be performed in these persons to identify treatment-related adverse effects including hypotension, syncope, electrolyte abnormalities, and acute kidney injury [Australian Hypertension Guidelines, 2016].
11. Adults aged 60 years and older with a SBP of 150 mm Hg and higher should have their SBP reduced to less than 150 mm Hg]. Adults aged 60 years and older with a history of stroke or transient ischemic attack should have their SBP reduced to less than 140 mm Hg. Adults aged 60 years and older at high cardiovascular risk should have their SBP reduced to less than 140 mm Hg [guideline from the American College of Physicians and the American Academy of Family Physicians, 2017].

BP Blood pressure, *SBP* Systolic blood pressure, *CKD* Chronic kidney disease, *DBP* Diastolic blood pressure
Reference (adapted from): Aronow [46]

elderly, especially in higher risk groups. Future guidelines may be affected by results of the SPRINT landmark study which demonstrates the benefits of intensive BP reduction in CV morbidity and mortality which extends to patients with CKD and prediabetes, and demonstrates no negative impact on cognition in those patients greater than or equal to 75 years of age.

Future Guidelines

Future hypertensive guidelines may be impacted by the robust outcomes from SPRINT and return the BP goals in elderly to less than 140 and perhaps even lower.

2017 American College of Cardiology/American Heart Association/American Academy of Physician Assistants/Association of Black Cardiologists/American College of Preventative Medicine/American Geriatrics Society/American Pharmacists Association/American Society of Hypertension/American Society for Preventative Cardiology/National Medical Association/Preventive Cardiovascular Nurses Association Guideline for the Prevention, Detection, Evaluation and Management of High Blood Pressure in Adults.

References

1. Benjamin EJ, Blaha MJ, Chiuve SE, Cushman M, Das SR, Deo R, et al. Heart disease and stroke statistics—2017 update: a report from the American Heart Association. Circulation. 2017;135;e146–e603. Available from https://doi.org/10.1161/CIR.0000000000000485
2. Bromfield SG, Bowling CB, Tanner RM, Peralta CA, Odden MC, Oparil S, Muntner P. Trends in hypertension prevalence, awareness, treatment, and control among US adults 80 years and older, 1988-2010. J ClinHypertens (Greenwich). 2014;16:270–6. https://doi.org/10.1111/jch.12281.
3. Aronow WS, Fleg JL, Pepine CJ, Artinian NT, Bakris G, Brown AS, et al. ACCF/AHA 2011 expert consensus document on hypertension in the elderly: a report of the American College of Cardiology Foundation Task Force on clinical expert consensus documents developed in collaboration with the American Academy of Neurology, American Geriatrics Society, American Society for Preventive Cardiology, American Society of Hypertension, American Society of Nephrology, Association of Black Cardiologists, and European Society of Hypertension. J Am Coll Cardiol. 2011;57(20):2037–114.
4. Oparil S. Sy 11-3 hypertension in women: more dangerous than in men? J Hypertens. 2016;34:e366.
5. Lloyd-Jones DM, Evans JC, Levy D. Hypertension in adults across the age spectrum: current outcomes and control in the community. JAMA. 2005;294:466–72.
6. Ashman JJ, Rui P, Schappert SM. Age differences in visits to office-based physicians by adults with hypertension: United States, 2013, NCHS data brief, no 263. Hyattsville: National Center for Health Statistics; 2016.
7. Bumgarner J. The health of the presidents: the 41 United States Presidents through 1993 from a physician's point of view. Jefferson: McFarland & Company, Inc; 1994.
8. Wang Ji G, Staessen JA, Franklin SS, et al. Systolic and diastolic blood pressure lowering as determinants of cardiovascular outcome. Hypertension. 2005;45:907–13.
9. O'Rourke MF, Nichols WW. Aortic diameter, aortic stiffness, and wave reflection increase with age and isolated systolic hypertension. Hypertension. 2005;45:652–8.
10. Franklin SS, Jacobs MJ, Wong ND, et al. Predominance of isolated systolic hypertension among middle-aged and elderly US hypertensives: analysis based on National Health and Nutrition Examination Survey (NHANES) III. Hypertension. 2001;37:869–74.
11. Liu X, Rodriguez CJ, Wang K. Prevalence and trends of isolated systolic hypertension among untreated adults in the United States. J Am Soc Hypertens. 2015;9(3):197–205.
12. Choi HY, Park HC, Ha SK. Salt sensitivity and hypertension: a paradigm shift from kidney malfunction to vascular endothelial dysfunction. Electrolytes Blood Press. 2015;13(1):7–16.
13. Chisholm P, Anpalahan M. Orthostatic hypotension: pathophysiology, assessment, treatment and the paradox of supine hypertension. Intern Med J. 2017;47:370–9.
14. FDA Consumer report website. Accessed 5 Aug 2017.: https://www.fda.gov/ForConsumers/ConsumerUpdates/ucm402287.htm#cuff.
15. Pickering TG, Hall JE, Appel LJ, Falkner BE, Graves J, Hill MN, et al. Recommendations for blood pressure measurement in humans and experimental animals: part 1: blood pressure measurement in humans: a statement for professionals from the Subcommittee of Professional and Public Education of the American Heart Association Council on High Blood Pressure Research. Hypertension. 2005;142–61(5):45.
16. Million Hearts. Available at: http://millionhearts.hhs.gov., 2017.
17. Centers for Disease Control and Prevention. Self-measured blood pressure monitoring: actions steps for clinicians. Atlanta: Centers for Disease Control and Prevention, US Dept of Health and Human Services;

2014. https://millionhearts.hhs.gov/files/MH_SMBP_Clinicians.pdf.
18. Leung AA, Nerenberg K, Daskalopoulou SS, McBrien K, Zarnke KB, Dasgupta K, Cloutier L, Gelfer M, Lamarre-Cliche M, Milot A, Bolli P. Hypertension Canada's 2016 Canadian Hypertension Education Program Guidelines for blood pressure measurement, diagnosis, assessment of risk, prevention, and treatment of hypertension. Can J Cardiol. 2016;32(5):569–88.
19. Kang Y-Y, Wang J-G. The J-curve phenomenon in hypertension. Pulse. 2016;4(1):49–60. https://doi.org/10.1159/000446922.
20. McEvoy JW, Chen Y, Rawlings A, Hoogeveen RC, Ballantyne CM, Blumenthal RS, Coresh J, Selvin E. Diastolic blood pressure, subclinical myocardial damage, and cardiac events: implications for blood pressure control. J Am Coll Cardiol. 2016;68(16):1713–22.
21. Amery A, Birkenhager W, Brixko P, Bulpitt C, Clement D, de Leeuw P, et al. Influence of antihypertensive drug treatment on morbidity and mortality in patients over the age of 60 years. EWPHE results: sub-group analysis based on entry stratification. J Hypertens. 1986;4:S642–7.
22. Staessen J, Bulpitt C, Clement D, De Leeuw P, Fagard R, Fletcher A, et al. Relation between mortality and treated blood pressure in elderly patients with hypertension: report of the European working party on high blood pressure in the elderly. BMJ. 1989;298:1552–6. https://doi.org/10.1136/bmj.298.6687.1552.
23. Dahlöf B, Hansson L, Lindholm LH, Schersten B, Ekbom T, Wester PO. Morbidity and mortality in the Swedish trial in old patients with hypertension (STOP-hypertension). Lancet. 1991;338(8778):1281–5.
24. SHEP Cooperative Research Group. Prevention of stroke by antihypertensive drug treatment in older persons with isolated systolic hypertension. Final results of the systolic hypertension in the elderly program (SHEP). JAMA. 1991;265:3255–64. https://doi.org/10.1001/jama.265.24.3255.
25. Party MW. Medical Research Council trial of treatment of hypertension in older adults: principal results. BMJ. 1992;304(6824):405–12.
26. Staessen JA, Fagard R, Thijs L, Celis H, Arabidze GG, Birkenhäger WH, Bulpitt CJ, De Leeuw PW, Dollery CT, Fletcher AE, Forette F. Randomised double-blind comparison of placebo and active treatment for older patients with isolated systolic hypertension. Lancet. 1997;350(9080):757–64.
27. Beckett NS, Peters R, Fletcher AE, Staessen JA, Liu L, Dumitrascu D, et al. Treatment of hypertension in patients 80 years of age or older. N Engl J Med. 2008;358:1887–98. https://doi.org/10.1056/NEJMoa0801369.
28. Verdecchia P, Staessen JA, Angeli F, et al. Usual versus tight control of systolic blood pressure in non-diabetic patients with hypertension (Cardio-Sis): an open-label randomised trial. Lancet. 2009;374:525–33.
29. James PA, Oparil S, Carter BL, et al. 2014 evidence-based guideline for the management of high blood pressure in adults: report from the panel members appointed to the Eighth Joint National Committee (JNC 8). JAMA. 2013;311:507–20.
30. Wenger NK, Ferdinand KC, Merz CN, Walsh MN, Gulati M, Pepine CJ. Women, hypertension, and the systolic blood pressure intervention trial. Am J Med. 2016;129(10):1030–6.
31. Qaseem A, Wilt TJ, Rich R, Humphrey LL, Frost J, Forciea MA, et al. Pharmacologic treatment of hypertension in adults aged 60 years or older to higher versus lower blood pressure targets: a clinical practice guideline from the American College of Physicians and the American Academy of family physicians. Ann Intern Med. 2017;166:430–7. https://doi.org/10.7326/M16-1785.
32. Wright JT Jr, Williamson JD, Whelton PK, et al. SPRINT research group. A randomized trial of intensive versus standard blood-pressure control. N Engl J Med. 2015;373(22):2103–16.
33. Williamson JD, Supiano MA, Applegate WB, et al. Intensive vs standard blood pressure control and cardiovascular disease outcomes in adults aged ≥75 years: a randomized clinical trial. JAMA. 2016;315(24):2673–82.
34. Padwal R, Rabi DM, Schiffrin EL. Recommendations for intensive blood pressure lowering in high-risk patients, the Canadian view- point. Hypertension. 2016;68:3–5.
35. Bress AP, King JB, Kreider KE, Beddhu S, Simmons DL, Cheung AK, SPRINT Research Group et al. Effect of intensive versus standard blood pressure treatment according to baseline prediabetes status: a post Hoc Analysis of a Randomized Trial. Diabetes Care. 2017. pii: dc170885. https://doi.org/10.2337/dc17-0885.
36. Cheung AK, Rahman M, Reboussin DM, Craven TE, Greene T, Kimmel PL, SPRINT Research Group, et al. Effects of intensive BP control in CKD. J Am Soc Nephrol JASN. 2017;28:2812–23 . ASN2017020148; published ahead of print June 22, 2017. https://doi.org/10.1681/ASN.2017020148.
37. Forette F, Seux ML, Staessen JA, et al. The prevention of dementia with antihypertensive treatment. New evidence from the Systolic Hypertension in Europe (SYST-EUR) study. Arch Intern Med. 2002;162:2046–52.
38. Tzourio C, Anderson C, Chapman N, et al. Effects of blood pressure lowering with perindopril and indapamide therapy on dementia and cognitive decline in patients with cerebrovascular disease. Arch Intern Med. 2003;163:1069–75.
39. Peters R, Beckett N, Forette F, et al. Incident dementia and blood pressure lowering in the hypertension in the very elderly trial cognitive function assessment (HYVET-COG): a double-blind, placebo controlled trial. Lancet Neurol. 2008;7:683–9.
40. Hajjar I, Rosenberger KJ, Kulshreshtha A, et al. Association of JNC-8 and SPRINT systolic blood

pressure levels with cognitive function and related racial disparity. JAMA Neurol. 2017.;Epub ahead of print;74:1199–205.

41. Benetos A, Bulpitt CJ, Petrovic M, Ungar A, Rosei EA, Cherubini A, Redon J, Grodzicki T, Dominiczak A, Strandberg T, Mancia G. An expert opinion from the European Society of Hypertension–European Union Geriatric Medicine Society Working Group on the management of hypertension in very old, frail subjects. Hypertension. 2016;67(5):820–5.
42. Mancia G, Fagard R, Narkiewicz K, et al. ESH/ESC guidelines for the management of arterial hypertension. J Hypertens. 2013;31:1281–357.
43. The ALLHAT Officers and Coordinators for the ALLHAT Collaborative Research Group. Major outcomes in high-risk hypertensive patients randomized to angiotensin-converting enzyme inhibitor or calcium channel blocker vs diuretic: he Antihypertensive and Lipid-Lowering Treatment to Prevent Heart Attack Trial (ALLHAT). JAMA. 2002;288:2981–97.
44. Dahlöf B, Sever PS, Poulter NR, et al. Prevention of cardiovascular events with an antihypertensive regimen of amlodipine adding perindopril as required versus atenolol adding bendroflumethiazide as required, in the Anglo-Scandinavian cardiac outcomes trial-blood pressure lowering arm (ASCOT-BPLA): a multicentre randomized control trial. Lancet. 2005;366:895–906.
45. Yoon SS, Fryar CD, Carroll MD. Hypertension prevalence and control among adults: United States, 2011–2014, NCHS data brief, no 220. Hyattsville: National Center for Health Statistics; 2015.
46. Aronow WS. Managing hypertension in the elderly: What is different, what is the same? Curr. Cardiovasc Risk Rep. 2017;11(8):22.
47. Wright JT, Fine LJ, Lackland DT, Ogedegbe G, Dennison Himmelfarb CR. Evidence supporting a systolic blood pressure goal of less than 150 mm Hg in patients aged 60 years or older: the minority view. Ann Intern Med. 2014;160:499–503.
48. Krakoff LR, Gillespie RL, Ferdinand KC, et al. Hypertension recommendations from the eighth joint national committee panel members raise concerns for elderly black and female populations. J Am Coll Cardiol. 2014;64(4):394–402.

Management of Hypertension in Diabetes Mellitus

7

Michael Doumas and George L. Bakris

Introduction

Diabetes mellitus is a progressive metabolic disease with severe macrovascular (coronary artery disease, heart failure, stroke, peripheral artery disease) and microvascular (nephropathy, retinopathy) complications. Diabetes mellitus is associated with a two-fold to three-fold increased risk for cardiovascular events and is the leading cause of chronic kidney disease with almost half of end-stage renal disease cases being attributed to diabetes [1, 2]. The prevalence of type 2 diabetes mellitus increased dramatically during the last decades reaching epidemic dimensions, with even more disappointing projections for the near future [3, 4]. This increase in incidence around most of the world is primarily due to the increase in global obesity. The findings of two recent studies generate even greater concerns. The incidence of both type 1 and type 2 diabetes increased significantly among youths in the US during the last decade, especially in minority populations [5]. Moreover, a large Swedish Registry revealed that although mortality and cardiovascular morbidity declined significantly during the last decade, fatal outcomes declined significantly less in diabetic compared to control individuals [6].

Arterial hypertension is a major public health problem with more than 1 billion affected individuals worldwide, a number that is expect to climb to 1.5 billion in 2025 [7]. Hypertension is a major cardiovascular risk factor and overwhelming observational data demonstrate a linear relationship between blood pressure levels even in the normal range and the risk of cardiovascular events [8]. Elevated blood pressure levels affect the heart (myocardial infarction, heart failure, left ventricular hypertrophy, atrial fibrillation), the brain (stroke, transient ischaemic attack, vascular dementia), the kidneys (chronic kidney disease), and the eyes (hypertensive retinopathy). Hypertension is among the most studied conditions and numerous randomized controlled studies have established the benefits of antihypertensive therapy on all cardiovascular and renal outcomes. Hypertension is very frequently encountered in diabetic patients and its prevalence depends on the type of diabetes, age, race, gender, and body mass index. Overall, more than half of diabetic patients have elevated blood pressure levels, which are associated with both macro- and micro-vascular diabetic complications.

This chapter summarizes the guideline recommendations for the management of elevated blood pressure in patients with type 2 diabetes

M. Doumas
Second Propedeutic Department of Internal Medicine, Aristotle University, Thessaloniki, Greece

Veteran Affairs Medical Center and George Washington University, Washington, DC, USA

G. L. Bakris (✉)
Comprehensive Hypertension Center, Department of Medicine, University of Chicago, Chicago, IL, USA
e-mail: gbakris@uchicago.edu

V. Papademetriou et al. (eds.), *Management of Hypertension*,
https://doi.org/10.1007/978-3-319-92946-0_7

mellitus, presents the landmark studies in this field and the relevant meta-analyses that paved the way for these recommendations, and finally critically evaluates currently available data and provides future perspectives for the management of arterial hypertension in diabetic patients, especially on when to initiate therapy, at what blood pressure goal and the more appropriate drugs to attain it.

The Guidelines

Several scientific societies from many specialties (hypertension, diabetology, endocrinology, nephrology, cardiology) at different parts of the world have issued guideline recommendations for the management of arterial hypertension in patients with diabetes mellitus. The exhaustive presentation of all guidelines is beyond the scope of this chapter, so the most representative guidelines will be summarized.

American Diabetes Association (ADA)

The ADA updates its recommendations at the beginning of each year. While the 2017 update is not substantially different from the 2016 guidelines [9], the ADA BP Consensus report was just published and will result in a major change in the 2018 guidelines [10]. Examples of updates will be the mandate to measure standing pressure on initial visit, using of home blood pressure monitoring to assess adherence and presence of white coat hypertension and many other more subtle differences. The blood pressure goal of less than 140 mmHg for systolic and less than 90 mmHg for diastolic is recommended for all patients with diabetes mellitus and hypertension who can tolerate this level (level of evidence A). A lower blood pressure goal of <130/80 mmHg is recommended for higher-risk patients if it can be achieved without undue treatment burden (level of evidence B). Initiation of antihypertensive therapy is recommended for blood pressure values of 140/90 mmHg or greater in addition to lifestyle therapy (level of evidence A). Patients with a blood pressure > 160/100 mmHg should be initially treated with combination therapy of a renin angiotensin system blocker with either a thiazide-like diuretic or a calcium antaagonist (level of evidence A) [11]. RAS-inhibitors are considered treatment of choice for patients with very high or macro-albuminuria (level of evidence A). The new ADA BP consensus report does NOT mandate their use in microalbuminuria or normotension in diabetes since there has been a failure of outcome data for prevention of events in this setting [10]. Lifestyle modification is recommended for patients with blood pressure levels >120/80 mmHg (level of evidence B).

Expert Panel Report (JNC8)

The Eighth Joint National Committee released its evidence-based recommendations for the management of high blood pressure in adults in 2014 [12]. It is recommended initial pharmacological therapy at blood pressure levels >140 mmHg for systolic and >90 mmHg for diastolic blood pressure. Likewise, the blood pressure goal with antihypertensive therapy is set at <140 mmHg for systolic and <90 mmHg for diastolic blood pressure (Grade E – Expert Opinion recommendation). The same thresholds apply for adult patients with chronic kidney disease as well. Initial antihypertensive therapy should include a thiazide-type diuretic, calcium antagonist, ACE-inhibitor, or ARB in nonblack diabetic patients (Grade B, Moderate recommendation), while in black patients a thiazide-type diuretic or a calcium antagonist should be used as initial therapy (Grade C – Weak recommendation for black patients with diabetes mellitus). These guidelines were NOT well accepted and the most recent guidelines released in November of 2017 are radically different from the Expert Panel Report.

There are too many differences to highlight in this article. Major differences from previous guidelines include: (a) a new staging system shown in Table 7.1, (b) new blood pressure goals for most people including most people over 65 years of age to be <130/80 mmHg and (c) a focus on not only how to measure blood pressure

Table 7.1 Categories of BP in Adults[a]

BP Category	SBP		DBP
Normal	<120 mmHg	And	<80 mmHg
Elevated	120–129 mmHg	And	<80 mmHg
Hypertension			
Stage 1	130–139 mmHg	Or	80–89 mmHg
Stage 2	140–159 mmHg	Or	90–99 mmHg
Stage 3	≥160 mmHg	Or	≥100 mmHg

[a]Individuals with SBP and DBP in 2 categories should be designated to the higher BP category

in the office but a major emphasis on home blood pressure [13]. The spirit of these new guidelines is to look at blood pressure in the context of a >10% 10-year cardiovascular risk. If present one has to be more aggressive about lowering the blood pressure and achieving goal. For those with diabetes the guideline is similar to the new ADA recommendations only more stringent. Specific guidelines for those with hypertension and diabetes mellitus: In adults with diabetes mellitus and hypertension, antihypertensive drug treatment should be initiated at a blood pressure greater than or equal to 130/80 mmHg with a treatment goal of less than 130/80 mmHg (level A). In adults with diabetes mellitus and hypertension, all classes of antihypertensive agents are useful and effective (level A). In adults with diabetes mellitus and hypertension, ACE inhibitors or ARBs may be considered in the presence of albuminuria (level B) [13].

European Society of Hypertension

The most recent guidelines for the management of arterial hypertension by the European Society of Hypertension and the European Society of Cardiology will be published in 2018 and are available online [14]. These guidelines devote a specific section for the management of hypertension in patients with diabetes mellitus. Ambulatory blood pressure measurement is considered useful to unveil masked hypertension in diabetic patients. Initiation of antihypertensive therapy is considered mandatory at systolic blood pressure values >160 mmHg; moreover, it is strongly recommended in diabetic patients with stage I hypertension (systolic blood pressure 140–160 mmHg), while initiation at lower blood pressure levels is not recommended. Regarding blood pressure targets in patients with diabetes mellitus, a systolic blood pressure goal of <140 mmHg is recommended, while the corresponding goal for diastolic blood pressure is <85 mmHg. Regarding the type of antihypertensive therapy, all classes can be used and are recommended for the management of hypertension in diabetic patients; it is also recommended that individual therapy should take comorbidities into account. RAS blockers may be preferred in diabetic patients, especially in the presence of macro-albuminuria, while the simultaneous administration of two RAS blockers should be avoided. Finally, systolic blood pressure values <130 mmHg are strongly suggested in the presence of overt proteinuria, provided that renal function is closely monitored.

The Landmark Studies

A large body of epidemiological evidence demonstrates the role of blood pressure elevation on diabetic macro- and micro-vascular complications, while numerous randomized controlled studies verified the benefits of antihypertensive therapy on cardiovascular and renal outcomes. Here we summarize the findings of the more important studies in this field.

UKPDS

The United Kingdom Prospective Diabetes Study (UKPDS) evaluated the macro- and micro-vascular effects of tight (blood pressure goal <150/85 mmHg with captopril or atenolol) and less stringent (blood pressure goal <180/105 mmHg) blood pressure control in patients with newly diagnosed type 2 diabetes mellitus [15]. A total of 1148 mostly middle-aged (mean age: 56 years) participants with uncontrolled blood pressure (mean baseline blood pressure: 160/94 mmHg) were randomly assigned (2:1 ratio) to tight or less stringent blood pressure control for a median follow-up period of 8.4 years. Blood pressure levels were significantly different in the two groups during the follow-up period of the study (144/82 mmHg vs 154/87 mmHg in the tight and less stringent group, respectively, $p < 0.0001$). Tight blood pressure control was associated with significant macro- and micro-vascular benefits compared with less stringent blood pressure control. In particular, a 34% reduction in relative risk ($p = 0.019$) for macro-vascular events (combined myocardial infarction, sudden death, stroke, and peripheral vascular disease) and a 37% reduction in risk ($p = 0.0092$) for micro-vascular events (retinopathy requiring photocoagulation, vitreous hemorrhage, fatal or nonfatal renal failure) were observed with tight compared to less stringent blood pressure control. Furthermore, stroke was reduced by 44%, heart failure declined by 56%, diabetes-related end-points were reduced by 24%, and diabetes related deaths were reduced by 32% with tight blood pressure control. On the other hand, no statistically significant benefits were observed with tight blood pressure control in all-cause mortality, fatal and nonfatal myocardial infarction, proteinuria, renal function deterioration, and diabetic neuropathy.

ACCORD

The Action to Control Cardiovascular Risk in Diabetes (ACCORD) trial evaluated whether intensive antihypertensive therapy (systolic blood pressure goal <120 mmHg) is superior to standard therapy (systolic blood pressure goal <140 mmHg) in patients with type 2 diabetes mellitus at high risk for cardiovascular events [16]. A total of 4733 middle-aged and elderly (mean age: 62.2 years) participants with long-standing diabetes (mean duration: 10 years) and rather controlled blood pressure (mean baseline blood pressure: 139.2/76.0 mmHg) were randomly assigned to intensive or standard antihypertensive therapy for 4.7 years. Blood pressure differed significantly between the two groups from the first months of therapy, and an average between-group difference of 14.2/6.1 mmHg was achieved early in the study (133.5/70.5 mmHg vs 119.3/64.4 mmHg for the intensive and standard therapy group, respectively). The study failed to reach its primary endpoint (a composite of nonfatal myocardial infarction, nonfatal stroke, and cardiovascular death) and most secondary endpoints (all-cause and cardiovascular mortality, nonfatal myocardial infarction, major coronary disease event, and fatal or nonfatal heart failure). Note however, that both nonfatal stroke and any stroke rates were significantly lower with intensive compared with standard therapy (HR: 0.63, 95% CI: 0.41–0.96, $p = 0.03$; and HR: 0.59, 95% CI: 0.39–0.89, $p = 0.01$, respectively). On the other hand, serious adverse events (mainly hypotension, syncope, bradycardia or arrhythmia, and hyperkalemia) occurred at a higher rate with intensive compared to standard therapy (3.3% vs 1.3%, $p < 0.001$, respectively); in addition, deterioration of renal function was significantly more frequent with intensive therapy ($p < 0.001$).

More recent updates and long term follow-up of ACCORD (ACCORDION) demonstrate that the difference in blood pressure was not sustained resulting in only a 4 mmHg difference in systolic blood pressure between group (Fig. 7.1) with a resultant elimination of the stroke benefit in the intensive group. Hence, there is NO legacy effect of blood pressure on outcomes. Additionally, an analysis performed after the ACCORD showed a major interaction between the intensive glycemic control group and the intensive blood pressure group, such that people died from hypoglycemia and hence, could not be evaluated in the intensive blood pressure arm [17]. Looking at the group that remained however shows a benefit in the lower blood pressure group on cardiovascular outcome.

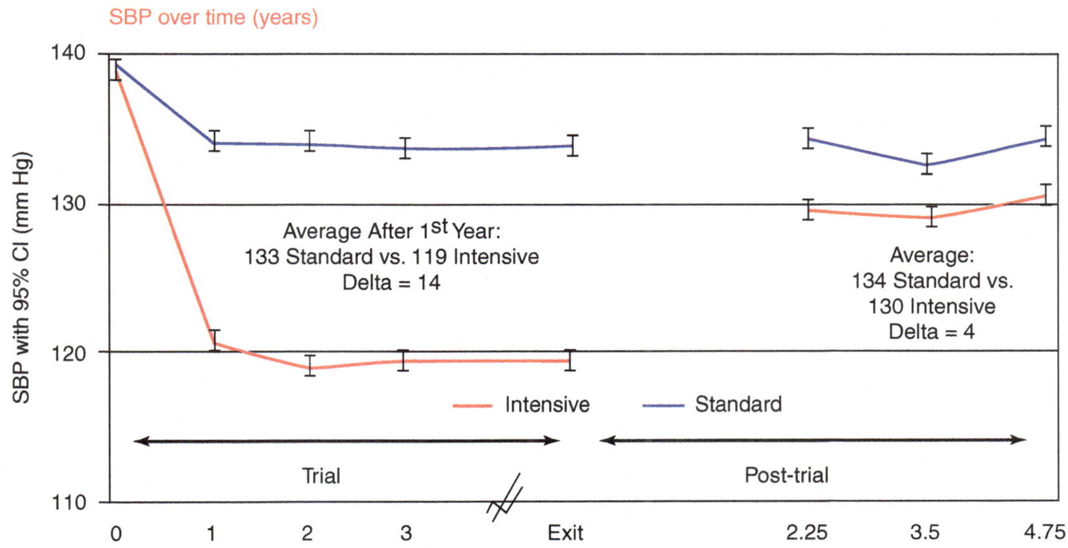

Mean number of medications prescribed:

Intensive	3.2	3.4	3.4	3.4	2.3	2.2	2.1
Standard	1.9	2.1	2.1	2.2	2.0	1.9	1.9
Intensive N =	2174	2071	1973	2019	1132	1223	1147
Standard N =	2208	2136	2077	2062	1218	1279	1196

Fig. 7.1 Blood pressure values over the ACCORD and ACCORDION studies. (Presented as late breaking trial American heart Assoc. 2015)

ADVANCE

The Action in Diabetes and Vascular disease: preterAx and diamicroN-MR Controlled Evaluation (ADVANCE) trial evaluated the effect of combination therapy with an ACE-inhibitor and a diuretic on serious vascular events in patients with type 2 diabetes mellitus, irrespective of baseline blood pressure or use of other antihypertensive drugs [18]. A total of 11,140 middle-aged and elderly (mean age: 66 years) high-risk participants with long-standing diabetes mellitus (mean duration: 8 years) and rather controlled blood pressure (mean baseline blood pressure: 145/81 mmHg) were randomly assigned to a fixed combination of perindopril and indapamide or matching placebo for a mean follow-up period of 4.3 years. A significant difference in blood pressure levels of 5.6/2.2 mmHg in average during the study was observed between the two groups. The relative risk of combined macro- and micro-vascular events was reduced by 9% (HR: 0.91; 95% CI: 0.83–1.00, p = 0.04), while the separate reductions in macro- and micro-vascular events were similar but not independently significant. Of major importance, active therapy was associated with a significant survival benefit; the relative risk for cardiovascular mortality was reduced by 18% (HR: 0.82, 95% CI: 0.68–0.98, p = 0.03) and for all-cause mortality was reduced by 14% (HR: 0.86, 95% CI: 0.75–0.98, p = 0.03). It was estimated that 79 patients need to be treated for 5 years with the fixed combination of perindopril and indapamide to prevent one death in high-risk patients with diabetes mellitus.

ABCD – Hypertensive Arm

The Appropriate Blood Pressure Control in Diabetes (ABCD) hypertensive trial evaluated the effects of intensive (diastolic blood pressure goal: 75 mmHg) versus moderate (diastolic blood pressure goal: 80–89 mmHg) blood pressure control, with nisoldipine or enalapril, on the incidence and progression of type 2 diabetic complications [19]. A total of 470 patients with type 2 diabetes mellitus and hypertension were randomly assigned to intensive therapy or moderate blood pressure control for 5.3 years. No difference were observed between the two groups in creatinine clearance changes (the primary outcome), and the same was evident regarding enalapril and nisoldipine therapy. Likewise, the progression rates from normo- to micro-albuminuria and from micro- to macro-albuminuria were similar between the two therapeutic strategies (intensive vs moderate) and between the two drugs (nisoldipine vs enalapril). Furthermore, no differences in diabetic retinopathy and diabetic neuropathy were observed between study groups. In contrast, all-cause mortality rates were significantly lower with intensive compared with moderate antihypertensive therapy (5.5 vs 10.7%, p = 0.037).

HOT

The Hypertension Optimal treatment (HOT) trial assessed the optimum target diastolic blood pressure in patients with arterial hypertension [20]. A total of 18,790 middle-aged and elderly (mean age: 61.5 years) participants with uncontrolled hypertension (mean baseline diastolic blood pressure: 105 mmHg) were randomly assigned to three group with a diastolic blood pressure goal of ≤90, ≤85, and ≤80 mmHg, respectively. Marked blood pressure reductions were achieved (26.2/20.3, 28.9/22.3, and 29.9/24.3 mmHg, in the three groups, respectively). However, the between group differences in achieved blood pressure values were smaller than anticipated (achieved mean diastolic blood pressure: 85.2 mmHg, 83.2 mmHg, and 81.1 mmHg, respectively) for a mean of 2 instead of 5 mmHg. No statistically significant differences were observed for the primary and secondary outcomes between the three groups. The lowest incidence of major cardiovascular events occurred at 82.6 mmHg and the lowest risk of cardiovascular mortality occurred at 86.5 mmHg for diastolic blood pressure. Of major clinical importance, statistically significant benefits with more aggressive antihypertensive therapy were observed among the 1501 study participants with diabetes mellitus at baseline. Major cardiovascular events and myocardial infarctions were halved in the most aggressively (≤80 mmHg) than in the least aggressively (≤90 mmHg) treated group, and cardiovascular mortality was also significantly lowered. In detail, compared to the most aggressively treated group, participants in the least aggressively treated group had a relative risk of 2.06 (95% CI: 1.24–3.44) for major cardiovascular events, of 2.01 (95% CI: 0.81–4.97) for fatal and nonfatal myocardial infarction, and of 3.0 (95% CI: 1.28–7.08) for cardiovascular mortality, while total mortality and stroke followed a trend towards the same direction. However, the results regarding patients with diabetes mellitus need to be viewed with caution due to the inherent limitations of subgroup analysis; they are, at best, hypothesis generating rather than definitive results.

Landmark Studies in Special Populations

Along with studies evaluating blood pressure reduction on outcomes in the general population of patients with diabetes, some studies evaluated the effects of antihypertensive therapy in special populations: normotensive individuals (ABCD-normotensive arm), patients with isolated systolic hypertension (SHEP, Syst-Eur), patients with prior cerebrovascular disease (PROGRESS), and patients with advanced diabetic kidney disease (RENAAL, IDNT). The findings of these studies are very informative and useful for the management of diabetic patients in everyday clinical practice.

ABCD – Normotensive Arm

The Appropriate Blood Pressure Control in Diabetes (ABCD) trial evaluated the effects of intensive (10 mmHg below the baseline diastolic blood pressure) versus moderate (80–89 mmHg) diastolic blood pressure control in normotensive patients with type 2 diabetes mellitus [21]. It was a pilot study focused on nephropathy prevention. A total of 480 diabetic patients with normal blood pressure (<140/90 mmHg) were randomly assigned to nisoldipine or enalapril in the intensive therapy group or matching placebo in the moderate therapy group for 5.3 years. Mean blood pressure was significantly lower in the intensive than in the moderate therapy group (128/75 mmHg vs 137/81 mmHg, $p < 0.0001$). The study failed to reach its primary endpoint (change in creatinine clearance); there were no significant differences in creatinine clearance changes and serum creatinine changes between the intensive and moderate therapy groups or between nisoldipine and enalapril within the intensive therapy group. However, the progression rates from normo- to micro-albuminuria and from micro- to macro-albuminuria were significantly lower with intensive compared with moderate therapy ($p = 0.012$ and $p = 0.028$, respectively). Intensive blood pressure control was associated with less progression of diabetic retinopathy ($p = 0.019$) and lower stroke rates ($p = 0.03$), irrespective of assignment to enalapril or nisoldipine.

SHEP – Syst-Eur

The Systolic Hypertension in the Elderly Program (SHEP) and the Systolic Hypertension in Europe (Syst-Eur) trials evaluated the effects of antihypertensive therapy in elderly patients with isolated systolic hypertension. Chlorthalidone was compared with placebo for 5 years in SHEP, while nitrendipine was compared to placebo for 2 years in Syst-Eur. A small portion of participants in these two trials had type 2 diabetes mellitus at baseline: 583/4736 in SHEP and 492/4695 in Syst-Eur. In SHEP, the absolute risk reduction with active therapy was twice as great for diabetic than in nondiabetic participants, probably due to the higher cardiovascular risk conferred by diabetes mellitus [22]. On average, blood pressure was significantly lower with active therapy than with placebo by 9.8/2.2 mmHg in diabetic patients. The relative risk reduction with active therapy in diabetic participants was 34% for major cardiovascular events (RR: 0.66, 95% CI: 0.46–0.94), 54% for fatal and nonfatal myocardial infarction (RR: 0.46, 95% CI: 0.24–0.88), and 56% for major coronary heart disease events (RR: 0.44, 95% CI: 0.25–0.77), while stroke and all-cause mortality rates moved towards the same direction but did not reach statistical significance [22]. In Syst-Eur, blood pressure was significantly lower with active therapy than with placebo by 8.6/3.9 mmHg in diabetic participants [23]. The morbidity and mortality benefits of active therapy were greater in diabetic than in nondiabetic participants. In diabetics, active therapy was associated with a relative risk reduction by 70% for cardiovascular mortality (95% CI: 19–89), by 62% for all cardiovascular events (95% CI: 19–80), and by 69% for stroke (95% CI: 14–89), while the reductions in cardiac events and all-cause mortality were towards the same direction but did not reach statistical significance [23]. It has to be acknowledged however once again that these findings need to be interpreted with caution, first because they come from subgroup analysis and second because the diabetic subgroup was rather small in both studies, not permitting for definitive conclusions.

PROGRESS

The Perindopril Protection Against Recurrent Stroke Study (PROGRESS) evaluated the effects of antihypertensive therapy (perindopril ± indapamide) for 3.9 years on stroke in patients with established cerebrovascular disease. Among 6105 study participants, 761 patients had type 2 diabetes mellitus at baseline [24]. The risk of recurrent stroke was significantly increased (by 35%) in diabetic compared to nondiabetic study participants. Blood pressure was significantly lower with active therapy than with placebo, for a difference of 9.5/4.6 mmHg in diabetic participants.

The relative risk reduction for stroke in diabetic patients was 38% (HR: 0.62, 95% CI: 0.42–0.92) and was slightly greater than the reduction in nondiabetic participants (HR: 0.72, 95% CI: 0.61–0.84). It was estimated that 16 diabetic patients with prior stroke need to be treated with antihypertensive therapy for 5 years to prevent a recurrent stroke [24].

Diabetic Kidney Disease Studies

RENAAL

The Reduction of Endpoints in Non-insulin dependent diabetes mellitus with the Angiotensin II Antagonist Losartan (RENAAL) trial evaluated the effects of losartan on renal and cardiovascular outcomes in patients with type 2 diabetes mellitus and nephropathy [25]. A total of 1513 patients were randomly assigned to losartan or matching placebo on top of conventional therapy for a mean follow-up period of 3.4 years. Study participants were mostly middle-aged and elderly (mean age: 60 years) with rather uncontrolled hypertension (mean baseline blood pressure: 152/82 mmHg) and were diagnosed with diabetic nephropathy. Active therapy was associated with a relative risk reduction of 16% (95% CI: 2–28, $p = 0.02$) for the primary outcome (a composite of a doubling of the baseline serum creatinine concentration, end-stage renal disease, or death). Significant benefits with active therapy were also observed when renal outcomes were assessed separately: the relative risk reduction for end-stage renal disease was 28% (95% CI: 11–42, $p = 0.002$) and for doubling of serum creatinine concentration was 25% (95% CI: 8–39, $p = 0.006$). In addition, proteinuria was reduced by 35% with active therapy ($p < 0.001$) and the rate of decline in renal function was reduced by 18% ($p = 0.01$) in the actively treated study participants. Cardiovascular morbidity and mortality was similar in the two groups, except for a relative risk reduction of 32% ($p = 0.005$) for heart failure hospitalization with active therapy.

Irbesartan Diabetic Nephropathy Trial (IDNT)

The (IDNT) evaluated the ability of an angiotensin II receptor blocker or a calcium antagonist to attenuate the progression of nephropathy in patients with type 2 diabetes mellitus and nephropathy [26]. A total of 1715 patients with diabetic nephropathy and hypertension were randomly assigned to irbesartan, amlodipine, or placebo for 2.6 years. The mean age of study participants was 59.3 years, the mean baseline blood pressure was 160/87 mmHg and the mean serum creatinine concentration was 1.67 mg/dl. The mean blood pressure was significantly lower (by 3.3 mmHg) in the two actively treated groups than in the placebo group, with no significant differences between the two therapies. Irbesartan therapy was associated with a significant relative risk reduction for the primary outcome (a composite of a doubling of the baseline serum creatinine concentration, the development of end-stage renal disease, or both) by 20% compared with placebo ($p = 0.02$) and by 23% compared with amlodipine ($p = 0.006$). When renal outcomes were assessed separately, the relative risk reduction for doubling of serum creatinine levels with irbesartan was 33% when compared to placebo ($p = 0.003$) and 37% when compared to amlodipine ($p < 0.001$). Likewise, irbesartan therapy was associated with a 23% lower relative risk for end-stage renal disease compared with placebo or amlodipine ($p = 0.07$ for both comparisons). There were no significant differences in the rates of cardiovascular outcomes or all-cause mortality between the three groups.

Meta-analyses

During the last decade many meta-analyses have been performed evaluating the effects of antihypertensive therapy on cardiovascular and renal outcomes in patients with diabetes mellitus. Some of them explored optimal blood pressure targets in diabetic patients and some others sought to identify potential differences between the various categories of antihypertensive drugs. Here we summarize the most important meta-analyses that specifically addressed the effects of antihypertensive therapy in patients with diabetes mellitus.

The Cochrane Collaboration meta-analysis by Arguedas et al. pooled data from 5 randomized studies with more than 7300 participants with type 2 diabetes mellitus, and assessed whether lower blood pressure targets (<130/85 mmHg) are associated with reduction in morbidity and mortality compared with standard blood pressure targets (<140–160 mmHg) [27]. For this meta-analysis, only the blood pressure arm of the ACCORD trial satisfied the inclusion criteria for systolic blood pressure comparisons, so the findings of the meta-analysis for systolic blood pressure targets are identical with the findings of ACCORD-BP and do not favor a lower systolic blood pressure goal. Four trials (ABCD-H, ABCD-N, ABCD-2 V, and HOT) with more than 2500 participants fulfilled the inclusion criteria regarding the diastolic blood pressure targets. There was no statistically significant difference between lower and standard blood pressure levels in myocardial infarction and in heart failure (RR: 0.95, 95% CI: 0.64–1.40; and RR: 1.06, 95% CI: 0.58–1.92, respectively), while a trend towards reductions in stroke and all-cause mortality was observed with lower blood pressure values (RR: 0.67, 95% CI: 0.42–1.05; and RR: 0.73, 95% CI: 0.53–1.01, respectively).

Bangalore et al. pooled data from 13 randomized trials with almost 40,000 participants with diabetes mellitus or impaired glucose tolerance, and assessed the differences between intensive (systolic blood pressure <135 mmHg) and standard antihypertensive therapy (systolic blood pressure <140 mmHg) [28]. Intensive blood pressure control (systolic blood pressure < 135 mmHg) was associated with significant benefits in stroke and all-cause mortality (17% and 10%, respectively; OR: 0.83, 95% CI: 0.73–0.95 and OR: 0.90, 95% CI: 0.83–0.98, respectively), in expense of a 20% increase of serious adverse events compared with standard therapy (systolic blood pressure <140 mmHg). Other macrovascular outcomes (apart from stroke) and microvascular outcomes (nephropathy, retinopathy, and neuropathy) were similar with intensive and standard blood pressure control. A continued stroke risk reduction was observed with systolic blood pressure levels down to 120 mmHg, the adverse events however increased by 40% at blood pressure levels <130/80 mmHg.

Emdin et al. pooled data from 49 trials with more than 100,000 participants and assessed the effects of systolic blood pressure lowering by 10 mmHg on the relative and absolute risk of vascular events [29]. It was found that each 10 mmHg lower systolic blood pressure was associated with a significant relative risk reduction by 13% for all-cause mortality (RR: 0.87, 95% CI: 0.78–0.96), by 11% for total cardiovascular events (RR: 0.89, 95% CI: 0.83–0.95), by 12% for coronary heart disease (RR: 0.88, 95% CI: 0.80–0.98), by 27% for stroke (RR: 0.73, 95% CI: 0.64–0.83), by 17% for albuminuria (RR: 0.83, 95% CI: 0.79–0.87), by 14% for heart failure (RR: 0.86, 95% CI: 0.74–1.00), and by 13% for retinopathy (RR:0.87, 95% CI: 0.76–0.99). The absolute risk reduction in events per 1000 patient years was 3.16 for all-cause mortality, 3.90 for total cardiovascular events, 1.81 for coronary heart disease, 4.06 for stroke, 9.33 for albuminuria, and 2.23 for retinopathy. Further analysis revealed that antihypertensive tehrapy reduced the risk for all outcomes when baseline blood pressure was equal to or over 140 mmHg, but reduced the risk only for stroke and albuminuria when baseline systolic blood pressure was lower than 140 mmHg. Likewise, antihypertensive therapy reduced the risk for all outcomes when achieved systolic blood pressure was >130 mmHg, but reduced the risk only for stroke and albuminuria when achieved systolic blood pressure was <130 mmHg. Finally, there were no differences between the various antihypertensive drug categories on the outcomes, except for a relative superiority of calcium antagonists on stroke and of diuretics on heart failure, and a relative inferiority of calcium antagonists and ACE-inhibitors on heart failure [29].

Thomopoulos et al. pooled data from 41 trials with more than 60,000 patients with type 2 diabetes mellitus and assessed the effects of blood pressure lowering to different systolic and diastolic blood pressure levels by various drugs in cardiovascular and renal outcomes [30]. It was found that in diabetic patients the standardized to a blood pressure difference of 10/5 mmHg relative risk was reduced by 27% for stroke (RR: 0.73, 95% CI: 0.63–0.86), by 29% for coronary heart disease (RR: 0.71, 95% CI: 0.61–0.81), by 25% for heart failure (RR: 0.75, 95% CI: 0.64–0.91), by 23% for cardiovascular mortality (RR: 0.77, 95% CI: 0.58–1.02), and by 18% for all-cause mortality (RR: 0.82, 95% CI: 0.72–0.93); the corresponding absolute risk reduction per 1000 patients for 5 years was 18, 19, 14, 13, and 18, respectively. An analysis of outcomes according to achieved systolic blood pressure (≥140, 130–140, <130 mmHg) in the treated group revealed greater relative risk reduction with higher blood pressure levels; the corresponding relative risk reductions in the three groups were: 48%, 24%, and 26% for stroke; 59%, 28%, and 14% for coronary heart disease, 55%, 23%, and 18% for heart failure, 44%, 33%, and + 28% for cardiovascular mortality, and 21%, 29%, and + 3% for all-cause mortality.

Likewise, the relative and the absolute risk reduction were greater with achieved diastolic blood pressure ≥ 80 mmHg compared to <80 mmHg; the relative risk was reduced by 53% and 28% for stroke, 49% and 28% for coronary heart disease, 76% and 20% for heart failure, 58% and 12% for cardiovascular mortality, and 20% and 18% for all-cause mortality, respectively. In an analysis of the individual antihypertensive categories it was found that diuretics were superior for heart failure prevention, beta-blockers were inferior for stroke prevention, and calcium antagonists were superior for stroke prevention and inferior for heart failure prevention, ACE-inhibitors were superior for coronary heart disease and heart failure prevention and angiotensin receptor blockers were superior for heart failure prevention, compared to other antihypertensive drugs. The relative risk for end-stage renal disease is reduced by 21% with antihypertensive therapy in diabetic patients and once again the greater risk reduction (relative and absolute) is observed with higher blood pressure values: 44% for achieved systolic blood pressure ≥140 mmHg and minimal if any for systolic blood pressure levels 130–140 mmHg and <140 mmHg [30].

Remonti et al. pooled data from 27 studies with almost 50,000 participants with type 2 diabetes mellitus and assessed the effects of antihypertensive drug categories on all-cause and cardiovascular mortality in patients with diabetes and hypertension [31]. There were no statistically significant differences in either all-cause or cardiovascular mortality with any antihypertensive drugs category compared with placebo. Likewise, no statistically significant mortality differences were observed when antihypertensive drug categories were compared with each other. The combination of ACE-inhibitors and calcium antagonists was associated with significant reductions in cardiovascular mortality compared with placebo, beta-blockers, calcium antagonists, angiotensin receptor blockers, and the combination of diuretics and beta-blockers. The combination of ACE-inhibitors with either calcium antagonists or diuretics was associated with significant reductions in all-cause mortality compared with the combination of diuretics and beta-blockers. However, the benefits of the ACE-inhibitor and calcium antagonist combination might be attributed to the lower blood pressure levels attained in the studies with this combination.

One possible exception to the aforementioned positive meta-analyses, one showing that systolic blood pressures below 130 mmHg did not result in fewer cardiovascular events was performed by Brunstrom and Carlberg. They pooled data from 49 trials with almost 75,000 participants with type 2 diabetes mellitus and assessed the impact of antihypertensive therapy at baseline systolic blood pressure >150 mmHg, 140–150 mmHg, and <140 mmHg on several outcomes [32]. At baseline systolic blood pressure levels >150 mmHg, antihypertensive therapy was associated with significant mortality and morbidity benefits, reducing the risk of all-cause mortality by 11% (RR: 0.89, 95% CI: 0.80–0.99), cardiovascular mortality by 25% (RR: 0.75, 95% CI: 0.57–0.99), myocardial infarction by 26% (RR: 0.74, 95% CI: 0.63–0.87), stroke by 23% (RR: 0.77, 95% CI: 0.65–0.91) and end-stage renal disease by 18% (RR: 0.82, 95% CI: 0.71–0.94).

At baseline, systolic blood pressure 140–150 mmHg the benefits of antihypertensive therapy were mostly maintained, with a relative risk reduction of 13% for all-cause mortality (RR: 0.87, 95% CI: 0.78–0.98), 16% for myocardial infarction (RR: 0.84, 95% CI: 0.76–0.93), and 20% for heart failure (RR: 0.80, 95% CI: 0.66–0.97). At baseline systolic blood pressure <140 mmHg, however the benefits disappeared, and a 15% increased risk for cardiovascular mortality (RR: 1.15, 95% CI: 1–00-1.32) and a tendency towards an increased risk for all-cause mortality (RR: 1.05, 95% CI: 0.95–1.16) were observed [32].

Critical Evaluation

Based on the aforementioned large randomized clinical trials, there is no doubt that antihypertensive therapy to levels below 130 mmHg systolic offers substantial benefits in patients with diabetes mellitus and hypertension, reducing cardiovascular morbidity and mortality and slowing renal function deterioration. Given the beneficial effects of antihypertensive drugs on macro- and micro-vascular complications of diabetes mellitus, three burning issues need to be addressed from the clinical point of view [33–39], in order to facilitate the management of diabetic patients in real life practice: (a) when to initiate antihypertensive drug therapy, (b) what is the optimal blood pressure goal and (c) which drugs are preferred for the achievement of these goals in patients with diabetes mellitus.

When to Initiate Antihypertensive Therapy

A wealth of evidence from large clinical trials demonstrated the benefits of blood pressure reduction at blood pressure levels >140/90 mmHg in patients with diabetes mellitus. However, more recent meta-analyses and long term follow-up of prospective clinical trials suggests blood pressure levels should be below 130/80 mmHg with new guidelines recommending people with >10% 10-year cardiovascular risk be treated with lifestyle intervention and monotherapy if blood pressure is 130–139 and/or 85–89 mmHg [13]. The ABCD-normotensive trial was woefully underpowered and hence, failed to show a benefit. Conversely, the ACCORDION study demonstrated in the intensive blood pressure group after censoring the intensive glycemic control group had a reduction in cardiovascular and stroke events. This was also born out in 3 other meta-analyses and captured in the updated ADA BP guidelines as well [10]. Likewise, antihypertensive therapy was associated with less progression of diabetic retinopathy and nephropathy (progression from normo- to micro-albuminuria and from micro- to macro-albuminuria) in the ABCD-normotensive trial. Note however, that the study was underpowered and failed to meet its primary endpoint (renal function) and to reduce all other cardiovascular outcomes (apart from stroke). Moreover, the study sample was rather small (n = 480), and the definition of normotension was based mainly on diastolic blood pressure (80–89 mmHg) permitting the inclusion of participants with systolic blood pressure up to 160 mmHg (the mean baseline systolic blood pressure was 137 mmHg), suggesting that some hypertensive patients were also included.

Indirect evidence from the ADVANCE mega-trial (n = 11,140) revealed significant benefits with antihypertensive therapy (a combination of ACE-inhibitor and diuretic) on combined macro- and micro-vascular events (9% reduction) as well as on cardiovascular and all-cause mortality (18% and 14% reduction, respectively) [18]. Of note, about one sixth of study participants had baseline blood pressure levels within the normotensive range (<140/90 mmHg) and the benefits on the primary outcome were identical among hypertensive and normotensive participants with diabetes mellitus (9% reduction for both groups).

Another factor to consider is the detrimental sequelae of elevated blood pressure, now Stage 1 hypertension (130–139/85–89 mmHg). Accumulating evidence indicates that Stage 1 hypertension (130–139/85–89 mmHg) is a precursor of more severe hypertension in a large proportion of individuals [13, 40]. Further blood pressure elevation is more likely in Stage 1 individuals with obesity and other comorbidities, including diabetes mellitus [41]. Even more importantly, Stage 1 hypertension is associated with increased risk for coronary, cerebrovascular, and chronic kidney disease, as well as cardiovascular mortality [42–45].

Collectively, these data while not conclusive suggest that the benefits of antihypertensive therapy in patients with diabetes mellitus are not limited in patients with blood pressure >140/90 mmHg but extend to people with blood pressure levels above 130/80 mmHg if at high cardiovascular risk. Therefore, it does seem clinically wise to consider the initiation of antihypertensive therapy in patients with diabetes and Stage 1 hypertension who have high cardiovascular risk (such as the participants in the ADVANCE trials) as the new ACC/AHA BP guideline recommends [13].

Which Is the Optimal Blood Pressure Goal?

The dogma 'the lower - the better' prevailed in the hypertension field for several decades, and was further re-enforced by the large meta-analysis of the Blood Pressure Trialists of more than one million individuals showing lower cardiovascular events at all ages with lower blood pressure values [8]. However, concerns regarding an excess of cardiovascular events with blood pressure reduction over a certain threshold (the so-called 'J-curve') have been expressed and revived by post-hoc analyses of several clinical trials, leading to the quest of the 'sweet spot', the optimal blood pressure levels that are associated with the largest reduction of cardiovascular events and beyond these levels cardiovascular events are increased instead of decreased [33–39]. However, this holds for people with coronary disease and not the general hypertensive population [46]. This is exemplified by a recent analysis of the VALUE trial, which demonstrated that patients in blood pressure strata ≥150/90 mmHg, but not those <130/70 mmHg, were at increased risk for adverse outcomes in this hypertensive, high-risk population; however, these were not generally people with diabetes [47]. In the ACCOMPLISH trial those with diabetes did demonstrate higher cardiovascular events and mortality at blood pressure levels below 115 mmHg [48].

Current guidelines continue to be aggressive and recommend blood pressure reduction to <130/80 mmHg in patients with diabetes mellitus or anyone with high cardiovascular risk >10% in 10 years, just like as in other high-risk patients (coronary artery disease, stroke, chronic kidney disease) [13]. Long term follow-up data from ACCORDION further solidify these findings now incorporated into diabetes guidelines and consensus reports [10].

Older clinical trials (UKPDS, SHEP, Syst-Eur, HOT) have clearly established the pronounced benefits of antihypertensive therapy in patients with diabetic mellitus [15, 20, 22, 23]. However, baseline blood pressure was very high in these studies (mean baseline systolic blood pressure: 160–175 mmHg) and achieved blood pressure was also high, above 140 mmHg (mean achieved systolic blood pressure: 144–153 mmHg). Therefore, these old studies did not permit for recommending blood pressure reduction in diabetic patients with what is now stage 2 hypertension and blood pressure targets below 145 mmHg. Of major clinical importance, one large clinical trial (ADVANCE), a smaller one (ABCD-HT) and one sub-study of a large trial (PROGRESS) showed significant benefits with further lowering of blood pressure (mean achieved systolic blood pressure: 132–134 mmHg) [18, 19, 24]. Based on these findings, it does not seem clinically unwise to consider lowering systolic blood pressure between 130 and 140 mmHg in patients with diabetes mellitus. Lastly, ACCORDION did achieve blood pressure levels well below 130 mmHg for an extended period of time, although in long term follow-up blood pressure levels rose such that there was only a 4 mmHg difference between groups (Fig. 7.1). As a result, the long term benefit of stroke, as seen in the main trial, was lost. Thus, blood pressure control does not have a legacy effect similar to glycemic control and thus, must be maintained for benefit.

The next question pops up immediately: can lower blood pressure targets be recommended? Recently a large observational study of more than 185,000 low-risk patients with type 2 diabetes mellitus in a Swedish registry revealed that the lowest risk of cardiovascular events was observed in participants within the lowest decile of systolic blood pressure (110–119 mmHg), although overall mortality and heart failure was increased in this group [49]. The current guidelines focus on high cardiovascular risk groups and not low risk groups. Moreover, almost all trials of lower blood pressure in low risk groups with diabetes have failed to show a benefit. The current guidelines however, focus on those with >10% 10-year risk of cardiovascular event, hence, the data in this subgroup is positive for blood pressure levels to be below 130/80 mmHg. There are no data or guidelines that support lower is better and most analyses show increased risk with blood pressure levels below 120 mmHg in people with diabetes [28, 30, 32].

The cardiovascular benefits of intensive therapy in UKPDS were noticed for each 10 mmHg reduction of systolic blood pressure down to 120 mmHg [50]. In the previously mentioned ABCD-normotensive study, the mean achieved systolic blood pressure was 128 mmHg and some benefits (stroke, urinary albumin excretion) were observed [21]. However, the study was small and the participants were normotensive at baseline, and thus the study is not representative of the general hypertensive population. The meta-analysis by Emdin et al. unveiled a significant benefit with every 10 mmHg decrease in systolic blood pressure [29]. Moreover, the two recent high-quality meta-analyses published in the Lancet in 2016 point towards lower targets as well [51, 52]. The meta-analysis by Xie et al. pooled data from 19 trials with almost 45,000 patients and found clear cardiovascular benefits with intensive blood pressure reduction and the greatest benefits were observed in clinical trials of high-risk participants, such as patients with diabetes mellitus, chronic kidney disease, and overt cardiovascular disease [51]. The meta-analysis by Ettehad et al. pooled data from 123 studies with more than 600,000 participants and found a 13% decline of total mortality and significant cardiovascular benefits for each 10 mmHg reduction of systolic blood pressure, even at levels <130 mmHg [52].

The most influential study in this field was the ACCORD-BP trial [16] but because of an interaction ($p = 0.03$) between the intensive glycemic control group and intensive blood pressure group failed to meet its primary end-point. This was due to a high rate of hypoglycemia resulting in death and hence, inability to assess blood pressure levels. As noted earlier the subsequent analysis of the intensive group censored showed a strong trend for a positive effect in the lower blood pressure group (Fig. 7.2) [17]. Any stroke and non-fatal stroke were pronouncedly decreased by 41% and 37% respectively. In addition, a non statistically significant trend towards lower nonfatal myocardial infarction rates was also observed (13% reduction, 95% CI: 0.68–1.10, $p = 0.25$). Can these benefits be neglected at all? Especially when one takes into account that stroke is the third cause of death with enormous financial burden and social consequences for the patient and his/her family.

Of even greater importance, the 2×2 factorial design of the study might have influenced the findings of the study, since intensively treated patients could be treated with either standard or intensive glycemic control. And there is some evidence that this parameter indeed influenced and confused the findings of the study. Among participants in the blood pressure arm of the study, the relative risk of the primary outcome was significantly lower with intensive blood pressure therapy (HR: 0.74, 95% CI: 0.55–1.00), intensive glycemia therapy (HR: 0.67, 95% CI: 0.50–0.91), or both (HR: 0.71, 95% CI: 0.52–0.96) than with combined standard blood pressure and glycemia therapy [17]. Among

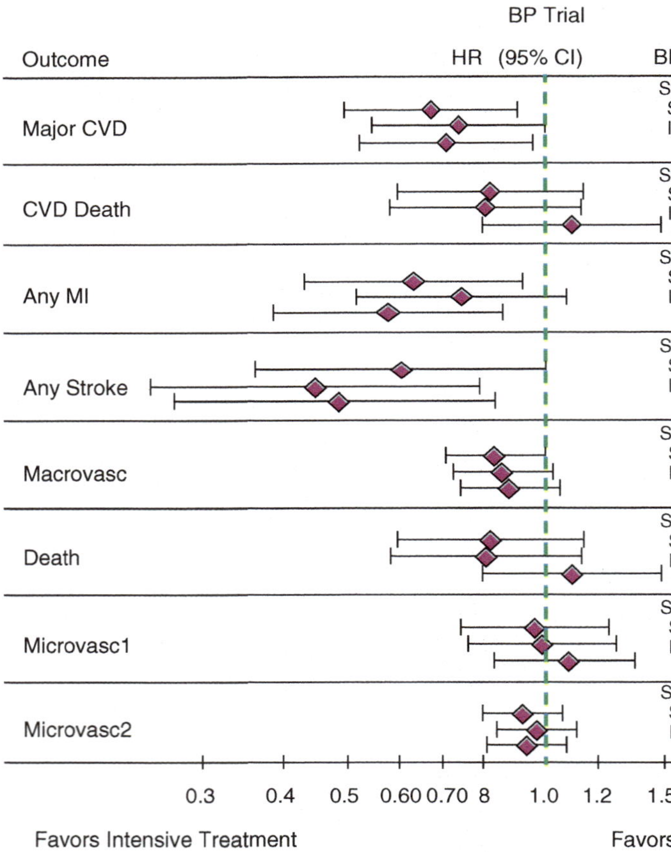

Outcome	BP/Gly	N	5 Yr Rate	HR	(95% CI)	p
Major CVD	Std/Std	102	(9.2%)	1.0		
	Std/Int	71	(8.1%)	0.87	(0.50-0.91)	0.011
	Int/Std	77	(8.9%)	0.74	(0.55-1.00)	0.049
	Int/Int	72	(6.5%)	0.71	(0.52-0.96)	0.025
CVD Death	Std/Std	23	(2.0%)	1.0		
	Std/Int	14	(1.2%)	0.82	(0.80-1.14)	0.251
	Int/Std	18	(1.5%)	0.81	(0.58-1.14)	0.224
	Int/Int	28	(2.2%)	1.09	(0.80-1.49)	0.575
Any MI	Std/Std	88	(5.9%)	1.0		
	Std/Int	43	(3.7%)	0.83	(0.43-0.93)	0.019
	Int/Std	50	(4.4%)	0.75	(0.52-1.08)	0.119
	Int/Int	38	(3.4%)	0.58	(0.39-0.88)	0.007
Any Stroke	Std/Std	24	(2.1%)	1.0		
	Std/Int	20	(1.7%)	0.81	(0.38-1.01)	0.054
	Int/Std	18	(1.4%)	0.44	(0.25-0.79)	0.006
	Int/Int	18	(1.4%)	0.48	(0.84-1.70)	0.011
Macrovasc	Std/Std	241	(23.9%)	1.0		
	Std/Int	214	(20.3%)	0.83	(0.70-0.98)	0.030
	Int/Std	205	(19.9%)	0.88	(0.73-1.02)	0.070
	Int/Int	217	(21.8%)	0.88	(0.74-1.04)	0.124
Death	Std/Std	51	(4.3%)	1.0		
	Std/Int	41	(3.4%)	0.82	(0.80-1.14)	0.251
	Int/Std	48	(3.8%)	0.81	(0.58-1.14)	0.224
	Int/Int	87	(5.8%)	0.08	(0.80-1.49)	0.575
Microvasc1	Std/Std	118	(11.1%)	1.0		
	Std/Int	118	(10.7%)	0.98	(0.75-1.24)	0.742
	Int/Std	115	(11.1%)	0.98	(0.78-1.27)	0.599
	Int/Int	122	(12.2%)	1.08	(0.83-1.38)	0.581
Microvasc2	Std/Std	398	(55.9%)	1.0		
	Std/Int	381	(53.8%)	0.92	(0.80-1.08)	0.280
	Int/Std	384	(53.4%)	0.97	(0.84-1.11)	0.829
	Int/Int	387	(53.8%)	0.94	(0.81-1.08)	0.379

Fig. 7.2 Five-year event rates comparing the three more intensively treated groups to the standard BP-lowering/standard glucose-lowering treatment group in ACCORD BP trial

participants with standard glycemia therapy, intensive compared with standard blood pressure therapy was associated with a statistically significant 56% reduction of stroke (HR: 0.44, 95% CI: 0.25–0.79); all other secondary outcomes were towards the same direction, without reaching however statistical significance: 25% reduction of any myocardial infarction (HR: 0.75, 95% CI: 0.52–1.08), 19% reduction of cardiovascular death (HR: 0.81, 95% CI: 0.58–1.14), and 19% reduction of total death (HR: 0.81, 95% CI: 0.58–1.14) [17].

The recent findings of the 'twin-study' in non-diabetic patients, the SPRINT trial, with impressive benefits of aggressive blood pressure control down to 120 mmHg add further fuel towards the more aggressive management of hypertension [53]. Moreover, the substantial survival benefits of aggressive therapy in SPRINT were evident in participants with pre-diabetes as well, providing further indirect evidence favoring lower targets [54]. Collectively, data suggesting lower blood pressure targets than currently recommended (<140/90 mmHg) are not robust and conclusive; however the direct cerebrovascular benefits in ACCORD-BP and the indirect evidence from the post-hoc analysis of the ACCORD-BP by Margolis combined with the extrapolations of the SPRINT trial pave the way for considering lower blood pressure targets in diabetic patients at high cardiovascular risk, when these targets can be well tolerated by the patients without any symptoms or signs of adverse events.

The new guidelines have reverted to very strong support for <140/90 mmHg but push for <130/80 mmHg in anyone with a >10% 10-year risk of cardiovascular events [10, 13]. Data from observational studies and large randomized controlled trials (mostly subgroup and/or post-hoc analyses) also supports the cardiovascular benefits of antihypertensive therapy are maintained at lower systolic blood pressure levels, even less than 130 mmHg. Therefore, a systolic blood pressure range of 125–130 mmHg might be the appropriate blood pressure goal in diabetic patients, if it is well-tolerated and devoid of symptoms or signs of cardiovascular and/or renal adverse effects.

Whether this systolic blood pressure range is the intersection where the greatest cardiovascular benefits meet with minimally increased adverse events, thus offering the best benefit/risk ratio remains to be verified. Moreover, it is of utmost clinical importance to identify whether lower blood pressure targets are appropriate for all patients with diabetes mellitus or different targets should be applied according to patient characteristics: baseline cardiovascular risk (high vs moderate vs low), age (very elderly vs elderly vs young), race, renal function, patients at high cerebrovascular risk (prior stroke, South East Asia, Eastern Europe), etc.

Which Are the Preferred Drugs?

A wealth of evidence indicates that the main benefits of antihypertensive therapy derive from the reduction of blood pressure *per se*, irrespective of the drugs used to attain blood pressure reduction [14]. Most guidelines recommend initiating therapy with either a calcium antagonist, a RAS blocker or a thiazide-like diuretic [13, 14]. Therefore, the main goal of hypertension management in patients with diabetes should be to lower the elevated blood pressure. Another factor to consider when first choosing drugs is that patients with diabetes need an average of three drugs to attain blood pressure control [9, 14]. Therefore, the question about the most appropriate first drug is actually deceptive and attention should be focused rather on preferred combinations than in first choice agents.

Given that, RAS-inhibitors offer superior nephroprotection when compared to placebo or other antihypertensive drugs, as shown in IDNT and RENAAL in type 2 diabetes mellitus with angiotensin receptor blockers [25, 26] and the older Collaborative Study Group trial in type I diabetes mellitus with ACE-inhibitors [55]. However, this class of drugs was used on background diuretics and CCBs in these trials. Therefore, RAS-inhibitors should be first choice drugs in patients with diabetes that have macro-albuminuria or very high albuminuria as well as reduced eGFR [10]. The newer recommendations do not mandate their use in microalbuminuric or normotensive people with diabetes. Moreover, RAS-inhibitors are very well combined with calcium antagonists and diuretics, showing enhanced efficacy, while minimizing the adverse effects of these drugs (ankle edema with calcium antagonists, and hypokalemia and metabolic alterations with diuretics), and should therefore be a component of combination therapy in the case that another drug has been selected as a first choice agent. This was clearly shown in the ACCOMPLISH trial [56].

Beta-blockers are associated with worsening of glycemic control and impaired feeling of hypoglycemia and should therefore be used in diabetic patients only when indicated, such as in congestive heart failure, in coronary artery disease and post-myocardial infarction. Vasodilating beta-blockers (carvedilol, nebivolol) do not share the adverse metabolic effects of traditional beta-blockers [57], as shown with carvedilol in the GEMINI trial [58], and could be preferred in diabetic patients.

Since the combination of RAS-inhibitors with calcium antagonists or diuretics are amongst the preferred ones, the question arises whether one of them is superior to the other. In the ACCOMPLISH trial, the combination of an ACE-inhibitor with a calcium antagonist conferred significantly greater reduction of cardiovascular events and mortality compared with the combination with a diuretic [59]. The superiority of a combination with a calcium antagonist was evident in diabetic patients as well, and was maintained even in high-risk diabetic patients [56]. Moreover, renal events were almost halved with this combination compared with the diuretic combination [60]. Therefore, in diabetic patients who need combination therapy (failure to achieve goal blood pressure with monotherapy or very high baseline blood pressure levels), it does not seem clinically unwise to recommend the combination of a RAS-inhibitor with a dihydropyridine calcium antagonist, unless diuretics are indicated or calcium antagonists are contra-indicated. When three drugs are needed, the combination of a RAS-inhibitor with a calcium antagonist and a diuretic seems the most attractive combination from the pathophysiologic point of view and is the most widely used combination in everyday clinical practice.

The combination of two RAS-inhibitors (ACE-inhibitors and angiotensin receptor blockers) should be avoided. The ONTARGET and the VA-NEPHRON trials showed that this combination not only does not confer any significant benefits but is also associated with increased adverse rates [61, 62], including acute kidney injury, a worsening of chronic kidney disease progression, and a higher incidence of hyperkalemia [63]. Similar findings were observed in the Aliskiren Trial in Type 2 Diabetes Using Cardiovascular and Renal Disease Endpoints (ALTITUDE) with the combination of an ACE-inhibitor with a direct renin inhibitor [64].

Another factor that needs to be addressed is the use of fixed combinations instead of liberal ones. The combination of two or even three drugs in one pill is associated with increased adherence to antihypertensive therapy. A meta-analysis by Bangalore et al. showed that adherence to therapy is improved by 26% when fixed combinations are used instead of liberal ones [65]. Better adherence to antihypertensive therapy is associated with significant reductions in cardiovascular morbidity [66] and significant survival benefits [67].

Conclusions

A large number of randomized controlled studies unequivocally demonstrate the benefits of antihypertensive therapy in patients with diabetes mellitus and hypertension. The substantial benefits of antihypertensive therapy are also evident in special patient populations, such as patients with diabetic nephropathy, diabetic patients with isolated systolic hypertension, diabetic patients with prior cerebrovascular disease, and in high-risk patients. All guidelines for the management of hypertension in diabetic patients recommend the initiation of antihypertensive therapy when blood pressure levels are above 140/90 mmHg and the newer ones have set a goal blood pressure of less than 130/80 mmHg, without any discrimination between diabetic and non-diabetic individuals. These recommendations are evidence-based and focus more on cardiovascular risk in the context of achieving blood pressure goal than just the number. Based on all the recent data it seems sound to adopt a more aggressive strategy for the management of elevated blood pressure in high-risk diabetic patients; supporting evidence exists and does not seem right to neglect it.

References

1. Stamler J, Vaccaro O, Neaton JD, et al. Diabetes, other risk factors, and 12-yr cardiovascular mortality for men screened in the Multiple Risk Factor Intervention Trial. Diabetes Care. 1993;16:434–44.
2. White SL, Chadban SJ, Jan S, et al. How can we achieve global equity in provision of renal replacement therapy? Bull World Health Organ. 2008;86:229–37.
3. Whiting DR, Guariguata L, Weil C, Shaw J. IDF diabetes atlas: global estimates on the prevalence of diabetes for 2011 and 2030. Diabetes Res Clin Pract. 2011;94:311–21.
4. Boyle JP, Thompson TJ, Gregg EW, Barker LE, Williamson DF. Projection of the year 2050 burden of diabetes in the US adult population: dynamic modelling of incidence, mortality, and prediabetes prevalence. Popul Health Metr. 2010;8:29.
5. Mayer-Davis EJ, Lawrence JM, Dabelea D, et al. Incidence trends of type 1 and type 2 diabetes among youths, 2002–2012. N Engl J Med. 2017;376:1419–29.
6. Rawshani A, Rawshani A, Franzen S, et al. Mortality and cardiovascular disease in type 1 and type 2 diabetes. New Engl J Med. 2017;376:1407–18.
7. Kearney PM, Whelton M, Reynolds K, et al. Global burden of hypertension: analysis of worldwide data. Lancet. 2005;365:217–23.
8. Lewington S, Clarke R, Qizibash N, Peto R, Collins R. Age specific relevance of usual blood pressure to vascular mortality: a meta-analysis of individual data for one million adults in 61 prospective studies. Lancet. 2002;360:1903–13.
9. American Diabetes Association. Cardiovascular disease and risk management. Diabetes Care. 2017;40:S75–87.

10. de Boer I, Bangalore S, Benetos A, et al. Diabetes and hypertension: a position statement by the American Diabetes Association. Diabetes Care. 2017;40:1273–84.
11. Gradman AH, Basile JN, Carter BL, Bakris GL. Combination therapy in hypertension. J Clin Hypertens. 2011;13:146–54.
12. James PA, Oparil S, Carter BL, Cushman WC, Dennison-Himmelfarb C, Handler J, et al. 2014 evidence-based guideline for the management of high blood pressure in adults: report from the panel members appointed to the Eighth Joint National Committee (JNC 8). JAMA. 2014;311:507–20.
13. Whelton PKCR, Aronow WS, Casey DE Jr, Collins KJ, Dennison- Himmelfarb C, DePalma SM, et al. 2017 ACC/AHA/AAPA/ABC/ACPM/AGS/APhA/ASH/ASPC/NMA/PCNA guideline for the prevention, detection, evaluation and management of high blood pressure in adults: a report of the American College of Cardiology/American Heart Association and Task Force on Clinical Practice guidelines. Hypertension. 2018;71:1269–324.
14. 2018 European Guidelines for the treatment of high blood pressure. In 2018. https://academic.oup.com/eurheartj/article/39/11/908/4934765. Accessed July 15, 2018.
15. UK Prospective Diabetes Study Group. Tight blood pressure control and risk of macrovascular and microvascular complications in type 2 diabetes: UKPDS 38. BMJ. 1998;317:703–13.
16. The ACCORD Study Group. Effects of intensive blood-pressure control in type 2 diabetes mellitus. N Engl J Med. 2010;362:1575–85.
17. Margolis KL, O'Connor PJ, Morgan TM, et al. Outcomes of combined cardiovascular risk factor management strategies in type 2 diabetes: the ACCORD randomized trial. Diabetes Care. 2014;37:1721–8.
18. ADVANCE Collaborative Group. Effects of a fixed combination of perindopril and indapamide on macrovascular and microvascular outcomes in patients with type 2 diabetes mellitus (the ADVANCE trial): a randomised controlled trial. Lancet. 2007;37:829–40.
19. Estacio RO, Jeffers BW, Gifford N, Schrier RW. Effect of blood pressure control on diabetic microvascular complications in patients with hypertension and type 2 diabetes. Diabetes Care. 2000;23:B54–64.
20. Hansson L, Zanchetti A, Carruthers SG, Dahlof B, Elmfeldt D, Julius S, et al. Effects of intensive blood pressure lowering and low-dose aspirin in patients with hypertension: principal results of the Hypertension Optimal Treatment (HOT) randomised trial. HOT Study Group Lancet. 1998;351:1755–62.
21. Schrier RW, Estacio RO, Esler A, Mehler P. Effects of aggressive blood pressure control in normotensive type 2 diabetic patients on albuminuria, retinopathy and strokes. Kidney Int. 2002;61:1086–97.
22. Curb JD, Pressel SL, Cutler JA, Savage PJ, Applegate WB, Black H, et al. Systolic Hypertension in the Elderly Program Cooperative Research Group. Effect of diuretic-based antihypertensive treatment on cardiovascular disease risk in older diabetic patients with isolated systolic hypertension. JAMA. 1996;276:1886–92.
23. Tuomilehto J, Rastenyte D, Birkenhäger WH, Thijs L, Antikainen R, Bulpitt CJ, et al. Effects of calcium-channel blockade in older patients with diabetes and systolic hypertension. N Engl J Med. 1999;340:677–84.
24. Berthet K, Neal BC, Chalmers JP, MacMahon SW, Bousser M-G, Colman SA, et al. Reductions in the risks of recurrent stroke in patients with and without diabetes: the PROGRESS trial. Blood Press. 2004;13:7–13.
25. Brenner BM, Cooper ME, de Zeeuw D, Keane WF, Mitch WE, Parving HH, et al. Effects of losartan on renal and cardiovascular outcomes in patients with type 2 diabetes and nephropathy. N Engl J Med. 2001;345:861–9.
26. Lewis EJ, Hunsicker LG, Clarke WR, Berl T, Pohl MA, Lewis JB, et al. Renoprotective effect of the angiotensin-receptor antagonist irbesartan in patients with nephropathy due to type 2 diabetes. N Engl J Med. 2001;345:851–60.
27. Arguedas JA, Leiva V, Wright JM. Blood pressure targets for hypertension in people with diabetes mellitus. Cochrane Database Syst Rev. 2013;10:CD008277.
28. Bangalore S, Kumar S, Lobach I, Messerli FH. Blood pressure targets in subjects with type 2 diabetes mellitus/impaired fasting glucose: observations from traditional and bayesian random-effects meta-analyses of randomized trials. Circulation. 2011;123:2799–810.
29. Emdin CA, Rahimi K, Neal B, Callender T, Perkovic V, Patel A. Blood pressure lowering in type 2 diabetes. A systematic review and meta-analysis. JAMA. 2015;313:603–15.
30. Thomopoulos C, Parati G, Zanchetti A. Effects of blood pressure lowering treatment on outcome incidence in hypertension: 10 – should blood pressure management differ in hypertensive patients with and without diabetes mellitus? Overview and meta-analyses of randomized trials. J Hypertens. 2017;35:922–44.
31. Remonti LR, Dias S, Leitao CB, et al. Classes of antihypertensive agents and mortality in hypertensive patients with type 2 diabetes–network meta-analysis of randomized trials. J Diabetes Complicat. 2016;30:1192–200.
32. Brunström M, Carlberg B. Effect of antihypertensive treatment at different blood pressure levels in patients with diabetes mellitus: systematic review and meta-analyses. BMJ. 2016;352:i717.
33. Dojki FK, Bakris G. Blood pressure goals in T2DM – time for a rethink? Nat Rev Endocrinol. 2016;12:629–30.
34. Glassock RJ, Bakris G. Impact of blood pressure lowering in type 2 diabetes. Nat Rev Nephrol. 2015;11:320–1.

35. Laffin LJ, Bakris G. Update on blood pressure goals in diabetes mellitus. Curr Cardiol Rep. 2015;17:37.
36. Yamout H, Bakris G. In search for the 'sweet spot' for blood pressure level in diabetes. Heart. 2014;100:1404–5.
37. Sternlicht H, Bakris G. Management of hypertension in diabetic nephropathy: how low should we go? Blood Purif. 2016;41:139–43.
38. Patney V, Whaley-Connell A, Bakris G. Hypertension management in diabetic kidney disease. Diabetes Spectr. 2015;28:175–80.
39. Yamout H, Lazich I, Bakris G. Blood pressure, hypertension, RAAS blockade, and drug therapy in diabetic kidney disease. Adv Chronic Kidney Dis. 2014;21:281–6.
40. Vasan RS, Larson MG, Leip EP, Kannel WB, Levy D. Assessment of frequency of progression to hypertension in non-hypertensive participants in the Framingham Heart Study: a cohort study. Lancet. 2001;358:1682–6.
41. Doumas M, Katsiki N, Mikhailidis D. Prehypertension, the risk of hypertension, and events. (in press).
42. Guo X, Zhang X, Guo L, Li Z, Zheng L, Yu S, Yang H, Zhou X, Zhang X, Sun Z, Li J, Sun Y. Association between pre-hypertension and cardiovascular outcomes: a systematic review and meta-analysis of prospective studies. Curr Hypertens Rep. 2013;15:703–16.
43. Li Y, Xia P, Xu L, Wang Y, Chen L. A meta-analysis on prehypertension and chronic kidney disease. PLoS One. 2016;11:e0156575.
44. Huang Y, Su L, Cai X, Mai W, Wang S, Hu Y, Wu Y, Tang H, Xu D. Association of all-cause and cardiovascular mortality with prehypertension: a meta-analysis. Am Heart J. 2014;167:160–8.
45. Wang S, Wu H, Zhang Q, Xu J, Fan Y. Impact of baseline prehypertension on cardiovascular events and all-cause mortality in the general population: a meta-analysis of prospective cohort studies. Int J Cardiol. 2013;168:4857–60.
46. Bangalore S, Messerli FH, Wun CC, et al. J-curve revisited: an analysis of blood pressure and cardiovascular events in the Treating to New Targets (TNT) trial. Eur Heart J. 2010;31:2897–908.
47. Kjeldsen SE, Berge E, Bangalore S, et al. No evidence for a J-shaped curve in treated hypertensive patients with increased cardiovascular risk: the VALUE trial. Blood Press. 2016;25:83–92.
48. Weber MA, Bloch M, Bakris GL, et al. Cardiovascular outcomes according to systolic blood pressure in patients with and without diabetes: an ACCOMPLISH substudy. J Clin Hypertens. 2016;18:299–307.
49. Adamsson Eryd S, Gudbjornsdottir S, Manhem K, et al. Blood pressure and complications in individuals with type 2 diabetes and no previous cardiovascular disease: national population based cohort study. BMJ. 2016;354:14070.
50. Adler AI, Stratton IM, Neil HA, et al. Association of systolic blood pressure with macrovascular and microvascular complications of type 2 diabetes (UKPDS 36): prospective observational study. BMJ. 2000;321:412–9.
51. Xie X, Atkins E, Lv J, et al. Effects of intensive blood pressure lowering on cardiovascular and renal outcomes: updated systematic review and meta-analysis. Lancet. 2016;387:435–43.
52. Ettehad D, Emdin CA, Kiran A, Anderson SG, Callender T, Emberson J, et al. Blood pressure lowering for prevention of cardiovascular disease and death: a systematic review and meta-analysis. Lancet. 2016;387:957–67.
53. The SPRINT Research Group. A randomized trial of intensive versus standard blood-pressure control. N Engl J Med. 2015;373:2103–16.
54. Bress A, Beddhu S, King J, et al. Intensive blood pressure control reduces cardiovascular events in patients with prediabetes. Presented at: American Diabetes Association 77th Scientific Sessions; June 9–13, 2017; San Diego, CA. Abstract 212-LB.
55. Lewis EJ, Hunsicker LG, Bain RP, Rohde RD. The effect of angiotensin-converting-enzyme inhibition on diabetic nephropathy. The Collaborative Study Group. N Engl J Med. 1993;329:1456–62.
56. Weber MA, Bakris GL, Jamerson K, Weir M, Kjeldsen SE, Devereux RB, et al. Cardiovascular events during differing hypertension therapies in patients with diabetes. J Am Coll Cardiol. 2010;56:77–85.
57. Manolis A, Doumas M. Erectile function in cardiovascular disease and hypertension: the role of nebivolol. J Hypertens. 2016;5:226.
58. Bakris GL, Fonseca V, Katholi RE, et al. Metabolic effects of carvedilol vs metoprolol in patients with type 2 diabetes mellitus and hypertension: a randomized controlled trial. JAMA. 2004;292:2227–36.
59. Jamerson K, Weber MA, Bakris GL, Dahlöf B, Pitt B, Shi V, et al. Benazepril plus amlodipine or hydrochlorothiazide for hypertension in high-risk patients. N Engl J Med. 2008;359:2417–28.
60. Bakris GL, Sarafidis PA, Weir MR, et al. Renal outcomes with different fixed-dose combination therapies in patients with hypertension at high risk for cardiovascular events (ACCOMPLISH): a prespecified secondary analysis of a randomized controlled trial. Lancet. 2010;375:1173–81.
61. ONTARGET Investigators. Telmisartan, ramipril, or both in patients at high risk for vascular events. N Engl J Med. 2008;358:1547–59.
62. Fried LF, Emanuele N, Zhang JH, et al. Combined angiotensin inhibition for the treatment of diabetic nephropathy. N Engl J Med. 2013;369:1892–903.
63. Mann J, Schmieder R, McQueen M, et al. Renal outcomes with telmisartan, ramipril or both in people at high vascular risk (the ONTARGET study): a multicentre, randomized, double-blind, controlled trial. Lancet. 2008;372:547–53.
64. ALTITUDE Investigators. Cardiorenal endpoints in a trial of aliskiren for type 2 diabetes. N Engl J Med. 2012;367:2204–13.

65. Bangalore S, Kamalakkannan G, Parkar S, Messerli FH. Fixed-dose combinations improve medication compliance. Am J Med. 2007;120:713–9.
66. Mazzaglia G, Ambrosioni E, Alacqua M, et al. Adherence to antihypertensive medications and cardiovascular morbidity among newly diagnosed hypertensive patients. Circulation. 2009;120: 1598–605.
67. Chowdhury R, Khan H, Heydon E, et al. Adherence to cardiovascular therapy: a meta-analysis of prevalence and clinical consequences. Eur Heart J. 2013;34:2940–8.

Chronic Kidney Disease and Hypertension

8

Pedro A. Jose and Van Anthony M. Villar

Hypertension can cause kidney disease and kidney disease can cause hypertension [1]. However, hypertension may cause progressive kidney disease only in genetically susceptible individuals [2, 3]. According to the National Kidney Foundation Kidney Disease Outcomes Quality Initiative (KDOQI) guidelines, chronic kidney disease is defined as abnormalities of the kidney structure or function that is present for ≥3 months (Table 8.1) [4, 5]. A surrogate end-point, decline in estimated glomerular filtration rate (GFR) of 30–40% over 2–3 years, has also been suggested as the definition of chronic kidney disease [6, 7]. The prevalence of chronic kidney disease is rising sharply worldwide and affects 13.1% of the population in the USA [8, 9]. Patients with chronic kidney disease represent a population not only at risk of progression to end-organ failure but are also at higher risk for cardiovascular diseases, including hypertension [1, 9]. Kidney failure is defined as GFR <15 ml/min or on dialysis, as per KDOQI guidelines [4, 5]. End-stage renal disease (ESRD), an administrative term in the United States, includes patients treated by dialysis or transplantation, irrespective of the level of GFR [10]. Relative to previous years, in 2013, the second most common cause of ESRD continues to be hypertension, the prevalence of which is about 30% [1, 9]. The incidence of hypertension in patients with kidney disease increases with decreasing GFR: 18.3% (GFR ≤90 ml/min/1.73 m^2); 41.0% (GFR 60–89 ml/min/1.73 m^2); 71.8% (GFR 45–59 ml/min/1.73m^2; 78.3% (GFR 30–44 ml/min/1.73 m2); and 82.1% (GFR < 30 ml/min/1.73 m^2) [9]. A recent meta-analysis reported that the incidence of hypertension is 84% in patients with estimated GFR <60 ml/min [11].

P. A. Jose (✉)
Division of Renal Diseases and Hypertension, The George Washington University School of Medicine and Health Sciences, Washington, DC, USA

Department of Medicine and Department of Pharmacology and Physiology, The George Washington University School of Medicine and Health Sciences, Washington, DC, USA

Department of Medicine, The George Washington University School of Medicine and Health Sciences, Washington, DC, USA
e-mail: pjose@mfa.gwu.edu

V. A. M. Villar
Division of Renal Diseases & Hypertension, The George Washington University School of Medicine and Health Sciences, Washington, DC, USA

Department of Medicine, The George Washington University School of Medicine and Health Sciences, Washington, DC, USA

History of Kidney Disease and Hypertension

In 1808, Thomas I. Young suggested in his Croonian Lecture on the functions of the heart and arteries that an increase in the hydrostatic pressure of the blood could distend the artery,

V. Papademetriou et al. (eds.), *Management of Hypertension*,
https://doi.org/10.1007/978-3-319-92946-0_8

Table 8.1 Criteria for Chronic Kidney Disease [4, 5]

Markers of kidney damage (one or more)	Albuminuria (AER ≥30 mg/24 hr.; ACR ≥30 mg/g (≥3 mg/mmol)) Urine sediment abnormalities Electrolyte and other abnormalities due to tubular disorders Abnormalities detected by histology Structural abnormalities detected by imaging History of kidney transplantation
Decreased GFR	GFR <60 ml/min/1.73 m^2

GFR glomerular filtration rate, *AER* albumin excretion rate, *ACR* albumin-to-creatinine ratio

making it weak and give way [12]. In 1836, Richard Bright noted an association between the heart and the kidney and that the blood vessels in the kidneys are chronically inflamed due to the presence of albumin in the urine [13]. In 1914, Volhard and Fahr classified kidney diseases into three groups, degenerative, inflammatory, and arteriosclerotic diseases [14]. They further divided nephrosclerosis into the benign and malignant form and suggested a role of increased blood pressure and inflammation in the pathogenesis of renal disease [14, 15].

Role of the Kidney in Hypertension

The kidney is crucial in the long-term regulation of blood pressure [16–47]. The kidney controls blood pressure by secretion of vasoactive hormones and regulation of water and electrolyte balance [16–30, 41–44]. Inherent renal arterial myogenic responses also modify the response of the kidney to increased blood pressure [46–49]. Therefore, many studies have focused on the abnormal renal handling of sodium in the pathogenesis of essential hypertension [16–30]. Renal sodium transport is increased in humans with essential hypertension and several animal models of essential hypertension [16–30]. The impaired renal sodium handling in essential hypertension may be the result of abnormal regulation of natriuretic and antinatriuretic pathways [16–30, 50]. The sympathetic nervous [16–18, 39, 40, 46, 51–53] and renin-angiotensin systems [16–18, 38, 41, 42, 46, 48] are antinatriuretic pathways. Products of arachidonic acid metabolism [16, 17, 46, 54], dopamine [16, 18, 28, 43, 46, 54], endothelin [55, 56], kallikrein-kinin [50], and nitric oxide [6, 17, 18, 46, 56], among others, provide important counter-regulatory natriuretic pathways.

Role of the kidney in hypertension: evidence from experimental models of hypertension Direct and indirect measurements (e.g., lithium clearance) have shown that sodium and fluid reabsorptions in the renal proximal tubule and thick ascending limb of Henle are increased in several rodent models of essential hypertension [16–18] (e.g., spontaneously hypertensive rat [SHR] [19, 20], Dahl salt-sensitive rat [21, 22], Milan hypertensive rat [23]) but distal tubule mechanisms may also be involved (e.g., Sabra hypertensive rat [23, 24]). Abnormal pressure-natriuresis is also observed early in the Lyon hypertensive rat [25]. Essential hypertension in humans is also associated with increased sodium transport in the renal proximal tubule and medullary thick ascending limb, although increased distal tubular transport has also been reported [26–29] . By contrast, monogenic hypertension is caused by increased sodium transport mainly in the distal nephron [30].

Direct proof of the importance of the kidney in the long-term regulation of blood pressure comes from renal transplantation studies. Several studies have shown that the transplantation of Wistar-Kyoto (WKY) kidneys into first-generation offspring from a cross of WKY and SHRs reduces or prevents the increase in blood pressure with age; conversely, transplantation of SHR kidneys into normotensive rats increases blood pressure [31]. Cross-transplantation experiments in genetically hypertensive rats have also demonstrated the importance of the kidney and the contribution of extrarenal factors to the long-term regulation of blood pressure [31–34]. The high blood pressure in the recipients of "hypertensive" kidneys is associated with sodium retention [35] and an elevated sensitivity of the blood pressure of SHRs to sodium intake has been previously documented [36, 37]. However, the fact that transplantation of WKY kidneys into SHRs does not always normalize blood pressure supports the notion that extrarenal mechanisms may also contribute to the long-term regulation of blood pressure [38]. Subsequent experiments showed that the contribution of the kidneys to hypertension, even in SHRs, is modified by extrarenal factors [39]. One example of an extrarenal contributor to blood pressure regulation is the sympathetic nervous system; the sensitivity of blood pressure to sodium intake is reduced by neonatal sympathectomy [40]. Cross-transplantation studies in mice also suggest that about 50% of blood pressure control is renal and about 50% is extra-renal, depending on the experimental model [41–43].

Role of the kidney in hypertension: evidence from humans with essential hypertension The importance of the kidney in the long-term regulation of blood pressure in humans was first supported by the studies of Curtis et al. [44]. They reported the normalization of blood pressure in six African Americans with malignant hypertension after renal transplantation. Subsequently, Guidi et al. reported that the ability of a transplanted "hypertensive" kidney to transmit hypertension was found only in those recipients without a family history of hypertension [45]. Surprisingly, this did not occur in renal transplant recipients with a positive family history of hypertension. The authors suggested that recipients with a family history of hypertension may have developed extra-renal mechanisms that counteract the renal pressor effect of the transplanted kidney.

Does Hypertension Cause Kidney Disease?

Hypertension and Kidney Disease: Experimental Evidence

Renal blood flow and GFR are independent of renal perfusion pressure over a defined range (80–180 mmHg) [46]. An increase in renal perfusion pressure above the upper limits of autoregulation or impaired autoregulation, secondary to impaired myogenic constriction, would allow the perfusion pressure to damage the renal arterioles and glomeruli and subsequently the renal tubules [46, 47]. Impaired myogenic constriction has been shown in experimental animals and humans with hypertension [47–49]. The impaired myogenic response in hypertension may be intrinsic or secondary to abnormalities in vasoconstrictor and constrictor hormones [46, 50].

The Dahl salt-sensitive rat [21, 22], Fawn-hooded hypertensive rat [57], Lyon hypertensive rat [25], Milan hypertensive rat [23], Sabra hypertension-prone rat [24], SHR [19, 20, 58, 59], salt-loaded stroke-prone SHR [57], and two-kidney, one-clip rat [60–62] are well-characterized models of hypertension, and the development of hypertension and hypertensive kidney damage in many of these models has been described. In the SHR, it is claimed that the renal damage is pressure-dependent; the vascular damage leads to a loss of autoregulation and arterial hypertrophy in the juxtamedullary cortex. The early vascular damage in the juxtamedullary nephrons causes tubular atrophy and interstitial fibrosis which progress along the vascular tree out into the outer cortex [59]. The similar pattern of renal damage in the SHR, salt-loaded stroke-prone SHR, and the nonclipped kidney after 24 weeks of two-kidney, one-clip hypertension is suggestive of a common genetic pathway [62]. The unclipped kidneys, which are exposed to high blood pressure for 11 weeks, develop glomerular and tubulointerstitial injury with tubulointerstitial cell proliferation and interstitial monocyte-macrophage infiltration. By contrast, clipped kidneys, protected from hypertension but with high local renin expression, have minimal abnormalities [60]. Attenuating the development and severity of hypertension prevents the development of end-organ damage in two-kidney, one-clip hypertensive rat model [61].

Hypertension and Kidney Disease: Clinical Evidence

Many but not all observational studies have shown a log-linear increase in the risk of kidney failure with high blood pressure levels [63–65], even those in the prehypertension range, especially in the elderly [65]. A group of investigators that found absence of an association between elevated blood pressure and accelerated decline in GFR [66] found in another study that ambulatory arterial stiffness, which is calculated from ambulatory blood pressure, is an independent risk factor for the accelerated age-related decline in GFR [67] in a middle-aged white population. In African-Americans, the risk of blood pressure-related ESRD is high, independent of age and sex [68]. Genetics may play a role because there is an association of coding variants of apolipoprotein L1 (*APOL1*) and mild kidney disease but not cardiovascular disease in African-Americans with hypertension [69, 70]. However, *APOL1* variants are not associated with the longitudinal increase in blood pressure [71]. Additional genes are probably involved in hypertension causing kidney disease and vice versa because there are no *APOL1* risk alleles in a remote living aboriginal group with high rates of chronic kidney disease and hypertension [72]. Indeed, loss of *GSTM1* (glutathione S-transferase Mu 1) is associated with accelerated progression of hypertensive kidney disease in the African American Study of Kidney Disease (AASK) [73]. African Americans with both *APOL1* high-risk alleles and *GSTM1* null have the highest risk of adverse renal outcomes [74]. Age has to be factored in these studies because about 20% of elderly (≥60 years) hypertensive patients without cardiovascular disease have moderate decrease in GFR [75]. Whereas hypertension is a frequent cause of kidney disease in the adult population, in the pediatric population, hypertension is usually caused by kidney disease [76]. In the adult population, strict blood pressure control many not always delay the progression of chronic kidney disease to ESRD and could increase the risk of death [77–82]. However, in the pediatric population, strict blood pressure control delays the progression of kidney disease [83]. In general, non-malignant hypertension is probably not an important *de novo* cause of renal insufficiency but rather a promoter of existing kidney disease [84].

Hypertensive nephrosclerosis is a non-specific clinical diagnosis given to patients with chronic kidney disease, low-level proteinuria, and elevated blood pressure [85]. However, this term is all encompassing of kidney diseases with hypertension, including the nephrosclerosis with aging, obesity, and atherosclerosis. It has been suggested to use the term "arterionephrosclerosis" as the clinical diagnosis of patients with chronic kidney disease and elevated blood pressure in patients without diabetic disease or known genetic cause. In patients with a known genetic cause, the term glomerulosclerosis preceded by the genetic cause should be used, e.g., *APOL1*-associated glomerulosclerosis [85, 86]. The main renal histological finding in nephrosclerosis is interstitial inflammatory fibrosis [85]. Oxidative stress also participates in the pathogenesis of nephrosclerosis, independently of blood pressure, in the SHR [87]. A reactive oxygen species scavenging drug, e,g., 3-dimercaptosuccinic acid, prevented the nephrosclerosis and rise in blood pressure in Dahl salt-sensitive rats [88]. The hypertensive nephropathy associated with angiotensin II-induced hypertension is due in part to oxidative stress and inflammation caused by CC chemokine receptor 2 activation [89]. Increased sodium chloride intake can cause not only essential hypertension [18–29] but also inflammation [90–95], oxidative stress [96–99], and kidney disease [100–103].

Conclusion

Inflammation and oxidative stress are important in the pathogenesis of hypertension and renal disease [104–108]. Inflammation can cause oxidative stress and vice versa [105, 109]. Sodium chloride can cause inflammation, oxidative stress, hypertension, and kidney disease [110, 111] (Fig. 8.1). It is likely that hypertension and kidney disease can have the same causes, e.g., increased sodium intake, products of metabolism, including uric acid [112], inflammation, oxidative stress, and environmental pollution [113–116], among others.

Acknowledgment This work is supported, in part, by grants from the National Institutes of Health: HL023081, HL092196, HL068686, HL068686, and DK039308.

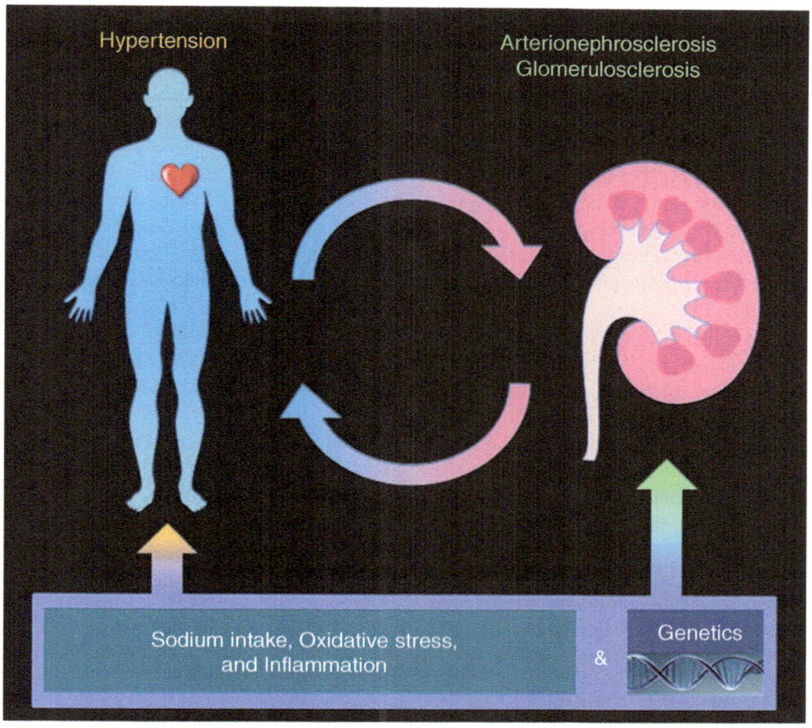

Fig. 8.1 Sodium chloride intake, oxidative stress, and inflammation interact with genetics to cause hypertensive kidney disease

References

1. Kopp JB. Rethinking hypertensive kidney disease: arterionephrosclerosis as a genetic, metabolic, and inflammatory disorder. Curr Opin Nephrol Hypertens. 2013;22:266–72.
2. O'Seaghdha CM, Fox CS. Genetics of chronic kidney disease. Nephron Clin Pract. 2011;118:c55–63.
3. Garrett MR, Pezzolesi MG, Korstanje R. Integrating human and rodent data to identify the genetic factors involved in chronic kidney disease. J Am Soc Nephrol. 2010;21:398–405.
4. Kidney Disease: Improving Global Outcomes (KDIGO) CKD Work Group. KDIGO 2012 clinical practice guideline for the evaluation and management of chronic kidney disease. Kidney Int Suppl. 2013;3:1–150.
5. KDIGO 2017. Clinical practice guideline update for the diagnosis, evaluation, prevention, and treatment of chronic kidney disease–mineral and bone disorder (CKD-MBD). Kidney Int Suppl. 2017;7:1–59.
6. Levey AS, Inker LA, Matsushita K, Greene T, Willis K, Lewis E, et al. GFR decline as an end point for clinical trials in CKD: a scientific workshop sponsored by the National Kidney Foundation and the US Food and Drug Administration. Am J Kidney Dis. 2014;64:821–35.
7. Chang WX, Asakawa S, Toyoki D, Nemoto Y, Morimoto C, Tamura Y, et al. Predictors and the subsequent risk of end-stage renal disease – usefulness of 30% decline in estimated GFR over 2 years. PLoS One. 2015;10:e0132927.
8. Coresh J, Selvin E, Stevens LA, Manzi J, Kusek JW, Eggers P, et al. Prevalence of chronic kidney disease in the United States. JAMA. 2007;298:2038–47.
9. U.S. Renal Data System. Atlas of Chronic Kidney Disease and End-Stage Renal Disease in the United States. Bethesda, MD: National Institutes of Health, National Institute of Diabetes and Digestive and Kidney Diseases; 2008. USRDS 2015 Annual Data Report. http://www.usrds.org/adr.aspx.
10. National Kidney Foundation. K/DOQI clinical practice guidelines for chronic kidney disease: evaluation, classification, and stratification. Am J Kidney Dis. 2002;39:S1–266.
11. Tangri N, Grams ME, Levey AS, Coresh J, Appel LJ, Astor BC, et al. Multinational assessment of accuracy of equations for predicting risk of kidney failure: a meta-analysis. JAMA. 2016;315:164–74.
12. Young TI. The Croonian lecture. On the functions of the heart and arteries. Phil Trans R Soc Lond. 1809;1:1–31.
13. Bright R. Tabular view of the morbid appearances in 100 cases connected with albuminous urine: with observations. Guys Hosp Rep. 1836;1:380–400.
14. Volhard F, Fahr T. Die Brightsche Nierenkrankheit. Klinik, Pathologie und Atlas. Berlin: Springer; 1914.
15. Heidland A, Gerabek W, Sebekova K. Franz Volhard and Theodor Fahr: achievements and controversies

in their research in renal disease and hypertension. J Hum Hypertens. 2001;15:5–16.
16. Hall JE, Granger JP, do Carmo JM, da Silva AA, Dubinion J, George E, et al. Hypertension: physiology and pathophysiology. Compr Physiol. 2012;2:2393–442.
17. Majid DS, Prieto MC, Navar LG. Salt-sensitive hypertension: perspectives on intrarenal mechanisms. Curr Hypertens Rev. 2015;11:38–48.
18. Ortiz PA, Garvin JL. Intrarenal transport and vasoactive substances in hypertension. Hypertension. 2001;38:621–4.
19. LaPointe MS, Sodhi C, Sahai A, Batlle D. Na+/H+ exchange activity and NHE-3 expression in renal tubules from the spontaneously hypertensive rat. Kidney Int. 2002;62:157–65.
20. Sonalker PA, Tofovic SP, Jackson EK. Cellular distribution of the renal bumetanide-sensitive Na-K-2Cl cotransporter BSC-1 in the inner stripe of the outer medulla during the development of hypertension in the spontaneously hypertensive rat. Clin Exp Pharmacol Physiol. 2007;34:1307–12.
21. Liu J, Yan Y, Liu L, Xie Z, Malhotra D, Joe B, et al. Impairment of Na/K-ATPase signaling in renal proximal tubule contributes to Dahl salt-sensitive hypertension. J Biol Chem. 2011;286:22806–13.
22. Roman RJ, Kaldunski ML. Enhanced chloride reabsorption in the loop of Henle in Dahl salt-sensitive rats. Hypertension. 1991;17:1018–24.
23. Ferrandi M, Salardi S, Parenti P, Ferrari P, Bianchi G, Braw R, et al. Na+/K+/Cl(−)-cotransporter mediated Rb+ fluxes in membrane vesicles from kidneys of normotensive and hypertensive rats. Biochim Biophys Acta. 1990;1021:13–20.
24. Yagil Y, Mekler J, Wald H, Popovtzer MM, Ben-Ishay D. Sodium handling by the Sabra hypertension prone (SBH) and resistant (SBN) rats. Pflugers Arch. 1986;407:547–51.
25. Miao CY, Liu KL, Benzoni D, Sassard J. Acute pressure-natriuresis function shows early impairment in Lyon hypertensive rats. J Hypertens. 2005;23:1225–31.
26. Aviv A, Hollenberg NK, Weder A. Urinary potassium excretion and sodium sensitivity in blacks. Hypertension. 2004;43:707–13.
27. Chiolero A, Maillard M, Nussberger J, Brunner HR, Burnier M. Proximal sodium reabsorption: an independent determinant of blood pressure response to salt. Hypertension. 2000;36:631–7.
28. Doris PA. Promoting regulatory gene variation in sodium reabsorption. Hypertension. 2008;52:623–4.
29. Strazzullo P, Galletti F, Barba G. Altered renal handling of sodium in human hypertension: short review of the evidence. Hypertension. 2003;41:1000–5.
30. Lifton RP, Wilson FH, Choate KA, Geller DS. Salt and blood pressure: new insight from human genetic studies. Cold Spring Harb Symp Quant Biol. 2002;67:445–50.
31. Bianchi G, Fox U, Di Francesco GF, Giovanetti AM, Pagetti D. Blood pressure changes produced by kidney cross-transplantation between spontaneously hypertensive rats and normotensive rats. Clin Sci Mol Med. 1974;47:435–48.
32. Morgan DA, DiBona GF, Mark AL. Effects of interstrain renal transplantation on NaCl-induced hypertension in Dahl rats. Hypertension. 1990;5:436–42.
33. Churchill PC, Churchill MC, Bidani AK, Kurtz TW. Kidney-specific chromosome transfer in genetic hypertension: the Dahl hypothesis revisited. Kidney Int. 2001;60:705–14.
34. Dahl LK, Heine M, Thompson K. Genetic influence of the kidneys on blood pressure. Evidence from chronic renal homografts in rats with opposite predispositions to hypertension. Circ Res. 1974;40:94–101.
35. Frey BA, Grisk O, Bandelow N, Wussow S, Bie P, Rettig R. Sodium homeostasis in transplanted rats with a spontaneously hypertensive rat kidney. Am J Physiol Regul Integr Comp Physiol. 2000;279:R10991104.
36. Calhoun DA, Zhu S, Wyss JM, Oparil S. Diurnal blood pressure variation and dietary salt in spontaneously hypertensive rats. Hypertension. 1994;24:1–7.
37. Ely DE, Thorén P, Wiegand J, Folkow B. Sodium appetite as well as 24-h variations of fluid balance, mean arterial pressure and heart rate in spontaneously hypertensive (SHR) and normotensive (WKY) rats, when on various sodium diets. Acta Physiol Scand. 1987;129:81–92.
38. Sander S, Rettig R, Ehrig B. Role of the native kidney in experimental post transplantation hypertension. Pflugers Arch. 1996;431:971–6.
39. Grisk O, Frey BAJ, Uber A, Rettig R. Sympathetic activity in early renal posttransplantation hypertension in rats. Am J Physiol Regul Integr Comp Physiol. 2000;279:R1737–44.
40. Grisk O, Rose HJ, Lorenz G, Rettig R. Sympathetic renal interaction in chronic arterial pressure control. Am J Physiol Regul Integr Comp Physiol. 2002;283:R441–50.
41. Crowley SD, Coffman TM. In hypertension, the kidney breaks your heart. Curr Cardiol Rep. 2008;10:470–6.
42. Crowley SD, Gurley SB, Herrera MJ, Ruiz P, Griffiths R, Kumar AP, et al. Angiotensin II causes hypertension and cardiac hypertrophy through its receptors in the kidney. Proc Natl Acad Sci U S A. 2006;103:17985–90.
43. Asico L, Zhang X, Jiang J, Cabrera D, Escano CS, Sibley DR, et al. Lack of renal dopamine D5 receptors promotes hypertension. J Am Soc Nephrol. 2011;22:82–9.
44. Curtis JJ, Luke RG, Dustan HP, Kashgarian M, Whelchel JD, Jones P, et al. Remission of essential hypertension after renal transplantation. N Engl J Med. 1983;309:1009–15.
45. Guidi E, Menghetti D, Milani S, Montagnino G, Palazzi P, Bianchi G. Hypertension may be transplanted with the kidney in humans: a long-term historical prospective follow-up of recipients grafted with kidneys coming from donors with or without hypertension in their families. J Am Soc Nephrol. 1996;7:1131–8.

46. Carlström M, Wilcox CS, Arendshorst WJ. Renal autoregulation in health and disease. Physiol Rev. 2015;95:405–511.
47. Vavrinec P, Henning RH, Goris M, Landheer SW, Buikema H, van Dokkum RP. Renal myogenic constriction protects the kidney from age-related hypertensive renal damage in the Fawn-Hooded rat. J Hypertens. 2013;31:1637–45.
48. Vettoretti S, Ochodnicky P, Buikema H, Henning RH, Kluppel CA, de Zeeuw D, et al. Altered myogenic constriction and endothelium-derived hyperpolarizing factor-mediated relaxation in small mesenteric arteries of hypertensive subtotally nephrectomized rats. J Hypertens. 2006;24:2215–23.
49. Schofield I, Malik R, Izzard A, Austin C, Heagerty A. Vascular structural and functional changes in type 2 diabetes mellitus: evidence for the roles of abnormal myogenic responsiveness and dyslipidemia. Circulation. 2002;106:3037–43.
50. Rhaleb NE, Yang XP, Carretero OA. The kallikrein-kinin system as a regulator of cardiovascular and renal function. Compr Physiol. 2011;1:971–93.
51. Osborn JW, Fink GD, Kuroki MT. Neural mechanisms of angiotensin II-salt hypertension: implications for therapies targeting neural control of the splanchnic circulation. Curr Hypertens Rep. 2011;13:221–8.
52. DiBona GF. Sympathetic nervous system and hypertension. Hypertension. 2013;61:556–60.
53. Young CN, Davisson RL. In vivo assessment of neurocardiovascular regulation in the mouse: principles, progress, and prospects. Am J Physiol Heart Circ Physiol. 2011;301:H654–62.
54. Fernandez MM, Gonzalez D, Williams JM, Roman RJ, Nowicki S. Inhibitors of 20-hydroxyeicosatetraenoic acid (20-HETE) formation attenuate the natriuretic effect of dopamine. Eur J Pharmacol. 2012;686:97–103.
55. Speed JS, Fox BM, Johnston JG, Pollock DM. Endothelin and renal ion and water transport. Semin Nephrol. 2015;35:137–44.
56. Hyndman KA, Dugas C, Arguello AM, Goodchild TT, Buckley KM, Burch M, et al. High salt induces autocrine actions of ET-1 on inner medullary collecting duct NO production via upregulated ETB receptor expression. Am J Physiol Regul Integr Comp Physiol. 2016;311:R263–71.
57. Kodavanti UP, Russell JC, Costa DL. Rat models of cardiometabolic diseases: baseline clinical chemistries, and rationale for their use in examining air pollution health effects. Inhal Toxicol. 2015;27(Suppl 1):2–13.
58. Watanabe Y, Yoshida M, Yamanishi K, Yamamoto H, Okuzaki D, Nojima H, et al. Genetic analysis of genes causing hypertension and stroke in spontaneously hypertensive rats: gene expression profiles in the kidneys. Int J Mol Med. 2015;36:712–24.
59. Hultström M. Development of structural kidney damage in spontaneously hypertensive rats. J Hypertens. 2012;30:1087–91.
60. Eng E, Veniant M, Floege J, Fingerle J, Alpers CE, Menard J, et al. Renal proliferative and phenotypic changes in rats with two-kidney, one-clip Goldblatt hypertension. Am J Hypertens. 1994;7:177–85.
61. Gudbrandsen OA, Hultstrøm M, Leh S, Monica Bivol L, Vågnes Ø, Berge RK, et al. Prevention of hypertension and organ damage in 2-kidney, 1-clip rats by tetradecylthioacetic acid. Hypertension. 2006;48:460–6.
62. Skogstrand T, Leh S, Paliege A, Reed RK, Vikse BE, Bachmann S, et al. Arterial damage precedes the development of interstitial damage in the nonclipped kidney of two-kidney, one-clip hypertensive rats. J Hypertens. 2013;31:152–9.
63. Klag MJ, Whelton PK, Randall BL, Neaton JD, Brancati FL, Ford CE, et al. Blood pressure and end-stage renal disease in men. N Engl J Med. 1996;334:13–8.
64. Tozawa M, Iseki K, Iseki C, Kinjo K, Ikemiya Y, Takishita S. Blood pressure predicts risk of developing end-stage renal disease in men and women. Hypertension. 2003;41:1341–5.
65. Garofalo C, Borrelli S, Pacilio M, Minutolo R, Chiodini P, De Nicola L, et al. Hypertension and prehypertension and prediction of development of decreased estimated GFR in the general population: a meta-analysis of cohort studies. Am J Kidney Dis. 2016;67:89–97.
66. Eriksen BO, Stefansson VT, Jenssen TG, Mathisen UD, Schei J, Solbu MD, et al. Blood pressure and age-related GFR decline in the general population. BMC Nephrol. 2017;18(1):77.
67. Eriksen BO, Stefansson VTN, Jenssen TG, Mathisen UD, Schei J, Solbu MD, et al. High ambulatory arterial stiffness index is an independent risk factor for rapid age-related glomerular filtration rate decline in the general middle-aged population. Hypertension. 2017;69:651–9.
68. Whelton PK, Klag MJ. Hypertension as a risk factor for renal disease. Review of clinical and epidemiological evidence. Hypertension. 1989;13(5 Suppl):I19–27.
69. Parsa A, Kao WH, Xie D, Astor BC, Li M, Hsu CY, et al. APOL1 risk variants, race, and progression of chronic kidney disease. N Engl J Med. 2013;369:2183–96.
70. Langefeld CD, Divers J, Pajewski NM, Hawfield AT, Reboussin DM, Bild DE, et al. Apolipoprotein L1 gene variants associate with prevalent kidney but not prevalent cardiovascular disease in the Systolic Blood Pressure Intervention Trial. Kidney Int. 2015;87:169–75.
71. Chen TK, Estrella MM, Vittinghoff E, Lin F, Gutierrez OM, Kramer H, et al. APOL1 genetic variants are not associated with longitudinal blood pressure in young black adults. Kidney Int. 2017;92(4):964–71. pii: S0085-2538(17)30231-4.
72. Hoy WE, Kopp JB, Mott SA, Winkler CA. Absence of APOL1 risk alleles in a remote living Australian Aboriginal group with high rates of CKD, hyperten-

sion, diabetes, and cardiovascular disease. Kidney Int. 2017;91:990.
73. Chang J, Ma JZ, Zeng Q, Cechova S, Gantz A, Nievergelt C, et al. Loss of GSTM1, a NRF2 target, is associated with accelerated progression of hypertensive kidney disease in the African American Study of Kidney Disease (AASK). Am J Physiol Renal Physiol. 2013;304:F348–55.
74. Bodonyi-Kovacs G, Ma JZ, Chang J, Lipkowitz MS, Kopp JB, Winkler CA, et al. Combined effects of GSTM1 null allele and APOL1 renal risk alleles in CKD progression in the African American Study of Kidney Disease and Hypertension Trial. J Am Soc Nephrol. 2016;27:3140–315.
75. Salvador-González B, Mestre-Ferrer J, Soler-Vila M, Pascual-Benito L, Alonso-Bes E, Cunillera-Puértolas O, et al. Chronic kidney disease in hypertensive subjects ≥60 years treated in Primary Care. Nefrologia. 2017;37:406–14.
76. Gallibois CM, Jawa NA, Noone DG. Hypertension in pediatric patients with chronic kidney disease: management challenges. Int J Nephrol Renovasc Dis. 2017;10:205–13.
77. Lv J, Ehteshami P, Sarnak MJ, Tighiouart H, Jun M, Ninomiya T, et al. Effects of intensive blood pressure lowering on the progression of chronic kidney disease: a systematic review and meta-analysis. CMAJ. 2013;185:949–57.
78. Ku E, Gassman J, Appel LJ, Smogorzewski M, Sarnak MJ, Glidden DV, et al. BP control and long-term risk of ESRD and mortality. J Am Soc Nephrol. 2017;28:671–7.
79. Kovesdy CP, Lu JL, Molnar MZ, Ma JZ, Canada RB, Streja E, et al. Observational modeling of strict vs conventional blood pressure control in patients with chronic kidney disease. JAMA Intern Med. 2014;174:1442–9.
80. Bansal N. Stricter systolic blood pressure control is associated with higher all-cause mortality in patients with chronic kidney disease. Evid Based Med. 2015;20:68.
81. Xie X, Atkins E, Lv J, Bennett A, Neal B, Ninomiya T, et al. Effects of intensive blood pressure lowering on cardiovascular and renal outcomes: updated systematic review and meta-analysis. Lancet. 2016;387:435–43.
82. Burgner A, Lewis JB. Hypertension: is it time to reconsider blood pressure guidelines? Nat Rev Nephrol. 2014;10:620–1.
83. ESCAPE Trial Group, Wühl E, Trivelli A, Picca S, Litwin M, Peco-Antic A, et al. Strict blood-pressure control and progression of renal failure in children. N Engl J Med. 2009;361:1639–50.
84. Hsu CY. Does non-malignant hypertension cause renal insufficiency? Evidence-based perspective. Curr Opin Nephrol Hypertens. 2002;11:267–72.
85. Freedman BI, Cohen AH. Hypertension-attributed nephropathy: what's in a name? Nat Rev Nephrol. 2016;12:27–36.
86. Meyrier A. Nephrosclerosis: a term in quest of a disease. Nephron. 2015;129:276–82.
87. Nishikimi T, Koshikawa S, Ishikawa Y, Akimoto K, Inaba C, Ishimura K, et al. Inhibition of Rho-kinase attenuates nephrosclerosis and improves survival in salt-loaded spontaneously hypertensive stroke-prone rats. J Hypertens. 2007;25:1053–63.
88. Gonick HC, Cohen AH, Ren Q, Saldanha LF, Khalil-Manesh F, Anzalone J, et al. Effect of 2,3-dimercaptosuccinic acid on nephrosclerosis in the Dahl rat. I. Role of reactive oxygen species. Kidney Int. 1996;50:1572–81.
89. Liao TD, Yang XP, Liu YH, Shesely EG, Cavasin MA, Kuziel WA, et al. Role of inflammation in the development of renal damage and dysfunction in angiotensin II-induced hypertension. Hypertension. 2008;52:256–63.
90. Sakata F, Ito Y, Mizuno M, Sawai A, Suzuki Y, Tomita T, et al. Sodium chloride promotes tissue inflammation via osmotic stimuli in subtotal-nephrectomized mice. Lab Investig. 2017;97:432–46.
91. Amara S, Ivy MT, Myles EL, Tiriveedhi V. Sodium channel γENaC mediates IL-17 synergized high salt induced inflammatory stress in breast cancer cells. Cell Immunol. 2016;302:1–10.
92. Yan SH, Zhao NW, Jiang WM, Wang XT, Zhang SQ, Zhu XX, et al. Hsp90β is involved in the development of high salt-diet-induced nephropathy via interaction with various signalling proteins. Hsp90β is involved in the development of high salt-diet-induced nephropathy via interaction with various signalling proteins. Open Biol. 2016;6:150159.
93. Hernandez AL, Kitz A, Wu C, Lowther DE, Rodriguez DM, Vudattu N, et al. Sodium chloride inhibits the suppressive function of FOXP3+ regulatory T cells. J Clin Invest. 2015;125:4212–22.
94. Binger KJ, Gebhardt M, Heinig M, Rintisch C, Schroeder A, Neuhofer W, et al. High salt reduces the activation of IL-4- and IL-13-stimulated macrophages. J Clin Invest. 2015;125:4223–38.
95. Wade B, Abais-Battad JM, Mattson DL. Role of immune cells in salt-sensitive hypertension and renal injury. Curr Opin Nephrol Hypertens. 2016;25:22–7.
96. Srivastava A, Singh A, Singh SS, Mishra AK. Salt stress-induced changes in antioxidative defense system and proteome profiles of salt-tolerant and sensitive Frankia strains. J Environ Sci Health A Tox Hazard Subst Environ Eng. 2017;52:420–8.
97. Leibowitz A, Volkov A, Voloshin K, Shemesh C, Barshack I, Grossman E. Melatonin prevents kidney injury in a high salt diet-induced hypertension model by decreasing oxidative stress. J Pineal Res. 2016;60:48–54.
98. Liu X, Wang W, Chen W, Jiang X, Zhang Y, Wang Z, et al. Regulation of blood pressure, oxidative stress and AT1R by high salt diet in mutant human dopamine D5 receptor transgenic mice. Hypertens Res. 2015;38:394–9.

99. Lai EY, Luo Z, Onozato ML, Rudolph EH, Solis G, Jose PA, et al. Effects of the antioxidant drug tempol on renal oxygenation in mice with reduced renal mass. Am J Physiol Renal Physiol. 2012;303: F64–74.
100. Wong MM, Arcand J, Leung AA, Raj TS, Trieu K, Santos JA, et al. The science of salt: a regularly updated systematic review of salt and health outcomes (August to November 2015). J Clin Hypertens (Greenwich). 2016;18:1054–62.
101. McMahon EJ, Campbell KL, Bauer JD, Mudge DW. Altered dietary salt intake for people with chronic kidney disease. Cochrane Database Syst Rev. 2015;18:CD010070.
102. Mahajan A, Rodan AR, Le TH, Gaulton KJ, Haessler J, Stilp AM, et al. Trans-ethnic fine mapping highlights kidney-function genes linked to salt sensitivity. Am J Hum Genet. 2016;99:636–46.
103. Ahn SY, Kim S, Kim DK, Park JH, Shin SJ, Lee SH, et al. Urinary sodium excretion has positive correlation with activation of urinary renin angiotensin system and reactive oxygen species in hypertensive chronic kidney disease. J Korean Med Sci. 2014;29(Suppl 2):S123–30.
104. Harrison DG, Guzik TJ, Lob HE, Madhur MS, Marvar PJ, Thabet S, et al. Inflammation, immunity, and hypertension. Hypertension. 2011;57:132–40.
105. Guzik TJ, Touyz RM. Oxidative stress, inflammation, and vascular aging in hypertension. Hypertension. 2017; pii: HYPERTENSIONAHA.117.07802.
106. Cuevas S, Villar VA, Jose PA, Armando I. Renal dopamine receptors, oxidative stress, and hypertension. Int J Mol Sci. 2013;14:17553–72.
107. Banday AA, Lokhandwala MF. Oxidative stress causes renal angiotensin II type 1 receptor upregulation, Na+/H+ exchanger 3 overstimulation, and hypertension. Hypertension. 2011;57:452–9.
108. Loperena R, Harrison DG. Oxidative stress and hypertensive diseases. Med Clin North Am. 2017; 101:169–93.
109. Vlassara H, Torreggiani M, Post JB, Zheng F, Uribarri J, Striker GE. Role of oxidants/inflammation in declining renal function in chronic kidney disease and normal aging. Kidney Int Suppl. 2009;2009:S3–S11.
110. Frame AA, Wainford RD. Renal sodium handling and sodium sensitivity. Kidney Res Clin Pract. 2017;36(2):117–31.
111. Foss JD, Kirabo A, Harrison DG. Do high-salt microenvironments drive hypertensive inflammation? Am J Physiol Regul Integr Comp Physiol. 2017;312(1):R1–4.
112. Kanbay M, Segal M, Afsar B, Kang DH, Rodriguez-Iturbe B, Johnson RJ. The role of uric acid in the pathogenesis of human cardiovascular disease. Heart. 2013;99(11):759–66.
113. Yang BY, Qian ZM, Vaughn MG, Nelson EJ, Dharmage SC, Heinrich J, et al. Is prehypertension more strongly associated with long-term ambient air pollution exposure than hypertension? Findings from the 33 Communities Chinese Health Study. Environ Pollut. 2017;229:696–704.
114. Xu X, Wang G, Chen N, Lu T, Nie S, Xu G, et al. Long-term exposure to air pollution and increased risk of membranous nephropathy in China. J Am Soc Nephrol. 2016;27(12):3739–46.
115. Lipfert FW. Long-term associations of morbidity with air pollution: a catalogue and synthesis. J Air Waste Manag Assoc. 2018;68:12–28.
116. Al Suleimani YM, Al Mahruqi AS, Al Za'abi M, Shalaby A, Ashique M, Nemmar A, et al. Effect of diesel exhaust particles on renal vascular responses in rats with chronic kidney disease. Environ Toxicol. 2017;32:541–9.

Hypertension Management in African Americans: The AASK and Other Landmark Trial Application

9

Ping Li, Annise K. Chung, Samir S. Patel, and Vasilios Papademetriou

Introduction

Hypertension is a major public health challenge and affects 120 million adults in the United States. Recent hypertension trial outcomes indicate that further lowering of blood pressure below the standard target may reduce mortality [1] which is now reflected in the latest treatment guidelines that have lowered the target blood pressure to 130/80 mmHg [2]. The excess burden of hypertension among African-Americans was recognized in the early twentieth century and largely contributes to the excessive morbidity and mortality seen in this population compared to other racial/ethnic groups. It is well documented that hypertension in African-Americans is more prevalent, has an earlier onset, increased severity and results in more complications than other populations [3]. Despite treatment advances, improved access to health care, and similar control rates across most racial groups, African-Americans continue to experience high rates of hypertension attributable complications such as end stage renal disease (ESRD), heart failure and stroke. A comprehensive approach for effective management of hypertension in the African-American population is crucial to address this important health disparity. The pathogenesis, new hypertension guidelines and clinical trial outcomes related to African-Americans, specifically the African American Study of Kidney Disease and Hypertension (AASK) trial, will be discussed in this chapter. The term "African-American" or "Black" patients will refer to all people of African ancestry living in the USA.

Epidemiology

Hypertension has been recognized as the most potent risk to cardiovascular health of African Americans and is the leading cause of

P. Li
Washington Veterans Affairs Medical Center, Washington, DC, USA

Georgetown University Hospital, Washington, DC, USA

George Washington University School of Medicine, Washington, DC, USA

A. K. Chung
Georgetown University Hospital, Washington, DC, USA

S. S. Patel
Washington Veterans Affairs Medical Center, Washington, DC, USA

George Washington University School of Medicine, Washington, DC, USA

V. Papademetriou (✉)
Georgetown University and VA Medical Center, Washington, DC, USA

V. Papademetriou et al. (eds.), *Management of Hypertension*,
https://doi.org/10.1007/978-3-319-92946-0_9

cardiovascular and end stage renal disease. The recent National Health and Nutrition Survey (NHANES) 2011–2012 [4] indicated the age-adjusted prevalence of hypertension was higher among non-Hispanic blacks (42.4%) than non-Hispanic whites (28%), non-Hispanic Asians (24.9%) or Hispanic (25.9%) adults. Relative to whites, African Americans have more blood pressure elevations above conventional hypertension thresholds (140/90 mmHg), experience earlier onset hypertension, manifest greater blood pressure elevation (>180/110 mmHg), and have more comorbid conditions such as diabetes and left ventricular hypertrophy that augment risk for poor clinical outcomes [5]. The prevalence rates of hypertension are steadily increasing in all racial groups and African women have the highest hypertension prevalence at 46.1%, compared to black men (44.9%) and non-Hispanic and Hispanic women (30%). Awareness, treatment and control rates of hypertension have increased over time in all racial groups [6]. The hypertension control rate (blood pressure < 140/90 mmHg) was higher among non-Hispanic whites (55.7%), than non-Hispanic blacks (48.5%), non-Hispanic Asian (43.5%), or Hispanic (47.4%) adults. Despite some treatment advances, hypertension attributable morbidity and mortality in African Americans remain high with 30% more nonfatal stroke, 80% more fatal stroke, 50% more cardiovascular disease, and fourfold more kidney disease compared to other populations [7, 8]. In addition, the Coronary Artery Risk Development in Young Adults (CARDIA) study, showed that African Americans have a 20-fold higher rate of incident heart failure before the age of 50 compared to White Americans, which is considered directly related to hypertension [9]. Further, Black – White differences in hypertension-related hospitalization rates increased from 2004 to 2009 with threefold higher rates among African Americans compared to White Americans [10]. Overall, hypertension is thought to account for 50% of the Black-White mortality disparity in the USA.

Pathogenesis of Hypertension

There are no unique risk factors or biomarkers for hypertension between racial/ethnic groups. However, some pathophysiological mechanisms that are etiologically linked to the development of hypertension do tend to be disproportionately prevalent in selected racial/ethnic groups. In 2017, Musemwa and Gadegbeku [11] proposed that the excess burden of hypertension in African Americans is likely due to interactions of biological, environmental, and social factors superimposed on a genetically-susceptible population (Fig. 9.1).

Roles of Genetic Contribution in the Development of Hypertension in African Americans

Multiple genetic variations with intermediate phenotypes unique to African Americans have been extensively identified, but the results are not conclusive and not linked to hypertension burden in this special population. In a recent study with more than 1000 African Americans, a genome-wide association study (GWAS) using pathway-based analysis identified two potential blood pressure regulation candidate genes associated with systolic blood pressure, SLC24A4 (sodium/potassium/calcium exchanger) and CACNA1H (a voltage-dependent calcium channel) with replication of some their findings in a West African cohort [12]. Unfortunately, these new results could not be replicated in an independent Milwaukee cohort of nearly 2500 African Americans [13]. The Continental Origins and Genetic Epidemiology Network (COGENT) performed the largest blood pressure GWAS including individuals of African (29, 000), European (69,000), and East Asian (19,000) ancestries and found common blood pressure loci across ethnic groups [14]. In contrast, the excess burden of non-diabetic kidney disease has been explained in part by genetic high risk variants in the apolipoprotein 1 (APOL1) gene among African

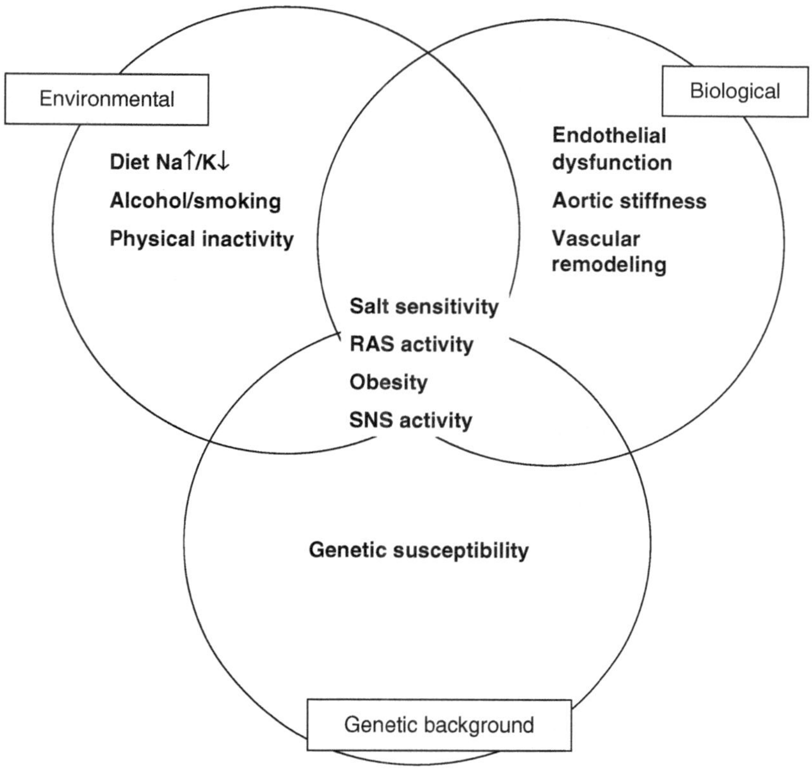

Fig. 9.1 Proposed excess burden of hypertension in African Americans. (Adapted from Ref. [12])

Americans [15, 16]. However, there is conflicting data whether the APOL1 genetic mutations are associated with the increased cardiovascular risk. APOL1 risk alleles have recently been linked to higher systolic blood pressure and earlier onset of hypertension in young African Americans prior to the decline in renal function [17], but these findings were not duplicated in the AASK trial cohort [18]. In summary, these inconclusive race-specific findings using the state-of-the-art genetic investigational tools did not find unique blood pressure regulation genes in African Americans and further research is needed to explore the complex question.

Obesity

Body mass index (BMI) positively correlates with blood pressure and is well documented in all racial/ethnic groups. Obesity is more prevalent in African Americans, particularly in African American women compared to White or Hispanic populations. In obesity, hypertension along with dyslipidemia, and insulin resistance often composes a health risk cluster: metabolic syndrome which is a significant cardiovascular risk. One in six African American women is considered to be extremely obese (BMI > 40 kg/m^2) and this prevalence is almost fourfold higher than that in white or Hispanic women [5]. Obesity impacts blood pressure through multiple mechanisms including increasing sympathetic nerve activity, salt sensitivity, and activation of renal angiotensin aldosterone system (RAAS), and glomerular hypertrophy which has been implicated in subsequent renal injury [19].

Salt-Sensitivity

Salt sensitivity is more common in normotensive and hypertensive African Americans than the general population. Higher rates of obesity and lower oral potassium intake contribute to the excess prevalence of salt sensitivity in this population [20, 21]. Both weight loss and increases in potassium intake ameliorate salt sensitivity with a reversal of the pressor effects of sodium in salt sensitive African Americans. Importantly, salt sensitivity is linked to a reduced dipping in nocturnal blood pressure, microalbuminuria, and other pressure related target organ injury [22, 23].

Renin-Angiotensin-Aldosterone System

It is well observed that African Americans have low circulating levels of renin as well as a lower response to monotherapy with angiotensin converting enzyme (ACE) inhibitors compared to diuretics. Clinical evidence suggests that low renin levels in the circulation reflect high local tissue angiotensin II production rather than high volume status. Increased tissue angiotensin II promotes inflammation and fibrosis in the kidney leading to excess salt retention [24, 25]. In a salt-sensitive and low-renin African American population, urinary angiotensinogen, a marker of intra-renal RAAS activation, was associated with elevated blood pressure [26]. In addition, circulating the aldosterone level is increased in African Americans. Collectively, RAAS activation plays an important role in hypertension and pressure-related target organ damage that is not reflected by hormonal activity in the circulation.

Vascular Dysfunction

Enhanced peripheral vascular resistance is the primary contributor to the maintenance of hypertension. A review of vascular studies in normotensive Black and White individuals concludes that African Americans have enhanced adrenergic vascular reactivity and attenuated vasodilator response [27]. The scientific literature suggests the vasodilatory impairment is due to both endothelium-dependent and non-endothelium -dependent mechanisms. Reduced nitric oxide (NO) bioavailability largely contributes to endothelium dependent vasodilation [5]. Dysregulation of oxygen derived free radicals, and endothelin-1 may potentiate the imbalance of vasoactive hormones that leads to elevated blood pressure and vascular remodeling [28]. Recent evidence suggests that central aortic pressure better reflects the load on target organs than brachial pressure. Central pressures are more predictive of cardiovascular outcomes and may partially explain racial differences in cardiovascular outcomes despite equivalent rates of hypertension control [29, 30]. In an important recent study, healthy young black men with similar clinical characteristics as young white men, including brachial blood pressure, were found to have higher central blood pressures, enhanced augmentation of central blood pressure, increased central arterial stiffness, increased carotid intima-media thickness, and reduced endothelial function [31]. Similar findings of greater carotid arterial stiffness was observed in the Black population of the Atherosclerosis Risk in Communities (ARIC) study when compared to the White population at baseline analysis [32]. Therefore, vascular dysfunction occurs earlier and may not be clinically apparent in the African American population versus White population. The above findings regarding differences in vasculature may be an important clue to the in the cause and consequences of hypertension in African American population.

Social Behavior and Environmental Risk Factors

There are many studies linking dietary habits and other lifestyle indicators to inadequate blood pressure control in the African American population [33]. Higher prevalent rates of obesity, excess dietary intake of sodium, and inadequate dietary intake of potassium are well recognized in African Americans. Physical inactivity rates are higher among the Hispanic and African American adults compared to White

Americans. The consumption of large amounts of alcohol (>210 g/week) is associated with higher risk of hypertension in adults, but the risk is observed at low to moderate amounts (1–209 g/per week) of alcohol in black men in high stress environments and with low socioeconomic status [34]. However, a cross-sectional study of NHANES data from 2001–2006 concluded that health behaviors do not fully explain the existing racial disparities in hypertension prevalence and control rate in this special population [35].

Application of Clinical Trial Results and Guidelines to African American Hypertensive Patients

African American Study of Kidney Disease and Hypertension (AASK) Trial

The African American Study of Kidney disease and Hypertension (AASK) study [36] was the first large scale trial to investigate the effects of three different anti-hypertensive drug classes as well as the effects of two levels of blood pressure (Intensive vs Standard) on decline in kidney function in an African American hypertensive population with chronic kidney disease using a 3 × 2 factorial design. The study enrolled 1094 African Americans aged 18–70 years with hypertensive renal disease (GFR: 20–65 ml/min/per 1.73 m^2) and followed for 3–6.4 years. Open label antihypertensive agents were added to the groups to reach the blood pressure goal. In 2002, final results of the AASK trial showed the ACE inhibitor, ramipril, was better than the β blocker, metoprolol, or the dihydropyridine calcium channel blocker (CCB), amlodipine, in slowing glomerular filtration rate (GFR) decline in African American hypertensive patients with mild to moderate hypertensive kidney disease. Metoprolol was not different from the amlodipine in the clinical outcomes. Of note, there was no difference between the intensive blood pressure (MAP: 92 mmHg) and standard blood pressure (MAP: 102–107 mmHg) groups in regards to the kidney function decline and the secondary clinical composite outcome. The secondary clinical composite end point in the AASK trial comprised of a decrease in GFR ≥50%, or ≤25 ml/min/1.73 m^2, ESRD or death. The final results from the AASK trial suggest that reduction in blood pressure to levels below those currently advocated for cardiovascular risk reduction did not provide additional renal protective benefits to African Americans with hypertensive nephrosclerosis. This conclusion must be considered in the setting of the relatively limited follow up time period and that only one third of the subjects in the original AASK trial had a urinary protein excretion >220 mg/g creatinine. The low level of urinary protein excretion for the majority of subjects would argue against significant loss of kidney function over the several years of the clinical trial. In the long-term follow up, AASK trial participants were invited to enroll into cohort phase after completing trial phase in which blood pressure target was less than 130/80 mmHg in the intensive blood pressure group and all patients were followed up to 8.8–12.2 years [37]. There was no significant difference between two blood pressure groups in slowing the progression of chronic kidney disease and primary outcome which includes doubling of serum creatinine and ESRD or death. However, in patients with proteinuria ≥220 mg/g, the intensive blood pressure control provided significant renal protection in this special group of patients as compared with standard blood pressure control. Another long term (up to 14.4 years) follow up study with AASK trial participants [38] found the strict blood pressure control did not delay the onset of ESRD, but may reduce the relative risk of death in African American hypertensive patients with chronic kidney disease. Cardiovascular outcomes were also studied in AASK trial participants with mean follow up of 4.1 years. The cardiovascular events rate (cardiac death, myocardial infarction, stroke, and heart failure) was not different among the three anti-hypertensive drug classes or two blood pressure control levels. However, the AASK trial was not powered for cardiovascular events thereby limiting conclusions regarding intensive versus standard blood pressure regimens [39]. Importantly, the final AASK trial results provide the fundamental basis for the use of ACE inhibitor in the hypertensive African American population with mild to moderate chronic kidney disease. The relative superiority of the ACE inhibitor as initial therapy in African American with non-diabetic kidney disease is ironic given the long-hold belief that CCBs were preferred anti-hypertensive agents for African Americans [40]. The AASK trial findings were consistent with renal outcomes in other populations with non-diabetic hypertensive kidney disease.

Antihypertensive and Lipid-Lowering Treatment to Prevent Heart Attack Trial (ALLHAT)

ALLHAT trial was the largest hypertensive trial in recent years and this study enrolled over 33,357 hypertensive patients with age >50 years and at least one other cardiovascular risk factor from 623 North American Centers during 1994 through 2002 [41, 42] in which 35% of patients are African American. The ALLHAT trial was designed to determine whether CCB or ACE inhibitor is superior to a thiazide diuretic in reduction of cardiovascular outcomes. Other anti-hypertensive agents were added to achieve blood pressure <140/90 mmHg in all groups. The final trial results demonstrated the primary cardiovascular end points (fatal coronary heart disease and non-fatal myocardial infarction) were not different among treatment groups. The diuretic, chlorthalidone, was associated with greater reductions in blood pressure then the ACE inhibitor, lisinopril. Chlorthalidone was also associated with a relative reduction in heart failure and stroke compared with lisinopril [43]. However, the higher stroke risk relative to chlorthalidone in the lisinopril group was experienced only in African American patients and can plausibly be explained by the lesser blood pressure reduction in lisinopril treatment group, where systolic blood pressure was on average 4 mmHg higher. The blood pressure differences were likely even larger between the lisinopril and chlorthalidone treatment groups in preceding study years.

The ALLHAT design employed a rather restrictive sequence of treatment scheme, which was not practical in clinical practice since African American patients with hypertension are more required using a diuretic as add on agent for hypertension treatment which was not permitted in ALLHAT trial. In this high risk population, the ALLHAT trial also showed amlodipine was comparable to chlorthalidone and lisinopril for the renal events rate as well as for an estimated rate of decline of renal function in an elderly population. This was an unexpected result, because the dihydropridine CCBs provide good anti-hypertensive therapy but, not renal protective effects beyond those anticipated with blood pressure reduction.

Systolic Blood Pressure Interventional Trial (SPRINT)

The SPRINT trial was a latest randomized large trial to evaluate the impact of intensive blood pressure control (systolic blood pressure < 120mmHg) vs standard blood pressure control (systolic blood pressure < 140 mmHg) on the incident cardiovascular, renal and neurological outcomes in a diverse population [1]. More than 9000 non-diabetic patients with cardiovascular risk and chronic kidney were enrolled in the trial in which 30% participants are African American. The trial results revealed intensive blood pressure control reduced cardiovascular composite outcomes by 25% in the high risk patients as compared with standard treatment. These results differ from the Action to Control Cardiovascular Risk in Diabetes (ACCORD) trial [44] which did not see a difference with intensive blood pressure therapy in a smaller population with type 2 diabetes. A sub-analysis study [45] further revealed similar treatment benefits exist in African American racial/ethnicity groups as compared with other racial groups with intensive blood pressure management group, although the African American population required an average of 0.3 more medications to achieve the systolic blood pressure goal of <120 mmHg. The above trials highlight the current uncertainty of the ideal blood pressure target of hypertension treatment. However, the large SPRINT trial demonstrated some beneficial outcomes and no significant harm thereby effectively opening the door for more aggressive therapy in high risk populations such as hypertensive African Americans.

International Society of Hypertension in Blacks Consensus Statement (ISHIB)

The 2010 International Society of Hypertension in Blacks (ISHIB) Consensus panel updated recommendations for more aggressive hypertension therapy than proposed by other guidelines for African American population. The ISHIB panel endorsed blood pressure target of <135/85 mmHg for primary prevention, and <130/80 for secondary prevention and initiation of lifestyle modifications at blood pressure ≥115/75 mmHg [46]. The guideline focused on the risk stratified treatment and early use of two drug combination therapy and initial therapy agents with diuretics or CCBs.

The optimal blood pressure target of hypertension treatment in general population has been debated many years, general population guidelines worldwide agree that treatment is warranted for stage 1 hypertension (blood pressure ≥140/90 mmHg) [47–51]. However, the guidelines vary in blood pressure targets in older persons in the general population (Table 9.1). The JNC 8 convened an expert panel in 2014 and recommended raising the blood pressure target in patients >60 years without diabetes and chronic kidney disease to 150/90 mmHg [52]. The newly published ACC/AHA guideline in 2017 [2] recommends to relax the blood pressure target to 130/80 mmHg in the general population regardless ages and racial/ethnicity. Those new hypertension treatment guidelines are consistent with the 2010 ISHIB Consensus panel recommendations and endorses target blood pressure is <130/80 mmHg in African American population with hypertension (Table 9.2).

Table 9.1 Comparison of initial drug therapy by race in hypertension consensus panels

Guidelines	Initial therapy in non-Blacks	Initial therapy in Blacks
ISHIB (2010)	–	Diuretics or CCB
NICE (2011)	<55 years ACEI, ARB; >55 years CCB	CCB
ESH/ESC (2013)	Any class	Diuretics or CCB
AHA/ACC/CDC (2014)	Thiazide, ACEI, ARB, CCB	–
ASH/ISH (2014)	Thiazide, ACEI, ARB, CCB	Thiazide or CCB
2014 JNC VIII	Thiazide, ACEI, ARB, CCB	Thiazide or CCB
CHEP (2016)	Thiazide, ACEI, ARB, CCB	Thiazide, CCB, ARB, BB if <60 years
AHA/ACC (2017)	Thiazide, ACEI, ARB, CCB	Thiazide, CCB, ACEI, ARB

Abbreviations: ISHB International Society of Hypertension in Blacks, *NICE* National Institute for Health and Clinical Evidence, *ESH/ESC* European Society of Hypertension/European Society of Cardiology, *AHA* American Heart Association, *ACC* American College of Cardiology, *CDC* United States Centers for Disease Control and Prevention, *ASH/ISH* American Society of Hypertension/International Society of Hypertension, *JNC VIII* the Eighth Join National Committee, *CHEP* Canadian Hypertension Education Program

Table 9.2 Blood pressure targets by hypertension consensus panels

Guidelines	Blood pressure target	Age-specific blood pressure target	Diabetes	Chronic kidney disease	Combination blood pressure threshold
ISHIB (2010)	<135/85	–	<130/80	<130/80	<15/10
NICE (2011)	<140/90	<150/90	<140/90	<140/90	–
ESH/ESC (2013)	<140/90	<140 or 150/90	<140/85	<140/90	Preferred
AHA/ACC/ CDC (2014)	<140/90	<140–145/90	<140/90	<140/90	<20/10
ASH/ISH (2014)	<140/90	<150/90	<140/90	<140/90	<20/10
JNC VIII (2014)	<140/90	<150/90	<140/90	<140/90	<20/10
CHEP (2016)	<140/90	<150/90	<130/80	<140/80	<20/10
AHA/ACC (2017)	<130/80	<130/80	<130/80	<130/80	–

Age specific blood pressure targets: NICE, ESH/ESC, AHA/ACC/CDC, ASH/ISH, CHEP are for any age >80 years; 2014 JNC VIII for age >60 years
ESH/ESC, combination preferred for markedly high blood pressure or high risk patients
AHA/ACC/CDC, blood pressure goal, if tolerated
JNC VIII, if blood pressure below target and well tolerated, no need to adjust
Optional alternative
CHEP, optional

Conclusion

Despite advances in hypertension treatment, the prevalence of hypertension in African Americans is higher when compared to other racial/ethnic populations. Hypertension develops at an earlier age in African Americans than Whites and is associated with more severe hypertension related complications, including chronic kidney disease, end stage renal disease, stroke, heart failure and cardiovascular disease. Hypertension may account for 50% of the Black-White mortality disparity in the USA. Therefore, it is crucial to address the unique risks in this specific population. The pathogenesis of hypertension in African Americans is multifactorial, and a multi-pronged approach may be necessary to address hypertension control. Addressing health disparities, such as social and environmental risks, that contribute to the development of hypertension in African American patients can have an important impact on treatment. Modifiable risk factors such as salt intake, obesity, and physical inactivity should be addressed routinely during clinic visits. Based on the latest recommendations, combination drug therapy with diuretics and RAAS inhibitors is preferred in this special population. It remains to be seen whether this population has specific genetic predisposition to hypertension. Overall, the needs of African Americans are diverse, and a comprehensive treatment plan should address each of these pathogenetic mechanisms.

References

1. Group SR, Wright JT Jr, Williamson JD, Whelton PK, Snyder JK, Sink KM, et al. A randomized trial of intensive versus standard blood-pressure control. N Engl J Med. 2015;373(22):2103–16.
2. Whelton PK, Carey RM, Aronow WS, Casey DE Jr, Collins KJ, Dennison Himmelfarb C, et al. 2017 ACC/AHA/AAPA/ABC/ACPM/AGS/APhA/ASH/ASPC/NMA/PCNA guideline for the prevention, detection, evaluation, and management of high blood pressure in adults: a report of the American College of Cardiology/American Heart Association Task Force on Clinical Practice Guidelines. Hypertension. 2018;71:e13–e115.
3. Flack JM, Okwuosa T, Sudhakar R, Ference B, Levy P. Should African Americans have a lower blood pressure goal than other ethnic groups to prevent organ damage? Curr Cardiol Rep. 2012;14(6):660–6.
4. Nwankwo T, Yoon SS, Burt V, Gu Q. Hypertension among adults in the United States: national health and nutrition examination survey, 2011–2012. NCHS Data Brief. 2013;(133):1–8.

5. Flack JM, Nasser SA, Levy PD. Therapy of hypertension in African Americans. Am J Cardiovasc Drugs. 2011;11(2):83–92.
6. Fletcher RD, Amdur RL, Kolodner R, McManus C, Jones R, Faselis C, et al. Blood pressure control among US veterans: a large multiyear analysis of blood pressure data from the Veterans Administration Health Data Repository. Circulation. 2012;125(20):2462–8.
7. Go AS, Mozaffarian D, Roger VL, Benjamin EJ, Berry JD, Blaha MJ, et al. Heart disease and stroke statistics–2014 update: a report from the American Heart Association. Circulation. 2014;129(3):e28–e292.
8. Carnethon MR, Pu J, Howard G, Albert MA, Anderson CAM, Bertoni AG, et al. Cardiovascular health in African Americans: a scientific statement from the American Heart Association. Circulation. 2017;136(21):e393–423.
9. Bibbins-Domingo K, Pletcher MJ, Lin F, Vittinghoff E, Gardin JM, Arynchyn A, et al. Racial differences in incident heart failure among young adults. N Engl J Med. 2009;360(12):1179–90.
10. Will JC, Nwaise IA, Schieb L, Zhong Y. Geographic and racial patterns of preventable hospitalizations for hypertension: Medicare beneficiaries, 2004–2009. Public Health Rep. 2014;129(1):8–18.
11. Musemwa N, Gadegbeku CA. Hypertension in African Americans. Curr Cardiol Rep. 2017;19(12):129.
12. Adeyemo A, Gerry N, Chen G, Herbert A, Doumatey A, Huang H, et al. A genome-wide association study of hypertension and blood pressure in African Americans. PLoS Genet. 2009;5(7):e1000564.
13. Kidambi S, Ghosh S, Kotchen JM, Grim CE, Krishnaswami S, Kaldunski ML, et al. Non-replication study of a genome-wide association study for hypertension and blood pressure in African Americans. BMC Med Genet. 2012;13:27.
14. Franceschini N, Fox E, Zhang Z, Edwards TL, Nalls MA, Sung YJ, et al. Genome-wide association analysis of blood-pressure traits in African-ancestry individuals reveals common associated genes in African and non-African populations. Am J Hum Genet. 2013;93(3):545–54.
15. Parsa A, Kao WH, Xie D, Astor BC, Li M, Hsu CY, et al. APOL1 risk variants, race, and progression of chronic kidney disease. N Engl J Med. 2013;369(23):2183–96.
16. Tin A, Grams ME, Estrella M, Lipkowitz M, Greene TH, Kao WH, et al. Patterns of kidney function decline associated with APOL1 genotypes: results from AASK. Clin J Am Soc Nephrol. 2016;11(8):1353–9.
17. Nadkarni GN, Wyatt CM, Murphy B, Ross MJ. APOL1: a case in point for replacing race with genetics. Kidney Int. 2017;91(4):768–70.
18. Chen TK, Appel LJ, Grams ME, Tin A, Choi MJ, Lipkowitz MS, et al. APOL1 risk variants and cardiovascular disease: results from the AASK (African American Study of Kidney Disease and Hypertension). Arterioscler Thromb Vasc Biol. 2017;37(9):1765–9.
19. Landsberg L, Aronne LJ, Beilin LJ, Burke V, Igel LI, Lloyd-Jones D, et al. Obesity-related hypertension: pathogenesis, cardiovascular risk, and treatment–a position paper of the The Obesity Society and The American Society of Hypertension. Obesity (Silver Spring). 2013;21(1):8–24.
20. Madhavan S, Alderman MH. Ethnicity and the relationship of sodium intake to blood pressure. J Hypertens. 1994;12(1):97–103.
21. Weinberger MH. Salt sensitivity of blood pressure in humans. Hypertension. 1996;27(3 Pt 2):481–90.
22. Bankir L, Bochud M, Maillard M, Bovet P, Gabriel A, Burnier M. Nighttime blood pressure and nocturnal dipping are associated with daytime urinary sodium excretion in African subjects. Hypertension. 2008;51(4):891–8.
23. Sanders PW. Dietary salt intake, salt sensitivity, and cardiovascular health. Hypertension. 2009;53(3):442–5.
24. Price DA, Fisher ND. The renin-angiotensin system in blacks: active, passive, or what? Curr Hypertens Rep. 2003;5(3):225–30.
25. Boddi M, Poggesi L, Coppo M, Zarone N, Sacchi S, Tania C, et al. Human vascular renin-angiotensin system and its functional changes in relation to different sodium intakes. Hypertension. 1998;31(3):836–42.
26. Michel FS, Norton GR, Maseko MJ, Majane OH, Sareli P, Woodiwiss AJ. Urinary angiotensinogen excretion is associated with blood pressure independent of the circulating renin-angiotensin system in a group of african ancestry. Hypertension. 2014;64(1):149–56.
27. Taherzadeh Z, Brewster LM, van Montfrans GA, VanBavel E. Function and structure of resistance vessels in black and white people. J Clin Hypertens (Greenwich). 2010;12(6):431–8.
28. Campia U, Cardillo C, Panza JA. Ethnic differences in the vasoconstrictor activity of endogenous endothelin-1 in hypertensive patients. Circulation. 2004;109(25):3191–5.
29. Roman MJ, Devereux RB, Kizer JR, Lee ET, Galloway JM, Ali T, et al. Central pressure more strongly relates to vascular disease and outcome than does brachial pressure: the Strong Heart Study. Hypertension. 2007;50(1):197–203.
30. Safar ME, Blacher J, Pannier B, Guerin AP, Marchais SJ, Guyonvarc'h PM, et al. Central pulse pressure and mortality in end-stage renal disease. Hypertension. 2002;39(3):735–8.
31. Heffernan KS, Jae SY, Wilund KR, Woods JA, Fernhall B. Racial differences in central blood pressure and vascular function in young men. Am J Physiol Heart Circ Physiol. 2008;295(6):H2380–7.
32. Din-Dzietham R, Couper D, Evans G, Arnett DK, Jones DW. Arterial stiffness is greater in African Americans than in whites: evidence from the Forsyth County, North Carolina, ARIC cohort. Am J Hypertens. 2004;17(4):304–13.

33. Ferdinand KC, Ferdinand DP. Race-based therapy for hypertension: possible benefits and potential pitfalls. Expert Rev Cardiovasc Ther. 2008;6(10):1357–66.
34. Fuchs FD, Chambless LE, Whelton PK, Nieto FJ, Heiss G. Alcohol consumption and the incidence of hypertension: the Atherosclerosis Risk in Communities Study. Hypertension. 2001;37(5):1242–50.
35. Redmond N, Baer HJ, Hicks LS. Health behaviors and racial disparity in blood pressure control in the national health and nutrition examination survey. Hypertension. 2011;57(3):383–9.
36. Wright JT Jr, Bakris G, Greene T, Agodoa LY, Appel LJ, Charleston J, et al. Effect of blood pressure lowering and antihypertensive drug class on progression of hypertensive kidney disease: results from the AASK trial. JAMA. 2002;288(19):2421–31.
37. Appel LJ, Wright JT Jr, Greene T, Agodoa LY, Astor BC, Bakris GL, et al. Intensive blood-pressure control in hypertensive chronic kidney disease. N Engl J Med. 2010;363(10):918–29.
38. Ku E, Gassman J, Appel LJ, Smogorzewski M, Sarnak MJ, Glidden DV, et al. BP control and long-term risk of ESRD and mortality. J Am Soc Nephrol. 2017;28(2):671–7.
39. Norris K, Bourgoigne J, Gassman J, Hebert L, Middleton J, Phillips RA, et al. Cardiovascular outcomes in the African American Study of Kidney Disease and Hypertension (AASK) Trial. Am J Kidney Dis. 2006;48(5):739–51.
40. Flack JM, Sica DA. Therapeutic considerations in the African-American patient with hypertension: considerations with calcium channel blocker therapy. J Clin Hypertens (Greenwich). 2005;7(4 Suppl 1):9–14.
41. Officers A, Coordinators for the ACRGTA, Lipid-Lowering Treatment to Prevent Heart Attack T. Major outcomes in high-risk hypertensive patients randomized to angiotensin-converting enzyme inhibitor or calcium channel blocker vs diuretic: the Antihypertensive and Lipid-Lowering Treatment to Prevent Heart Attack Trial (ALLHAT). JAMA. 2002;288(23):2981–97.
42. Wright JT Jr, Dunn JK, Cutler JA, Davis BR, Cushman WC, Ford CE, et al. Outcomes in hypertensive black and nonblack patients treated with chlorthalidone, amlodipine, and lisinopril. JAMA. 2005;293(13):1595–608.
43. Leenen FH, Nwachuku CE, Black HR, Cushman WC, Davis BR, Simpson LM, et al. Clinical events in high-risk hypertensive patients randomly assigned to calcium channel blocker versus angiotensin-converting enzyme inhibitor in the antihypertensive and lipid-lowering treatment to prevent heart attack trial. Hypertension. 2006;48(3):374–84.
44. Group AS, Cushman WC, Evans GW, Byington RP, Goff DC Jr, Grimm RH Jr, et al. Effects of intensive blood-pressure control in type 2 diabetes mellitus. N Engl J Med. 2010;362(17):1575–85.
45. Still CH, Rodriguez CJ, Wright JT Jr, Craven TE, Bress AP, Chertow GM, et al. Clinical outcomes by race and ethnicity in the Systolic Blood Pressure Intervention Trial (SPRINT): a randomized clinical trial. Am J Hypertens. 2017;31(1):97–107.
46. Flack JM, Sica DA, Bakris G, Brown AL, Ferdinand KC, Grimm RH Jr, et al. Management of high blood pressure in Blacks: an update of the International Society on Hypertension in Blacks consensus statement. Hypertension. 2010;56(5):780–800.
47. Jones DW, Hall JE. Seventh report of the Joint National Committee on Prevention, Detection, Evaluation, and Treatment of High Blood Pressure and evidence from new hypertension trials. Hypertension. 2004;43(1):1–3.
48. McManus RJ, Caulfield M, Williams B, National Institute for H, Clinical E. NICE hypertension guideline 2011: evidence based evolution. BMJ. 2012;344:e181.
49. Go AS, Bauman MA, Coleman King SM, Fonarow GC, Lawrence W, Williams KA, et al. An effective approach to high blood pressure control: a science advisory from the American Heart Association, the American College of Cardiology, and the Centers for Disease Control and Prevention. Hypertension. 2014;63(4):878–85.
50. Weber MA, Schiffrin EL, White WB, Mann S, Lindholm LH, Kenerson JG, et al. Clinical practice guidelines for the management of hypertension in the community: a statement by the American Society of Hypertension and the International Society of Hypertension. J Clin Hypertens (Greenwich). 2014;16(1):14–26.
51. Leung AA, Nerenberg K, Daskalopoulou SS, McBrien K, Zarnke KB, Dasgupta K, et al. Hypertension Canada's 2016 Canadian hypertension education program guidelines for blood pressure measurement, diagnosis, assessment of risk, prevention, and treatment of hypertension. Can J Cardiol. 2016;32(5):569–88.
52. James PA, Oparil S, Carter BL, Cushman WC, Dennison-Himmelfarb C, Handler J, et al. 2014 evidence-based guideline for the management of high blood pressure in adults: report from the panel members appointed to the Eighth Joint National Committee (JNC 8). JAMA. 2014;311(5):507–20.

Comparison Therapies in the Treatment of Hypertension. The ASCOT and ACCOMPLISH Trial

10

Nikolaos Magkas, Athanasia Kapota, and Costas Tsioufis

Abbreviations

ABPM	Ambulatory blood pressure monitoring
ACC	American College of Cardiology
ACCOMPLISH	Avoiding Cardiovascular events through Combination therapy in Patients Living with Systolic Hypertension
ACEI	Angiotensin-converting enzyme inhibitor
AF	Atrial fibrillation
AHA	American Heart Association
AIx	Augmentation index
ALLHAT	Antihypertensive and Lipid-Lowering Treatment to Prevent Heart Attack Trial
ARB	Angiotensin receptor blocker
ASCOT	Anglo-Scandinavian Cardiac Outcomes Trial
ASCOT-BPLA	Anglo-Scandinavian Cardiac Outcomes Trial- Blood Pressure Lowering Arm
ASCOT-LLA	Anglo-Scandinavian Cardiac Outcomes Trial- Lipid Lowering Arm
ASH	American Society of Hypertension
BB	Beta-blocker
BHS	British Hypertension Society
BMI	Body mass index
BNP	Brain natriuretic peptide
BP	Blood pressure
CAFE	Conduit Artery Function Evaluation
CCB	Calcium channel blockers
CHD	Coronary heart disease
CI	Confidence interval
CKD	Chronic kidney disease
CV	Cardiovascular
CVD	Cardiovascular disease
eGFR	Estimated glomerular filtration rate
ESC	European Society of Cardiology
ESH	European Society of Hypertension
ESRD	End-stage renal disease
HDL	High-density lipoprotein
HF	Heart failure
HFrEF	Heart failure with reduced ejection fraction
HOPE	Heart Outcomes Prevention Evaluation
HR	Hazard ratio
HTN	Hypertension
ISH	International Society of Hypertension
JNC	Joint National Committee

N. Magkas
First Cardiology Clinic, Medical School, National and Kapodistrian University of Athens, Hippokration Hospital, Athens, Greece

A. Kapota
Hipporcration General Hospital of Athens, Athens, Greece

C. Tsioufis (✉)
First Cardiology Clinic, University of Athens, Hippokration Hospital, Athens, Greece

Georgetown University, Washington, DC, USA

V. Papademetriou et al. (eds.), *Management of Hypertension*,
https://doi.org/10.1007/978-3-319-92946-0_10

LIFE	Losartan Intervention for Endpoint reduction in hypertension
LV	Left ventricle/left ventricular
LVH	Left ventricular hypertrophy
MI	Myocardial infarction
MRA	Mineralocorticoid receptor antagonist
NICE	National Institute for Health and Clinical Excellence
ONTARGET	ONgoing Telmisartan Alone and in Combination with Ramipril Global Endpoint Trial
PAD	Peripheral artery disease
PWV	Pulse wave velocity
RAAS	Renin-angiotensin-aldosterone system
RCT	Randomized controlled trial
SD	Standard deviation
SHEP	Systolic Hypertension in the Elderly Program
STEMI	ST-segment elevation myocardial infarction
VALUE	Valsartan Antihypertensive Long-term Use Evaluation

Introduction

Combination therapy has been successfully tried in many trials with hypertensive patients, is strongly recommended by international guidelines for the management of hypertension and is widely used in everyday clinical practice, as it seems necessary for achieving the recommended goal of blood pressure (BP) values (140/90 mmHg in most cases) in the majority of hypertensives [1]. It has been associated with better BP control and improved cardiovascular outcomes when used as initial therapy in newly diagnosed hypertension (HTN) [2, 3]. At least 75% of the overall hypertensive population will require combination therapy in order to achieve BP target [4], especially patients with grade 2 or grade 3 HTN (systolic BP > 160 mmHg and/or diastolic BP > 100 mmHg). Indeed, relevant guidelines recommend that it should be the first choice for individuals in whom BP values are markedly above the target (>20 mmHg for systolic or >10 mmHg for diastolic BP) or for those at high risk for cardiovascular events including diabetics [1, 5].

The theoretical basis for combination therapy relies on the assumption that, since several mechanisms are involved in the pathophysiology of HTN, optimal BP control often requires blockade of more than one physiological pathways. Moreover, the inhibition of one factor that contributes to high BP usually triggers a compensatory response from another one resulting in inadequate BP reduction. Therefore, in most cases it is necessary to target more than one mechanisms, which can be achieved only with multiple antihypertensive agents [4]. The main advantage of combination therapy compared to monotherapy is its greater efficacy, since adding a second agent results in much larger BP reduction than increasing the dose of the first drug [1, 4, 6]. Furthermore, more patients are likely to achieve BP control quickly when the initial therapy is a combination of antihypertensive agents, which could be beneficial, especially for high-risk individuals [1]. Furthermore, combination therapy, when administered at fixed doses in a single tablet, favors better compliance [1, 7–9]. Another advantage is the fewer adverse events, probably due to lower doses of each agent required for blood pressure control and to the fact that one agent may counterbalance the side effects of the other. The main disadvantage is that sometimes it is difficult to assess the effectiveness and tolerability of each specific agent in case treatment changes are needed due to inefficacy or adverse events. Additionally, combination therapy may result in exposing a number of hypertensives to an unnecessary agent [1, 5].

According to the European Society of Hypertension/European Society of Cardiology (ESH/ESC) 2013 Guidelines for the management of arterial hypertension, there are five classes of first-line antihypertensive agents: thiazide diuretics, angiotensin-converting enzyme inhibitors (ACEIs), angiotensin receptor blockers (ARBs), calcium channel blockers (CCBs) and beta-blockers (BB). All combinations between them are considered proper for the treatment of hypertension (with some limitations), except for the combination ACEI + ARB [1], which was associated with significantly worse renal outcomes in the ONgoing Telmisartan Alone and in Combination with Ramipril Global Endpoint

Trial (ONTARGET) [10]. The combination of BB and non-dihydropyridine CCB (verapamil, diltiazem) should also be avoided due to the risk of bradyarrythmias. Moreover, the combination of beta-blocker and diuretic should be used with caution, if not at all, in patients with metabolic syndrome and/or glucose intolerance [1], as there is evidence that it increases the onset of diabetes mellitus [11–14]. Based on the results of large clinical trials, ESH-ESC 2013 Guidelines suggest that the preferred two-drug combinations are ACEI + CCB, ARB + CCB, ACEI + thiazide diuretic, ARB + thiazide diuretic and CCB + thiazide diuretic. In any case, the selection of antihypertensive agents in combination therapy should also be individualized, according to each patient's comorbidities, as some drugs have provided larger benefits in specific conditions [1].

Despite the wide use of combination therapy in many randomized controlled trials (RCTs), in most of them the second or third agent was added after the failure of monotherapy to achieve BP control and it was usually not prespecified. Thus, most of the available data about the efficacy of combination therapy and the comparison between different combinations are indirect. Among the large number of RCTs in hypertension, two of them are considered to be the landmarks in the comparison of combination therapies in terms of cardiovascular outcomes: the Anglo-Scandinavian Cardiac Outcomes Trial (ASCOT) [14] and the Avoiding Cardiovascular events through Combination therapy in Patients Living with Systolic Hypertension (ACCOMPLISH) trial. The ACCOMPLISH trial directly compared two combinations; the one arm was treated with an ACEI and a CCB and the other with the same ACEI and a diuretic [15]. In ASCOT, despite the fact that the initial treatment in both groups was monotherapy (a CCB vs a BB), 78% of the patients were on two or more drugs by the end of the trial and patients from each arm were receiving the prespecified combinations for at least 50% of the time throughout the trial (50% for the CCB + ACEI regimen and 55% for the BB + diuretic regimen) [14]. Taking into account that ASCOT was one of the larger RCTs in hypertension, its results, although indirect, had a great impact on the use of combination therapies in hypertension.

The ASCOT

The Anglo-Scandinavian Cardiac Outcomes Trial was an independent, investigator-led, multicenter, prospective, randomized controlled trial that was conducted from February 1998 to June 2005 in seven countries (United Kingdom, Ireland, Sweden, Norway, Denmark, Finland and Iceland). The rationale of the trial was to compare two antihypertensive regimens in the prevention of cardiovascular disease (CVD), one composed of the 'newer' (for that era) drugs, i.e. ACEIs and CCBs, and the other composed of the 'older' drugs, i.e. beta-blockers and thiazide diuretics; the BB + diuretic regimen was the most frequent combination at that time. Up to then, there was a lack of data about the comparison of combination therapies in hypertension or the clinical benefit obtained from the use of ACEIs and CCBs. Moreover, a shortfall in the efficacy of antihypertensive therapy to prevent coronary heart disease (CHD) had been observed with the older drugs, as the rates of reduction of CHD incidence achieved in randomized trials were remarkably lower than those that had been predicted from observational data for similar BP reduction. An emerging debate was in progress about the adverse effects of diuretics and beta-blockers that potentially attenuated the benefit from their antihypertensive action. On the other hand, there were data suggesting that the 'newer' agents, mainly ACEIs (or ARBs) and, to a lesser extent CCBs, might confer benefits 'beyond BP lowering' due to their pleiotropic actions. Thereby, a large trial comparing a regimen composed of a CCB and an ACEI with a regimen composed of a BB and a diuretic seemed necessary in order to provide new information in the field of treatment of hypertension [16].

ASCOT enrolled 19,257 hypertensive subjects aged 40–79 years old with at least three other factors for CHD; in contrast to most hypertension trials, patients with previous myocardial infarction (MI) were excluded. Participants were randomly assigned to receive either amlodipine 5–10 mg plus perindopril 4–8 mg if required (CCB-based regimen, n = 9639) or atenolol 50–100 mg adding bendroflumethiazide 1.25–2.5 mg if required (BB-based regimen, n = 9618). The second drug was added if monotherapy was inadequate to

Table 10.1 Treatment algorithm in ASCOT [14]

	CCB-based regimen	BB-based regimen
Step 1	Amlodipine 5 mg	Atenolol 50 mg
Step 2	Amlodipine 10 mg	Atenolol 100 mg
Step 3	Amlodipine 10 mg + perindopril 4 mg	Atenolol 100 mg + bendroflumethiazide 1.25 mg + potassium
Step 4	Amlodipine 10 mg + perindopril 8 mg (2 × 4 mg)	Atenolol 100 mg + bendroflumethiazide 2.5 mg + potassium
Step 5	Amlodipine 10 mg + perindopril 8 mg (2 × 4 mg) + doxazosin gastrointestinal transport system 4 mg	Atenolol 100 mg + bendroflumethiazide 2.5 mg + potassium + doxazosin gastrointestinal transport system 4 mg
Step 6	Amlodipine 10 mg + perindopril 8 mg (2 × 4 mg) + doxazosin gastrointestinal transport system 8 mg	Atenolol 100 mg + bendroflumethiazide 2.5 mg + potassium + doxazosin gastrointestinal transport system 8 mg

achieve BP control (BP > 140/90 mmHg). Doxazocin was added as a third drug in both groups if necessary and further treatment could be given according to physicians' preferences as required (Table 10.1). This was the blood-pressure lowering arm (ASCOT-BPLA), which was the main part of the study. Patients with total cholesterol within the 'normal' range (<6.5 mmol/l or approximately <250 mg/dl, n = 10,305) were further randomized to atorvastatin 10 mg or placebo and that was the lipid lowering arm of the study (ASCOT-LLA) [17]. Patients were well-matched between groups without significant differences in the basic demographic and clinical characteristics. The primary endpoint was non-fatal MI (including silent MI) and fatal CHD. The study also had many secondary endpoints, the most important of which were all-cause mortality, cardiovascular mortality, stroke, heart failure (HF), peripheral artery disease (PAD), new-onset diabetes and development of renal impairment.

The ASCOT-BPLA was terminated prematurely by the data safety monitoring board after 5.5 years of median follow-up and 106,153 patient-years of observation, as patients in the calcium channel blocker-based regimen had better outcomes. Although the difference was not significant, fewer patients in the amlodipine-based regimen compared to those in the atenolol-based regimen met the primary endpoint [429 vs 474 events, unadjusted hazard ratio (HR): 0.90, 95% confidence interval (CI): 0.79–1.02, p = 0.1052]. The difference of the two regimens in preventing non-fatal MI or fatal CHD would probably have achieved statistical significance, if the trial had not been terminated prematurely, as it was powered for 1150 patients to have such events, whereas only 903 had met the primary endpoint at the time of the termination of the study. Moreover, individuals in the CCB-based regimen had significantly better outcomes in several crucial secondary endpoints, such as all-cause mortality (738 vs 820 deaths, unadjusted HR: 0.89, 95% CI: 0.81–0.99, p = 0.025), total cardiovascular events and procedures (1362 vs 1602 events, unadjusted HR: 0.84, 95% CI: 0.78–0.90, p < 0.0001), stroke (327 vs 422 strokes, unadjusted HR: 0.77, 95% CI: 0.66–0.89, p = 0,0003) and incidence of new-onset diabetes (567 vs 799 cases, unadjusted HR: 0,70, 95% CI: 0,63–0.78, p < 0.0001), as shown in Table 10.2 and Figs. 10.1 and 10.2. The superiority of the CCB-based regimen appeared in all 18 subgroups of the study, including the subgroup of diabetic patients (n = 5137) [14, 18]. Incidentally, ASCOT-LLA was also ended prematurely after 3.3 years of median follow-up, as the primary outcome was significantly lower in the atorvastatin group (100 vs 154 events, HR: 0.64, 95% CI: 0.50–0.80, p = 0.0005 with similar BP values in both groups), as well as the secondary outcomes of total cardiovascular events (389 vs 486 events, HR: 0.79, 95% CI: 0.69–0.90, p = 0.0005), and stroke (89 vs 121 strokes, HR:0.73, 95% CI: 0.56–0.96, p = 0.024) [17].

The large majority of participants (78%) in ASCOT-BPLA were taking at least two antihy-

Table 10.2 Effect of treatment on all endpoints in ASCOT

	Amlodipine-based regimen (n = 9639)		Atenolol-based regimen (n = 9618)			
	Number (%)	Rate per 1000	Number (%)	Rate per 1000	Unadjusted HR (95% CI)	p
Primary endpoints						
Non-fatal myocardial infarction (including silent)-fatal CHD	429 (5%)	8-2	474 (5%)	9-1	0.90 (0.79-1.02)	0.1052
Secondary endpoints						
Non-fatal myocardial infarction (excluding silent)+fatal CHD	390 (4%)	7-4	444 (5%)	8-5	0.87 (0.76-1.00)	0.0458
Total coronary endpoint	753 (8%)	14-6	852 (9%)	16-8	0.87 (0.79-0.96)	0.0070
Total cardiovascular events and procedures	1362 (14%)	27-4	1602 (17%)	32-8	0.84 (0.78-0.90)	<0.0001
All-cause mortality	738 (8%)	13-9	820 (9%)	15-5	0.89 (0.81-0.99)	0.0247
Cardiovascular mortality	263 (3%)	4-9	342 (4%)	6-5	0.76 (0.65-0.90)	0.0010
Fatal and non-fatal stroke	327 (3%)	6-2	422 (4%)	8-1	0.77 (0.66-0.89)	0.0003
Fatal and non-fatal heart failure	134 (1%)	2-5	159 (2%)	3-0	0.84 (0.66-1.05)	0.1257
Tertiary endpoints						
Silent myocardial infarction	42 (0.4%)	0-8	33 (0.3%)	0-6	1.27 (0.80-2.00)	0.3089
Unstable angina	73 (1%)	1-4	106 (1%)	2-0	0.68 (0.51-0.92)	0.0115
Chronic stable angina	205 (2%)	3-9	208 (2%)	4-0	0.98 (0.81-1.19)	0.8323
Peripheral arterial disease	133 (1%)	2-5	202 (2%)	3-9	0.65 (0.52-0.81)	0.0001
Life-threatening arrhythmias	27 (0.3%)	0-5	25 (0.3%)	0-5	1.07 (0.62-1.85)	0.8009
Development of diabetes mellitus	567 (6%)	11-0	799 (8%)	15-9	0.70 (0.63-0.78)	<0.0001
Development of renal impairment	403 (4%)	7-7	469 (5%)	9-1	0.85 (0.75-0.97)	0.0187
Post-hoc endpoints						
Primary endpoint+coronary revascularisation procedures	596 (6%)	11-5	688 (7%)	13-4	0.85 (0.77-0.96)	0.0058
Cardiovasular death+myocardial infarction+stroke	796 (8%)	15-4	937 (10%)	18-4	0.84 (0.76-0.92)	0.0003

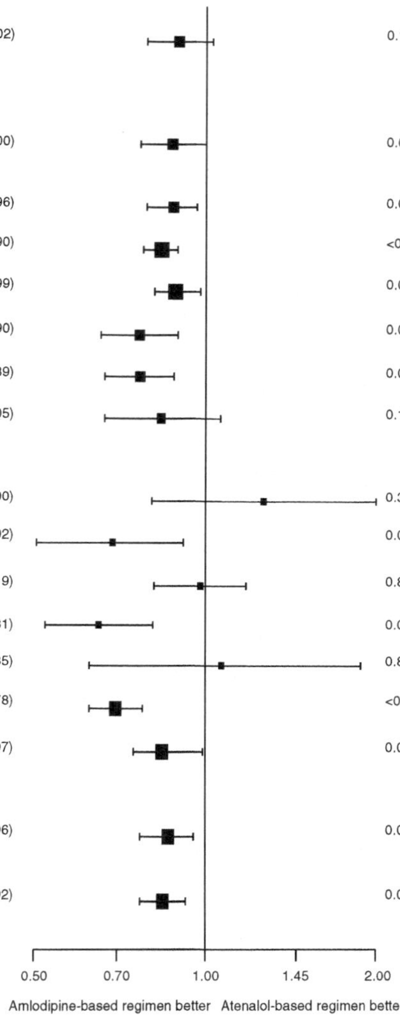

Rates per 1000 patient years [14]

pertensive drugs at the end of the study and, throughout the trial, patients in the amlodipine-based treatment arm were taking amlodipine and perindopril for a mean of 50% of the time and patients in the atenolol-based treatment arm were taking atenolol and bendroflumethiazide for a mean of 55% of the time (Table 10.3). Thus, although all patients were given monotherapy as initial treatment, the prespecified two-drug combinations were studied for a large proportion of the total patient-years of the trial. As a result, ASCOT was the first study to claim that one combination (a CCB plus an ACEI) may be better compared to another (a BB plus a diuretic), because it was found to be associated with lower all-cause and cardiovascular mortality, fewer cardiovascular events and lower incidence of new-onset diabetes [14].

Although it is generally accepted that the main objective in the treatment of hypertension is BP

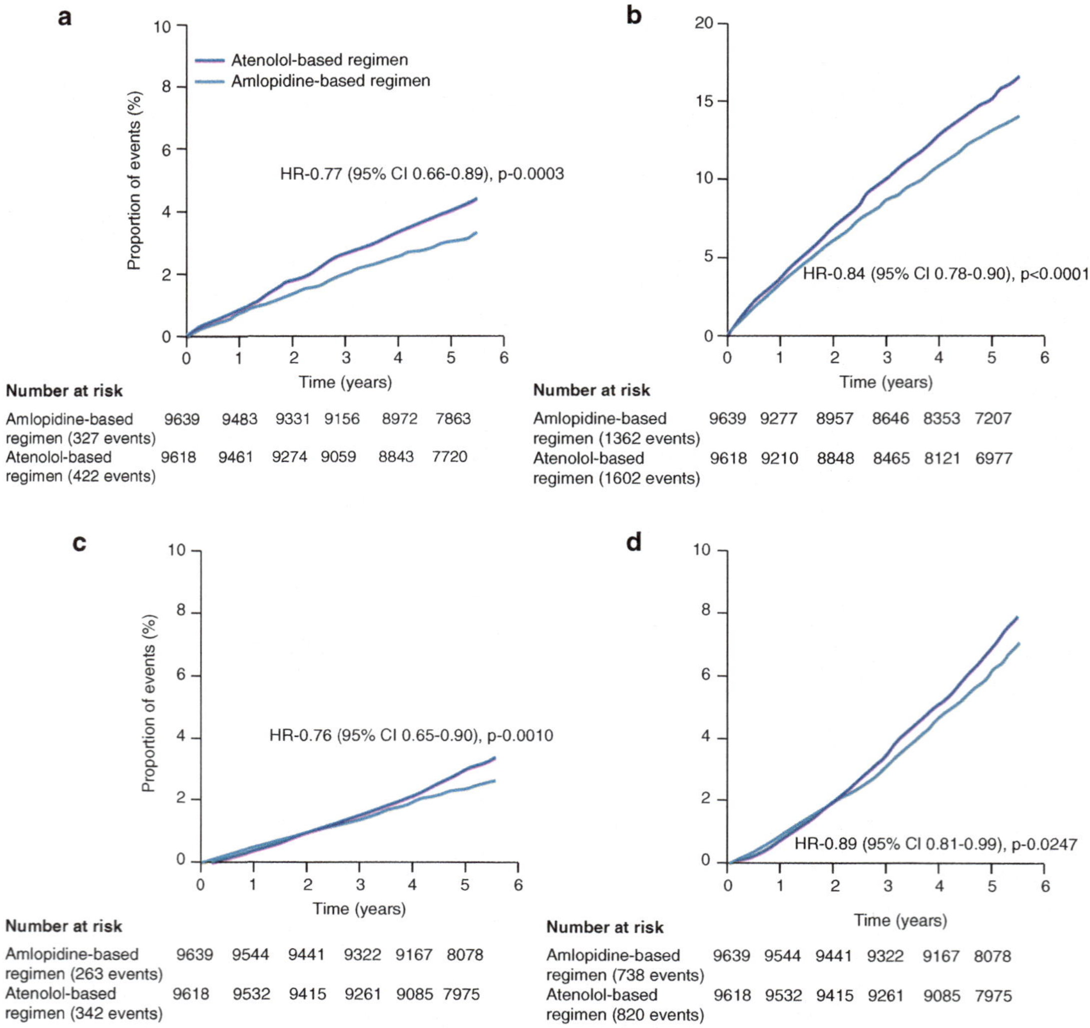

Fig. 10.1 Kaplan-Meier curves of cumulative incidence of fatal and non-fatal stroke (**a**), total cardiovascular events and procedures (**b**), cardiovascular mortality (**c**), and all-cause mortality (**d**) in ASCOT. (Dahlöf et al. [14])

reduction, large controversy and conflicting data exist about a possible superiority of some antihypertensive agents over others either in specific groups or in the entire population of hypertensives [1]. The results of ASCOT had an important impact on clinical practice establishing the CCB + ACEI combination as a safe, effective, well-tolerated and, in many cases, preferable combination. Moreover, this trial contributed to the cleaning of the suspicion that CCBs are less effective than other agents in the prevention of CHD in hypertensives [1, 19]. However, diuretics were still considered the cornerstone of the treatment of hypertension in the general population, as they had been proven beneficial in the prevention of cardiovascular disease. The Antihypertensive and Lipid-Lowering Treatment to Prevent Heart Attack Trial (ALLHAT), the largest trial ever conducted in hypertension, where a diuretic was found to be non-inferior, if not superior, to an ACEI and a CCB, had just been published [20] and diuretics had received a 'preferred initial agent' recommendation from the 7th report of the Joint National Committee (JNC-7) [21]. As a result, beta-blockers, the main component of the regimen, were deemed to be

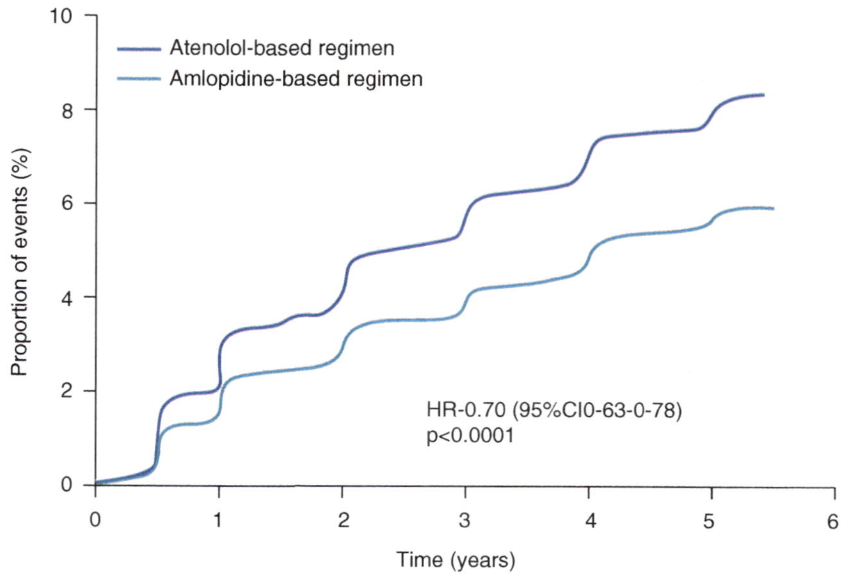

Number at risk

Amlopidine-based regimen (567 events)	9639	9383	9165	8966	8726	7618
Atenolol-based regimen (799 events)	9618	9295	9014	8735	8455	7319

Fig. 10.2 Kaplan-Meier curves of cumulative incidence of new-onset diabetes mellitus in ASCOT. (Dahlöf et al. [14])

Table 10.3 Mean percentage of time on the prespecified treatment regimens in each arm of ASCOT during every year of follow-up and throughout the study [14]

Year	1	2	3	4	5	≥6	All study
Randomised to amlodipine							
Amlodipine	88.2	83.1	81.5	80.8	80.0	79.2	82.5
Perindopril	46.2	58.7	61.6	63.4	64.1	64.0	58.5
Amlodipine + perindopril	39.1	49.6	52.2	53.8	54.2	54.2	49.5
Randomised to atenolol							
Atenolol	87.4	81.3	78.4	76.4	74.9	73.9	79.4
Bendroflumethiazide	56.6	68.2	69.0	69.3	69.0	68.6	65.7
Atenolol + bendroflumethiazide	49.1	58.0	57.6	57.3	56.4	55.7	54.9

the factor that was mainly responsible for the inferiority of the BB + diuretic combination either as a separate antihypertensive agent or in combination with thiazides. This argument was further strengthened by the Losartan Intervention for Endpoint Reduction in Hypertension (LIFE) trial, which compared an ARB(losartan)-based regimen with a BB(atenolol)-based regimen. The study reported that the composite primary end-point of cardiovascular morbidity and death occurred in significantly fewer patients in the ARB-based treatment group (HR: 0.87, 95% CI: 0.77–0.98, p = 0.021) [22]. Relevant meta-analyses that were published at that time also concluded that beta-blockers were less effective than other drugs in preventing cardiovascular events in hypertensives [23–25], which is in accordance with the results of a recent large meta-analysis [26]. On the other hand, it should be noticed that (i) other data claim that BBs have no significant difference compared to other agents in hard clinical endpoints [27, 28], (ii) atenolol, a vasoconstrictive BB, was mainly used in these studies (including ASCOT); thus, the effect of vasodilating BBs, which are probably superior in terms of cardiovascular outcomes [1], was not actually assessed.

Many possible explanations were given for the findings of the trial. First of all, the amlodipine ± perindopril regimen achieved larger BP reduction than the atenolol ± bendroflumethiazide regimen. Mean BP reduction was 27.5/17.7 mmHg and 25.7/15.6 mmHg respectively, with an average difference of 2.7/1.9 mmHg in BP rates between groups throughout the trial (Fig. 10.3). However, even though this difference was significant, the ASCOT investigators claimed that it was too low to explain fully the better outcomes in the CCB-based regimen, as similar rates of BP reduction generally provide fewer clinical benefits than those observed in ASCOT. Thus, they concluded, there should be other factors besides better BP control that favored the amlodipine ± perindopril combination over the atenolol ± bendroflumethiazide regimen [14, 29]. On the contrary, data from a meta-analysis suggest that the difference of 2.7/1.9 mmHg may be enough to explain the improved outcomes of the CCB ± ACEI group [30]. Other authors suggested that the dose of bendroflumethiazide (1.25–2.5 mg) was too low and was the main cause of the inferior antihypertensive effect of this regimen [31]. It was also argued that the dose of 100 mg of atenolol increased the regimen's side effects without a corresponding benefit in its antihypertensive action [32]. Regarding BP values, differences between treatment arms were more pronounced at the first months of the trial, especially in the first 3 months, where the largest differences (5.9/2.4 mmHg) were observed (Fig. 10.3). Early BP control, especially in high-risk patients, could confer an additional benefit, as shown in VALUE trial [33], and might be a cause for the better outcomes in this treatment regimen. Another hemodynamic parameter that probably influenced the outcomes is the within-individual BP variability, which is considered to be a risk factor for cardiovascular events [34]. Blood pressure variability was significantly lower in the CCB-based regimen; moreover, it decreased over time in the amlodipine-based group, while in increased over time in the atenolol-based group [35]. In addition, patients in the CCB-based treatment group had a lower incidence of resistant hypertension, indicating another advantage of this regimen [36].

The association of beta-blockers, diuretics and, to a larger extent, their combination with glucose intolerance and new-onset diabetes mellitus [1, 5] was probably an important factor that favored the CCB + ACEI combination and

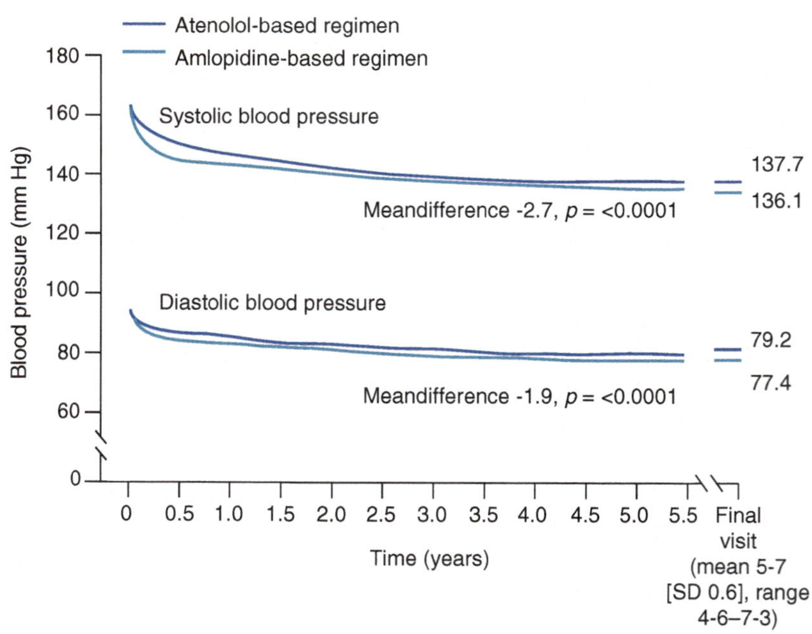

Fig. 10.3 Blood pressure over time by treatment group in ASCOT. (Dahlöf et al. [14])

contributed to the results of ASCOT. The presence of diabetes was significantly higher in the BB ± diuretic group at the end of the study (same base line incidence of diabetes at both groups) [14] and the use of these agents was found to be a major determinant of new-onset diabetes in a subsequent analysis [37]. Furthermore, patients in this group had significantly higher levels of fasting glucose and triglycerides, higher body mass index (BMI) and lower levels of high-density lipoprotein (HDL), indicating that this regimen exerts adverse effects not only on glucose metabolism but also on the other components of the metabolic syndrome [14]. These findings are in consistency with several studies and meta-analyses that have demonstrated the dysmetabolic actions of b-blockers, diuretics and their combination, especially in predisposed patients [12, 13, 38–41]. Beta-blockers are considered to cause insulin resistance and diabetes mellitus through peripheral vasoconstriction, that diminishes cellular glucose uptake, inhibition of lipolysis and blockade of insulin secretion from the pancreatic cells [42]. Diuretics are believed to play a diabetogenic role through hypokalemia, which also reduces insulin secretion [5, 43]. On the other hand, ACEIs and CCBs are considered not to worsen, or even improve, insulin sensitivity [1]. Since diabetes and metabolic syndrome increase the risk for cardiovascular morbidity and mortality, the adverse metabolic effects of beta-blockers and diuretics may attenuate the benefit from their antihypertensive action and explain the observed inferiority of their combination compared to the combination of a CCB plus an ACEI in the prevention of cardiovascular disease. Indeed, the difference in HDL concentration was found to have an important impact on the cardiovascular outcomes between ASCOT treatment groups [28]. Regarding beta-blockers, it should also be noticed that their diabetogenic action seems to be less intense when using vasodilating BBs, such as nebivolol, carvedilol and celiprolol. Anyhow, ESH-ESC Guidelines recommend that BBs, diuretics or their combination should be used only as additional drugs and with great caution in hypertensives with metabolic syndrome, while ACEIs, ARBs and CCBs are clearly preferable [1].

ASCOT study also reported that participants treated with the CCB ± ACEI combination had significantly lower rates of renal impairment (403 vs 469 cases, HR: 0.85, 95% CI: 0.75–0.97, $p = 0.02$) and lower concentrations of creatinine [14]. This finding may also be related to the better outcomes of this group, as it is well-known that chronic kidney disease (CKD) is a major risk factor for cardiovascular disease [44] as well as for death from other causes. The antiproteinuric effect and the nephroprotective properties of ACEIs (and ARBs) in both diabetic and non-diabetic nephropathy are well established and have placed these drugs in the first line of treatment of hypertension in patients with renal disease and/or proteinuria [1, 45]. Therefore, the use of perindopril as a second drug is an obvious reason for the better renal function observed in this group. Another factor that probably contributed to the higher concentrations of creatinine in the atenolol-based regimen is the use of diuretics, which can cause renal dysfunction, mainly due to depletion of intravascular volume and reduction of renal blood flow [46].

ASCOT investigators claimed that the results of ASCOT-BPLA may be associated with the differences in the outcomes between the two treatment arms of ASCOT-LLA. Indeed, there were numerical differences in the risk reduction produced by atorvastatin between the amlodipine-based and the atenolol-based regimen. The primary end point of non-fatal MI and fatal CHD was reduced by 53% in the CCB-based treatment group compared to placebo vs a 16% reduction in the BB-based treatment group (difference between risk reductions of borderline significance) and total CV events and endpoints were reduced by 27% in the CCB-based treatment group vs a 15% reduction in the BB-based treatment group (difference non-significant). Thus, it was proposed that there might have been a synergistic effect between CCBs, ACEIs or their combination with atorvastatin, a possible and positive interaction that inhibits the atherosclerotic process, promotes plaque stabilization, improves endothelial function and, eventually, enlarges the benefit provided by each drug alone. A potential synergy between amlodipine and atorvastatin is further supported by the fact that the benefits from the use of atorvastatin were observed within the first 3 months of the trial, while most patients in the CCB-based regimen were still on monotherapy with amlodipine [47]. A similar interaction between ACEIs and statins has also been reported by a Greek study [48].

Another important issue in ASCOT was that significantly fewer serious adverse events attributed to the antihypertensive therapy were observed in the CCB-based treatment arm (2% or 162 of 9639 patients vs 3% or 254 of 9618 patients, $p < 0.0001$), although the total adverse events were similar in both groups [14]. Adverse events are the most usual reason for treatment discontinuation and non-adherence, which is very high in hypertension and obviously a risk factor for poor BP control [1]. It is a common belief among physicians, but as well has been demonstrated in clinical trials [49], that adverse events are more common with BBs and diuretics than with ACEIs and CCBs. Moreover, the most frequent side effect of ACEIs, cough, can be easily managed with the replacement of the ACEI with an ARB, which is considered an equivalent drug in most cases, while the most frequent side effect of CCBs, peripheral edema, is largely attenuated when a CCB is combined with an ACEI [1, 4, 50, 51]. Even if compliance with treatment has not been reported to be different in the two groups of the ASCOT, since adherence is generally high in clinical trials due to close follow-up, in real life this is an essential issue which may justify a preference for ACEIs (or ARBs) and CCBs.

In addition to the above findings directly extracted from ASCOT, it seems likely (but not certain) that the so-called pleiotropic actions of the 'newer' drugs exerted a beneficial effect 'beyond BP lowering' in the respective treatment arm. There are many data suggesting that ACEIs and CCBs have anti-atherogenic and cardioprotective properties and they are probably more effective than beta-blockers and diuretics in the prevention or delay of several forms of cardiovascular disease. This refers mostly to ACEIs due to their ability to inhibit the renin-angiotensin-aldosterone system (RAAS) [52–54]. Treatment with ACEIs has been associated with improved outcomes in many trials, e.g. the Heart Outcomes Prevention Evaluation (HOPE) study, where ramipril reduced cardiovascular events in high-risk patients independently of the presence of hypertension (reported BP reduction attributable to ramipril 3–4/1–2 mmHg) [55], supporting the 'benefits beyond BP lowering' hypothesis. Similar anti-atherogenic actions have been attributed to CCBs, mainly amlodipine [56, 57], though to a lesser extent. Combination therapy with ACEI + CCB could provide additional benefits in vascular function [54, 58, 59]. Therefore, it is reasonable to assume that the vasoprotective and cardioprotective properties of ACEIs and CCBs contributed to the better cardiovascular outcomes in the group treated with this regimen.

ASCOT Sub-studies

Concurrently with ASCOT, several other sub-studies were conducted providing further possible explanations for the results of the main study. The Conduit Artery Function Evaluation (CAFE) study was a sub-study that examined the effect of the antihypertensive regimens given in ASCOT on the morphology of the aortic pressure waveform, central aortic pressures, augmentation index (AIx) and other hemodynamic indexes ($n = 2199$ patients already recruited in ASCOT) [60]. The aortic pressure waveform is a composite of a forward pulse wave created by ventricular contraction and a reflected wave coming from the periphery of the arterial tree. Two peaks of the aortic pressure waveform can be identified: the first peak due to the forward wave and the second peak due to the composition of the forward and the reflected wave, which represents the central aortic systolic pressure [1]. AIx is defined as the ratio of the difference between central aortic systolic pressure and pressure at the first peak of the aortic pulse wave to central aortic pulse pressure The CAFE study demonstrated that, while brachial systolic blood pressure was reduced to a similar extent in both treatment arms, there was a significantly larger reduction in central aortic systolic blood pressure, central aortic pulse

Table 10.4 Central pressures and other hemodynamic indices in the two treatment groups of the CAFE study [62]

Parameter	Atenolol	Amlodipine	Difference (atenolol-amlodipine)	p value
Peripheral SBP, mm Hg	133.9 (133, 134.7)	133.2 (132.5, 133.8)	0.7 (−0.4, 1.7)	0.2
Peripheral DBP, mm Hg	78.6 (78.1, 79.1)	76.9 (76.4, 77.4)	1.6 (0.9, 2.4)	<0.0001
Peripheral PP, mm Hg	55.3 (54.6, 56)	56.2 (55.6, 56.9	−0.9 (−1.9, 0)	0.06
Heart rate, BPM	58.6 (58, 59.2)	69.3 (68.6, 69.9)	−10.7 (−11.5, −9.8)	<0.0001
Central SBP, mm Hg	125.5 (124.7, 126.3)	121.2 (120.5, 121.9	4.3 (3.3, 5.4)	<0.0001
Central DBP, mm Hg	79.1 (78.6, 79.6)	77.8 (77.3, 78.3)	1.4 (0.6, 2.1)	0.0002
Central PP, mm Hg	46.4 (45.7, 47.1)	43.4 (42.8, 44)	3.0 (2.1, 3.9)	<0.0001
Augmentation index, %	31.9 (31.3, 32.4)	25.3 (24.8, 25.9)	6.5 95.8, 7.3)	<0.0001
Augmentation, mm Hg	15.4 (14.9, 15.8)	11.5 (11.2, 11.9)	3.8 (3.3, 3.4)	<0.0001

pressure and augmentation index in the CCB ± ACEI treatment arm (Table 10.4). These results were consistent with time throughout the trial and correspond with other studies that have reported a more beneficial effect of angiotensin-converting enzyme inhibitors and calcium channel blockers on central aortic pressures compared to beta-blockers and diuretics [61–65]. Furthermore, the inferiority of atenolol-based regimen in reducing central pressures persisted even if vasodilating drugs were added, suggesting that all combinations that include atenolol are less effective in improving central hemodynamics. The CAFE Investigators proposed that, first, ACEIs and CCBs reduce the pressure of reflection waves through vasodilation and, second, the slower heart rate due to beta-blockade prolongs the systolic ejection time, delays the peak of the forward wave and therefore increases the probability that the reflected wave will augment the systolic aortic pressure. Moreover, central aortic pulse pressure was found to be significantly associated with a post hoc–defined composite outcome of total cardiovascular events and worsening of renal function in the patients of CAFE study, indicating that the larger improvement in hemodynamic indexes with the amlodipine-based regimen may provide an explanation for the improved clinical outcomes observed in this group at the main study [60]. This is in accordance with the mechanistic point of view that central pressures represent the actual hemodynamic load imposed on heart, kidneys, brain and large arteries more reliably than brachial BP as well as with other studies and meta-analyses, at which central hemodynamics have been independently associated with cardiovascular and all-cause mortality [66, 67].

Patients in the CCB ± ACEI regimen were also found to have better cardiac diastolic function (assessed by conventional and tissue Doppler imaging echocardiography) compared to patients in the BB ± diuretic regimen according to another ASCOT sub-study with 1006 patients [68, 69]. This could be another factor that favored the CCB ± ACEI regimen, although the secondary endpoint of heart failure was only numerically and not significantly lower in this group [14]. This sub-study had an important limitation, as base-line echocardiographic data were not available, however, several indexes of diastolic function were better in the amlodipine-based regimen as well as the rates of brain natriuretic peptide (BNP). The explanation of these findings is not clear since significant regression of left ventricular hypertrophy (LVH) was observed in both groups, but the anti-fibrotic action of ACEIs through the suppression of RAAS might have played a role [68, 69].

During ASCOT, ambulatory blood pressure monitoring (ABPM) was performed in 1905 participants in order to assess the impact of the treatment regimens on ambulatory BP and whether ambulatory BP values were related to cardiovascular outcomes. Daytime BP was slightly higher in the amlodipine-based treatment arm (by 1.1/1.6 mmHg), night-time systolic BP was higher in the atenolol-based treatment arm by 2.2 mmHg and 24-h systolic BP was similar in both groups [70]. In accordance with other reports [71], higher nocturnal SBP was significantly associated with worse cardiovascular outcomes to a larger extent than clinic BP or daytime BP, concluding that this might have contributed to the results of the whole ASCOT study in favor of the CCB ± ACEI treatment arm. The lower rates of nocturnal BP in these patients were attributed to the longer half-life time of amlodipine [70]; CCBs are generally considered to achieve a more uniform blood pressure control compared with other agents [1].

Another ASCOT sub-study with 720 patients showed favorable results of the amlodipine-based regimen in indexes of retinal microcirculation compared to the atenolol-based one. These findings may reflect a beneficial impact of this regimen on the microvasculature in total, mainly through vasodilation and regression of small arteries remodeling. Impaired microcirculation results in reduced blood flow and is associated with target-organ damage and cardiovascular morbidity, while other data suggest a possible link between microvascular with macrovascular disease. Thus, the improvement in indexes of retinal microcirculation, which serve as markers of better function of microvasculature, may be a therapeutic target and the results of this sub-study indicate another potential advantage of the CCB ± ACEI regimen compared to the BB ± diuretic regimen in the main ASCOT study [72].

Although irrelevant with the comparison of combination therapies, ASCOT also provided valuable information about the treatment of hypertension with antihypertensive agents beyond the five main classes, i.e. ACEIs, ARBs, CCBs, BBs and diuretics. Doxazocin, an alpha-blocker, and spironolactone, a mineralocorticoid receptor antagonist (MRA) were successfully used as add-on therapies when BP target was not obtained with the prespecified two-drug combination. Doxazosin was, by design, the third drug to be added if BP was uncontrolled and 10,069 participants were treated with it. Doxazosin appeared to be well-tolerated, safe and effective. It produced a mean BP reduction of 11.7/6.9 mmHg with relatively low rates of discontinuation (7.5%) [73]. Most importantly, the association of the use of doxazosin with heart failure, which was observed in ALLHAT [74] and was the main concern for this drug, was not confirmed, as the rates of HF were low in this population [73]. Furthermore, ASCOT contributed to the establishment of MRAs as additional therapy in resistant hypertension, since spironolactone, which was used as fourth-line therapy (1411 patients with a dose of 25–50 mg), was as well safe and effective. It provided even larger mean BP reduction (21.9/9.5 mmHg) with low rates of discontinuation and adverse events [75]. Of course, these data are non-randomized and not placebo-controlled and should be interpreted with caution. Nevertheless, they are useful for the selection of the most appropriate combination in cases of resistant hypertension.

Finally, an important sub-study of ASCOT evaluated the response of patients of different ethnicities and the results were interesting, despite the important limitation that the large majority of patients (>90%) were whites. While the response to amlodipine monotherapy and to the addition of diuretic (on top of atenolol) were similar in all groups, blacks showed a lower response to beta-blocker monotherapy and blacks and South Asians showed a lower response to the addition of perindopril (on top of amlodipine). Lower activation of the RAAS and larger plasma volume are the proposed mechanisms for these findings [76]. These results are in accordance with other studies, such as ALLHAT [77], and international guidelines that recommend CCBs and diuretics to be preferred in black hypertensives [1, 45, 78].

The ACCOMPLISH Trial

The ACCOMPLISH trial is considered the second (after ASCOT) landmark trial in the comparison of combination therapies in hypertension. It was a multicenter, prospective, randomized, double-blinded, controlled trial that was conducted from October 2003 to January 2008 in five countries (United States of America, Denmark, Norway, Sweden and Finland). The trial recruited 11,506 hypertensive patients at high risk for cardiovascular events, i.e. with a history of CHD, stroke, peripheral artery disease, renal disease, diabetes mellitus or LVH. The ACCOMPLISH trial was the first trial to compare directly two combinations of antihypertensive agents, since a two-drug regimen was the initial treatment for all participants. Patients were randomly assigned to receive either benazepril 20–40 mg plus amlodipine 5–10 mg (n = 5744 patients) or benazepril 20–40 mg plus hydrochlorothiazide 12.5–25 mg (n = 5762 patients) in order to achieve BP control. If two-drug therapy failed to achieve BP control, other classes of antihypertensive agents, such as beta-blockers, alpha-blockers, clonidine or spironolactone, were added. Mean age was 68 years old, 60.4% of participants were diabetics; baseline BP rates and basic demographic and clinical characteristics were similar in both groups. The primary endpoint was a composite of cardiovascular events and death from cardiovascular causes [15]. The rationale of the study was to compare the efficacy of two combinations that were composed of the three most widely used classes of antihypertensive agents at that time: angiotensin-converting enzyme inhibitors, calcium channel blockers and thiazide diuretics. Beta-blockers had fallen back in the treatment of hypertension in the light of data (including ASCOT) that were questioning their ability to prevent cardiovascular disease to the same degree with the other drugs. Diuretics were still considered a first-line antihypertensive agent, as they had proven their efficacy in several trials, including ALLHAT, where a diuretic was found to be non-inferior, if not superior, compared to an ACEI and a CCB [22]. ACEIs and CCBs appeared as the new, attractive, safe and effective drugs with the possible benefits beyond blood pressure lowering, at least at specific populations (especially the ACEIs). Therefore, a comparison of an ACEI + CCB vs an ACEI + diuretic combination seemed a reasonable aim for a large study [15] and a direct test of the JNC-7 recommendation of a diuretic as a preferred agent for initial treatment (either as monotherapy or in combination therapy) in hypertensive patients [21, 79].

Similarly to ASCOT, the ACCOMPLISH trial was ended prematurely by the data and safety monitoring committee after a mean follow-up of 3 years, as there was a difference in the outcomes between the two treatment groups that exceeded the boundary of the prespecified stopping rule. Significantly fewer patients in the benazepril plus hydrochlorothiazide group had a primary-outcome event compared to the benazepril plus amlodipine group (552 patients or 9.6% vs 679 patients or 11.8%), representing a relative risk reduction of 19.6% (HR:0.80, 95% CI: 0.72 to 0.90, $p < 0.001$), as shown in Fig. 10.4. Regarding the components of the primary endpoint, patients in the ACEI + CCB group had significantly fewer MIs (HR: 0.78, 95% CI: 0.62–0.99, $p = 0.04$) and coronary revascularization procedures (HR: 0.86, 95%CI: 0.74–1.00, $p = 0.04$) and there was also a trend towards fewer cardiovascular deaths (HR: 0.80, 95% CI:0.62–1.03, $p = 0.08$), which would probably have achieved statistical significance if the study had not been terminated prematurely (Fig. 10.5). The difference in all-cause mortality was non-significant (HR: 0.90, 95% CI:0.76–1.07, $p = 0.24$). In contrast to ALLHAT, the rate of hospitalization for heart failure was similar in the diuretic-based and the CCB-based regimen (HR:1.04,95% CI: 0.79–1.38, $p = 0.77$). These results were observed in both diabetics and non-diabetics and in both younger and older patients of the study. The difference between the two groups in mean BP values was small, i.e. 0.9 mmHg for systolic BP and 1.1 mmHg for diastolic BP, both in favor of the ACEI + CCB group (131.6/73.3 mmHg in the ACEI + CCB group and 132.5/74.4 mmHg in the ACEI + diuretic group). The majority of participants in both groups (approximately 70%) were on the prespecified treatment regimen at the end of the study and 32.3% of patients received additional antihypertensive agents. It is noteworthy that approximately 75% of patients of both groups achieved BP control (defined as BP < 140/90 mmHg), which is the best rate ever seen in a large trial, while only 37.3% had their BP controlled at the beginning of the study [15]. The high rates of BP control partially explain the relatively low, compared to other trials, rates of cardiovascular events at a high-risk population and indicate the value of achieving BP targets in terms of CVD prevention [80].

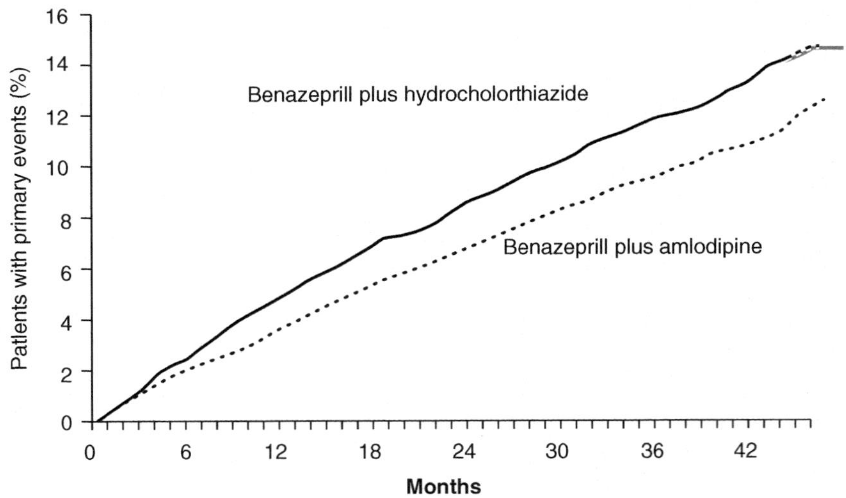

No. at risk

Benazepril plus amlodipine	5512	5317	5141	4959	4739	2826	1447
Benazepril plus hydrochlorothiazide	5483	5274	5082	4892	4655	2749	1390

Fig. 10.4 Kaplan–Meier curves for time to first primary composite end point in ACCOMPLISH. There were 552 patients with events (9.6%) in the benazepril–amlodipine group, as compared with 679 patients with events (11.8%) in the benazepril–hydrochlorothiazide group; HR: 0.80, 95% CI: 0.72 to 0.90, p < 0.001. (Jamerson et al. [15])

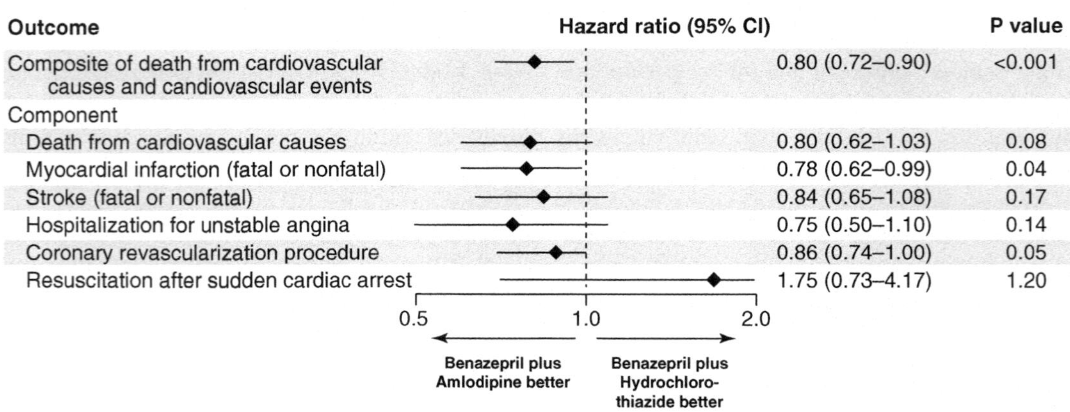

Fig. 10.5 Hazard ratios for the primary outcome and the individual components in ACCOMPLISH trial. (Jamerson et al. [15])

The ACCOMPLISH trial was actually a comparison between a CCB (amlodipine) and a diuretic (hydrochlorothiazide) as add-on drugs to an ACEI-based regimen. Up to then, no study had ever shown a superiority of a CCB-based over a diuretic-based regimen [1]. Thereby, the ACCOMPLISH results had an important impact on the emerging debate about which regimens are more beneficial, especially in high-risk individuals, and whether diuretics should remain a preferred choice for initial treatment.

There is general agreement that the findings of ACCOMPLISH cannot be attributed to the difference in the mean BP between the two treatment arms, which was rather small (0.9/1.1 mmHg), though still statistically significant (Fig. 10.6). Additionally, a sub-study of ACCOMPLISH with 573 patients demonstrated that there were no

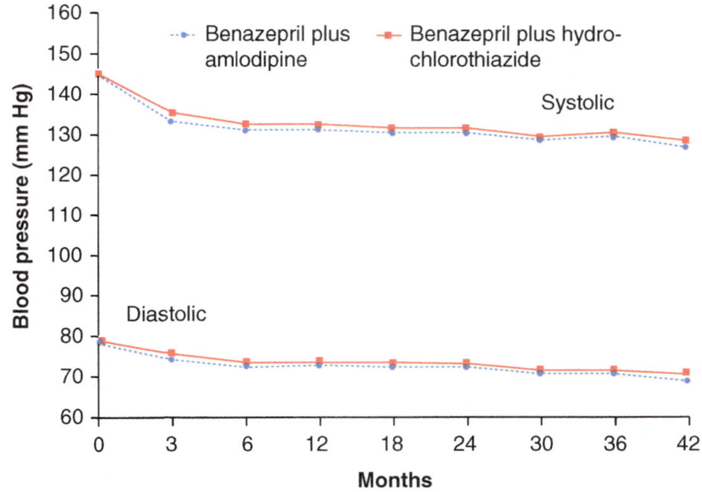

No. at risk

Benazepril plus amlodipine	5740	5517	5404	5178	5010	4866	4298	2804	1074
Benazepril plus hydrochloro-thiazide	5757	5537	5408	5222	5033	4825	4299	2529	1042

Fig. 10.6 Effects of treatment on systolic and diastolic blood pressure over time in ACCOMPLISH. (Jamerson et al. [15])

major differences in 24-h mean blood pressure between treatment arms; in fact, the small differences observed were in favor of the hydrochlorothiazide-based regimen [81]. It is not clear whether the higher percentage of BP control achieved in the ACEI+CCB group (75.4% vs 72.4%) contributed to the results or whether the numerically but non-significantly lower rate of drug discontinuation in the same group (28.8% vs 31.2%) affected treatment compliance and consequently the observed outcomes [15]. Some authors suggested that the choice of hydrochlorothiazide as component of the ACEI + diuretic regimen might have favored the ACEI + CCB combination, since chlorthalidone was the diuretic used in the large trials, e.g. the ALLHAT [20] and the Systolic Hypertension in the Elderly Program (SHEP) trial [82] that established this class of agents as first-line treatment in hypertension. It was also claimed that, since chlorthalidone is twice as potent (mg for mg) as hydrochlorothiazide and it was used at the dose of 12.5–25 mg in ALLHAT and SHEP, the dose of hydrochlorothiazide 12.5–25 mg used in ACCOMPLISH was suboptimal and might have underestimated the antihypertensive effect of this drug. Moreover, hydrochlorothiazide has a shorter half-life time compared to either chlorthalidone or amlodipine, which was used in the other treatment arm of ACCOMPLISH, thus, it is probably less effective in lowering BP throughout the full 24-h dosing period [58, 83]. The ACCOMPLISH Investigators argued that the choice of hydrochlorothiazide at the dose of 12.5–25 mg reflected broad clinical practice, as it is the most commonly prescribed thiazide diuretic, and that the antihypertensive effect of the drug was adequate, since the differences in mean BP and 24-h ambulatory BP were small [15, 81].

Other authors indicated that the fact that a large proportion of the participants had a history of coronary artery disease favored the amlodipine-based regimen due to the anti-ischemic actions of this agent [80]. Indeed, events from the coronary vasculature were significantly fewer in this treatment group. Nevertheless, this benefit was not limited in the reduction of coronary revascularization procedures, where CCBs were already known to be useful as first-line treatment of stable angina [84], but was extended to the incidence of myocardial infarction, whose rate was as well significantly lower in the amlodipine-based group [15].

Similarly to ASCOT, the superiority of the CCB + ACEI combination in ACCOMPLISH was attributed to physiological actions of the treatment regimens beyond BP lowering. Since an ACEI (benazepril) was contained in both treatment regimens of ACCOMPLISH, the debate was mostly referring to the physiological effects of a CCB (amlodipine) and a diuretic (hydrochlorothiazide) either when added to an ACEI or as separate agents. There is evidence suggesting that CCBs have vasoprotective and anti-atherosclerotic properties [56, 57], which might be more intense when these agents are combined with ACEIs [54, 58, 59], while diuretics are considered to have limited, if any, nonhemodynamic vascular benefits [15, 85]. Furthermore, diuretics exert metabolic adverse effects as they cause hypokalemia and other electrolytic disturbances, that may result in severe arrhythmias and worse prognosis [86], impair glucose and lipid metabolism and increase serum uric acid levels [12, 41, 87]. Diuretics also stimulate the RAAS through intravascular volume contraction [4], resulting in exposure of heart and vessels to the deleterious consequences of RAAS activation [52, 53]. These adverse effects may attenuate the benefit from their antihypertensive action [88] and could be partially responsible for the shortfall in the prevention of CHD with antihypertensive treatment that was observed in the first hypertension trials, where diuretics and BBs were mainly used [16]. It was also stated that when baseline BP levels are near to target, such as in ACCOMPLISH (mean baseline BP levels approximately 145/80 mmHg), benefits from BP lowering are expected to be reduced compared to populations with higher baseline BP levels, therefore adverse effects from antihypertensive therapy will be more apparent [88].

Some other factors that contributed to the results of the ASCOT were also present at the ACCOMPLISH trial. A prespecified secondary renal endpoint, defined as doubling of serum creatinine or progression to end-stage renal disease (ESRD), was significantly worse in the diuretic-based regimen (3.7% vs 2.0% of patients, HR: 0.52, 95% CI: 0.41–0.65, $p < 0.0001$-Table 10.5) and partly explains the worse cardiovascular outcomes at the same group, as renal disease predisposes to cardiovascular events. Since both groups were treated with an ACEI and CCBs are not known to affect renal function significantly, the use of a diuretic was probably related to renal impairment due to volume depletion and/or hypotension resulting in reduced renal blood flow. Indeed, hypotension and dizziness were significantly more frequent in the ACEI + diuretic group in non-CKD patients. It should also be noticed that these results were observed despite the fact that albuminuria was reduced to a larger extent in the benazepril + hydrochlorothiazide group; the significance of this finding is unclear,

Table 10.5 Renal outcomes by treatment arm in the intention-to-treat population (n = 11,506) in ACCOMPLISH trial [48]

	Benazepril plus amlodipine (n = 5744)	Benazepril plus hydrochlorothiazide (n = 5762)	Hazard ratio (95% CI)	p value
Main endpoint of progression of chronic kidney disease	113 (1.97%)	215 (3.73%)	0.52 (0.41–0.65)	<0.0001
Doubling of serum creatinine concentration	105 (1.83%)	208 (3.61%)	0.51 (0.39–0.63)	<0.0001
Dialysis	7 (0.12%)	13 (0.23%)	0.53 (0.21–1.35)	0.180
eGFR <15 mL/min/1·73 m^2	18 (0.31%)	17 (0.30%)	1.06 (0.54–2.05)	0.868
Progression of chronic kidney disease and cardiovascular death	220 (3.83%)	345 (5.99%)	0.63 (0.53–0.74)	<0.0001
Progression of chronic kidney disease and all-cause mortality	346 (6.02%)	465 (8.07%)	0.73 (0.64–0.84)	<0.0001

because only a small proportion (~5%) of participants had macro-albuminuria at the beginning of the study [46].

As in ASCOT, the superiority of the ACEI + CCB regimen may as well have occurred due to a better ability of this combination to reduce central pressures. CCBs are generally considered more effective than diuretics in improving central hemodynamics either as separate agents [61, 62, 65] or when used on top of a RAAS inhibitor [89, 90], probably due to more intense vasodilation. In addition, an ARB + CCB combination has been reported to achieve larger aortic pulse wave velocity (PWV) reduction compared to an ARB + diuretic [89]. An ACEI + CCB regimen was also found superior to an ACEI + diuretic regimen in improving indices of microvascular structure in a small study [91]. Moreover, the ARB + CCB combination has been shown to achieve larger reduction in blood pressure variability compared to the ARB + diuretic regimen [92], CCBs have been reported to be more effective in reducing BP variability compared to other antihypertensive agents [93, 94] and are considered to exert a more uniform BP reduction [1].

An interesting sub-analysis of ACCOMPLISH trial suggested that the clinical response to antihypertensive treatment and, consequently, the cardiovascular outcomes could be associated with body weight and BMI. This analysis showed that rates of the primary endpoint were similar in obese patients (BMI > 30 kg/m^2, n = 5709) of both treatment groups, while in overweight (25 kg/m^2 < BMI < 30 kg/m^2, n = 4157) and normal-weight (BMI < 25 kg/m^2, n = 1616) the primary endpoint was significantly lower in the benazepril + amlodipine group (Table 10.6). The results were similar for the secondary endpoints as well and no major differences in BP values were observed among body weight groups [95]. These findings indicated that

Table 10.6 Comparison of event rates within obese, overweight, and normal weight categories in the population of ACCOMPLISH trial

	Benazepril and amlodipine	Benazepril and hydrochlorothiazide	Hazard ratio (95%CI)	p value
Obese				
Primary endpoint	142/2887 (5%)	152/2822 (5%)	0.89 (0.71–1.12)	0.3189
Cardiovascular death	48/2887 (2%)	47/2822 (2%)	0.97 (0.65–1.45)	0.8844
Total myocardial infarction	67/2887 (2%)	66/2822 (2%)	0.97 (0.68–1.36)	0.8426
Total stroke	52/2887 (2%)	51/2822 (2%)	0.99 (0.67–1.46)	0.9541
Overweight				
Primary endpoint	103/2059 (5%)	137/2098 (7%)	0.76 (0.59–0.94)	0.0369
Cardievascular death	38/2059 (2%)	53/2098 (3%)	0.73 (0.48–1.11)	0.1372
Total myocardial infarction	44/2059 (2%)	65/2098 (3%)	0.69 (0.47–1.00)	0.0522
Total stroke	43/2059 (2%)	54/2098 (3%)	0.81 (0.54–1.21)	0.2953
Normal				
Primary endpoint	43/791 (5%)	75/825 (9%)	0.57 (0.39–0.84)	0.0037
Cardievascular death	21/791 (3%)	34/825 (4%)	0.62 (0.36–1.07)	0.0853
Total myocardial infarction	14/791 (2%)	28/825 (3%)	0.50 (0.26–0.96)	0.0364
Total stroke	17/791 (2%)	28/825 (3%)	0.60 (0.33–1.11)	0.1025

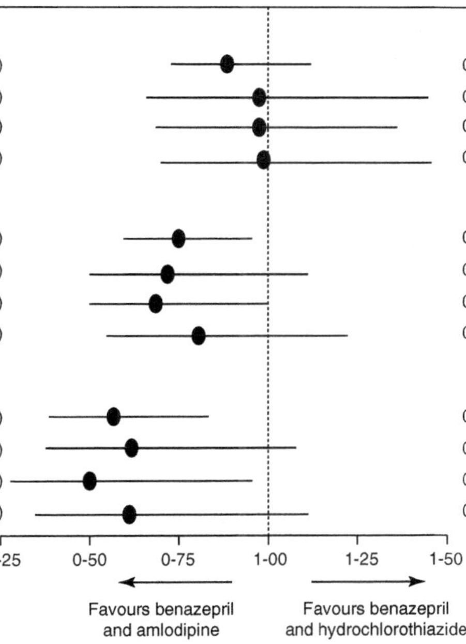

Mancia et al. [95]
Hazard ratio was calculated by Cox's regression and adjusted for age, sex, diabetes, and previous history of cardiovascular events, stroke, or chronic kidney disease

diuretic therapy was less protective in non-obese hypertensives, while it provided adequate cardiovascular protection in obese patients; a similar observation was also extracted from an analysis of the SHEP trial [96]. There is evidence suggesting that hypertension in obese individuals is mostly mediated by volume overload and in lean ones mostly by vasoconstriction and intrinsic vascular pathology and the ACCOMPLISH Investigators argued that this point of view could explain their findings. Additionally, it is not clear whether and to what extent the so-called 'obesity paradox' (better cardiovascular outcomes in patients with increased BMI) is also implicated. In any case, the ACCOMPLISH Investigators concluded that diuretics may not be the best choice for non-obese patients [95]. Of course, diuretics should be used with caution in obese patients due to their potential diabetogenic action [1]. Thus, the results of this analysis should be interpreted rather as a discouragement in diuretic use in non-obese hypertensives than as a signal of potential beneficial action of these drugs in obese patients, where they are already known to exert adverse metabolic effects.

Comparing Antihypertensive Combinations

ASCOT and ACCOMPLISH, the two most important trials in combination therapy in hypertension, suggested a possible superiority of the ACEI + CCB regimen compared to diuretic + beta-blocker and ACEI + diuretic respectively [14, 15]. These two RCTs, in conjunction with other studies, established the ACEI + CCB combination as a safe, well-tolerated and effective in the prevention of CVD regimen that preserves the advantages of both ACEIs and CCBs and potentially confers benefits beyond BP lowering, especially in high-risk hypertensives. Indeed, this combination causes relatively few serious side effects [14], as the one component may offset the side effects of the other [4], and provides adequate, prompt and uniform blood pressure reduction with a favorable effect on several hemodynamic parameters besides clinic BP, such as BP variability, nocturnal BP and central pressures [14, 35, 60, 70]. Furthermore, it exerts anti-atherosclerotic and anti-proliferative effects [52–54], thereby it is a preferable regimen for hypertensives with LVH, peripheral artery disease or coronary artery disease [97]. Another advantage of the ACEI + CCB combination is its nephroprotective properties [14, 15], thereby it is a first-line regimen for patients with kidney disease (including uncomplicated proteinuria). Additionally, it is the combination of choice for patients with metabolic syndrome, because it prevents, or at least does not cause, new-onset diabetes in contrast to BB- or diuretic-based regimens, and it is also suitable for diabetics with hypertension, where a RAAS inhibitor should be included in the antihypertensive regimen [1].

The ACEI + thiazide combination is as well a popular regimen, since it has been proven effective in reducing BP and preventing from cardiovascular disease. It shares the same advantages with all ACEI-based combinations and the RAAS blockade exerted by ACEIs offsets the RAAS activation induced by diuretics [4, 87]; furthermore, hypokalemia and hyperglycemia caused by diuretics are attenuated when an ACEI is added [4, 11]. Therefore, it is an appropriate regimen for hypertensives with vascular disease, diabetes or chronic kidney disease, even if renal outcomes were better with the ACEI + CCB combination in ACCOMPLISH [15]. The ACEI + diuretic combination is very useful in hypertensives with systolic HF (where a beta-blocker and an MRA should also be added). On the other hand, it may exert the adverse metabolic effects of diuretics, i.e. new-onset diabetes, hypokalemia and other electrolytic disturbances, impairment of renal function, hyperuricemia and worsening of lipidemic profile, albeit they are less common when a thiazide is combined with an ACEI. Moreover, an ACEI + diuretic combination might be less effective than an ACEI + CCB regimen for the delay of the atherosclerotic process, as diuretics generally produce minor, if any, non-hemodynamic benefits in vascular function [15, 85].

The thiazide diuretic + beta-blocker combination was the most widely used regimen during the past decades at the first trials in hypertension [5] and before the admission of ACEIs and CCBs in everyday clinical practice. It is effective in achieving BP control and generally reduced the rates of CVD in older trials, however, a shortfall in the prevention of CVD, mainly of coronary events, was observed with this regimen compared with the reduction expected from observational studies [16], findings consistent with the results of ASCOT [14]. Taking into account the results of other studies with BBs [22–25] and the fact that solid data supported the efficacy of diuretics in the prevention of CVD [21], BBs were considered responsible for the lower than expected improvement in outcomes. Furthermore, the dysmetabolic effects of the components of this regimen, mainly the development of new-onset diabetes, seem to be enlarged when they are combined and this combination is recommended to be avoided, unless there are compelling indications, in patients with metabolic syndrome [1, 5]. The diuretic + BB combination also seems to be less effective than other regimens in reducing central pressures [60] and less tolerable with increased rates of discontinuation [14, 49]. Even if there are data indicating that these disadvantages may be attenuated with the use of vasodilating BBs [1], this combination and BB-based regimens overall have fallen back in the treatment of uncomplicated hypertension [1, 45]. Nevertheless, ESH/ESC Guidelines still recommended it as a possible combination and its main use is in hypertensives with systolic HF (along with an ACEI or ARB and an MRA) [1] and in patients who do not tolerate RAAS inhibitors and CCBs.

The CCB + thiazide diuretic combination is generally safe and effective and has widely and successfully been used in clinical trials [5, 98, 99]. Moreover, the addition of a diuretic may attenuate the CCB-induced peripheral edema [100]. However, its additive BP reduction is rather moderate [4], while direct data about comparison of this regimen with other combinations are lacking. It is a preferable and convenient regimen for black hypertensives who have no compelling indication for another class [78] and for hypertensives who cannot tolerate an ACEI or an ARB. The ACEI + BB and the dihydropyridine CCB + BB combination are proper but less studied regimens, while the non-dihydropyridine CCB + BB combination should generally be avoided due to the risk of bradyarrythmias, even if it seems attractive for rate control in patients with atrial fibrillation (AF) [1]. An ACEI + BB regimen is the best choice for hypertensives with coronary heart disease and concomitant systolic LV dysfunction, previous ST-segment elevation myocardial infarction (STEMI), stable angina or asymptomatic myocardial ischaemia and is obligatory for all patients with heart failure with reduced ejection fraction (HFrEF), with the addition of an MRA and, if needed, a diuretic [1, 97, 101–103]. The main disadvantage of this combination is its relatively low additional BP reduction compared to ACEI and BB monotherapy [4]. The dihydropyridine CCB + BB combination is mainly used in hypertensives with stable angina that requires more than one anti-anginal agents [1, 97] or in patients with hypertension who do not tolerate or have contraindications for RAAS inhibitors and diuretics.

Finally, regarding ARB-based combinations, the same principles that apply for ACEIs are generally valid for ARBs, since these two classes are generally considered equivalent [1, 4, 45, 50, 51]. Thus, the ARB + CCB and the ARB + thiazide diuretic regimens are recommended as preferred two-drug combinations and the ARB + BB is considered a possible but less studied regimen. The ACEI + ARB combination is absolutely contraindicated due to increased risk of serious adverse effects [1] as reported in ONTARGET study. In this large trial (n = 25,620 patients at high risk for CV events) participants were randomly assigned to receive ramipril, telmisartan or their combination. All cardiovascular outcomes were similar in the three groups. However, the primary renal outcome, a composite of dialysis, doubling of serum creatinine and death, occurred in significantly more patients in the combination group (HR 1.09, 95%: 1.01–1.18, p = 0.037 compared to ramipril), despite the larger reduction in proteinuria observed in the same arm. Syncope and hypotension were also significantly more frequent in the combination group [10, 51]. An important advantage of ARB-based combinations is their better tolerance compared to ACEI-based ones, since dry cough, a frequent side effect of ACEIs, is uncommon with ARBs [87]. The most important trial that successfully used an ARB-based combination was LIFE, where most patients in the ARB-based group received hydrochlorothiazide added on losartan and cardiovascular morbidity and mortality were significantly lower in the losartan-based treatment arm compared to the atenolol-based group [22].

The Impact of ASCOT, ACCOMPLISH on HTN Guidelines Recommendations

Selecting the most appropriate treatment regimen either as monotherapy or as combination therapy remains probably the most challenging and, concurrently, controversial issue in hypertension [104]. Although there is a vast amount of data from RCTs and meta-analyses, the results are in many cases conflicting. It should also be taken into account that most of the trials in hypertension enrolled high-risk patients, because demonstrating significant differences in hard endpoints in lower risk populations would require an extremely long follow-up [105]. Thereby, it is not certain whether the results of these studies can be extrapolated to all hypertensives. Regarding combination therapy, the evidence is rather scarce; despite the fact that many trials did use more than one agents in order to achieve BP targets in most participants, few of them intended, by design, to compare different combinations (with ASCOT and ACCOMPLISH being the most important ones). The large number of potential combinations makes the issue even more complex. Most experts and guidelines recommendations agree that BP control is the main treatment target and that in conditions like CHD, HFrEF, PAD, LVH, CKD, diabetes, metabolic syndrome and black ethnicity specific regimens should be preferred. However, there is no unanimity on whether specific regimens provide further cardiovascular benefits beyond blood pressure lowering in the general population of hypertensives independent of each individual's comorbidities and, consequently, which regimen should be preferred for the treatment of uncomplicated hypertension [1, 45, 106–109]. These concerns refer mainly to a possible superiority of ACEIs, ARBs and, to a lesser extent, CCBs over other drugs due to their pleiotropic actions, with some data being supportive [14, 15, 22, 104, 110, 111] and other rejective [28, 30, 104, 112, 113] to this assumption.

The results of ASCOT and ACCOMPLISH had an important impact on hypertension guidelines published after the termination of these studies. The ESC/ESH 2007 Guidelines did not classify the diuretic + BB combination as 'preferred' (as in previous guidelines) and suggested that BBs, especially in combination with a thiazide diuretic, should be avoided in patients with the metabolic syndrome or at high risk for diabetes. Nevertheless, they maintained BBs as first-line agents [5]. The JNC-8 downgraded both BBs and diuretics not only as a combination, but also as separate agents for the treatment of uncomplicated hypertension. Thiazide-type diuretics are no longer recommended as preferred initial choice but as equal drugs with ARBs, ACEIs and CCBs, while BBs are no longer considered to be equally effective agents compared to ACEIs, ARBs and CCBs and should be used as fourth-line therapy, after initiating an ACEI or ARB, a CCB and a diuretic. Consequently, diuretic-based combinations are no longer considered superior but equal to combinations based on ACEIs, ARBs and CCBs. It is also stated that the benazepril + amlodipine is considered superior to benazepril + hydrochlorothiazide in patients >55 years old for the outcomes that ACCOMPLISH showed better results in the respective treatment arm [45]. The British Hypertension Society – National Institute for Health and Clinical Excellence (BHS-NICE) Guidelines published a rapid update soon after the results of ASCOT (in June 2006), where BBs were downgraded as fourth-line therapy (after

ACEIs, CCBs and thiazide-type diuretics alone or in combinations) and ACEIs were recommended as initial therapy for patients <55 years old [114]. Moreover, NICE 2011 guidelines, obviously influenced by the results of ACCOMPLISH, recommend a CCB as initial therapy in hypertensives >55 years instead of a CCB or a thiazide-type diuretic, as suggested in the previous NICE guidelines, and clearly upgrade the ACEI (or ARB) + CCB regimen as first-choice two-drug combination. They also state that if a diuretic is to be used, chlorthalidone should be preferred over hydrochlorothiazide [108]. Finally, the successful use of spironolactone as third or fourth drug in ASCOT largely contributed to the establishment of MRAs as a reliable additional therapy, when drugs from the main classes fail to achieve BP control [1, 45, 108].

As a result of different interpretation of data that are in many cases conflicting, current recommendations for the treatment of hypertension are not uniform among hypertension societies. ESH/ESC 2013 Guidelines suggest that ACEIs, ARBs, CCBs, BBs and thiazide-type diuretics should be considered equal for monotherapy treatment of uncomplicated hypertension in the general (non-black) population while specific agents should be preferred in specific conditions [1]. The JNC-8 considers ACEIs, ARBs, CCBs and thiazide-type diuretics as first-line agents in non-black patients and CCBs and thiazides in blacks, while BBs are to be used as fourth-line therapy [45]. Similar recommendations are provided by the American College of Cardiology/American Heart Association (AHA/ACC) 2017 Guidelines: thiazide-type diuretics, CCBs, ACEIs and ARBs should be preferred in the general population and CCBs and thiazide-type diuretics in black hypertensives [109]. NICE 2011 Guidelines recommend ACEIs and ARBs as initial therapy for non-blacks <55 years old and CCBs are the first choice followed by thiazide-type diuretics for non-blacks >55 years old and all black hypertensives. BBs are not recommended for initial therapy and may be considered only in younger patients who cannot receive an ACEI or ARB or have evidence of increased activity of the sympathetic system [108]. The American Society of Hypertension – International Society of Hypertension (ASH-ISH) 2014 Guidelines have similar recommendations with NICE, with the exceptions of equal eligibility of CCBs and thiazides in older and black patients and a slightly different boundary for the distinction between older and younger patients (60 instead of 55 years old) [107]. The Hypertension Canada's 2017 Guidelines consider ACEIs, ARBs, CCBs and thiazide-type diuretics as suitable drugs for initial therapy; the same recommendation also applies for BBs, but only for patients <60 years old [106]. The new edition of joint ESH/ESC guidelines is under preparation and they are expected to be presented in June 2018.

Regarding two-drug combination therapy in hypertensives without compelling indication for a specific regimen, all Guidelines consider the combination ACEI + ARB absolutely contraindicated [1, 45, 106–108, 114]. ESH/ESC 2013 Guidelines classify the ACEI + thiazide, ARB + thiazide, ACEI + CCB, ARB + CCB, CCB + thiazide combinations as 'preferred'. The BB + thiazide combination is considered useful, with the limitation that non-vasodilating BBs and diuretics should be used only as additional drugs in hypertensives with the metabolic syndrome and/or prediabetes. The ACEI + BB, ARB + BB, dihydropyridine CCB + BB combinations are considered possible but less studied regimens and the non-dihydropyridine CCB + BB should be avoided (Fig. 10.7) [1]. Similar to ESH/ESC, the JNC-8 recommends the same five two-drug combinations as preferred in non-blacks, while the CCB + thiazide combination is considered preferable in blacks. BBs are not recommended to be included in a two-drug combination [45]. ACC/AHA 2017 Guidelines make no specific recommendation for combination therapy, thus, it should be assumed that all two-drug combinations that consist of the first-line agents (thiazide-type diuretics, CCBs, ACEIs and ARBs), with the exception of the ACEI + ARB combination, are considered equal [109]. NICE guidelines suggest that the ACEI + CCB or the ARB + CCB regimens are the best choices for non-blacks, followed by ACEI + thiazide-type diuretic or

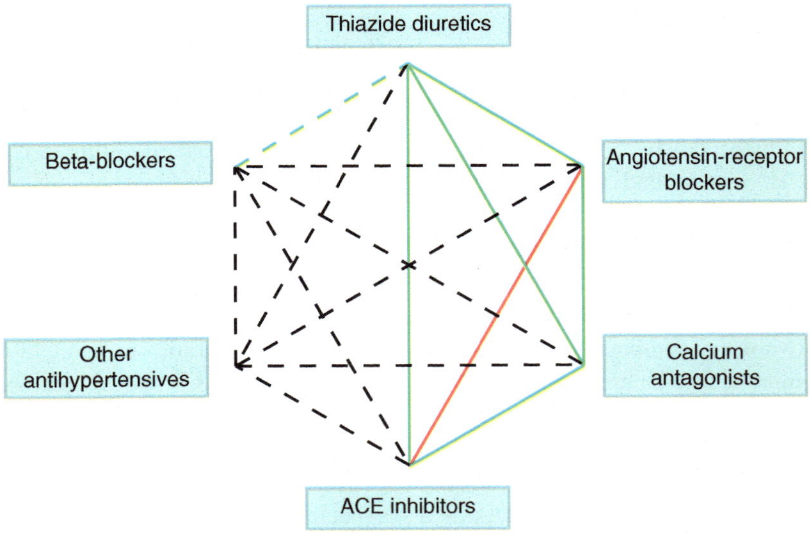

Fig. 10.7 Possible combinations of classes of antihypertensive drugs according to ESC/ESH Guidelines. Green continuous lines: preferred combinations; green dashed line: useful combination (with some limitations); black dashed lines: possible but less well-tested combinations; red continuous line: not recommended combination. Although verapamil and diltiazem are sometimes used with a beta-blocker to improve ventricular rate control in permanent atrial fibrillation, only dihydropyridine calcium antagonists should normally be combined with beta-blockers. (Mancia et al. [1])

ARB + thiazide-type diuretic, while an ARB + CCB should be offered in blacks [108]. The ASH-ISH Guidelines recommend the ACEI + CCB, ARB + CCB, ACEI + thiazide, ARB + thiazide combinations as first-line regimens [107] and the Canadian Guidelines consider all combinations of the first-line agents (including BBs), except from the ACEI + ARB regimen, suitable for two-drug therapy [106]. It is concluded from the above recommendations that if BP is uncontrolled with two drugs and a third agent should be added, ESH/ESC, JNC-8, NICE and ASH-ISH Guidelines agree that the ACEI or ARB + CCB + thiazide-type diuretic combination should be the first-line regimen [1, 45, 107, 108], while Canadian Guidelines consider all combinations that do not include both an ACEI an ARB proper [106]. If additional therapy is required, BBs, MRAs (mainly spironolactone), higher dose of thiazide diuretics, potassium-sparing diuretics and alpha-blockers are the next choices. Direct vasodilators, centrally acting agents and referral to hypertension expert are the last options if BP is still uncontrolled [1, 45, 106–108].

Conclusions

In conclusion, combination therapy in hypertension is safe and more effective compared to monotherapy for an increasing number of patients in order to achieve BP control and obtain maximum cardiovascular protection in hypertensive individuals. Moreover, current guidelines recommend it as initial therapy in patients with high baseline BP values and/or at high risk for cardiovascular events. ASCOT and ACCOMPLISH are the landmark trials in the comparison of different combinations of antihypertensive agents and demonstrated a superiority of an ACEI + CCB combination over a BB + diuretic and an ACEI + diuretic combination respectively in terms of cardiovascular outcomes [14, 15]. These trials established this combination as a safe, effective and, in many cases, preferable regimen for the treatment of hypertension and had a significant impact on guidelines for the management of hypertension [1, 45, 108, 113] as well as on everyday clinical practice. Most importantly, the relatively low rates of events in ACCOMPLISH, where BP control was the best ever observed in a large trial [15], emphasized the great importance of adequate BP reduction, which remains the main treatment target.

References

1. Mancia G, Fagard R, Narkiewicz K, Redón J, Zanchetti A, Böhm M, et al. 2013 ESH/ESC Guidelines for the management of arterial hypertension: the Task Force for the management of arterial hypertension of the European Society of Hypertension (ESH) and of the European Society of Cardiology (ESC). J Hypertens. 2013;31(7):1281–357. https://doi.org/10.1097/01.hjh.0000431740.32696.cc.
2. Byrd JB, Zeng C, Tavel HM, Magid DJ, O'Connor PJ, Margolis KL, et al. Combination therapy as initial treatment for newly diagnosed hypertension. Am Heart J. 2011;162(2):340–6. https://doi.org/10.1016/j.ahj.2011.05.010. Epub 2011 Jul 18.
3. Corrao G, Nicotra F, Parodi A, Zambon A, Heiman F, Merlino L, et al. Cardiovascular protection by initial and subsequent combination of antihypertensive drugs in daily life practice. Hypertension. 2011;58(4):566–72. https://doi.org/10.1161/HYPERTENSIONAHA.111.177592.
4. Gradman AH, Basile JN, Carter BL, Bakris GL. American Society of Hypertension Writing Group. Combination therapy in hypertension. J Clin Hypertens (Greenwich). 2011;13(3):146–54. https://doi.org/10.1111/j.1751-7176.2010.00397.x.
5. Mancia G, De Backer G, Dominiczak A, Cifkova R, Fagard R, Germano G, et al. 2007 Guidelines for the management of arterial hypertension: the Task Force for the Management of Arterial Hypertension of the European Society of Hypertension (ESH) and of the European Society of Cardiology (ESC). J Hypertens. 2007;25(6):1105–87.
6. Wald DS, Law M, Morris JK, Bestwick JP, Wald NJ. Combination therapy versus monotherapy in reducing blood pressure: meta-analysis on 11,000 participants from 42 trials. Am J Med. 2009;122(3):290–300.
7. Corrao G, Parodi A, Zambon A, Heiman F, Filippi A, Cricelli C, et al. Reduced discontinuation of antihypertensive treatment by two-drug combination as first step. Evidence from daily life practice. J Hypertens. 2010;28(7):1584–90.
8. Claxton AJ, Cramer J, Pierce C. A systematic review of the associations between dose regimens and medication compliance. Clin Ther. 2001;23(8):1296–310.
9. Gupta AK, Arshad S, Poulter NR. Compliance, safety, and effectiveness of fixed-dose combinations of antihypertensive agents: a meta-analysis. Hypertension. 2010;55(2):399–407. https://doi.org/10.1161/HYPERTENSIONAHA.109.139816. Epub 2009 Dec 21.
10. Mann JF, Schmieder RE, McQueen M, Dyal L, Schumacher H, Pogue J, et al. Renal outcomes with telmisartan, ramipril, or both, in people at high vascular risk (the ONTARGET study): a multicentre, randomised, double-blind, controlled trial. Lancet. 2008;372(9638):547–53. https://doi.org/10.1016/S0140-6736(08)61236-2.
11. Kalra S, Kalra B, Agrawal N. Combination therapy in hypertension: an update. Diabetol Metab Syndr. 2010;2(1):44. https://doi.org/10.1186/1758-5996-2-44.
12. Elliott WJ, Meyer PM. Incident diabetes in clinical trials of antihypertensive drugs: a network meta-analysis. Lancet. 2007;369(9557):201–7.
13. Mancia G, Grassi G, Zanchetti A. New-onset diabetes and antihypertensive drugs. J Hypertens. 2006;24(1):3–10.
14. Dahlöf B, Sever PS, Poulter NR, Wedel H, Beevers DG, Caulfield M, et al. Prevention of cardiovascular events with an antihypertensive regimen of amlodipine adding perindopril as required versus atenolol adding bendroflumethiazide as required, in the Anglo-Scandinavian Cardiac Outcomes Trial-Blood Pressure Lowering Arm (ASCOT-BPLA): a multicentre randomised controlled trial. Lancet. 2005;366(9489):895–906.
15. Jamerson K, Weber MA, Bakris GL, Dahlöf B, Pitt B, Shi V, et al. Benazepril plus amlodipine or hydrochlorothiazide for hypertension in high-risk patients. N Engl J Med. 2008;359(23):2417–28. https://doi.org/10.1056/NEJMoa0806182.
16. Sever PS, Dahlöf B, Poulter NR, Wedel H, Beevers G, Caulfield M, et al. Rationale, design, methods and baseline demography of participants of the Anglo-Scandinavian Cardiac Outcomes Trial. ASCOT investigators. J Hypertens. 2001;19(6):1139–47.
17. Sever PS, Dahlöf B, Poulter NR, Wedel H, Beevers G, Caulfield M, et al. Prevention of coronary and stroke events with atorvastatin in hypertensive patients who have average or lower-than-average cholesterol concentrations, in the Anglo-Scandinavian Cardiac Outcomes Trial–Lipid Lowering Arm (ASCOT-LLA): a multicentre randomised controlled trial. Lancet. 2003;361(9364):1149–58.
18. Ostergren J, Poulter NR, Sever PS, Dahlöf B, Wedel H, Beevers G, et al. The Anglo-Scandinavian Cardiac Outcomes Trial: blood pressure-lowering limb: effects in patients with type II diabetes. J Hypertens. 2008;26(11):2103–11. https://doi.org/10.1097/HJH.0b013e328310e0d9.
19. Pahor M, Psaty BM, Alderman MH, Applegate WB, Williamson JD, Cavazzini C, et al. Health outcomes associated with calcium antagonists compared with other first-line antihypertensive therapies: a meta-analysis of randomised controlled trials. Lancet. 2000;356(9246):1949–54.
20. ALLHAT Officers and Coordinators for the ALLHAT Collaborative Research Group. The Antihypertensive and Lipid-Lowering Treatment to Prevent Heart Attack Trial. Major outcomes

in high-risk hypertensive patients randomized to angiotensin-converting enzyme inhibitor or calcium channel blocker vs diuretic: the Antihypertensive and Lipid-Lowering Treatment to Prevent Heart Attack Trial (ALLHAT). JAMA. 2002;288(23):2981–97.
21. Chobanian AV, Bakris GL, Black HR, Cushman WC, Green LA, Izzo JL Jr, et al. The seventh report of the joint national committee on prevention, detection, evaluation, and treatment of high blood pressure: the JNC 7 report. JAMA. 2003;289(19):2560–72.
22. Dahlöf B, Devereux RB, Kjeldsen SE, Julius S, Beevers G, de Faire U, et al. Cardiovascular morbidity and mortality in the Losartan Intervention for Endpoint reduction in hypertension study (LIFE): a randomised trial against atenolol. Lancet. 2002;359(9311):995–1003.
23. Lindholm LH, Carlberg B, Samuelsson O. Should beta blockers remain first choice in the treatment of primary hypertension? A meta-analysis. Lancet. 2005;366(9496):1545–53.
24. Bradley HA, Wiysonge CS, Volmink JA, Mayosi BM, Opie LH. How strong is the evidence for use of beta-blockers as first-line therapy for hypertension? Systematic review and meta-analysis. J Hypertens. 2006;24(11):2131–41.
25. Carlberg B, Samuelsson O, Lindholm LH. Atenolol in hypertension: is it a wise choice? Lancet. 2004;364(9446):1684–9.
26. Wiysonge CS, Bradley HA, Volmink J, Mayosi BM, Opie LH. Beta-blockers for hypertension. Cochrane Database Syst Rev. 2017;1:CD002003. https://doi.org/10.1002/14651858.CD002003.pub5.
27. Pepine CJ, Handberg EM, Cooper-DeHoff RM, Marks RG, Kowey P, Messerli FH, et al. A calcium antagonist vs a non-calcium antagonist hypertension treatment strategy for patients with coronary artery disease. The International Verapamil-Trandolapril Study (INVEST): a randomized controlled trial. JAMA. 2003;290(21):2805–16.
28. Law MR, Morris JK, Wald NJ. Use of blood pressure lowering drugs in the prevention of cardiovascular disease: meta-analysis of 147 randomised trials in the context of expectations from prospective epidemiological studies. BMJ. 2009;338:b1665. https://doi.org/10.1136/bmj.b1665.
29. Poulter NR, Wedel H, Dahlöf B, Sever PS, Beevers DG, Caulfield M, et al. Role of blood pressure and other variables in the differential cardiovascular event rates noted in the Anglo-Scandinavian Cardiac Outcomes Trial-Blood Pressure Lowering Arm (ASCOT-BPLA). Lancet. 2005;366(9489):907–13.
30. Turnbull F, Blood Pressure Lowering Treatment Trialists' Collaboration. Effects of different blood-pressure-lowering regimens on major cardiovascular events: results of prospectively-designed overviews of randomised trials. Lancet. 2003;362(9395):1527–35.
31. Ritter J, Warren J. ASCOT–old or new drugs for blood pressure? Br J Clin Pharmacol. 2006;61(3):363.
32. Burrill PD. ASCOT: a tale of two treatment regimens: is ASCOT-BPLA being hyped-up? BMJ. 2005;331(7523):1022.
33. Weber MA, Julius S, Kjeldsen SE, Brunner HR, Ekman S, Hansson L, et al. Blood pressure dependent and independent effects of antihypertensive treatment on clinical events in the VALUE Trial. Lancet. 2004;363(9426):2049–51.
34. Hastie CE, Jeemon P, Coleman H, McCallum L, Patel R, Dawson J, et al. Long-term and ultra long-term blood pressure variability during follow-up and mortality in 14,522 patients with hypertension. Hypertension. 2013;62(4):698–705. https://doi.org/10.1161/HYPERTENSIONAHA.113.01343.
35. Rothwell PM, Howard SC, Dolan E, O'Brien E, Dobson JE, Dahlöf B, et al. Effects of beta blockers and calcium-channel blockers on within-individual variability in blood pressure and risk of stroke. Lancet Neurol. 2010;9(5):469–80. https://doi.org/10.1016/S1474-4422(10)70066-1.
36. Gupta AK, Nasothimiou EG, Chang CL, Sever PS, Dahlöf B, Poulter NR, et al. Baseline predictors of resistant hypertension in the Anglo-Scandinavian Cardiac Outcome Trial (ASCOT): a risk score to identify those at high-risk. J Hypertens. 2011;29(10):2004–13. https://doi.org/10.1097/HJH.0b013e32834a8a42.
37. Gupta AK, Dahlof B, Dobson J, Sever PS, Wedel H, Poulter NR, Anglo-Scandinavian Cardiac Outcomes Trial Investigators. Determinants of new-onset diabetes among 19,257 hypertensive patients randomized in the Anglo-Scandinavian Cardiac Outcomes Trial–Blood Pressure Lowering Arm and the relative influence of antihypertensive medication. Diabetes Care. 2008;31(5):982–8. https://doi.org/10.2337/dc07-1768.
38. Grimm C, Köberlein J, Wiosna W, Kresimon J, Kiencke P, Rychlik R. New-onset diabetes and antihypertensive treatment. GMS Health Technol Assess. 2010;6:Doc03. https://doi.org/10.3205/hta000081.
39. Sharma AM, Pischon T, Hardt S, Kunz I, Luft FC. Hypothesis: beta-adrenergic receptor blockers and weight gain: a systematic analysis. Hypertension. 2001;37(2):250–4.
40. Fonseca VA. Effects of beta-blockers on glucose and lipid metabolism. Curr Med Res Opin. 2010;26(3):615–29. https://doi.org/10.1185/03007990903533681.
41. Musini VM, Nazer M, Bassett K, Wright JM. Blood pressure-lowering efficacy of monotherapy with thiazide diuretics for primary hypertension. Cochrane Database Syst Rev. 2014;(5):CD003824. https://doi.org/10.1002/14651858.CD003824.pub2.
42. Ladage D, Schwinger RH, Brixius K. Cardio-selective beta-blocker: pharmacological evidence and their influence on exercise capacity. Cardiovasc Ther. 2013;31(2):76–83. https://doi.org/10.1111/j.1755-5922.2011.00306.x.
43. Zillich AJ, Garg J, Basu S, Bakris GL, Carter BL. Thiazide diuretics, potassium, and the develop-

ment of diabetes: a quantitative review. Hypertension. 2006;48(2):219–24.
44. Piepoli MF, Hoes AW, Agewall S, Albus C, Brotons C, Catapano AL, et al. 2016 European Guidelines on cardiovascular disease prevention in clinical practice: The Sixth Joint Task Force of the European Society of Cardiology and Other Societies on Cardiovascular Disease Prevention in Clinical Practice (constituted by representatives of 10 societies and by invited experts) Developed with the special contribution of the European Association for Cardiovascular Prevention & Rehabilitation (EACPR). Eur Heart J. 2016;37(29):2315–81. https://doi.org/10.1093/eurheartj/ehw106.
45. James PA, Oparil S, Carter BL, Cushman WC, Dennison-Himmelfarb C, Handler J, et al. 2014 evidence-based guideline for the management of high blood pressure in adults: report from the panel members appointed to the Eighth Joint National Committee (JNC 8). JAMA. 2014;311(5):507–20. https://doi.org/10.1001/jama.2013.284427.
46. Bakris GL, Sarafidis PA, Weir MR, Dahlöf B, Pitt B, Jamerson K, et al. Renal outcomes with different fixed-dose combination therapies in patients with hypertension at high risk for cardiovascular events (ACCOMPLISH): a prespecified secondary analysis of a randomised controlled trial. Lancet. 2010;375(9721):1173–81. https://doi.org/10.1016/S0140-6736(09)62100-0.
47. Sever P, Dahlöf B, Poulter N, Wedel H, Beevers G, Caulfield M, et al. Potential synergy between lipid-lowering and blood-pressure-lowering in the Anglo-Scandinavian Cardiac Outcomes Trial. Eur Heart J. 2006;27(24):2982–8.
48. Athyros VG, Mikhailidis DP, Papageorgiou AA, Bouloukos VI, Pehlivanidis AN, Symeonidis AN, et al. Effect of statins and ACE inhibitors alone and in combination on clinical outcome in patients with coronary heart disease. J Hum Hypertens. 2004;18(11):781–8.
49. Veronesi M, Cicero AF, Prandin MG, Dormi A, Cosentino E, Strocchi E, et al. A prospective evaluation of persistence on antihypertensive treatment with different antihypertensive drugs in clinical practice. Vasc Health Risk Manag. 2007;3(6):999–1005.
50. Bangalore S, Fakheri R, Toklu B, Ogedegbe G, Weintraub H, Messerli FH. Angiotensin-converting enzyme inhibitors or angiotensin receptor blockers in patients without heart failure? Insights from 254,301 patients from randomized trials. Mayo Clin Proc. 2016;91(1):51–60. https://doi.org/10.1016/j.mayocp.2015.10.019.
51. ONTARGET Investigators, Yusuf S, Teo KK, Pogue J, Dyal L, Copland I, et al. Telmisartan, ramipril, or both in patients at high risk for vascular events. N Engl J Med. 2008;358(15):1547–59. https://doi.org/10.1056/NEJMoa0801317.
52. Cowan BR, Young AA. Left ventricular hypertrophy and renin-angiotensin system blockade. Curr Hypertens Rep. 2009;11(3):167–72.
53. Montecucco F, Pende A, Mach F. The renin-angiotensin system modulates inflammatory processes in atherosclerosis: evidence from basic research and clinical studies. Mediat Inflamm. 2009;2009:752406. https://doi.org/10.1155/2009/752406.
54. Jamerson KA, Avoiding Cardiovascular Events Through Combination Therapy in Patients Living with Systolic Hypertension Trial. The first hypertension trial comparing the effects of two fixed-dose combination therapy regimens on cardiovascular events: Avoiding Cardiovascular events through Combination therapy in Patients Living with Systolic Hypertension (ACCOMPLISH). J Clin Hypertens (Greenwich). 2003;5(4 Suppl 3):29–35.
55. Heart Outcomes Prevention Evaluation Study Investigators, Yusuf S, Sleight P, Pogue J, Bosch J, Davies R, et al. Effects of an angiotensin-converting-enzyme inhibitor, ramipril, on cardiovascular events in high-risk patients. N Engl J Med. 2000;342(3):145–53.
56. Mason RP. Mechanisms of plaque stabilization for the dihydropyridine calcium channel blocker amlodipine: review of the evidence. Atherosclerosis. 2002;165(2):191–9.
57. Mason RP. Atheroprotective effects of long-acting dihydropyridine-type calcium channel blockers: evidence from clinical trials and basic scientific research. Cerebrovasc Dis. 2003;16(Suppl 3):11–7.
58. Cohen DL, Townsend RR. Will the results of the ACCOMPLISH trial affect the recommendations of JNC 8? J Clin Hypertens (Greenwich). 2009;11(2):100–1. https://doi.org/10.1111/j.1751-7176.2009.00075.x.
59. Ferrari R. Angiotensin converting enzyme inhibitor-calcium antagonist combination: an alliance for cardioprotection? J Hypertens Suppl. 1997;15(2):S109–17.
60. Williams B, Lacy PS, Thom SM, Cruickshank K, Stanton A, Collier D, et al. Differential impact of blood pressure-lowering drugs on central aortic pressure and clinical outcomes: principal results of the Conduit Artery Function Evaluation (CAFE) study. Circulation. 2006;113(9):1213–25.
61. Dudenbostel T, Glasser SP. Effects of antihypertensive drugs on arterial stiffness. Cardiol Rev. 2012;20(5):259–63. https://doi.org/10.1097/CRD.0b013e31825d0a44.
62. Protogerou AD, Stergiou GS, Vlachopoulos C, Blacher J, Achimastos A. The effect of antihypertensive drugs on central blood pressure beyond peripheral blood pressure. Part II: evidence for specific class-effects of antihypertensive drugs on pressure amplification. Curr Pharm Des. 2009;15(3):272–89.
63. Boutouyrie P, Achouba A, Trunet P, Laurent S, EXPLOR Trialist Group. Amlodipine-valsartan combination decreases central systolic blood pressure more effectively than the amlodipine-atenolol combination: the EXPLOR study. Hypertension.

2010;55(6):1314–22. https://doi.org/10.1161/HYPERTENSIONAHA.109.148999.
64. Jiang XJ, O'Rourke MF, Zhang YQ, He XY, Liu LS. Superior effect of an angiotensin-converting enzyme inhibitor over a diuretic for reducing aortic systolic pressure. J Hypertens. 2007;25(5):1095–9.
65. Manisty CH, Hughes AD. Meta-analysis of the comparative effects of different classes of antihypertensive agents on brachial and central systolic blood pressure, and augmentation index. Br J Clin Pharmacol. 2013;75(1):79–92. https://doi.org/10.1111/j.1365-2125.2012.04342.x.
66. Vlachopoulos C, Aznaouridis K, O'Rourke MF, Safar ME, Baou K, Stefanadis C. Prediction of cardiovascular events and all-cause mortality with central haemodynamics: a systematic review and meta-analysis. Eur Heart J. 2010;31(15):1865–71. https://doi.org/10.1093/eurheartj/ehq024.
67. Safar ME, Blacher J, Pannier B, Guerin AP, Marchais SJ, Guyonvarc'h PM, et al. Central pulse pressure and mortality in end-stage renal disease. Hypertension. 2002;39(3):735–8.
68. Tapp RJ, Sharp A, Stanton AV, O'Brien E, Chaturvedi N, Poulter NR, et al. Differential effects of antihypertensive treatment on left ventricular diastolic function: an ASCOT (Anglo-Scandinavian Cardiac Outcomes Trial) substudy. J Am Coll Cardiol. 2010;55(17):1875–81. https://doi.org/10.1016/j.jacc.2009.11.084.
69. Barron AJ, Hughes AD, Sharp A, Baksi AJ, Surendran P, Jabbour RJ, et al. Long-term antihypertensive treatment fails to improve E/e' despite regression of left ventricular mass: an Anglo-Scandinavian cardiac outcomes trial substudy. Hypertension. 2014;63(2):252–8. https://doi.org/10.1161/HYPERTENSIONAHA.113.01360.
70. Dolan E, Stanton AV, Thom S, Caulfield M, Atkins N, McInnes G, et al. Ambulatory blood pressure monitoring predicts cardiovascular events in treated hypertensive patients–an Anglo-Scandinavian cardiac outcomes trial substudy. J Hypertens. 2009;27(4):876–85. https://doi.org/10.1097/HJH.0b013e328322cd62.
71. Hansen TW, Li Y, Boggia J, Thijs L, Richart T, Staessen JA. Predictive role of the nighttime blood pressure. Hypertension. 2011;57(1):3–10. https://doi.org/10.1161/HYPERTENSIONAHA.109.133900.
72. Thom S, Stettler C, Stanton A, Witt N, Tapp R, Chaturvedi N, et al. Differential effects of antihypertensive treatment on the retinal microcirculation: an Anglo-Scandinavian Cardiac Outcomes Trial substudy. Hypertension. 2009;54(2):405–8. https://doi.org/10.1161/HYPERTENSIONAHA.109.133819.
73. Chapman N, Chang CL, Dahlöf B, Sever PS, Wedel H, Poulter NR, et al. Effect of doxazosin gastrointestinal therapeutic system as third-line antihypertensive therapy on blood pressure and lipids in the Anglo-Scandinavian Cardiac Outcomes Trial. Circulation. 2008;118(1):42–8. https://doi.org/10.1161/CIRCULATIONAHA.107.737957.
74. The ALLHAT Officers and Coordinators for the ALLHAT Collaborative Research Group. Major cardiovascular events in hypertensive patients randomized to doxazosin vs chlorthalidone: the antihypertensive and lipid-lowering treatment to prevent heart attack trial (ALLHAT). JAMA. 2000;283(15):1967–75.
75. Chapman N, Dobson J, Wilson S, Dahlöf B, Sever PS, Wedel H, et al. Effect of spironolactone on blood pressure in subjects with resistant hypertension. Hypertension. 2007;49(4):839–45.
76. Gupta AK, Poulter NR, Dobson J, Eldridge S, Cappuccio FP, Caulfield M, et al. Ethnic differences in blood pressure response to first and second-line antihypertensive therapies in patients randomized in the ASCOT Trial. Am J Hypertens. 2010;23(9):1023–30. https://doi.org/10.1038/ajh.2010.105.
77. Wright JT Jr, Dunn JK, Cutler JA, Davis BR, Cushman WC, Ford CE, et al. Outcomes in hypertensive black and nonblack patients treated with chlorthalidone, amlodipine, and lisinopril. JAMA. 2005;293(13):1595–608.
78. Flack JM, Sica DA, Bakris G, Brown AL, Ferdinand KC, Grimm RH Jr, et al. Management of high blood pressure in Blacks: an update of the International Society on Hypertension in Blacks consensus statement. Hypertension. 2010;56(5):780–800. https://doi.org/10.1161/HYPERTENSIONAHA.110.152892.
79. Byrd JB, Bakris G, Jamerson K. The contribution of the ACCOMPLISH trial to the treatment of stage 2 hypertension. Curr Hypertens Rep. 2014;16(3):419. https://doi.org/10.1007/s11906-014-0419-y.
80. McAlister FA, Herman RJ, Khan NA, Rabkin SW, Campbell N, Canadian Hypertension Education Program. Putting ACCOMPLISH into context: management of hypertension in 2010. CMAJ. 2010;182(15):1600–1. https://doi.org/10.1503/cmaj.092142.
81. Jamerson KA, Devereux R, Bakris GL, Dahlöf B, Pitt B, Velazquez EJ, et al. Efficacy and duration of benazepril plus amlodipine or hydrochlorothiazide on 24-hour ambulatory systolic blood pressure control. Hypertension. 2011;57(2):174–9. https://doi.org/10.1161/HYPERTENSIONAHA.110.159939.
82. SHEP Cooperative Research Group. Prevention of stroke by antihypertensive drug treatment in older persons with isolated systolic hypertension. Final results of the Systolic Hypertension in the Elderly Program (SHEP). JAMA. 1991;265(24):3255–64.
83. Ernst ME, Carter BL, Basile JN. All thiazide-like diuretics are not chlorthalidone: putting the ACCOMPLISH study into perspective. J Clin Hypertens (Greenwich). 2009;11(1):5–10. https://doi.org/10.1111/j.1751-7176.2008.00009.x.
84. Fox K, Garcia MA, Ardissino D, Buszman P, Camici PG, Crea F, et al. Guidelines on the management of stable angina pectoris: executive summary: the Task Force on the Management of Stable Angina Pectoris of the European Society of Cardiology. Eur Heart J. 2006;27(11):1341–81.
85. Zhou MS, Schulman IH, Jaimes EA, Raij L. Thiazide diuretics, endothelial function, and vascular oxidative stress. J Hypertens. 2008;26(3):494–500. https://doi.org/10.1097/HJH.0b013e3282f3e39d.

86. Franse LV, Pahor M, Di Bari M, Somes GW, Cushman WC, Applegate WB. Hypokalemia associated with diuretic use and cardiovascular events in the Systolic Hypertension in the Elderly Program. Hypertension. 2000;35(5):1025–30.
87. Mancia G, Laurent S, Agabiti-Rosei E, Ambrosioni E, Burnier M, Caulfield MJ, et al. Reappraisal of European guidelines on hypertension management: a European Society of Hypertension Task Force document. J Hypertens. 2009;27(11):2121–58. https://doi.org/10.1097/HJH.0b013e328333146d.
88. Giles TD, Houston MC. Do diuretics diminish the predicted benefits on ischemic heart disease events of lowering blood pressure in hypertension? Messages from ALLHAT, ACCOMPLISH, and ACCORD. J Clin Hypertens (Greenwich). 2010;12(7):469–71. https://doi.org/10.1111/j.1751-7176.2010.00327.x.
89. Matsui Y, Eguchi K, O'Rourke MF, Ishikawa J, Miyashita H, Shimada K, et al. Differential effects between a calcium channel blocker and a diuretic when used in combination with angiotensin II receptor blocker on central aortic pressure in hypertensive patients. Hypertension. 2009;54(4):716–23. https://doi.org/10.1161/HYPERTENSIONAHA.109.131466.
90. Ghiadoni L, Bruno RM, Cartoni G, Stea F, Magagna A, Virdis A, et al. Combination therapy with lercanidipine and enalapril reduced central blood pressure augmentation in hypertensive patients with metabolic syndrome. Vasc Pharmacol. 2017;92:16–21. https://doi.org/10.1016/j.vph.2015.06.004.
91. De Ciuceis C, Salvetti M, Rossini C, Muiesan ML, Paini A, Duse S, et al. Effect of antihypertensive treatment on microvascular structure, central blood pressure and oxidative stress in patients with mild essential hypertension. J Hypertens. 2014;32(3):565–74. https://doi.org/10.1097/HJH.0000000000000067.
92. Matsui Y, O'Rourke MF, Hoshide S, Ishikawa J, Shimada K, Kario K. Combined effect of angiotensin II receptor blocker and either a calcium channel blocker or diuretic on day-by-day variability of home blood pressure: the Japan Combined Treatment With Olmesartan and a Calcium-Channel Blocker Versus Olmesartan and Diuretics Randomized Efficacy Study. Hypertension. 2012;59(6):1132–8. https://doi.org/10.1161/HYPERTENSIONAHA.111.189217.
93. Webb AJ, Fischer U, Mehta Z, Rothwell PM. Effects of antihypertensive-drug class on interindividual variation in blood pressure and risk of stroke: a systematic review and meta-analysis. Lancet. 2010;375(9718):906–15. https://doi.org/10.1016/S0140-6736(10)60235-8.
94. Zhang Y, Agnoletti D, Safar ME, Blacher J. Effect of antihypertensive agents on blood pressure variability: the Natrilix SR versus candesartan and amlodipine in the reduction of systolic blood pressure in hypertensive patients (X-CELLENT) study. Hypertension. 2011;58(2):155–60. https://doi.org/10.1161/HYPERTENSIONAHA.111.174383.
95. Weber MA, Jamerson K, Bakris GL, Weir MR, Zappe D, Zhang Y, et al. Effects of body size and hypertension treatments on cardiovascular event rates: subanalysis of the ACCOMPLISH randomised controlled trial. Lancet. 2013;381(9866):537–45. https://doi.org/10.1016/S0140-6736(12)61343-9.
96. Wassertheil-Smoller S, Fann C, Allman RM, Black HR, Camel GH, Davis B, et al. Relation of low body mass to death and stroke in the systolic hypertension in the elderly program. The SHEP Cooperative Research Group. Arch Intern Med. 2000;160(4):494–500.
97. Task Force Members, Montalescot G, Sechtem U, Achenbach S, Andreotti F, Arden C, et al. 2013 ESC Guidelines on the management of stable coronary artery disease: the Task Force on the management of stable coronary artery disease of the European Society of Cardiology. Eur Heart J. 2013;34(38):2949–3003. https://doi.org/10.1093/eurheartj/eht296.
98. Julius S, Kjeldsen SE, Weber M, Brunner HR, Ekman S, Hansson L, et al. Outcomes in hypertensive patients at high cardiovascular risk treated with regimens based on valsartan or amlodipine: the VALUE randomised trial. Lancet. 2004;363(9426):2022–31.
99. Rimoldi SF, Messerli FH, Chavez P, Stefanini GG, Scherrer U. Efficacy and safety of calcium channel blocker/diuretics combination therapy in hypertensive patients: a meta-analysis. J Clin Hypertens (Greenwich). 2015;17(3):193–9. https://doi.org/10.1111/jch.12462.
100. Jadhav U, Hiremath J, Namjoshi DJ, Gujral VK, Tripathi KK, Siraj M, et al. Blood pressure control with a single-pill combination of indapamide sustained-release and amlodipine in patients with hypertension: the EFFICIENT study. PLoS One. 2014;9(4):e92955. https://doi.org/10.1371/journal.pone.0092955. eCollection 2014.
101. Authors/Task Force Members, Windecker S, Kolh P, Alfonso F, Collet JP, Cremer J, et al. 2014 ESC/EACTS Guidelines on myocardial revascularization: the Task Force on Myocardial Revascularization of the European Society of Cardiology (ESC) and the European Association for Cardio-Thoracic Surgery (EACTS). Developed with the special contribution of the European Association of Percutaneous Cardiovascular Interventions (EAPCI). Eur Heart J. 2014;35(37):2541–619. https://doi.org/10.1093/eurheartj/ehu278.
102. Ibanez B, James S, Agewall S, Antunes MJ, Bucciarelli-Ducci C, Bueno H, et al. 2017 ESC Guidelines for the management of acute myocardial infarction in patients presenting with ST-segment elevation. The Task Force for the management of acute myocardial infarction in patients presenting with ST-segment elevation of the European Society of Cardiology (ESC). Eur Heart J. 2017;39:119–77. https://doi.org/10.1093/eurheartj/ehx393.
103. Ponikowski P, Voors AA, Anker SD, Bueno H, Cleland JG, Coats AJ, et al. 2016 ESC Guidelines for the diagnosis and treatment of acute and chronic heart failure: the Task Force for the diagnosis and treatment of acute and chronic heart failure of the European Society of Cardiology (ESC) . Developed

with the special contribution of the Heart Failure Association (HFA) of the ESC. Eur Heart J. 2016;37(27):2129–200. https://doi.org/10.1093/eurheartj/ehw128.
104. Sever PS, Poulter NR, Elliott WJ, Jonsson MC, Black HR. Blood pressure reduction is not the only determinant of outcome. Circulation. 2006;113(23):2754–72. discussion 2773-4
105. Weder AB. The Avoiding Cardiovascular events through COMbination therapy in Patients Living with Systolic Hypertension (ACCOMPLISH) trial: a comparison of first-line combination therapies. Expert Opin Pharmacother. 2005;6(2):275–81.
106. Leung AA, Daskalopoulou SS, Dasgupta K, McBrien K, Butalia S, Zarnke KB, et al. Hypertension Canada's 2017 Guidelines for diagnosis, risk assessment, prevention, and treatment of hypertension in adults. Can J Cardiol. 2017;33(5):557–76. https://doi.org/10.1016/j.cjca.2017.03.005.
107. Weber MA, Schiffrin EL, White WB, Mann S, Lindholm LH, Kenerson JG, et al. Clinical practice guidelines for the management of hypertension in the community: a statement by the American Society of Hypertension and the International Society of Hypertension. J Clin Hypertens (Greenwich). 2014;16(1):14–26. https://doi.org/10.1111/jch.12237.
108. National Institute for Health and Care Excellence (NICE) Clinical Guidelines. Hypertension: clinical management of primary hypertension in adults. NICE Clinical Guideline 127. 2011. www.nice.org.uk/guidance/CG127
109. Whelton PK, Carey RM, Aronow WS, Casey DE Jr, Collins KJ, Dennison Himmelfarb C, et al. 2017 ACC/AHA/AAPA/ABC/ACPM/AGS/APhA/ASH/ASPC/NMA/PCNA guideline for the prevention, detection, evaluation, and management of high blood pressure in adults: executive summary: a report of the American College of Cardiology/American Heart Association Task Force on Clinical Practice Guidelines. Hypertension. 2017. pii: HYP.0000000000000066; https://doi.org/10.1161/HYP.0000000000000066.
110. van Vark LC, Bertrand M, Akkerhuis KM, Brugts JJ, Fox K, Mourad JJ, et al. Angiotensin-converting enzyme inhibitors reduce mortality in hypertension: a meta-analysis of randomized clinical trials of renin-angiotensin-aldosterone system inhibitors involving 158,998 patients. Eur Heart J. 2012;33(16):2088–97. https://doi.org/10.1093/eurheartj/ehs075. Epub 2012 Apr 17.
111. Costanzo P, Perrone-Filardi P, Petretta M, Marciano C, Vassallo E, Gargiulo P, et al. Calcium channel blockers and cardiovascular outcomes: a meta-analysis of 175,634 patients. J Hypertens. 2009;27(6):1136–51. https://doi.org/10.1097/HJH.0b013e3283281254.
112. Turnbull F, Neal B, Algert C, Chalmers J, Chapman N, Cutler J, et al. Effects of different blood pressure-lowering regimens on major cardiovascular events in individuals with and without diabetes mellitus: results of prospectively designed overviews of randomized trials. Arch Intern Med. 2005;165(12):1410–9.
113. Xue H, Lu Z, Tang WL, Pang LW, Wang GM, Wong GW, et al. First-line drugs inhibiting the renin angiotensin system versus other first-line antihypertensive drug classes for hypertension. Cochrane Database Syst Rev. 2015;1:CD008170. https://doi.org/10.1002/14651858.CD008170.pub2.
114. National Institute for Health and Clinical Excellence. Hypertension: management of hypertension in adults in primary care. (Clinical guideline 34). 2006. www.nice.org.uk/CG034.

Outcomes of Different Antihypertensive Regimens

11

Takeshi Fujiwara and Kazuomi Kario

Introduction

Current major hypertension guidelines [1–6] recommend diuretics, β-blockers, angiotensin-converting enzyme (ACE) inhibitors, Ca channel blockers (CCBs), and angiotensin II receptor blockers (ARBs) for both the initiation and maintenance phase of antihypertensive treatment. Among these antihypertensive medication classes, diuretics and β-blockers have been available since the 1950s and 1960s, respectively, and thus are considered classical antihypertensive drugs. Newer classes of antihypertensive medication, such as ACE inhibitors, CCBs, and ARBs, were developed in the 1970s, 1980s, and 1990s, respectively. Along with the development of the newer drugs, clinical data on the efficacy of antihypertensive drugs for the management of hypertension have also accumulated. In this review, we will introduce the main results from nine historical and landmark clinical trials that had a major impact on the current guidelines for the management of hypertension.

T. Fujiwara
Division of Cardiovascular Medicine, Department of Medicine, Jichi Medical University School of Medicine, Shimotsuke, Japan

Higashiagatsuma-machi National Health Insurance Clinic, Gunma, Japan

K. Kario (✉)
Division of Cardiovascular Medicine, Department of Medicine, Jichi Medical University School of Medicine, Tochigi, Japan
e-mail: kkario@jichi.ac.jp

Focus on the Landmark Trials

TOMHS: Treatment of Mild Hypertension Study [7]

Background At the time of this clinical trial, the efficacy of diuretics and β-blockers had already been reported, but the effectiveness of newer drug treatment, i.e., α-blockers, CCBs and ACE inhibitors, was not clear. In addition, nutritional-hygienic therapy had not been compared with antihypertensive drug treatment in clinical trials.

Objective To compare six antihypertensive interventions (placebo, diuretic, β-blocker, α-blocker, CCB, ACE inhibitor) for the treatment of mild hypertension.

Design A prospective, randomized, double-blind, multicenter, placebo-controlled clinical trial.

Patients Hypertensive patients (n = 902, 61.8% male, 20% black), aged 45 to 69 years (mean 54.8 ± 6.4 years) and not taking antihypertensive medication, with diastolic blood pressure (DBP) of 90 to 99 mmHg (mean 90.5 ± 3.4 mmHg).

V. Papademetriou et al. (eds.), *Management of Hypertension*,
https://doi.org/10.1007/978-3-319-92946-0_11

Treatment All patients received intensive nutritional-hygienic intervention aimed at weight reduction by means of a fat-modified diet, reductions in dietary sodium and alcohol intake, and increase in leisure-time physical activity. Eligible patients were randomized to receive nutritional-hygienic intervention plus one of the following six additional treatments at the indicated starting dose: (1) placebo (n = 234); (2) diuretic (chlorthalidone, 15 mg/day, n = 136); (3) β-blocker (acebutolol, 400 mg/day, n = 132); (4) α-blocker (doxazosin, 2 mg/day, n = 134); (5) CCB (amlodipine, 5 mg/day, n = 131); (6) ACE inhibitor (enalapril, 5 mg/day, n = 135). In this manuscript, the first group is referred to as the placebo group and the other groups are referred to as the drug-treatment groups.

Major clinical outcomes (1) death from coronary heart disease (CHD); (2) death from other cardiovascular disease (CVD) including stroke; (3) death from other causes; (4) nonfatal myocardial infarction (MI); (5) nonfatal stroke; (6) congestive heart failure (HF); (7) surgery for aortic aneurysm; (8) coronary artery bypass surgery; (9) coronary angioplasty; (10) thrombolytic therapy; or (11) hospitalization for unstable angina.

Follow-up Median follow-up was 4.4 years for the analyses of time to death or nonfatal CVD events.

Results

Blood Pressure Systolic blood pressure (SBP) and DBP were significantly decreased in the drug-treatment groups (−6.8 and − 3.7 mmHg, respectively) compared to the placebo group (both $p < 0.001$). The largest decrease in SBP was for patients assigned to the chlorthalidone group (−17.7 mmHg); the smallest decrease was for patients assigned to the doxazosin group (−14.2 mmHg). Trends for DBP were similar but

Table 11.1 Average blood pressure (BP) change from baseline at 48 months and based on all follow-up measurements for TOMHS participants by treatment group[a]

	Treatment groups						
	Acebutolol	Amlodipine maleate	Chlorthalidone	Doxazosin mesylate	Enalapril maleate	All drug treatments	Placebo
Systolic BP, mm Hg							
Change at 48 mo (SE)[b]	−13.9(1.3)	−14.1(1.3)	−14.6(1.5)	−13.4(1.2)	−11.3(1.3)	−13.4(0.6)	−8.6(1.1)
Change based on all follow-up BP measurements (SE)[c]	−17.0(1.0)	−15.6(0.9)	−17.7(1.0)	−14.2(0.9)	−14.7(0.9)	−15.9(0.4)	−9.1(0.7)
Diastolic BP, mm Hg							
Change at 48 mo (SE)[d]	−11.5(0.6)	−12.2(0.7)	−11.1(0.7)	−11.2(0.7)	−9.7(0.7)	−11.1(0.3)	−8.6(0.6)
Change based on all follow-up BP measurements (SE)[e]	−13.1(0.5)	−12.9(0.4)	−12.3(0.5)	−11.7(0.5)	−11.5(0.5)	−12.3(0.2)	−8.6(0.4)

[a]Number of participants in each treatment group who attended the 48-month visit were as follows: 126, acebutolol; 114, amiodipine; 117, chlorthalidone; 121, doxazosin; 119, emalapril; and 207, placebo. All but 10 participants had at least one follow-up BP measurement. TOMHS indicates Treatment of Mild Hypertension Study

[b]*P*<.01 for acebutolol, amiodipine, chlorthalidone, and doxazosin vs placebo; and all active drug treatments combined vs placebo

[c]*P*<.01 for each active drug treatment vs placebo; acebutolol vs doxazosin; chlorthalidone vs doxazosin and emalapril; and all active drug treatments combined vs placebo based on longitudinal analysis

[d]*P*<.01 for acebutolol, amiodipine, chlorithalidone, and doxazosin vs placebo; and all active drug treatments combined vs placebo

[e]*P*<.01 for each active drug treatment vs placebo; and all active drug treatments combined vs placebo based on longitudinal analysis

did not reach the level of statistical significance ($p = 0.10$) (Table 11.1).

Clinical events Table 11.2 shows the numbers and percentages of patients who experienced at least one clinical event during the follow-up period. The estimated relative risk (RR) (drug treatment vs. placebo) for a first major clinical event including non-CVD death was 0.69 ($p = 0.21$). This advantage for the drug-treatment groups was evident after approximately 1 year of follow-up (Fig. 11.1). The corresponding RR for a first major or other clinical event was 0.66 ($p = 0.03$).

Table 11.2 Number and percentage of TOMHS participants experiencing at least one clinical event during 4.4 years of follow-up[a]

	Treatment groups			
	All drug treatments (n = 668), no. of events (%)	Placebo (n = 234), no. of events (%)	Relative risk[b] (95% confidence interval)	*P*
Major CHD events[c]	26 (3.89)	12 (5.13)	0.76 (0.38–1.50)	.42
Major CHD or CVD events[d]	30 (4.49)	16 (6.84)	0.64 (0.35–1.18)	.15
All major clinical events				
Including non-CVD deaths[e]	34 (5.09)	17 (7.25)	0.69 (0.39–1.23)	.21
Major and other clinical events[f]	74 (11.08)	38 (16.24)	0.66 (0.44–0.97)	.03

[a]TOMHS indicates treatment of mild hypertension study

[b]Relative risk of specified event for drug treatment compared with placebo derived from proportional-hazards regression model that considered time to first event stratified by clinical center and use of antihypertensive medication at initial screen.

[c]The number of participants experiencing each major coronary heart disease (CHD) event were as follows: CHD death, three; nonfatal myocardial infarction, 16; congestive heart failure, two; surgery for aortic aneurysm, two; coronary artery bypass surgery, nine; coronary artery angioplasty. 17; thrombolytic therapy, six; and hospitalization for unstable 15. Some participants experienced multiple events

[d]AISO includes other cardiovascular disease (CVD) deaths (one death) and nonfatal stroke (participants)

[e]Also includes non-CVD deaths (five deaths)

[f]Also includes hospitalization for transient ischemic attack (seven participants); definite Rose angina (56 participants); Rose intermittent claudication (16 participants); and peripheral arterial occlusive disease (five participants)

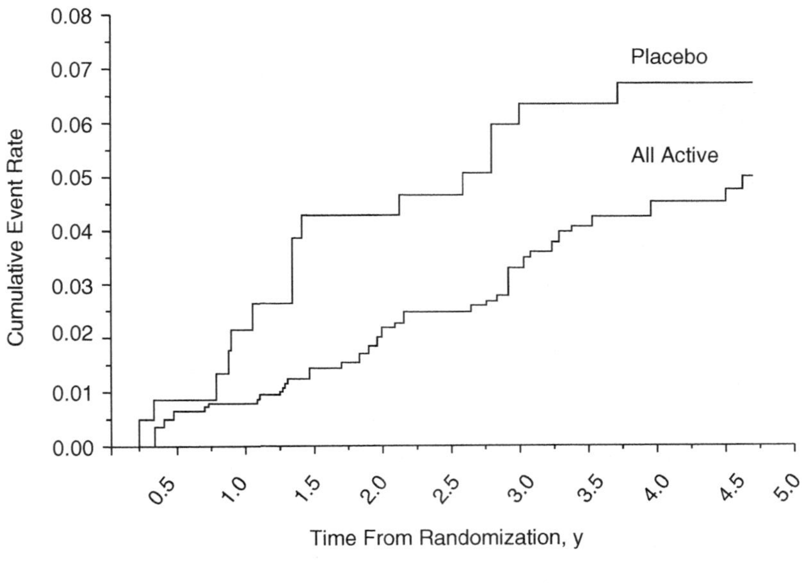

Fig. 11.1 Cumulative percentage of major clinical events for treatment of mild hypertension study participants randomly assigned to drug treatment and nutritional-hygienic intervention (all active) or to nutritional-hygienic intervention alone (placebo) (difference not significant)

Change in echocardiographically determined LV mass and incidence of LVH There were no significant differences in left ventricle (LV) mass on echocardiogram decline among the five drug-treatment groups ($p = 0.05$). In addition, incident rates for left ventricle hypertrophy (LVH) based on the echocardiogram did not vary among the five drug-treatments ($p = 0.45$) or between all drug-treatment groups combined and the placebo group ($p = 0.83$).

ECG abnormality In resting electrocardiography (ECG), the incidence was significantly lower for all drug-treatments combined compared with placebo for LVH ($p = 0.02$) and tall R waves ($p < 0.01$). On the other hand, in ambulatory ECG, there were no significant differences among drug-treatment groups in the incidence of ST-segment depression ($p = 0.32$) or between all drug-treatment groups combined and the placebo group ($p = 0.60$).

Quality of life and side effects The overall test for the combined seven quality-of-life indexes indicated that there was significantly greater improvement in quality of life for patients given acebutolol ($p < 0.001$) and chlorthalidone ($p = 0.008$) than for patients given placebo. The differences between all drug-treatment groups combined and the placebo group for the overall summary test was significant ($p = 0.007$).

The overall side-effect severity score based on 55 symptoms determined at each follow-up visit indicated that symptoms were more common among patients given placebo ($p = 0.05$). There were no significant differences in the side-effect severity score among the drug-treatment groups.

Comments The main findings of this study were as follows. First, intensive nutritional-hygienic intervention resulted in substantial BP reduction. This result indicated that an initial treatment involving only efforts at lifestyle improvement should be recommended for patients with hypertension. Second, there were substantial differences in BP reduction between the drug-treatment groups and the placebo group. Patients given nutritional-hygienic intervention and drug medication showed well-controlled BP (average 124/78 mmHg) and lower rates of CHD and CVD than those assigned to receive nutritional-hygienic intervention alone. Third, there were only modest differences in BP change among the drug-treatment groups. However, the number of patients in each drug-treatment group was quite small. Much larger clinical trials are needed to evaluate the ability of newer classes of drugs (α-blockers, CCBs and ACE inhibitors) to prevent major clinical events compared with classical drugs (diuretics and β-blockers).

INSIGHT: International Nifedipine GIST Study: Intervention as a Goal in Hypertension Treatment [8]

Background In the clinical trials of the 1970s and 1980s, diuretics and β-blockers, now considered the classical drugs, were mainly used as antihypertensive medications. After that period, newer drugs such as CCBs were developed. However, the information has been quite limited regarding the efficacy of the newer antihypertensive drugs for preventing cardiovascular outcomes.

Objective To compare the efficacy in preventing major complications from hypertension of nifedipine (CCB) administered in a long-acting gastrointestinal-transport-system (GIST) formulation and co-amilozide, a common and effective combination of the diuretics hydrochlorothiazide and amiloride.

Design A prospective, randomized, double-blind, multicenter clinical trial.

Patients Hypertensive patients (n = 6321, 46.3% male, mainly white), aged 55 to 80 years (mean 65 years), with SBP/DBP ≥ 150/95 mmHg or SBP ≥ 160 mmHg. In addition to hypertension, all patients had at least 1 additional risk factor for CVD events. The risk factors included hypercholesterolaemia, smoking, family history of MI in a parent or sibling before age 50 years, current LVH by echocardiography, CHD (including angina), LV strain confirmed by ECG strain pattern, or peripheral vascular disease.

Treatments Patients were randomly assigned nifedipine 30 mg/day or co-amilozide (hydrochlorothiazide 25 mg/day + amiloride 2.5 mg/day). If patients showed a fall in BP of <20/10 mmHg or a final BP of >140/90 mmHg, four optional dose-titration steps were used as follows: (1) dose-doubling of the randomized drug; (2) addition of atenolol 25 mg/day (or enalapril 5 mg/day if atenolol was contraindicated); (3) dose-doubling of the additional drugs; (4) addition of any other antihypertensive drug (other than CCBs or diuretics).

Major clinical outcomes The primary outcomes were as follows: (1) composite of death from any cardiovascular or cerebrovascular cause; (2) non-fatal stroke; (3) MI; and (4) HF. The secondary outcomes were as follows: (1) total mortality; (2) death from a vascular cause; and (3) non-fatal vascular events including transient ischemic attacks (TIA), angina (new or worsening), and renal failure.

Follow-up Four years.

Results

Blood pressure By the end of the titration phase, mean BP had fallen from 173/99 mmHg to 138/82 mmHg in the total treatment group (Fig. 11.2). The proportions of patients who received monotherapy or reached BPs lower than 140/90 mmHg differed slightly between the nifedipine and the co-amilozide group.

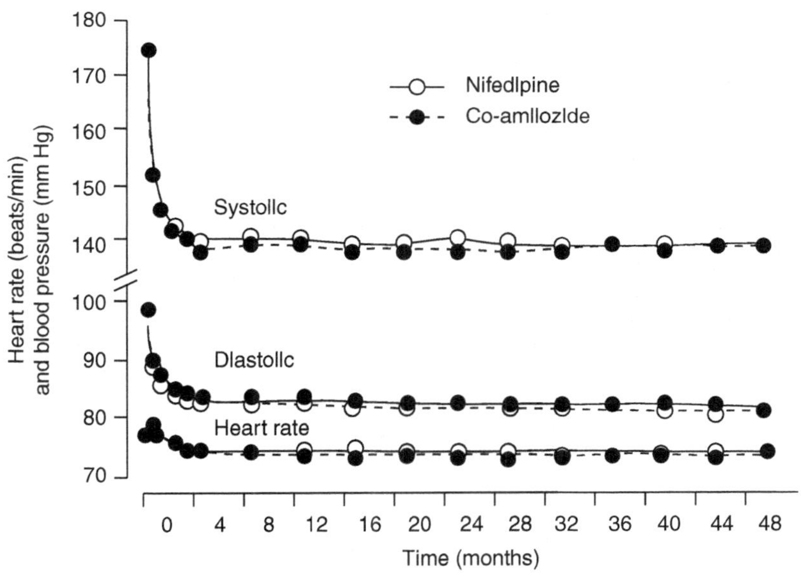

Patients remaining on treatment

Month	0	4	12	24	36	48
Nifedipine	3157	2735	2498	2234	2058	831
Monotherapy (%)		72	68	66	63	69
Blood pressure controlled (%)		56	54	54	56	58
Co-amilozide (n)	3164	2877	2693	2469	2288	944
Monotherapy (%)		66	66	65	63	72
Blood pressure controlled (%)		59	57	59	57	57

Fig. 11.2 Blood-pressure response to study drugs

Clinical events There were no significant differences in the primary outcomes between the nifedipine and the co-amilozide groups (6.3% vs. 5.8%, 18.2 vs. 16.5 events per 1000 patients-year, $p = 0.34$) (Table 11.3). Groups did not differ with respect to all-cause mortality, non-fatal outcomes, or the combined primary and secondary outcomes. The patients in the nifedipine group showed significantly higher risk of fatal MI compared to those in the co-amilozide group (0.5% vs. 0.2%, odds ratio [OR] 3.22, 95% CI 1.18–8.80, $p = 0.017$). Also, the patients in the nifedipine group showed significantly higher risk of non-fatal HF compared to those in the co-amilozide group (0.8% vs. 0.3%, OR 2.20, 95% CI 1.07–4.49, $p = 0.028$) (Table 11.3).

Adverse events 725 patients in the nifedipine group and 518 patients in the co-amilozide group withdrew because of adverse events ($p < 0.0001$). There was an early excess of withdrawals in the nifedipine group because of peripheral edema in 255 patients during dose titration. More patients on co-amilozide than on nifedipine had metabolic disorder: hypokalaemia (6.2% vs. 1.9%, $p < 0.0001$), hyponatraemia (1.9% vs. 0.3%, $p < 0.0001$), hyperuricaemia (6.4% vs. 1.3%, $p < 0.0001$), hyperglycaeia (7.7% vs. 5.6%, $p = 0.0001$), and renal impairment (4.6% vs. 1.8%, $p < 0.0001$). There was a significantly higher percentage of patients with new diabetes in the co-amilozide than the nifedipine group (5.6% vs. 4.3%, $p = 0.02$). There were fewer serious adverse events (defined as life-threatening,

Table 11.3 Individual outcomes

	Nifedipine	Co-amilozide	Odds ratio (95% CI)	*p*
Primary outcomes				
Composite	200 (6–3%)	182 (5–8%)	1–11 (0.90–1.36)	0.34[a]
Myocardial infarction				
Non-fatal	61 (1.9)	56 (1.8)	1.09 (0.76–1.58)	0.52
Fatal	16 (0.5)	5 (0.2)	3.22 (1.18–8.80)	0.017
Sudden death	17 (0.5)	23 (0.7)	0.74 (0.39–1.39)	0.43
Stroke				
Non-fatal	55 (1.7)	63 (2.0)	0.87 (0.61–1.26)	0.52
Fatal	12 (0.3)	11 (0.3)	1.09 (0.48–2.48)	0.84
Heart failure				
Non-fatal	24 (0.8)	11 (0.3)	2.20 (1.07–4.49)	0.028
Fatal	2 (0.1)	1 (<0.1)	2.01 (0.18–22.13)	0.63
Other cardiovascular death	13 (0.4)	12 (0.4)	1.09 (0.50–2.38)	0.85
Secondary outcomes				
Composite[c]	383 (12.1)	397 (12.5)	0.96 (0.83–1.12)	0.62
Deaths				
All (first event)[a]	153 (4.8)	152 (4.8)	1.01 (0.80–1.27)	0.95
Non-cardiovascular	71 (2.2)	66 (2.1)	1.08 (0.77–1.52)	0.67
Unknown cause	22 (0.7)	34 (1.1)	0.65 (0.38–1.11)	0.14
Cardiovascular	60 (1–9)	52 (1–6)	1.16 (0.80–1.69)	0.45
Non-fatal cardiovascular events	230 (7.3)	245 (7.7)	0.94 (0.78–1.13)	0.50
Primary events	140 (4.4)	130 (4.1)	1.08 (0.85–1.38)	0.53
Angina (worsening or new)	57 (1.8)	77 (0.4)	0.74 (0.52–1.04)	0.10
Transient ischaemic attacks	25 (0.8)	25 (0.8)	1.00 (0.57–1.75)	1.0
Renal failure	8 (0.3)	13 (0.4)	0.62 (0.26–1.49)	0.38

[a]Myocardial infarction, stroke, heart failure, and cardiovascular death
[b]Primary outcomes plus non-cardiovascular deaths, renal failure, angina, and transient
[c]23 additional in nifedipine group and 20 in co-amilozide group occurred after a previous endpoint

disabling, or leading to hospital admission) in the nifedipine group than in the co-amilozise group ($p = 0.02$).

Comments This study revealed that nifedipine and co-amilozide had a similar efficacy for cardiovascular outcomes. And in both groups, about 70% of patients received monotherapy at the end of the study period, with about 60% reaching BP of lower than 140/90 mmHg, suggesting that these agents were suitable for the management of hypertension in high-risk patients. However, nifedipine had a better effect on several metabolic markers than did co-amilozide, and showed fewer serious adverse events and less need for biochemical monitoring, indicating that nifedipine was better tolerated compared with co-amilozide. This study thus demonstrated that CCBs showed greater ease-of-use in daily clinical practice compared with diuretics.

LIFE: Losartan Intervention for Endpoint Reduction in Hypertension [9]

Background This study was designed in the early 1990s to address several findings and developments as follows. (1) β-blockers and diuretics had failed to return the rates of cardiovascular morbidity and mortality to normal in hypertensive patients. (2) LVH was known to be a cardinal manifestation of preclinical cardiovascular disease and an independent risk factor for all cardiovascular complications in hypertension, but no study had investigated whether reversal of LVH improved the cardiovascular prognosis in hypertensive patients. (3) Angiotensin II had been associated with development of LVH, and thus it was thought that blocking angiotensin II might be effective in reversing LVH. (4) Losartan was the first available ARB, but information was limited regarding the effectiveness of losartan for cardiovascular protection.

Objective To test the hypothesis that losartan would be more effective than atenolol (a β-blocker) in reducing cardiovascular morbidity and mortality in patients with essential hypertension.

Design A prospective, randomized, double-blind, multicenter, parallel-group clinical trial.

Patients Hypertensive patients (n = 9193, 54% female, 92% white), aged 55 to 80 years (mean 66.9 years), with previously treated or untreated hypertension and ECG signs of LVH. Patients with SBP ≥ 160–200 mmHg and/or DBP ≥ 95–115 mmHg after 1–2 weeks of placebo were randomized to a treatment group. The Cornell product ([QRS×(RaVL+SV3)] mm×mm) or Sokolow-Lyon ([SV1 + RV5 or V6] mm) were used as ECG-LVH criteria.

Treatments Patients were randomly assigned losartan 50 mg/day (n = 4605) or atenolol 50 mg/day (n = 4588). The target BP level was SBP/DBP ≤ 140/90 mmHg. In the case of insufficient BP reduction, the following dose-titration steps were used: (1) addition to hydrochlorothiazide 12.5 mg/day after 2 months; (2) dose-doubling of losartan or atenolol (each 100 mg/day) after 4 months; (3) dose-doubling of hydrochlorothiazide (25 mg/day) or addition of other antihypertensive medications after 6 months.

Major clinical outcomes The primary endpoints were as follows: (1) cardiovascular morbidity and death; (2) a composite outcome of cardiovascular death, MI, and stroke. Other outcomes were as follows: (1) total mortality; (2) angina pectoris or HF requiring admission to a hospital; (3) coronary or peripheral revascularization procedures; (4) resuscitated cardiac arrest; and (5) new-onset diabetes mellitus.

Follow-up The mean follow-up was 4.8 years.

Results

Blood pressure BP levels at the end of follow-up or at last visit before a primary outcome occurred fell by 30.2/16.6 mmHg and 29.1/16.8 mmHg in the losartan and atenolol groups, respectively ($p = 0.017/0.37$). Target BP of SBP/DBP ≤ 140/90 mmHg was achieved in 49% and 46% of losartan and atenolol patients, respectively. Heart rate decreased more in patients assigned to atenolol than losartan (−7.7 and − 1.8 bpm, respectively, $p < 0.0001$).

Primary outcomes The primary composite endpoint was reached in 508 (11%; rate per 1000 patient-years: 23.8) and 588 (13%; rate per 1000 patient-years: 27.9) patients in the losartan and atenolol group, respectively (HR 0.87, 95% CI 0.77–0.98, $p = 0.021$) (Table 11.4). There were no significant differences in cardiovascular mortality and MI between the two groups. On the other hand, losartan significantly decreased stroke events compared with atenolol (HR 0.75, 95% CI 0.63–0.89, $p = 0.001$) (Table 11.4).

Other outcomes There was a 25% lower incidence of new-onset diabetes in the losartan than the atenolol group (Table 11.4). In addition, losartan significantly improved the ECG-LVH sign compared with atenolol (Fig. 11.3a).

Medication adherence and adverse events Patients remained on the study drugs for 84% and 80% of the follow-up period in the losartan and atenolol group, respectively. Discontinuations as a result of all adverse events, drug-related adverse events, and serious drug-related adverse events were significantly less common in the patients receiving losartan than those receiving atenolol (Fig. 11.3b).

Comments Losartan was better than atenolol in reducing the frequency of the primary composite endpoint despite the small difference in BP reduction. In particular, losartan significantly reduced stroke events compared with atenolol, which meant than losartan could have a significant effect on stroke events over and above BP reduction. In this study, the rate of new-onset diabetes was significantly lower and the ECG-LVH

Table 11.4 Endpoints

	Losartan (n = 4605)		Atenolol (n = 4588)		Adjusted hazard ratio		Unadjusted hazard ratio	
Endpoint	n	Rate[a]	n	Rate	(95% CI)[b]	p	(95% CI)	p
Primary composite endpoint[c]	508 (11%)	23.8	588 (13%)	27.9	0.87 (0.77–0.98)	0.021	0.85 (0.76–0.96)	0.009
Cardiovascular mortality	204 (4%)	9.2	234 (5%)	10.6	0.89 (0.73–1.07)	0.206	0.87 (0.72–1.05)	0.136
Stroke	232 (5%)	10.8	309 (7%)	14.5	0.75 (0.63–0.89)	0.001	0.74 (0.63–0.88)	0.0006
Myocardial infarction	198 (4%)	9.2	188 (4%)	8.7	1.07 (0.88–1.31)	0.491	1.05 (0.86–1.28)	0.628
Other prespecified endpoints								
Total mortality	383 (8%)	17.3	431 (9%)	19.6	0.90 (0.78-1.03)	0.128	0.88 (0.77-1.01)	0.077
Admitted to hospital for:								
Angina pectoris	160 3(%)	7.4	141 (3%)	6.6	1.16 (0.92–1.45)	0.212	1.13 (0.90–1.42)	0.284
Heart failure	153 (3%)	7.1	161 (4%)	7.5	0.97 (0.78–1.21)	0.765	0.95 (0.76–1.18)	0.622
Revascularisation	261 (6%)	12.2	284 (6%)	13.3	0.94 (0.79–1.11)	0.441	0.91 (0.77–1.08)	0.292
Resuscitated cardiac arrest	9 (0.2%)	0.4	5 (0.1%)	0.2	1.91 (0.64–5.72)	0.250	1.80 (0.60–5.36)	0.294
New-onset diabetes[d]	241 (6%)	13.0	319 (8%)	17.4	0.75 (0.63–0.88)	0.001	0.75 (0.63–0.88)	0.001

[a]Per 1000 patient-years of follow-up
[b]For degree of left ventricular hypertrophy and Framingham risk score at randomisation
[c]Cardiovascular mortality, stroke, and myocardial infarction (numbers of patients with a first primary event)
[d]In patients without diabetes at randomisation (losartan, n = 4019; atenolol, n = 3979)

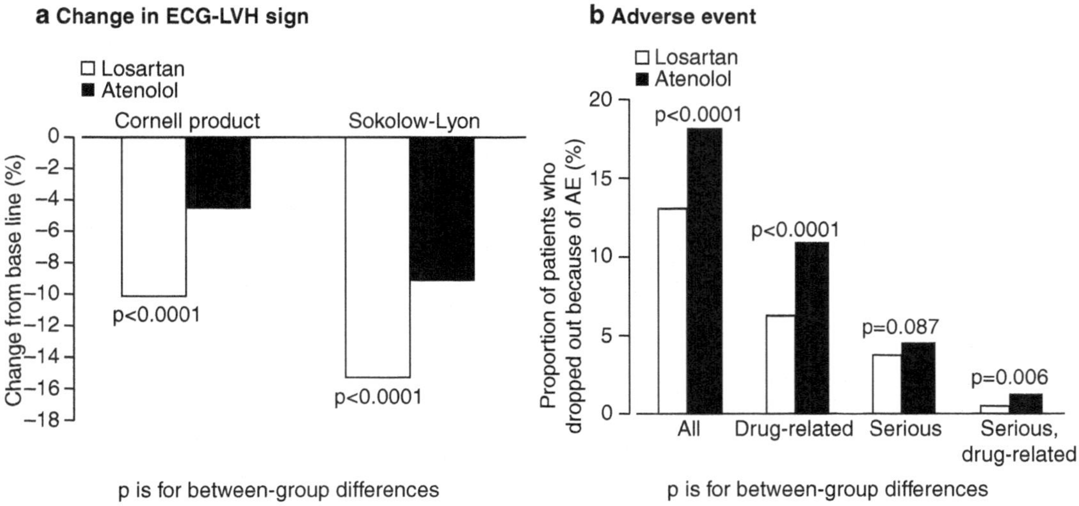

Fig. 11.3 Other outcomes (**a**) change in ECG-LVH sign (**b**) adverse event

sign was significantly improved in the losartan group compared to the atenolol group. These two results seemed to have had some effects on the reduction of stroke events. From the point of view of drug adherence, the lower rate of adverse events with losartan resulted in greater tolerability of losartan than atenolol. The LIFE was the first study demonstrating the efficacy of an ARB, and indicated that losartan had a greater clinical benefit in high-risk patients and enhanced tolerability.

ALLHAT: The Antihypertensive and Lipid-Lowering Treatment to Prevent Heart Attack Trial [10]

Background The benefits of diuretics and β-blockers for lowering BP levels had been established in earlier clinical trials. After these trials, newer classes of antihypertensive agents, such as CCBs and ACE inhibitors, became available. However, there was considerable uncertainty regarding the ability of these agents to lower the incidence of CHD in high-risk hypertensive subgroups such as older patients, black patients, and patients with diabetes. And the optimal first-step therapy for lowering the incidence of CHD had been unknown until this clinical trial.

Objective To determine whether treatment with a CCB or an ACE inhibitor lowers the incidence of CHD or other CVD events vs. treatment with a diuretic in high-risk hypertensive patients.

Design A prospective, randomized, double-blind, multicenter, active-controlled clinical trial.

Patients Stage 1 or 2 hypertensive patients (n = 33,357, 47% female, 35% black), aged 55 years or older (mean 67 years), with at least 1 additional risk factor for CHD events. The risk factors included previous (>6 months) MI or stroke, LVH demonstrated by ECG or echocardiography, history of type 2 diabetes, current smoking, high-density lipoprotein cholesterol of less than 35 mg/dL, or documentation of other atherosclerotic CVD.

Treatments Eligible patients were randomly assigned to the step 1 dosage as follows: (1) diuretic (chlorthalidone, 12.5–25 mg/day, n = 15,255); (2) CCB (amlodipine, 2.5–10 mg/day, n = 9048); (3) ACE inhibitor (lisinopril, 10–40 mg/day, n = 9054). The dose of study-supplied open-label step 2 drugs were 25–100 mg/day of atenolol; 0.05–0.2 mg/day of reserpine; or 0.1–0.3 mg twice a day of clonidine; step 3 was 25–100 mg twice a day of hydralazine. The goal BP in each randomized group was less than

140/90 mmHg and was achieved by titrating the assigned study drug (step 1) and adding open-label agents (step 2 or 3) when necessary.

Major clinical endpoints The primary outcome was fatal CHD or nonfatal MI combined. The secondary outcomes were as follows: (1) all-cause mortality; (2) fatal and nonfatal stroke; (3) combined CHD (the primary outcome, coronary revascularization, hospitalized angina); (4) combined CVD (combined CHD, stroke, other treated angina, HF, and peripheral arterial disease); (5) coronary revascularization; (6) cancer; (7); incident electrocardiographic LVH; (8) end-stage renal disease (ESRD); and (9) increase of the serum creatinine level. Two major safety outcomes were as follows: (1) angioedema; (2) hospitalization for gastrointestinal bleeding.

Follow-up Mean (SD) follow-up was 4.9 (1.4) years.

Results

Medication adherence Among patients in the chlorthalidone group, 87.1% were taking chlorthalidone or another diuretic at 1 year, decreasing to 80.5% at 5 years. Among patients in the amlodipine group, 87.6% were taking amlodipine or another CCB at 1 year, decreasing to 80.4% at 5 years. Among patients in the lisinopril group, 82.4% were taking lisinopril or another ACE inhibitor at 1 year, decreasing to 72.6% at 5 years.

Among patients with available medication information at 1 year, 26.7%, 25.9%, and 32.6% of those assigned to receive chlorthalidone, amlodipine, and lisinopril, respectively, were taking a step 2 or step 3 drug. At 5 years, the corresponding percentages were 40.7%, 39.5%, and 43.0%, respectively.

Blood pressure Among patients in the chlorthalidone group, the SBP/DBP levels were 146.2/84.0 mmHg at baseline, 136.9/79.3 mmHg at 1 year, and 133.9/75.4 mmHg at 5 years. The percentage of patients who achieved the BP goal of <140/90 mmHg at 5 years was 68.2%. Among patients in the amlodipine group, the SBP/DBP levels were 146.2/83.9 mmHg at baseline, 138.5/78.7 mmHg at 1 year, and 134.7/74.6 mmHg at 5 years. The percentage of patients who achieved the BP goal of <140/90 mmHg at 5 years was 66.3%. Among patients in the lisinopril group, the SBP/DBP levels were 146.4/84.1 mmHg at baseline, 140.0/79.9 mmHg at 1 year, and 135.9/75.4 mmHg at 5 years. The percentage of patients who achieved the BP goal of <140/90 mmHg at 5 years was 61.2%. Compared with the BP level at 5 years in patients treated with chlorthalidone, the patients in the amlodipine and lisinopril groups showed significantly higher SBP levels (amlodipine group, +0.8 mmHg, $p = 0.03$; lisinopril group, +2.0 mmHg, $p < 0.001$), and the patients with amlodipine showed significantly lower DBP levels (−0.8 mmHg, $p < 0.001$). Follow-up BPs in all 3 groups are shown in Fig. 11.4.

Primary and Secondary Outcomes

1. Amlodipine vs. chlorthalidone: No significant differences were observed between amlodipine and chlorthalidone for the primary outcome (6-year rate per 100 persons of amlodipine vs. chlorthalidone 11.3% vs. 11.5%, RR 0.98, 95% CI 0.90–1.07) (Fig. 11.5) or for the secondary outcomes. The amlodipine group showed significantly higher risk of HF (10.2% vs. 7.7%, RR 1.38, 95% CI 1.25–1.52) and hospitalized/fatal HF (8.4% vs. 6.5%, RR 1.35, 95% CI 1.21–1.50) compared with the chlorthalidone group. The treatment effects for all outcomes were consistent across the predefined subgroups (Fig. 11.6).
2. Lisinopril vs. chlorthalidone: No significant differences were observed between lisinopril and chlorthalidone for the primary outcome (6-year rate per 100 persons of lisinopril vs. chlorthalidone 11.4% vs. 11.5%, RR 0.99, 95% CI 0.91–1.08) (Fig. 11.5) or for the secondary outcomes. The lisinopril group showed significantly higher risk of stroke (6.3% vs. 5.6%, RR 1.15, 95% CI 1.02–1.30), combined CVD (33.3% vs. 30.9%, RR 1.10, 95% CI 1.05–1.16), HF (8.7% vs. 7.7%, RR 1.19,

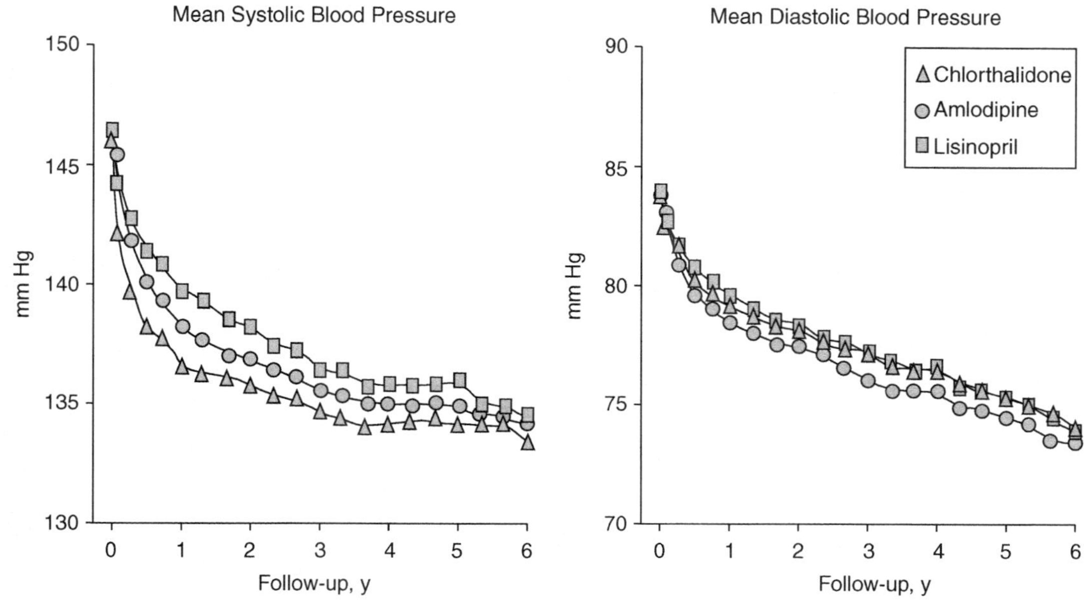

Fig. 11.4 Mean systolic and diastolic blood pressure by year during follow-up

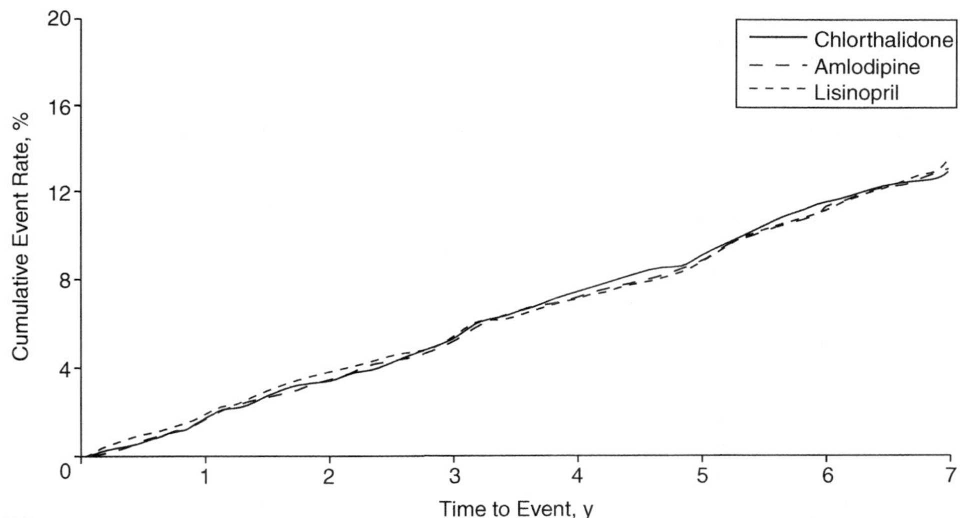

No. at Risk								
Chlorthalidone	15255	14477	13820	13102	11362	6340	2956	209
Amlodipine	9048	8576	8218	7843	6824	3870	1878	215
Lisinopril	9054	8535	8123	7711	6662	3832	1770	195

No significant difference was observed for amlodipine (relative risk [RRJ. 0.98; 95% confidence interval [CI], 0.90-1.07; P= .65) or lisinopril (RR. 0.99; 95% CI , 0.91-1 .08; P=.81) vs chlorthalidone with a mean follow-up of 4.9 years.

Fig. 11.5 Cumulative events rates for the primary outcomes (fatal coronary heart disease or nonfatal myocardial infarction) by treatment group

95% CI 1.07–1.31), hospitalized/treated angina (13.6% vs. 12.1%, RR 1.11, 95% CI 1.03–1.20), and coronary revascularization (10.2% vs. 9.2%, RR 1.10, 95% CI 1.00–1.21) compared with the chlorthalidone group. The treatment effects for all outcomes were

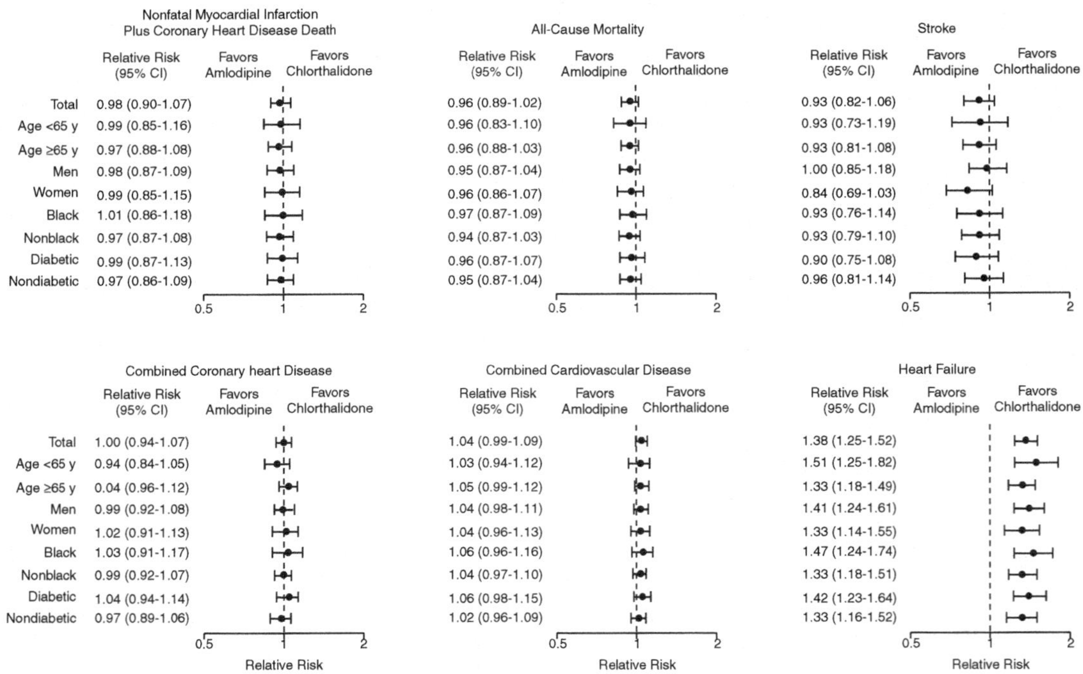

Fig. 11.6 Relative risk and 95% confidence intervals (CIs) for amlodipine/chlorthalidone comparisons in prespecified subgroups

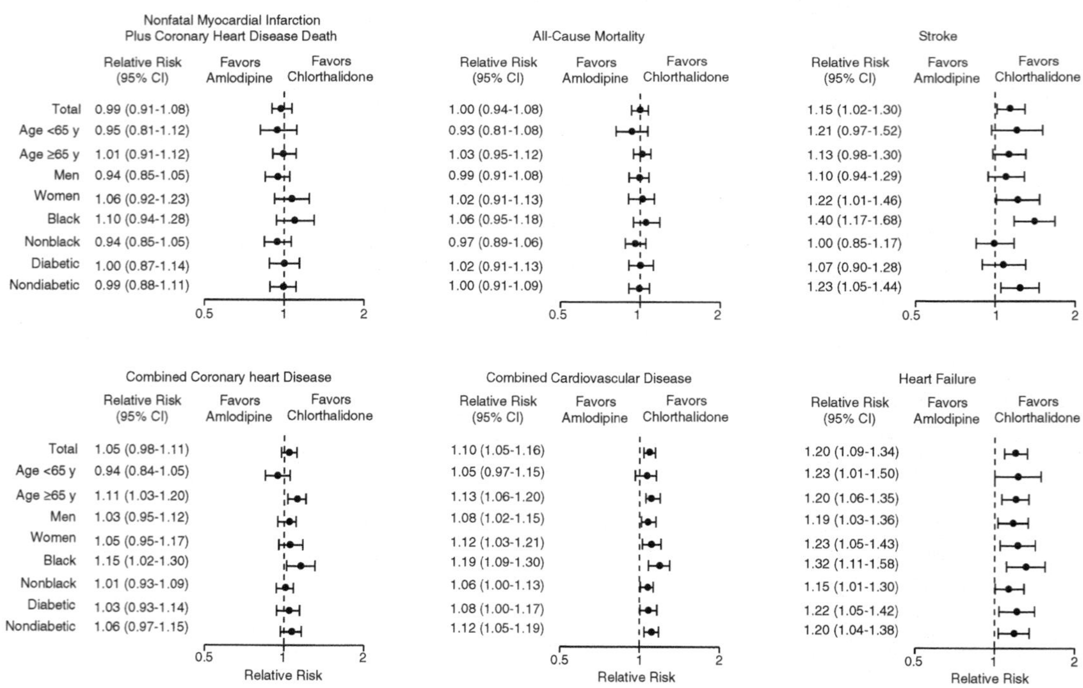

Fig. 11.7 Relative risk and 95% confidence intervals (CIs) for lisinopril/chlorthalidone comparisons in prespecified subgroups

consistent across subgroups by sex, diabetic status (Fig. 11.7), and baseline CHD status. For combined CHD, there was a significant differential effect by age ($p = 0.01$ for interaction) with RRs (lisinopril vs. chlorthalidone) of 0.94 (95% CI 0.84–1.05) for those less than 65 years vs. 1.11 (95% CI 1.03–1.20) in those 65 years or older. For stroke and combined CVD, there was a significant differential effect by race ($p = 0.01$ and $p = 0.04$ for interaction, respectively). The RRs (lisinopril vs. chlorthalidone) were 1.40 (95% CI 1.17–1.68) and 1.00 (95% CI 0.85–1.17) for stroke and 1.19 (95% CI, 1.09–1.30) and 1.06 (95% CI 1.00–1.13) for combined CVD in blacks and nonblacks, respectively (Fig. 11.7).

Primary safety outcomes Six-year rates of hospitalization for gastrointestinal bleeding occurred in 8.8%, 8.0%, and 9.6% of patients in the chlorthalidone, amlodipine, and lisinopril treatment groups, respectively, with no significant differences. Angioedema occurred in 0.1%, <0.1%, and 0.4% patients in the chlorthalidone, amlodipine, and lisinopril treatment groups, respectively. Significant differences were seen for the lisinopril vs. chlorthalidone comparison overall ($p < 0.001$), in blacks (<0.1% for chlorthalidone, 0.7% for lisinopril; $p < 0.001$), and in non-blacks (0.1% for chlorthalidone, 0.3% for lisinopril; $p = 0.002$).

Comments This study revealed that neither amlodipine nor lisinopril was superior to chlorthalidone in preventing major coronary events or increasing survival in high-risk hypertensive patients. The results of this study complemented the past two large active-controlled trials, SHEP (the Systolic Hypertension in the Elderly Program) [11] and Syst-Eur (Systolic Hypertension in Europe trial) [12]. These studies, together with ALLHAT, demonstrated that CCBs had equivalent ability to lower the incidence of CHD or other CVD events compared with diuretics, the efficacy of which had already been revealed in many clinical trials. We consider that the key point of the ALLHAT trial is its demonstration of the possible efficacy of CCBs for the management of high-risk hypertensive patients. Another important point, in terms of clinical practice, is that the cost of antihypertensive drugs cost could have a major impact on the nation's health care expenditures. This study indicated that the safety and efficacy were almost the same in the chlorthalidone, amlodipine, and lisinopril treatment groups. Taking these various factors into account, diuretics should be considered first for pharmacologic therapy in patients with hypertension. Diuretics are unsurpassed in lowering BP, reducing clinical events, and tolerability, and they are less costly. This study suggested that diuretics should be included in multi-antihypertensive regimens, if possible.

ABNP2: Second Australian National Blood Pressure Study [13]

Background Previous hypertension studies, most of which used primaly diuretics or β-blockers, demonstrated that the reduction of BP levels was associated with a reduced risk of cardiovascular events and death. Since those studies, newer classes of antihypertensive agents, including ACE inhibitors, CCBs, and ARBs, have become widely accepted into clinical practice. However, no data have been available in regard to the benefit of these newer agents in hypertensive patients. In addition, until this study was conducted, none of the studies involving ACE inhibitors or CCBs had yet demonstrated a clear difference in outcome between treatment groups.

Objective To compare the cardiovascular outcomes in older patients with hypertension who were treated with an ACE inhibitor with the outcomes in those treated with a diuretic.

Design A prospective, randomized, open-label, multicenter, clinical trial conducted at 1594 family practices throughout Australia.

Patients Hypertensive patients (n = 6083, 51% female, 95% white), aged 65–84 years (mean 71.9 years), with an average SBP >160 mmHg or DBP >90 mmHg (if the SBP was >140 mmHg), measured at the two study-entry visits, and with no recent cardiovascular events (within the previous 6 months).

Treatments The ACE inhibitor enalapril and the diuretic hydrochlorothiazide were recommended as initial therapy (the choice of the specific agent and dose was made by the family practitioner). The goal in each randomized group was to reduce the SBP by >20 mmHg to <160 mmHg (with a further reduction to <140 mmHg if tolerated), and to reduce DBP by >10 mmHg to <90 mmHg (with a further reduction to <80 mmHg if tolerated). To achieve the BP goal, the addition of β-blockers, CCBs, and α-blockers was recommended in both groups.

Major clinical outcomes The primary endpoint was all cardiovascular events or death from any cause. Cardiovascular events included the following: (1) coronary events, including MI; (2) sudden or rapid death from cardiac causes; (3) other death from coronary causes; (4) coronary events associated with therapeutic procedures involving the coronary arteries; (5) other cardiovascular events, including HF; (6) acute occlusion of a major feeding artery in any vascular bed other than cerebral or coronary; (7) death from non-coronary cardiac causes; (8) dissecting or ruptured aortic aneurysm; (9) death from vascular causes. Cerebrovascular events including stroke and TIA.

Follow-up Median follow-up was 4.1 years.

Results

Drug treatment The total of 6083 patients were randomly assigned to the ACE-inhibitor group (n = 3044) or the diuretic group (n = 3039). 65% of the patients in the ACE-inhibitor group and 67% of those in the diuretic group were receiving monotherapy. Concomitant antihypertensive medications included CCBs (in 22.9% of patients in the ACE-inhibitor group and 24.9% of patients in the diuretic group), β-blockers (10.8% and 13.7%, respectively), and ARBs (14.0% and 12.4%, respectively).

Blood pressure The baseline BP levels were 167/91 mmHg in the ACE-inhibitor group and 168/91 mmHg in the diuretic group. At year 1, BP had decreased by 20/9 mmHg in the ACE-inhibitor group and 22/9 mmHg in the diuretic group; at year 2, it had decreased by 23/10 mmHg in the ACE-inhibitor group and 24/10 mmHg in the diuretic group; at year 5, it had decreased by 26/12 mmHg in both groups. There were significant and clinically relevant reductions from the baseline values. In both men and women, the pattern of BP reduction was similar between the two treatments.

Primary outcomes The rate per 1000 patient-years of the ACE-inhibitor group was 56.1 and that of the diuretic group was 59.8. The hazard ratio (HR) for all cardiovascular events or death from any cause among patients in the ACE-inhibitor group as compared with those in the diuretic group was 0.89 (95% CI, 0.79–1.00; $p = 0.05$) (Table 11.5). There were almost twice as many events in male patients (907 events) as in female patients (524 events). The beneficial effects of ACE-inhibitor treatment were more evident in male patients (HR for both all cardiovascular events and first cardiovascular events, 0.83, 95% CI 0.71–0.97, $p = 0.02$). The P value for the interaction between sex and treatment-group assignment was 0.15 for all cardiovascular events or death from a cause and 0.14 for first cardiovascular events.

The HR for all first cardiovascular events in the ACE-inhibitor group as compared with the diuretic group was 0.88 (95% CI 0.77–1.01, $p = 0.07$) (Table 11.5). There was a significant reduction in the rate of first MI in the ACE-inhibitor group (HR 0.68, 95% CI 0.47–0.98, $p = 0.04$). In the cause-specific first fatal and nonfatal events (Table 11.6), the rate of fatal stroke was significantly higher with the ACE-inhibitor treatment (HR 1.91, 95% CI 1.04–3.50, $p = 0.04$). On the other hand, the rate of first nonfatal cardiovascular events was significantly lower with ACE-inhibitor treatment (HR 0.86, 95% CI 0.74–0.99, $p = 0.03$), especially the rate of MI (HR 0.68, 95% CI 0.47–0.99, $p = 0.05$).

Comments This study revealed that in elderly patients with hypertension, particularly among male patients, ACE-inhibitor-based therapy

Table 11.5 Primary end points and cause-specific first events[a]

Event	ACE-inhibitor group (*N* = 3044)		Diuretic group (*N* = 3039)		Hazard ratio (95% CI	*p* value
	No. of events	Rate per 1000 patient-yr	No. of events	Rate per 1000 patient-yr		
Primary end points						
All cardiovascular events or death from any cause	695	56.1	736	59.8	0.39 (0.79–1.00)	0.05
First cardiovascular event or death from any cause	490	41.9	529	45.7	0.89 (0.79–1.01)	0.06
Death from any cause	195	15.7	210	17.1	0.90 (0.75–1.09)	0.27
Cause-specific first events						
First cardiovascular event[b]	394	33.7	429	37.1	0.88 (0.77–1.01)	0.07
Coronary event	173	14.3	195	16.2	0.86 (0.70–1.06)	0.16
Myocardial infarction	58	4.7	82	6.7	0.68 (0.47–0.93)	0.04
Other cardiovascular event	134	11.0	144	11.9	0.90 (0.71–1.14)	0.36
Heart failure	69	5.6	78	6.4	0.85 (0.62–1.18)	0.33
Cerebrovascular event	152	12.5	163	13.6	0.90 (0.73–1.12)	0.35
Stroke	112	9.2	107	8.8	1.02 (0.78–1.33)	0.91

[a]Hazard ratios are for the event in the group assigned to angiotensin-converting–enzyme (ACE) inhibitors as compared with the diuretic group and are adjusted for age and sex. *CI* denotes confidence interval

[b]Myocardial infarction is a subcategory of coronary events; heart failure is a subcategory of other cardiovascular events; and stroke is a subcategory of cerebrovascular events. Patients were counted once for each type of first cardiovascular event they had, but patients who had more than one type of event were counted only once for the overall category of first cardiovascular event

Table 11.6 Cause-specific first events (Fatal and Nonfatal)[a]

Event	ACE-inhibitor group (*N* = 3044)		Diuretic group (*N* = 3039)		Hazard ratio (95% CI)	*P* value
	No. of events	Rate per 1000 patient-yr	No. of events	Rate per 1000 patient-yr		
Fatal events						
Cardiovascular	84	6.8	82	6.7	0.99 (0.72–1.35)	0.94
Coronary event	40	3.2	52	4.2	0.74 (0.49–1.11)	0.14
Myocardial infarction	9	0.7	11	0.9	0.79 (0.31–1.99)	0.61
Other cardiovascular event	15	1.2	15	1.2	0.95 (0.46–1.96)	0.89
Heart failure	2	0.2	8	0.7	0.24 (0.03–1.94)	0.18
Stroke	29	2.3	15	1.2	1.91 (1.04–3.50)	0.04
Noncardiovascular	111	9.0	128	10.4	0.84 (0.66–1.08)	0.18
Nonfatal cardiovascular events	338	28.9	380	32.8	0.86 (0.74–0.99)	0.03
Coronary event	141	11.6	149	12.4	0.92 (0.73–1.16)	0.49
Myocardial infarction	50	4.1	71	5.8	0.68 (0.47–0.99)	0.05
Other cardiovascular event	120	9.9	137	11.3	0.84 (0.66–1.07)	0.17
Heart failure	68	5.5	77	6.3	0.85 (0.62–1.17)	0.32
Stroke	91	7.5	94	7.8	0.93 (0.70–1.26)	0.65

[a]Myocardial infarction is a subcategory of coronary events; heart failure is a subcategory of other cardiovascular events. For non-fatal events, patients were counted once for each type of event they had, but patients who had more than one type of event were counted only once for the overall category of nonfatal cardiovascular events. Hazard ratios are for the event in the group assigned to angiotensin-converting–enzyme (ACE) inhibitors as compared with the diuretic group and are adjusted for age and sex. *CI* denotes confidence interval

resulted in an outcome advantage over a diuretic-based regimen, despite the similar reductions in BP levels. The results of this study were completely different from those of the ALLHAT [10]. However, caution is required in interpreting the disparate results between the two trials. First, there was a racial difference: 95% of the subjects in this study were white, while 35% of those in ALLHAT were blacks. Second, the baseline BP level was markedly higher in the patients of this study (168/91 mmHg) than in those of ALLHAT (146/84 mmHg). Third, the patients in this study were relatively healthy and active and had experienced few previous cardiovascular events. It would be expected that these differences in background greatly contributed to the different results. Finally, the strength of the ANBP2 study was that it was conducted in a family practice setting, and thus likely reflected the real-world effects of antihypertensive medications. Further studies will be needed to show the relative benefit of ACE-inhibitors in male patients.

CONVINCE: Controlled Onset Verapamil Investigation of Cardiovascular End Points [14]

Background At the time of this investigation, CCBs were often used in clinical practice, but the question of whether they had greater benefit than conventional antihypertensive agents such as β-blockers and diuretics remained controversial. In addition, there had been no study to investigate the timing of acute MI, cardiovascular event-related death, and stroke—all of which have their highest incidence during the early morning hours.

Objective To determine whether initial therapy with controlled-onset extended-release (CORE) verapamil was equivalent to a physician's choice of atenolol or hydrochlorothiazide in preventing cardiovascular disease.

Design A prospective, randomized, double-blind, multicenter, active-controlled clinical trial.

Patients Hypertensive patients (n = 16,602, 56% female, 84% white) aged 55 years or older (mean 66 years) with at least 1 other established risk factor for CVD (e.g., diabetes or smoking).

Treatments One group initially received CORE verapamil (n = 8241). The active-control group began with either hydrochlorothiazide (n = 3879) or atenolol (n = 4482).

Step 1 treatment: Patients received 2 bottles for initial treatment. One bottle contained tablets, 1 to be taken at bedtime, of either placebo or 180 mg of CORE verapamil. The other bottle contained tablets, 1 to be taken each morning, of placebo, 50 mg of atenolol, or 12.5 mg of hydrochlorothiazide. The dose of step 1 medication was doubled if SBP >140 mmHg and/or DBP > 90 mmHg.

Step 2 treatment: If BP levels still were not controlled after increasing the dose, 12.5 mg of hydrochlorothiazide could be added to the initial dose of either atenolol or CORE verapamil. Or 50 mg of atenolol could be added to the initial dose of hydrochlorothiazide. In addition, the dose of the added drug could be doubled if needed.

Step 3 treatment: Any additional antihypertensive agent (except a nondihydropyridine calcium antagonist, thiazide diuretic, or β-blocker) could be added (nonblinded) if needed. An ACE inhibitor was recommended.

Major clinical outcomes The primary endpoints were acute MI, stroke, or CVD-related death. Major secondary outcomes were as follows: (1) an expanded CVD end point, which included hospitalization for angina, cardiac revascularization or transplant, HF, TIA or carotid endarterectomy, accelerated or malignant hypertension, or renal failure in addition to the primary outcome; (2) all-cause mortality; (3) cancer; (4) hospitalization for bleeding (excluding hemorrhage stroke); and (5) incidence of primary endpoints occurring between 6 AM and noon.

Follow-up The median time receiving blinded treatment was 2.2 years.

Results

Adherence to study medication By the close of the trial, 39.4% of the CORE verapamil group and 39.7% of the atenolol or hydrochlorothiazide group had discontinued the blinded study medication. Patients assigned to receive CORE verapamil withdrew more often due to adverse signs or symptoms compared with those assigned atenolol or hydrochlorothiazide ($p = 0.02$); the most common reason was constipation (216 subjects in the CORE verapamil group compared with 28 in the atenolol or hydrochlorothiazide group). However, fewer patients assigned CORE verapamil (n = 115) withdrew because of poor BP control compared with those assigned atenolol or hydrochlorothiazide (n = 207) ($p < 0.001$).

Blood pressure control When averaged over the entire follow-up period, SBP/DBP was reduced by 13.6/7.8 mmHg and 13.5/7.1 mmHg from baseline in the CORE verapamil group and the atenolol or hydrochlorothiazide group, respectively. Both regimens lowered BP significantly.

Primary outcome There were 364 first primary events in the CORE verapamil group compared with 365 in the atenolol or hydrochlorothiazide group (Table 11.7). The HR for the CORE verapamil group compared with the atenolol or hydrochlorothiazide group was 1.02 (95% CI 0.88–1.18, $p = 0.77$). Also, there were no significant differences in each factor related to the

Table 11.7 Primary and secondary outcome by treatment assignment

	No. (%) of participants with event			
	COER verapamil	Atenolol or hydrochlorothiazide	Hazard ratio (95% confidence interval)	*P* value
Primary (composite) outcome[a]	364 (4.5)	365 (4.4)	1.02 (0.38–1.18)	.77
Fatal or nonfatal myocardial infarction	133 (1.6)	166 (2.0)	0.82 (0.65–1.03)	.09
Fatal or nonfatal stroke	133 (1.6)	118(1.4)	1.15 (0.90–1.48)	.26
Cardiovascular disease-related death	152 (1.9)	143(1.7)	1.09 (0.87–1.37)	.47
Primary event or cardiovascular hospitalization	793 (9.7)	775 (9.3)	1.05 (0.95–1.16)	.31
Angina pectoris	202 (2.5)	190 (2.3)	1.09 (0.89–1.33)	.39
Cardiac revascularization/cardiac transplant	163 (2.0)	166 (2.0)	1.01 (0.82–1.26)	.91
Heart failure	126 (1.5)	100 (1.2)	1.30 (1.00–1.69)	.05
Transient ischemic attack and/or carotid endarterectomy	89 (1.1)	105 (1.3)	0.87 (0.66–1.15)	.33
Accelerated/malignant hypertension	22 (0.3)	18 (0.2)	1.26 (0.67–2.34)	.47
Renal failure (acute/chronic)	27 (0.3)	34 (0.4)	0.81 (0.49–1.35)	.43
Death	337 (4.1)	319 (3.8)	1.08 (0.93–1.26)	.32
New cancer (excluding nonmelanoma skin cancer)	310 (3.8)	299 (3.6)	1.06 (0.91–1.24)	.46
Death	95 (1.2)	93 (1.1)	1.04 (0.79–1.39)	.76
Death or hospitalization due Lo bleeding[b]	118 (1.4)	79 (1.0)	1.54 (1.15–2.04)	.003
Deaths from bleeding	6 (0.1)	6 (0.1)	1.02 (0.33–3.17)	.97
Death or hospitalization due to serious adverse event	1381 (16.9)	1363 (16.4)	1.04 (0.97–1.12)	.29
Hospitalization for serious adverse event	1150 (14.1)	1143 (13.8)	1.03 (0.95–1.12)	.44

Abbreviation: *COER* controlled-onset extended-release

[a]First occurrence of stroke, myocardial infarction, or cardiovascular disease–related death

[b]Does not include intracerebral bleeding, which was counted as a primary and point (stroke)

primary outcome between the CORE verapamil group and the atenolol or hydrochlorothiazide group.

Secondary outcome The rate of hospitalization for HF was 30% higher with CORE verapamil compared with atenolol or hydrochlorothiazide (HR 1.30, 95% CI 1.00–1.69, p = 0.05). More patients assigned CORE verapamil (1.4%) than atenolol or hydrochlorothiazide (1.0%) died or were hospitalized for bleeding unrelated to stroke (HR 1.54, 95% CI 1.15–2.04, p = 0.003) (Table 11.7). For the primary outcome, treatment HRs did not vary significantly by time of day of the event (p = 0.43). In each treatment group, more patients had primary events between 6 AM and noon than any other 6-hour period (Fig. 11.8). The HR for the 6 AM to noon events was 1.15 (95% CI 0.86–1.53, p = 0.34).

Comments This study indicated that CORE verapamil was not equivalent to atenolol or hydrochlorothiazide in preventing cardiovascular disease-related events. When considered together with the results of ALLHAT [10], which found that a CCB (amlodipine) was not superior to a diuretic (chlorthalidone) in reducing the rate of CHD or stroke and was associated with a higher rate of HF, these results indicated that the effectiveness of CCB therapy in reducing CVD-related morbidity and mortality was similar but not better than that of diuretic or β-blocker treatment. The chronotherapeutic usage of antihypertensive agents was an attractive point in this study. However, additional investigations with larger numbers of patients and events were needed to verify the effectiveness of chronotherapy for reducing cardiovascular events.

VALUE: Valsartan Antihypertensive Long-Term Use Evaluation [15]

Background At the time of this study, renin-angiotensin-aldosterone system (RAAS) inhibitors, such as ACE inhibitors and ARBs, which were newer types of antihypertensive agent, were already being widely used in clinical practice. The LIFE [9] study showed the advantages of the ARB losartan over the β-blocker atenolol in hypertensive patients with LVH, with the primary advantage being a 25% reduction in stroke. Subsequently, the ANBP2 [13] reported fewer cardiovascular events in patients treated

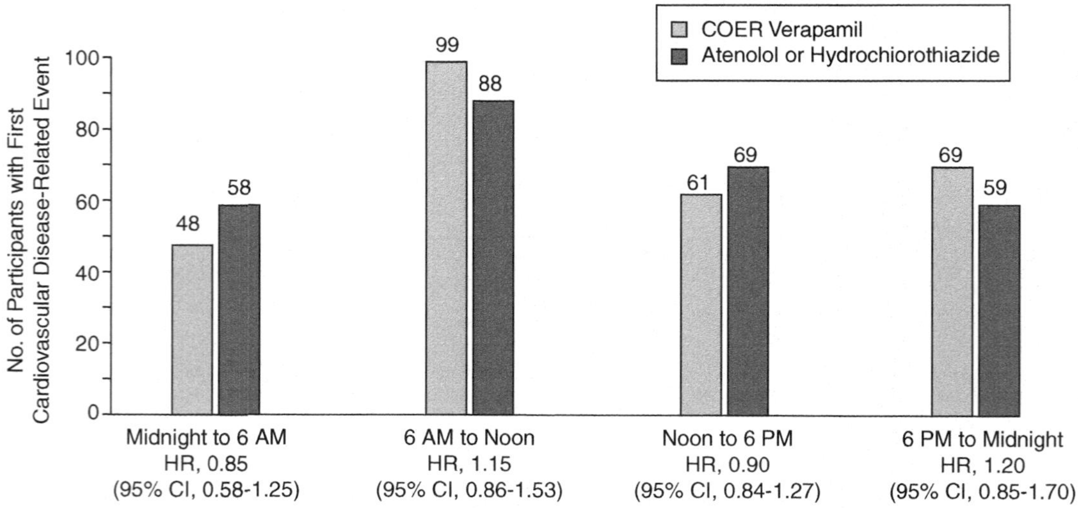

Time of onset of first cardiovascular disease-related event was determined for 2n participants in the controlled-onset extended-release (COER) verapamil group and 274 participants in the atenolol or hydrochlorothiazide group. There were 178 (24 %) events for which time of onset cou'd not be determined (87 among those randomized to COER verapamll and 91 among those randomized to atenolol or hydrochlorothiazide, hazard ratlo [HR]. 0.98; 95% confidence interval (CI], 0.73-1.32).

Fig. 11.8 Incidence of primary outcomes by treatment assignment and time of day with ACE inhibitors than in those given diuretics. However, the issue of whether the mechanism of action of antihypertensive drugs might influence their clinical effect remained unresolved. There was strong evidence suggesting that increased concentrations of angiotensin II were an independent risk factor for cardiac disease [16]. Valsartan was expected to reduce cardiac morbidity beyond its BP-lowering effect.

Objective To test the hypothesis that for the same level of BP control, valsartan-based treatment would be superior to amlodipine-based treatment for reduction of cardiac morbidity and mortality.

Design A prospective, randomized, double-blind, multicenter, active-controlled, parallel-group clinical trial.

Patients Hypertensive patients (n = 15,245, 42% female, 89% white), aged 50 years or older (mean 67 years), with untreated or previously treated hypertension and the presence of combinations of cardiovascular risk factors and cardiovascular disease. For previously untreated patients, hypertension was defined as a mean SBP between 160 and 210 mmHg, and a mean DBP <115 mmHg. The upper limit of BP for treated patients was SBP of 210 mmHg and/or DBP of 115 mmHg.

Treatments Patients were randomly assigned to receive valsartan 80 mg/day (n = 7649) or amlodipine 5 mg/day (n = 7596). The target BP level was SBP/DBP ≤ 140/90 mmHg. In cases with insufficient BP reduction, dose-titration steps were used once per month as follows: (1) valsartan and amlodipine were doubled in dose (valsartan 160 mg/day, amlodipine 10 mg/day); (2) hydrochlorothiazide 12.5 mg/day was added; (3) hydrochlorothiazide was doubled in dose (25 mg/day); (4) other antihypertensive medications were added. The baseline SBP/DBP levels were 154.5/87.4 mmHg and 154.8/87.6 mmHg in the valsartan and amlodipine group, respectively.

Major clinical outcomes The primary endpoint was the time to first cardiac event. This endpoint was a composite of sudden cardiac death, fatal MI, death during or after percutaneous coronary intervention or coronary artery bypass graft, death due to HF, and death associated with recent MI on autopsy, HF requiring hospital management, non-fatal MI, or emergency procedures to prevent MI. The secondary endpoints were fatal and non-fatal MI, fatal and non-fatal stroke, all-cause mortality, and new-onset diabetes.

Follow-up The mean follow-up was 4.2 years.

Results

Blood pressure At study end (72 months) or the final visit, the mean BP was 139.3/79.2 mmHg with valsartan-based regimens and 137.5/77.7 mmHg with amlodipine-based regimens. The amlodipine-based regimens significantly reduced the final BP levels compared with the valsartan-based regimens ($p < 0.0001$). After 1 month of treatment, BP in the amlodipine group was substantially (4.0/2.1 mmHg) lower than that in the valsartan group. At 6 months, the difference decreased to 2.1/1.6 mmHg. From the sixth month until the end of the study, BP decreased in both treatment groups: by 3.3/2.6 mmHg for the valsartan-based regimens, and 3.0/2.5 mmHg for the amlodipine-based regimens (Fig. 11.9). The target BP (SBP/DBP <140/90 mmHg) was achieved in 56% of patients in the valsartan group and 62% of those in the amlodipine group.

Major clinical outcomes The primary outcome, which was a composite of cardiac mortality and morbidity, occurred in 810 (10.6%, the rate per 1000 patient-years: 25.5) and 789 (10.4%, the rate per 1000 patient-years: 24.7) patients in the valsartan and amlodipine group, respectively (HR 1.04, 95% CI 0.94–1.15, $p = 0.49$) (Table 11.8). There were no significant differences in the primary outcome between the two groups. Of the secondary outcomes, MI was significantly more frequent in the valsartan group than in the amlodipine group (HR 1.19, 95% CI 1.02–1.38, $p = 0.02$). The rate of total cardiovascular events including stroke was 1074 in the valsartan vs. 1021 in the amlodipine group (HR 1.06, 95% CI 0.98–1.16, $p = 0.17$). The rate of all-cause death did not differ significantly

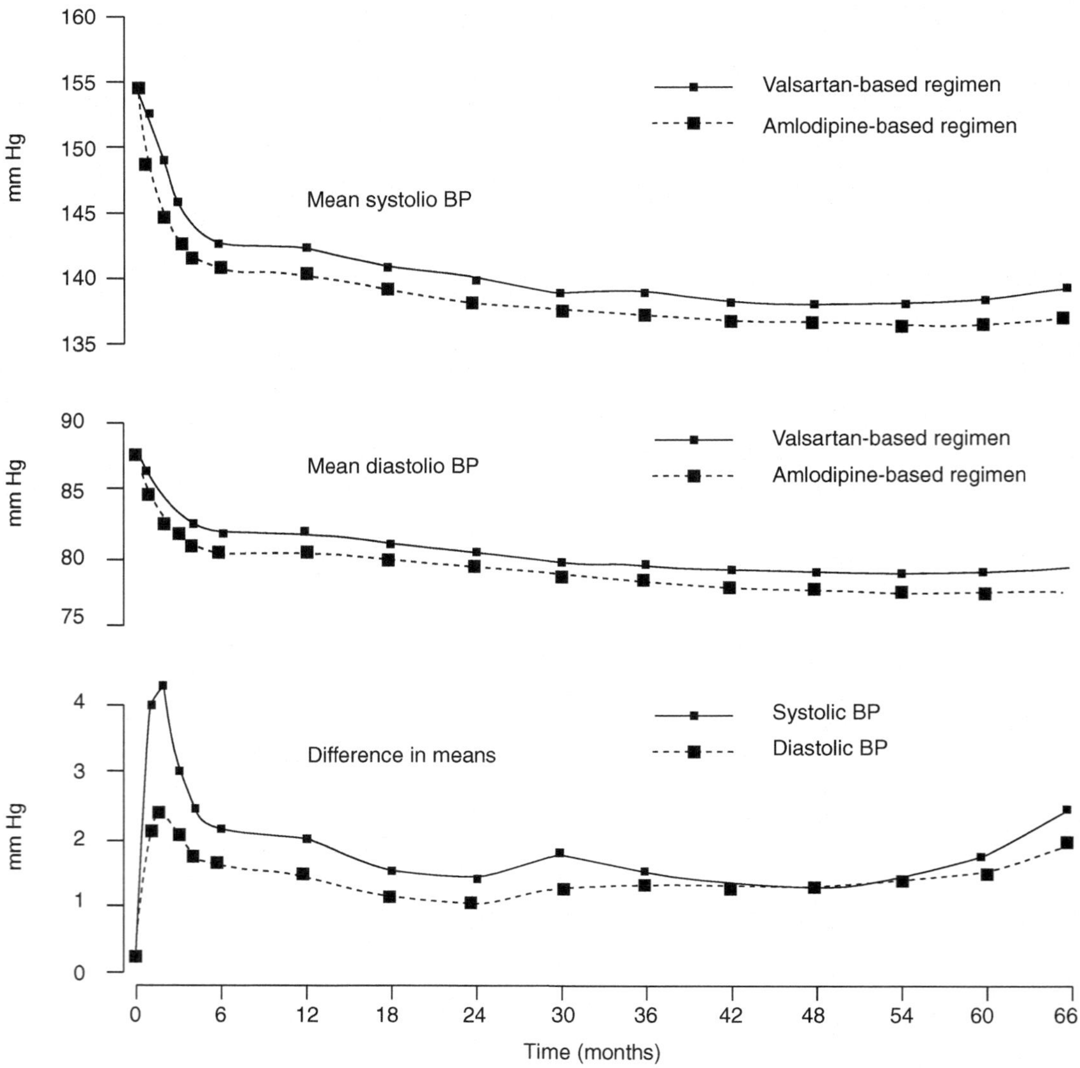

Fig. 11.9 BP difference between the two groups was significant (<0.000) at every time point. Overall differences in systolic BP=2.23 mm Hg (SE 0.18); overall differences in diastolic BP 1.59 mm Hg (SE 0.11). SDs of average BP at various time points in the amlodipine and valsartan groups are shown in Table 11.4

between the groups. New-onset diabetes arose in significantly fewer patients on valsartan than on amlodipine (32.1% vs. 41.1%, HR 0.77, 95% CI 0.69–0.86, $p < 0.0001$).

Table 11.9 show the BP differences and ORs over the time period of the trial for the primary and secondary endpoints. Higher ORs in favor of amlodipine were noted for all endpoints during the first 6 months, when BP differences between the treatment groups were greatest. In the following months, there was an attenuation in ORs.

Adherence to study medication Both treatment strategies were well tolerated with few severe adverse events. 73.7% of patients in the valsartan group and 74.9% of those in the amlodipine group remained on blinded study therapy throughout the entire follow-up period. 11.9% of patients in the valsartan group and 12.9% of those in the amlodipine group discontinued treatment because of adverse events. The most frequently reported adverse event was edema, which was twice as common in amlodipine-treated patients as in valsartan-treated patients (32.9% vs. 14.9%, $p < 0.0001$).

Table 11.8 Endpoints (first time occurrence in each category)

	Valsartan (n = 7649)		Amlodipine (n = 7596)			
	n (%)	Per 1000 patient years	n (%)	Per 1000 patient years	Hazard ratio (95% CI)	P
Primary composite	810 (10–6%)	25.5	789 (10–4%)	24.7	1.04 (0.94–1.15)	0.49
Cardiac mortality	304 (4–0%)	9.2	304 (4.0%)	9.2	1.01 (0.86–1.18)	0.90
Cardiac morbidity	586 (7–7%)	18–4	578 (7–6%)	18.1	1.02 (0.91–1.15)	0.71
Myocardial infarction[a]	369 (4–8%)	11–4	313 (4.1%)	9.6	1.19 (1.02-1.38)	0.02
Heart failure[a]	354 (4–6%)	11-0	400 (5–3%)	12.4	0.89 (0.77–1.03)	0.12
Stroke[a]	322 (4.2%)	10-0	281 (3.7%)	8.7	1.15 (0.98–1.35)	0.08
All-cause death	841 (11.0%)	25–6	818 (10.8%)	24.8	1.04 (0.94–1.14)	0.45
New onset diabetes	690 (13.1%)	32.1	845 (16-4%)	41.1	0.77[b] (0.69–0.86)	<0.0001

[a]Fatal and non-fatal
[b]Odds ratio, incidence rates and based on patients without diabetes at baseline

Table 11.9 Blood pressure and odds ratios throughout the study

	Mean blood pressure (SD)[a]		Time-specific interval odds ratios (95% CIs)				
Visit	Valsartan	Amlodipine	Primary endpoint	Stroke	Myocardial infarction	Heart failure	All-cause mortality
Baseline	154.5 (19.0)	154.8 (19.0)					
	87.4 (10.9)	87.6 (10.7)					
0–3 months	149.2 (19.5)	145.4 (16.1)	1.78 (1.22–2.60)	1.94 (1.10–3.42)	1.74 (0.94–3.22)	1.18 (0.70–2.00)	2.84 (1.51–5.34)
	84.8 (10.4)	82.6 (9.3)					
3–6 months	143.2 (16.8)	140.9 (14.3)	1.32 (0.89–1.96)	1.50 (0.82–2.72)	1.47 (0.76–2.83)	1.29 (0.73–2.28)	1.12 (0.70–1.81)
	82.1 (9.3)	80.4 (8.6)					
12 months	142.3 (16.9)	140.3 (14.4)	0.93 (0.69–1.26)	1.18 (0.71–1.95)	1.19 (0.74–1.90)	0.78 (0.49–1.24)	1.30 (0.93–1.83)
	81.7 (9.3)	80.2 (8.5)					
24 months	140.0 (16.2)	138.2 (13.8)	0.99 (0.80–1.24)	1.03 (0.73–1.45)	1.30 (0.94–1.80)	1.09 (0.78–1.50)	0.98 (0.78–1.23)
	80.4 (9.0)	79.2 (8-6)					
36 months	138.7 (16.1)	137.2 (13.5)	0.97 (0.78–1.19)	1.18 (0.83–1.68)	0.96 (0.69–1.34)	0.85 (0.63–1.16)	1.08 (0.88–1.33)
	79.5 (9.2)	78.1 (8-6)					
48 months	137.9 (15–6)	136.6 (13–6)	0.93 (0.745–1.15)	1.13 (0.79–1.61)	1.20 (0.86–1.67)	0.69 (0.51–0.94)	0.95 (0.78–1.15)
	78.8 (9.0)	77.5 (8.6)					
Study end	139.3 (17.6)	137.5 (15.0)	0.98 (0.74–1.29)	0.75 (0.45–1.25)	1.07 (0.72–1.59)	0.81 (0.53–1.22)	0.87 (0.70–1.09)
	79.2 (9.8)	77.7 (9.0)					

[a]Upper values systolic, lower values diastolic

Comments This study revealed that there were no significant differences between the valsartan-based regimens and amlodipine-based regimens with respect to cardiac morbidity and mortality. The most consistent significant difference between the groups was in BP control: the amlodipine-based regimens were significantly more efficacious in reducing BP, especially during the early treatment phase. Thus the study failed to confirm the authors' hypotheses, but rather found that amlodipine was more effective than valsartan. In this study, stroke incidence was lower in the amlodipine group than the valsartan group. On the other hand, The LIFE study [9] showed that losartan-based therapy was better than atenolol-based therapy in reducing strokes, despite the almost identical BP control of the two treatments. However, it could not be determined whether this reduction in stroke reflected the positive effects of the RAAS inhibitor. Especially with respect to stroke, even a small BP reduction would be important for preventing stroke events. The changes in the incidence of excess strokes over time in the valsartan group could be best explained by between-group differences in BP, which were largest in the first year. The results of this study provided new insight into the clinical importance of reaching the recommended BP goals within a relatively short period of time (weeks rather than months), at least in patients with hypertension who are at high cardiovascular risk.

CAFE: Conduit Artery Function Evaluation Within the Anglo-Scandinavian Cardiac Outcomes Trial (ASCOT-CAFE) [17]

Background At the time of this trial, emerging evidence had suggested that central aortic pressure may be an independent predictor of cardiovascular damage and clinical outcomes [18, 19]. In addition, in small studies, various classes of BP-lowering drugs showed different effects on central hemodynamic parameters, despite their similar effects on brachial artery pressure [20, 21]. However, there had been no information regarding the effects of BP-lowering drugs on central aortic hemodynamic parameters in large-scale clinical trials.

The CAFE study was designed as a large substudy within the Anglo-Scandinavian Cardiac Outcomes Trial (ASCOT) [22]. The CAFE study provided the first evaluation within a large cardiovascular outcomes trial of the impact of two different BP-lowering regimens on central aortic pressure.

Objective To test the hypothesis that different BP-lowering regimens would have different effects on central aortic pressure and cardiovascular outcomes despite their similar effects on brachial BP.

Design A prospective, randomized, open-label, multicenter, blinded end-point designed clinical trial.

Patients Hypertensive patients (n = 2073, 18% female, 86% white), aged 40–79 years (mean 63 years), with untreated or treated hypertension, and at least 3 additional cardiovascular risk factors: male, smoker, age > 55 years, LVH, ECG abnormalities of ischemic changes, type 2 diabetes, peripheral arterial disease, cerebrovascular disease, microalbuminuria or proteinuria, a ratio of plasma total cholesterol to HDL cholesterol of ≥6, or a family history of premature CHD. Hypertension was defined as follows: (1) in untreated hypertension, SBP ≥160 mmHg or DBP ≥100 mmHg; (2) in treated hypertension, SBP ≥140 mmHg or DBP ≥90 mmHg.

Recruitment into the CAFE study began 1 year after randomization into ASCOT to avoid the turbulence of the early BP changes and uptitration of treatment, so patients were studied when their treatment regimens were stable.

Treatments Patients were randomly assigned a regimen of either amlodipine plus a perindopril (amlodipine group, n = 1031) or an atenolol plus bendroflumethiazide K (atenolol group, n = 1042). The target BP level was SBP/DBP <140/90 mmHg for patients without diabetes and < 130/80 mmHg for patients with diabetes.

In cases with insufficient BP reduction, dose-titration steps were used every 6 months as follows: (1) at randomization, amlodipine 5 mg/day, atenolol 50 mg/day; (2) amlodipine and atenolol were doubled in dose (amlodipine 10 mg/day, atenolol 100 mg/day); (3) perindopril 4 mg/day was added in amlodipine group, and bendroflumethiazide K 1.25 mg/day was added in the atenolol group; (4) perindopril and bendroflumethiazide K were doubled in dose (perindopril 8 mg/day and bendroflumethiazide K 2.5 mg/day); (5) doxazosin gastrointestinal transport system 4 mg/day was added in both groups; (6) the doxazosin gastrointestinal transport system was doubled in both groups (doxazosin gastrointestinal transport system 8 mg/day). Baseline peripheral and central SBP/DBP levels were 133.2/76.9 mmHg and 121.2/77.8 mmHg in the amlodipine group and 133.9/78.6 mmHg and 125.5/79.1 mmHg in the atenolol group, respectively.

Peripheral and central BP measurements Peripheral BP was measured using a validated, semiautomated, oscillometric device (Omron 705CP; Omron). Central BP and other parameters were measured using a commercially available system (SphygmoCor). Aortic pressure waveforms were subjected to further analysis by using the SphygmoCor software to identify the time to the peak/shoulder of the first and second pressure wave component (T1, T2) during systole. The pressure at the peak/shoulder of the first component was identified as the P1 height (outgoing pressure wave), and the pressure differences between this point and the maximal pressure during systole (ΔP or augmentation) were identified as the reflected pressure wave occurring during systole (Fig. 11.10). The augmentation index (AIx), defined as the ratio of augmentation to central pulse pressure, was expressed as a percentage: AIx = (ΔP/PP) × 100,

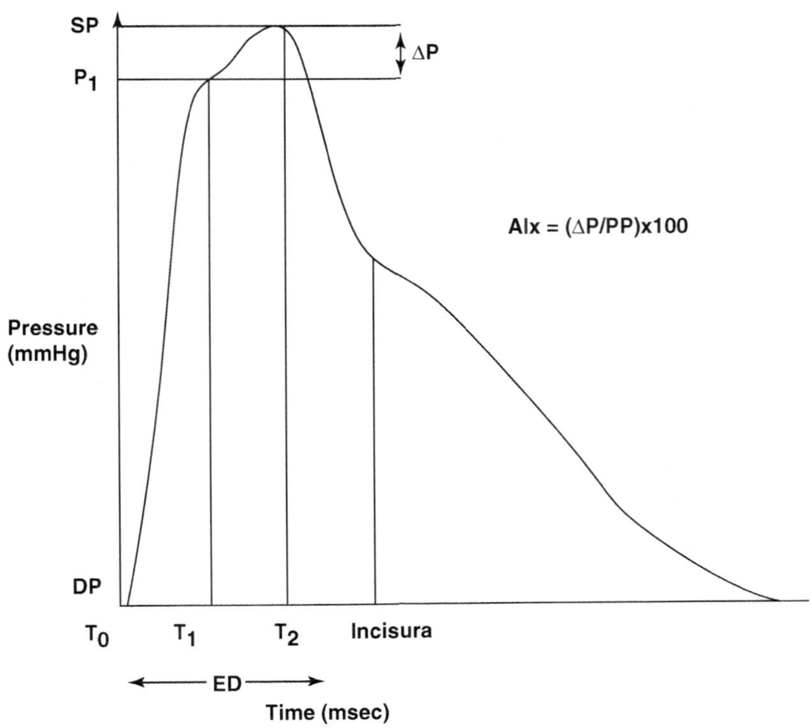

Fig. 11.10 Hemodynamic parameters derived by pulse wave analysis of the central aortic pressure wave. T0 indicates the time at the start of the waveform; T1, duration from start of waveform to the first peak/shoulder (outgoing pressure wave); T2, duration from start of waveform to the second peak/shoulder (reflected pressure wave); ED, ejection duration, or duration from start of waveform to closure of the aortic valve (incisura); SP, central aortic systolic pressure; DP, central aortic diastolic pressure; P1, P2 height difference between the minimum pressure and the pressure at the first peak/shoulder (T1); augmentation (ΔP), difference between maximal pressure (central aortic systolic pressure) and pressure at the first peak/shoulder (P1 height); PP pulse pressure, and Alx augmentation index

where P is pressure and PP is pulse pressure. Pulse pressure amplification (PPA) was expressed as the ratio of central pulse pressure (CPP) to peripheral (brachial) pulse pressure (PPP): PPA = PPP/CPP.

Major clinical outcomes The primary outcome was a comparison of the effects of the 2 treatment regimens on central aortic pressures derived from applanation tonometry. The secondary outcome was a composite clinical outcome comprising all cardiovascular events and renal impairment.

Follow-up The mean follow-up time after the initial tonometry measurement was 3 years.

Results

Hemodynamic data Most patients (95%) were taking at least 2 BP-lowering drugs, with 56% and 60% receiving the predefined combination therapy of amlodipine-perindopril, or atenolol-bendroflumethiazide, respectively. Only 7.0% (amlodipine) and 3.5% (atenolol) of patients remained on monotherapy throughout the CAFE study.

Figure 11.11 shows representative averaged radial artery waveforms and the resulting derived central aortic waveforms from individual patients with similar brachial BP. Atenolol monotherapy was associated with a broader peripheral

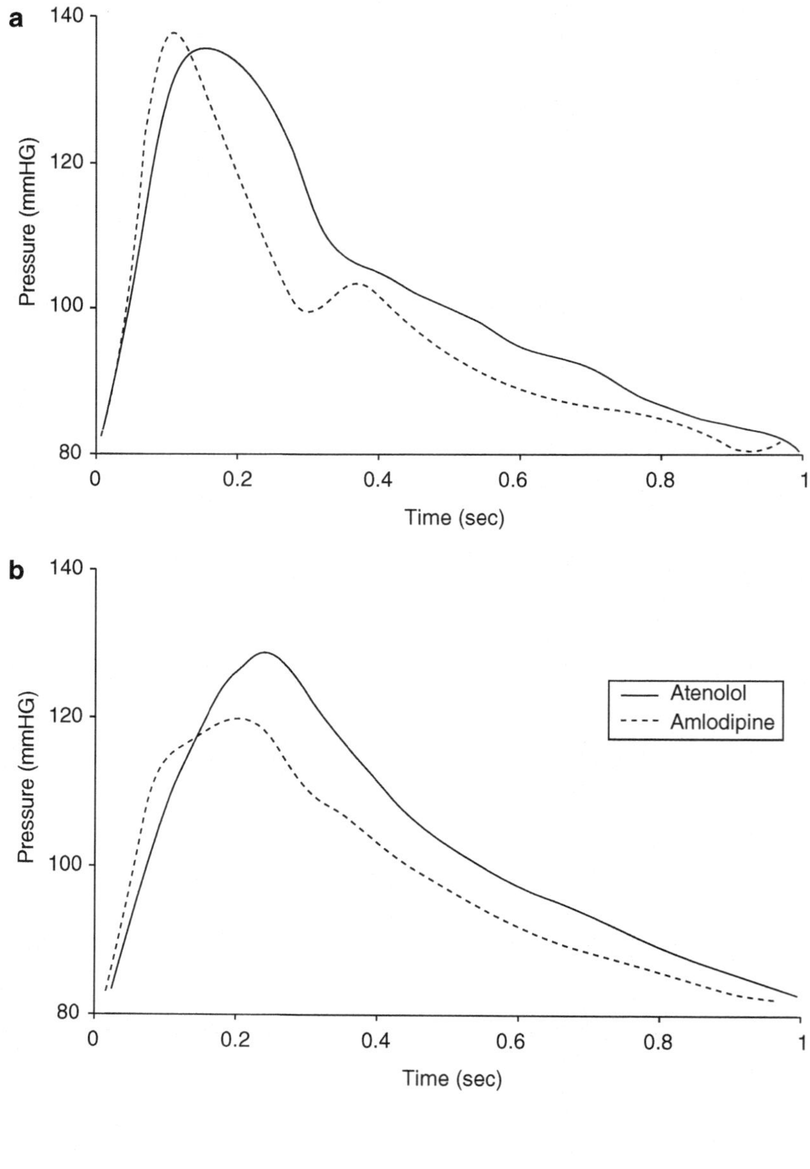

Fig. 11.11 Examples of peripheral (**a**) and corresponding derived central aortic (**b**) waveforms from patients of equal age treated with atenolol (solid line) or amlodipine (broken line) as mono-therapy achieving equivalent brachial blood pressures

waveform and a more prominent late systolic peak in the central aortic waveform.

Primary outcomes At the end of the CAFE study, brachial BPs were similar between the 2 groups and had fallen substantially from baseline: −27.8/−15.7 for amlodipine with/without perindopril vs. −26.0/−13.8 for atenolol with/without bendroflumethiazide. There were significant reductions of brachial DBP and central SBP/DBP in the amlodipine group compared to the atenolol group (Table 11.10).

A summary of the BP load for each treatment arm is also presented as the mean area under the curve (AUC) for each parameter. Despite the insignificant differences in brachial SBP (AUC difference, 0.7 mmHg; 95% CI −0.4–1.7; $p = 0.2$), derived central aortic systolic pressure was substantially lower in the amlodipine group (AUC difference, 4.3 mmHg; 95% CI 3.3–5.4; $p < 0.0001$; Table 11.10). There were small differences in central aortic diastolic pressure in favor of the amlodipine group (AUC difference, 1.4 mmHg; 95% CI 0.6–2.1; $p = 0.0002$; Table 11.10). Central aortic pulse pressure also was significantly lower in the amlodipine group compared with atenolol group (AUC difference, 3.0 mmHg; 95% CI 2.1–3.9; $p < 0.0001$; Table 11.10). Heart rate was significantly lower in the atenolol group (AUC difference, 10.7 bpm; 95% CI 9.8–11.5; $p < 0.0001$; Table 11.10).

P1 height was lower in the atenolol group (AUC difference, 0.8 mmHg; 95% CI 0.3–1.4; $p = 0.003$; Table 11.10). However, central aortic systolic pressure wave augmentation was markedly increased in the atenolol group compared with the amlodipine group (AUC difference, 3.8 mmHg; 95% CI 3.3–4.4; $p < 0.0001$; Table 11.10). The augmentation index was also increased in the atenolol group (AUC difference, 6.5%; 95% CI 5.8–7.3; $p < 0.0001$; Table 11.10).

Secondary outcomes Central aortic pulse pressure, central aortic pressure wave augmentation, and outgoing pressure wave height (P1 height), along with brachial pulse pressure, were significantly associated with the composite end-

Table 11.10 Hemodynamic and pulse wave analysis parameters by treatment arm for the CAFE cohort

Parameter	Atenoiol	Amlodipine	Difference (Atenoiol–Amlodipine)	Statistics *t* Test (*P*)
Peripheral SBP, mm Hg	133.9 (133, 134.7)	133.2 (132.5, 133.8)	0.7 (−0.4, 1.7)	0.2
Peripheral DBP, mm Hg	78.6 (78.1, 79.1)	76.9 (76.4, 77.4)	1.6 (0.9, 2.4)	<0.0001
Peripheral PP, mm Hg	55.3 (54.6, 56)	56.2 (55.6, 56.9)	−0.9(−1.9, 0)	0.06
Heart rate, bpm	58.6 (58, 59.2)	69.3 (68.6, 69.9)	−10.7 (−11.5, −9.8)	<0.0001
Central SBP, mm Hg	125.5 (124.7, 126.3)	121.2 (120.5, 121.9)	4.3 (3.3, 5.4)	<0.0001
Central DBP, mm Hg	79.1 (78.6, 79.6)	77.8 (77.3, 78.3)	1.4 (0.6, 2.1)	0.0002
Central PP, mm Hg	46.4 (45.7, 47.1)	43.4 (42.8, 44)	3.0 (2.1, 3.9)	<0.0001
Augmentation Index, %	31.9 (31.3, 32.4)	25.3 (24.8, 25.9)	6.5 (5.8, 7.3)	<0.0001
Augmentation, mm Hg	15.4 (14.9, 15.8)	11.5 (11.2, 11.9)	3.8 (3.3, 4.4)	<0.0001
P1 height, mm Hg	31 (30.6, 31.5)	31.9 (31.5, 32.3)	−0.8 (−1.4, −0.3)	0.003
Pulse pressure amplification, ratio	1.21 (1.2, 1.21)	1.31 (1.3, 1.32)	−0.11 (−0.12, −0.1)	<0.0001
T1, ms	109.2 (108.5, 109.9)	106.5 (106, 107)	2.7 (1.8, 3.5)	<0.0001
T2, ms	234.1 (232.8, 235.4)	215.2 (214, 216.4)	18.9 (17.1, 20.7)	<0.0001
ED, ms	322.5 (321, 324)	302.8 (301, 304)	19.7 (17.5, 22.0)	<0.0001
DD, ms	732.8 (724, 742)	588.1 (581, 595)	144.7 (133.1, 156.2)	<0.0001

T1 Indicates duration from start of waveform to the first peak/shoulder (outgoing pressure wave); T2, duration from start of waveform to the second peak/shoulder (reflected pressure wave); augmentation (ΔP), difference between maximal pressure and pressure at the first peak/shoulder (P1 Height); Aix, aortic augmentation index–proportion of the central pressure wave height attributable augmentation (ΔP)(Aix – (ΔP/PP) × 100); P1 Height, difference between the minimum pressure and the pressure at the first peak/shoulder (T1), *ED* ejection duration (duration from start of waveform to closure of the aortic wave [incisura]), and *DD* diastolic duration (duration from incisura to end of waveform) (see Fig. 11.2 for graphical representation) point ($p < 0.01$) in all models (Table 11.11). After adjustment, the central pulse pressure remained significantly associated with the composite clinical outcome in all 3 models. In addition, augmentation and/or peripheral pulse pressure were significantly associated with the

Table 11.11 Updated Cox proportional-hazards modeling for the composite clinical end point in the CAFE cohort

	χ^2	*P*	HR	95 % CI
Updated Cox proportional-hazards model unadjusted				
Model 1 (305 events)				
Peripheral PP	21.0	<0.0001	1.23	1.13–1.34
Central PP	17.8	<0.0001	1.22	1.12–1.34
Augmentation	7.1	0.008	1.24	1.06–1.47
P_1 height	19.0	<0.0001	1.43	1.22–1.69
Model 2 (245 events)				
Peripheral PP	19.7	<0.0001	1.24	1.13–1.36
Central PP	17.2	<0.0001	1.23	1.12–1.36
Augmentation	8.9	0.003	1.29	1.09–1.53
P_1 height	15.4	<0.0001	1.42	1.19–1.69
Model 3 (225 events)				
Peripheral PP	18.0	<0.0001	1.24	1.12–1.37
Central PP	15.5	<0.0001	1.23	1.11–1.36
Augmentation	7.7	0.005	1.28	1.08–1.53
P_1 height	14.3	<0.0001	1.42	1.19–1.71
Updated Cox proportional-hazards model adjusted for age and baseline risk factors				
Model 1 (305 events)				
Peripheral PP	3.83	0.050	1.10	1.00–1.22
Central PP	3.91	0.048	1.11	1.00–1.23
Augmentation	2.26	0.133	1.14	0.96–1.36
P_1 height	3.04	0.081	1.17	0.98–1.40
Model 2 (245 events)				
Peripheral PP	4.5	0.034	1.12	1.01–1.24
Central PP	5.0	0.026	1.13	1.02–1.26
Augmentation	4.2	0.040	1.21	1.01–1.45
P_1 height	2.5	0.114	1.16	0.96–1.40
Model 3 (225 events)				
Peripheral PP	4.1	0.044	1.12	1.00–1.25
Central PP	4.1	0.043	1.13	1.00–1.26
Augmentation	3.1	0.080	1.18	0.98–1.43
P_1 height	2.4	0.118	1.17	0.96–1.42

Cox proportional hazards regression models updated for blood pressure and hemodynamic Indices with time. Hazard ratios are presented per 10 mm Hg. The composite clinical outcome variable was all cardiovascular events and procedures plus development or renal impairment (see Data Supplement for details). Model 1 evaluates composite clinical outcomes in all patients from time or randomization into ASCOT. Model 2 evaluates composite clinical outcomes in all patients from time of first central aortic pressure measurement in CAFE. Model 3 evaluates composite clinical outcomes in all patients from time or first central aortic pressure measurement in CAFE excluding patients with events occurring prior to this time. Where indicated, models were adjusted for age and baseline risk factors including presence of peripheral vascular disease, diabetes mellitus, left ventricular hypertrophy on echocardiogram or ECG, ECG changes compatible with ischemic heart disease, history of cerebrovascular disease, microalbuminuria/proteinuria, plasma total:high-density lipoprotein cholesterol ratio greater than 6, family history of coronary artery disease, male sex, age over 55 years, or smoking status (current/recently). Blood pressures and hemodynamic factors were entered into the model individually and included brachial systolic blood pressure, central systolic blood pressure, difference between brachial and central systolic blood pressure, brachial pulse pressure, central pulse pressure, pulse pressure amplification, augmentation, augmentation index, and outgoing pressure wave height (P1 Height). Factors showing a significant association with the composite end point are shown composite clinical outcome after adjustment in models 2 and 3.

Comments The ASCOT-CAFE was the first study to investigate the effects of different antihypertensive agents on derived central aortic pressure/hemodynamics and cardiovascular outcomes. This study showed substantial and consistent differences in central aortic pressures and hemodynamics in favor of the amlodipine with/without perindopril-based therapy vs. atenolol with/without bendroflumethiazide-based therapy, despite the similar brachial SBP between the two treatment arms. These results indicated that the different BP-lowering drugs had different effects on the central aortic pressure/hemodynamics despite their similar effects on brachial BP, which in turn meant that brachial BP was not always a better surrogate for the effect of BP-lowering drugs on arterial hemodynamics than central aortic pressure. The greatest value of this study was its revelation that central aortic pressure was an important indicator for the management of hypertension. However, caution is required in interpreting the results of this study. It was usual to consider that there was no difference between peripheral PP and central PP in Model 1 of Table 11.11 (peripheral PP: HR 1.10, 95% CI 1.00–1.22, $p = 0.050$; central PP: HR 1.11, 95% CI 1.00–1.23, $p = 0.048$). Considering these results, it seemed that reducing the BP itself, including brachial and central BP, was the most important determinant for reducing the risk of cardiovascular outcomes.

ACCOMPLISH: Avoiding Cardiovascular Events Through Combination Therapy in Patients Living with Systolic Hypertension [23]

Background For patients at high-risk of CVD, treatment with multiple antihypertensive medications is often necessary to attain BP goals. At the time of this study, diuretics, CCBs, and ACE inhibitors/ARBs were often used in combination therapies, but the optimal combinations of antihypertensive medication were still unclear. Also around this time, the seventh report of the Joint National Committee on Prevention, Detection, Evaluation, and Treatment of High Blood Pressure (JNC7) [24] recommended that diuretics should be used in combination therapy. On the other hand, several other reports revealed that the combination of a CCB and an ACE inhibitor had better effects on organ damage compared with other antihypertensive combinations [25, 26]. Thus, the combination of an ACE inhibitor and a CCB was thought to be superior to the combination of an ACE inhibitor and a diuretic for the reduction of cardiovascular outcomes.

Objective To test the hypothesis that treatment with an ACE inhibitor combined with amlodipine would result in better cardiovascular outcomes than treatment with the same ACE inhibitor combined with a thiazide diuretic.

Design A prospective, randomized, double-blind, multicenter clinical trial.

Patients Hypertensive patients (n = 11,506, 39.5% female, 83% white), aged 60 years or older (mean 68.4 years), with an SBP ≥160 mmHg or currently on antihypertensive therapy and at high risk for CVD events; patients with a history of coronary events, myocardial infarction, revascularization, or stroke; and patients with impaired renal function; peripheral arterial disease; left ventricular hypertrophy; or diabetes mellitus. Patients aged 55–59 years were included if there was evidence of their having two or more of the CVD diseases or target-organ damages mentioned above [27].

Treatments Patients were randomly assigned a combination of 20 mg of benazepril and 5 mg of amlodipine (n = 5744) or a combination of 20 mg of benazepril and 12.5 mg of hydrochlorothiazide (n = 5762). The target BP level was SBP/DBP ≤ 140/90 mmHg (or a recommended target of SBP/DBP ≤ 130/80 mmHg for patients with diabetes or kidney disease). In cases of insufficient BP reduction, the benazepril component in both groups was increased to 40 mg daily 1 month after randomization. Thereafter, investigators increased the amlodipine dose to 10 mg daily and increased the hydrochlorothiazide dose to 25 mg daily, if necessary. The addition of other antihypertensive agents, including β-blockers, α-blockers, clonidine, and spironolactone, was permitted. Loop diuretics taken once daily were permitted for volume management. The dose-adjustment period was the initial 3 months. Baseline SBP/DBP levels were 145.3/80.1 mmHg and 145.4/80.0 mmHg in the benazepril-amlodipine and benazepril-hydrochlorothiazide group, respectively.

Major clinical outcomes The primary endpoint was the time to first cardiac event, which was defined as a composite of cardiovascular events and death from cardiovascular causes. Death from cardiovascular causes was defined as a death attributed to sudden death from cardiac causes, MI, stroke, coronary intervention, congestive HF, or other cardiovascular causes. A cardiovascular event was defined as a nonfatal MI, stroke, hospitalization for unstable angina, coronary revascularization, or resuscitation after sudden cardiac arrest. Secondary endpoints were a composite of cardiovascular events, defined as the primary endpoint excluding fatal events, and a composite of death from cardiovascular causes, nonfatal stroke, and nonfatal MI.

Follow-up The mean follow-up was 35.7 months for the benazepril-amlodipine group and 35.6 months for the benazepril-hydrochlorothiazide group.

Results

Drug treatment For the patients in the benazepril-amlodipine group, the mean (median) daily dose was 36.3 mg (39.4 mg) of benazepril and 7.7 mg (8.9 mg) of amlodipine; for patients in the benazepril-hydrochlorothiazide group, the mean (median) daily dose was 36.1 mg (39.4 mg) of benazepril and 19.3 mg (22.1 mg) of hydrochlorothiazide. In each group, 32.3% of the patients received approved antihypertensive agents in addition to the highest dose of study medication after 1 year in the study.

Blood pressure The mean BP after dose adjustment was 131.6/73.3 mmHg in the benazepril-amlodipine group and 132.5/74.4 mmHg in the benazepril-hydrochlorothiazide group. The mean difference in BP between the two groups was 0.9 mmHg systolic and 1.1 mmHg diastolic ($p < 0.001$ for both SBP and DBP). BP control, which was defined as SBP/DBP ≤ 140/90 mmHg, was attained in an average of 75.4% of patients in the benazepril-amlodipine group and 72.4% in the benazepril-hydrochlorothiazide group.

Major clinical outcomes The primary-outcome event occurred in 552 patients (9.6%) in the benazepril-amlodipine group as compared with 679 patients (11.8%) in the benazepril-hydrochlorothiazide group, representing an absolute risk reduction of 2.2 percentage points and a relative risk reduction of 19.6% (HR, 0.80; 95% CI, 0.72–0.90; $p < 0.001$) (Table 11.12). The primary event rates per 1000 patient-years were 32.3 in the benazepril-amlodipine group and 39.7 in the benazepril-hydrochlorothiazide group. For the secondary endpoint of cardiovascular events, there were 494 events (8.6%) in the benazepril-amlodipine group and 592 events (10.3%) in the benazepril-hydrochlorothiazide group, representing an absolute risk reduction of 1.7 percentage points and a relative risk reduction of 17.4% (HR, 0.83; 95% CI, 0.73–0.93; $p = 0.002$) (Table 11.12).

Adverse events The cumulative rate of discontinuation of a study drug was similar in the two groups (28.8% and 31.2% in the benazepril-amlodipine group and the benazepril-hydrochlorothiazide group, respectively). The most common reasons for discontinuation of the study medication were an adverse event or laboratory-test abnormality; 17.6% of the patients in the benazepril-amlodipine group and 18.4% of those in the benazepril-hydrochlorothiazide group discontinued the study medication for these reasons, with 13.4% and 14.3% of patients, respectively, discontinuing treatment due to adverse events alone.

Table 11.12 Hazard ratios for primary, secondary, and other prespecified end points, and results of the subgroup analysis

End Point	Benazepril–amlodipine group (*N* = 5744)	Benazepril–hydrochlorothiazide group (*N* = 5762)	Hazard ratio (95% CI)[a]	*P* value[b]
Primary				
Composite of cardiovascular events and death from cardiovascular causes — no. (%)	552 (9.6)	679 (11.8)	0.80 (0.72–0.90)	<0.001
Individual component — no (%)				
Death from cardiovascular causes	107 (1.9)	134 (2.3)	0.80 (0.62–1.03)	0.08
Fatal and nonfatal myocardial infarction	125 (2.2)	159 (2.8)	0.78 (0.62–0.99)	0.04
Fatal and nonfatal stroke	112 (1.9)	133 (2.3)	0.84 (0.65–1.08)	0.17
Hospitalization for unstable angina	44 (0.8)	59 (1.0)	0.75 (0.50–1.10)	0.14
Coronary revascularization procedure	334 (5.8)	386 (6.7)	0.86 (0.74–1.00)	0.04
Resuscitation after sudden cardiac arrest	14 (0.2)	8 (0.1)	1.75 (0.73–4.17)	0.20
Subgroup — no. with primary end point/total no. (%)				
Sex				
Male	365/3448 (10.6)	461/3515 (13.1)	0.80 (0.69–0.91)	0.001
Female	187/2296 (8.1)	218/2246 (9.7)	0.83 (0.68–1.01)	0.06
Age				
≥65 yr	336/3813 (10.1)	474/3827 (12.4)	0.81 (0.71–0.92)	0.002
≥70 yr	260/2363 (11.0)	323/2340 (13.8)	0.79 (0.67–0.93)	0.004
Presence of diabetes				
Yes	307/3478 (8.8)	383/3468 (11.0)	0.79 (0.68–0.92)	0.003
No	245/2266 (10.8)	296/2294 (12.9)	0.82 (0.69–0.97)	0.02
Secondary and other				
Composite of cardiovascular events — no. (%)	494 (8.6)	592 (10.3)	0.S3 (0.73–0.93)	0.002
Composite of death from cardiovascular events, non-fatal myocardial infarction, and nonfatal stroke — no. (%)	288 (5.0)	364 (6.3)	0.79 (0.67–0.92)	0.002
Death from any cause — no. (%)	236 (4.1)	262 (4.5)	0.90 (0.76–1.07)	0.24
Hospitalization for congestive heart failure — no. (%)	100 (1.7)	96 (1.7)	1.04 (0.79–1.38)	0.77
Primary end point plus hospitalization for congestive heart failure — no. (%)	617 (10.7)	738 (12.8)	0.83 (0.74–0.92)	0.0005

[a]Hazard ratios are for the benazepril–amlodipine group
[b]The P values are derived from a log-rank test

Comments This study revealed that combination treatment with benazepril plus amlodipine is superior to treatment with benazepril plus hydrochlorothiazide in reducing the risk of cardiovascular events and of death among high-risk patients with hypertension. These results appear surprising in light of the results of the ALLHAT [10], which indicated that amlodipine-based and chlorthalidone-based therapy had similar effects on mortality and on the rates of stroke and MI (Fig. 11.6). For some time, it remained unclear why the results were different between the two clinical trials. However, our previous study [28] might support the results of the ACCOMPLISH trial from the viewpoint of central hemodynamics. The Japan-Combined Treatment With Olmesartan and a Calcium Channel Blocker Versus Olmesartan and Diuretics Randomized Efficacy (J-CORE) study [28] demonstrated that the extent of the reduction in central SBP in the ARB/CCB (olmesartan/azelnidipine) combination was significantly greater than that in the ARB/diuretic (olmesartan/hydrochlorothiazide) combination, whereas the difference in the reduction in brachial SBP between the two groups was not significant. The reduction in aortic pulse wave velocity (PWV) was also significantly greater by the ARB/CCB combination than by the ARB/diuretic combination. Because the central SBP [17] and aortic PWV [29] have been reported to be independent predictors of cardiovascular morbidity in hypertensive patients, a beneficial effect of RAAS inhibitor/CCB treatment on central hemodynamics might lead to a more favorable effect on cardiovascular outcomes compared to the RAAS inhibitor/diuretic treatment. In addition, we recently demonstrated that the ARB/CCB (irbesartan/amlodipine) combination significantly reduced nocturnal BP, morning BP, and evening BP as measured by information and communication technology (ICT)-based home BP monitoring devices, and also office BP compared to the ARB/diuretic (irbesartan/trichlormethiazide) combination in the NOCTURNE study [30]. All these studies indicated that the RAAS inhibitor/CCB combination would be superior to the RAAS inhibitor/diuretic combination for the reduction of both office and out-of-office BP. Further studies are needed to establish the effectiveness of the RAAS inhibitor/CCB combination compared to the RAAS inhibitor/diuretic combination on perfect BP control.

Conclusion

We reviewed the nine historical hypertension clinical trials. The results of these clinical trials indicate the historical transition of antihypertensive medication therapies from classical drugs such as diuretics and β-blockers to newer agents such as CCBs, ACE inhibitors and ARBs. In addition, these trials confirmed the efficacy of diuretics in achieving substantial BP reductions. The most important points in the management of hypertension are to reduce the BP levels significantly in the early phase and to reach the BP goals without fail, as the VALUE [15] trial demonstrated, especially in high-risk patients with hypertensive complications. Among the approaches for realizing these objectives, intensive nutritional-hygienic intervention and the improvement of lifestyles are perhaps most essential for the management of hypertension, as clearly indicated by the results of the TOMHS [7], which was conducted in the 1980s–1990s. These remarkable advances in antihypertensive therapy have provided us with the ability to lower BP levels in hypertensive patients. Nevertheless, we must bear in mind that there remain many patients with uncontrolled BP levels [31] and the number of such patients will likely increase worldwide [32]. Therefore, we must focus our efforts on delivering the benefits of antihypertensive therapies to those particular patients for whom the cardiovascular outcomes are most likely to be improved, and the healthy life span extended.

References

1. Williams B, Williams H, Northedge J, Crimmins J, Caulfield M, Watts M, et al. Hypertension: the clinical management of primary hypertension in adults, Update of clinical guidelines 18 and 34. NICE clinical guideline no. 127. London: Published by the National

Clinical Guideline Centre at the Royal College of Physicians; 2011. http://guidance.nice.org.uk/CG127.
2. Mancia G, Fagard R, Narkiewixz K, Redon J, Zanchetti A, Böhm M, et al. 2013 ESH/ESC guidelines for the management of arterial hypertension: the Task Force for the Management of Arterial Hypertension of the European Society of Hypertension (ESH) and of the European Society of Cardiology (ESC). Eur Heart J. 2013;34:2159–219.
3. James PA, Oparil S, Carter BL, Cushman WC, Dennison-Himmelfarb C, Handler J, et al. 2014 evidence-based guideline for the management of high blood pressure in adults: report from the panel members appointed to the Eighth Joint National Committee (JNC 8). JAMA. 2014;311:507–20.
4. Weber MA, Schiffrin EL, White WB, Mann S, Lindholm LH, Kenerson JG, et al. Clinical practice guidelines for the management of hypertension in the community: a statement by the American Society of Hypertension and the International Society of Hypertension. J Clin Hypertens (Greenwich). 2014;16:14–26.
5. Shimamoto K, Ando K, Fujita T, Hasebe N, Higaki J, Horiuchi M, et al. The Japanese Society of Hypertension guidelines for the management of hypertension (JSH2014). Hypertens Res. 2014;37:253–392.
6. Daskalopoulou SS, Rabi DM, Zarnke KB, Dasgupta K, Nerenberg K, Cloutier L, et al. The 2015 Canadian Hypertension Education Program recommendations for blood pressure measurement, diagnosis, assessment of risk, prevention, and treatment of hypertension. Can J Cardiol. 2015;31:549–68.
7. Neaton JD, Grimm RH Jr, Prineas RJ, Stamler J, Grandits GA, Elmer PJ, et al. For the Treatment of Mild Hypertension Study Research Group. Treatment of Mild Hypertension Study. Final results. Treatment of Mild Hypertension Study Research Group. JAMA. 1993;270:713–24.
8. Brown MJ, Palmer CR, Castaigne A, de Leeuw PW, Mancia G, Rosenthal T, Ruilope LM. Morbidity and mortality in patients randomized to double-blind treatment with a long-acting calcium-channel blocker or diuretic in the International Nifedipine GIFT study: Interventional as a Goal in Hypertension Treatment (INSIGHT). Lancet. 2000;356:366–72.
9. Dahlöf B, Devereux RB, Kjeldsen SE, Julius S, Beevers G, de Faire U, LIFE Study Group, et al. Cardiovascular morbidity and mortality in the Losartan Intervention for Endpoint reduction in hypertension study (LIFE): a randomized trial against atenolol. Lancet. 2002;359:995–1003.
10. ALLHAT Officers and Coordinators for the ALLHAT Collaborative Research Group. The Antihypertensive and Lipid-Lowering Treatment to Prevent Heart Attack Trial. Major outcomes in high-risk hypertensive patients randomized to angiotensin-converting enzyme inhibitor or calcium channel blocker vs diuretic: the Antihypertensive and Lipid-Lowering Treatment to Prevent Heart Attack Trial (ALLHAT). JAMA. 2002;288:2981–97.
11. SHEP Cooperative Research Group. Prevention of stroke by antihypertensive drug treatment in older persons with isolated systolic hypertension: final results of the Systolic Hypertension in the Elderly Program (SHEP). JAMA. 1991;265:3255–64.
12. Staessen JA, Fagard R, Thijs L, Celis H, Arabidze GG, Birkenhäger WH, et al. Randomised double-blind comparison of placebo and active treatment for older patients with isolated systolic hypertension. The Systolic Hypertension in Europe (Syst-Eur) Trial Investigators. Lancet. 1997;350:757–64.
13. Wing LM, Reid CM, Ryan P, Beilin LJ, Brown MA, Jennings GL, Second Australian National Blood Pressure Study Group, et al. A comparison of outcomes with angiotensin-converting-enzyme inhibitors and diuretics for hypertension in the elderly. N Engl J Med. 2003;348:583–92.
14. Black HR, Elliott WJ, Grandits G, Grambsch P, Lucente T, White WB, CONVINCE Research Group, et al. Principal results of the Controlled Onset Verapamil Investigation of Cardiovascular End Points (CONVINCE) trial. JAMA. 2003;289:2073–82.
15. Julius S, Kjeldsen SE, Weber M, Brunner HR, Ekman S, Hansson L, VALUE trial group, et al. Outcome in hypertensive patients at high cardiovascular risk treated with regimens based on valsartan or amlodipine: the VALUE randomized trial. Lancet. 2004;363:2022–31.
16. Brunner HR. Experimental and clinical evidence that angiotensin II is an independent risk factor for cardiovascular disease. Am J Cardiol. 2001;87:3C–9C.
17. Williams B, Lacy PS, Thom SM, Cruickshank K, Stanton A, Collier D, CAFE Investigators; Anglo-Scandinavian Cardiac Outcomes Trial Investigators; CAFE Steering Committee and Writing Committee, et al. Differential impact of blood pressure-lowering drugs on central aortic pressure and clinical outcomes: principal results of the Conduit Artery Function Evaluation (CAFE) study. Circulation. 2006;113:1213–25.
18. Safar ME, Blacher J, Pannier B, Guerin AP, Marchais SJ, Guyonvarc'h PM, London GM. Central pulse pressure and mortality in end-stage renal disease. Hypertension. 2002;39:735–8.
19. Kingwell BA, Waddell TK, Medley TL, Cameron JD, Dart AM. Large artery stiffness predicts ischemic threshold in patients with coronary artery disease. J Am Coll Cardiol. 2002;40:773–9.
20. Kelly RP, Millasseau SC, Ritter JM, Chowienczyk PJ. Vasoactive drugs influence aortic augmentation index independently of pulse-wave velocity in health men. Hypertension. 2001;37:1429–33.
21. Hirata K, Vlachopoulos C, Adji A, O'Rourke MF. Benefits from angiotensin-converting enzyme inhibitor 'beyond blood pressure lowering': beyond blood pressure or beyond the brachial artery? J Hypertens. 2005;23:551–7.
22. Sever PS, Dahlöf B, Poulter NR, Wedel H, Beevers G, Caulfield M, et al. Rationale, design, methods and baseline demography of perticipants of the

Anglo-Scandinavian Cardiac Outcomes Trial. J Hypertens. 2001;19:1139–47.
23. Jamerson K, Weber MA, Bakris GL, Dahlöf B, Pitt B, Shi V, et al. Benazepril plus amlodipine or hydrochlorothiazide for hypertension in high-risk patients. N Engl J Med. 2008;359:2417–28.
24. Chobanian AV, Bakris GL, Black HR, Cushman WC, Green LA, Izzo JL Jr, National Heart, Lung, and Blood Institute Joint National Committee on Prevention, Detection, Evaluation, and Treatment of High Blood Pressure; National High Blood Pressure Education Program Coordinating Committee, et al. The seventh report of the Joint National Committee on prevention, detection, evaluation, and treatment of high blood pressure: the JNC 7 report. JAMA. 2003;289:2560–72.
25. Zhang X, Hintze TH. Amlodipine releases nitric oxide from canine coronary microvessels: an unexpected mechanism of action of a calcium channel-blocking agent. Circulation. 1998;97:576–80.
26. Neutel JM, Smith DH, Weber MA. Effect of antihypertensive monotherapy and combination therapy on arterial distensibility and left ventricular mass. Am J Hypertens. 2004;17:37–42.
27. Jamerson KA, Bakris GL, Wun CC, Dahlöf B, Lefkowitz M, Manfreda S, et al. Rationale and design of the avoiding cardiovascular events through combination therapy in patients living with systolic hypertension (ACCOMPLISH) trial: the first randomized controlled trial to compare the clinical outcome effects of first-line combination therapies in hypertension. Am J Hypertens. 2004;17:793–801.
28. Matsui Y, Eguchi K, O'Rourke MF, Ishikawa J, Miyashita H, Shimada K, Kario K. Differential effects between a calcium channel blocker and a diuretic when used in combination with angiotensin II receptor blocker on central aortic pressure in hypertensive patients. Hypertension. 2009;54:716–23.
29. Laurent S, Boutouyrie P, Asmar R, Gautier I, Laloux B, Guize L, et al. Aortic stiffness is an independent predictor of all-cause and cardiovascular mortality in hypertensive patients. Hypertension. 2001;37:1236–41.
30. Kario K, Tomitani N, Kanegae H, Ishii H, Uchiyama K, Yamagiwa K, et al. Comparative Effects of an Angiotensin II Receptor Blocker (ARB)/Diuretic vs. ARB/Calcium-Channel Blocker Combination on Uncontrolled Nocturnal Hypertension Evaluated by Information and Communication Technology-Based Nocturnal Home Blood Pressure Monitoring – The NOCTURNE Study. Circ J. 2017;81:948–57.
31. Chobanian AV. The hypertension paradox - more uncontrolled disease despite improved therapy. N Engl J Med. 2009;361:878–87.
32. Kearney PM, Whelton M, Reynolds K, Muntner P, Whelton PK, He J. Global burden of hypertension: analysis of worldwide data. Lancet. 2005;365:217–23.

Advantages and Disadvantages in Clinical Trials

12

William J. Kostis, Jeanne M. Dobrzynski, and John B. Kostis

Introduction and History

Describing the strengths and limitations of clinical trials in a chapter of this book is difficult because of the complexity of the issues, the large number of relevant publications and the accelerating rate of new developments in the field. For these reasons, this chapter is somewhat eclectic in including important items especially those pertaining to current developments. Making clinical decisions on individual patients after consideration of all strengths and limitations of clinical trials is difficult. As Hippocrates stated in the Aphorisms, Life is short, and art long, opportunity fleeting, experience misleading, and judgment difficult. Ὁ βίος βραχύς, ἡ δὲ τέχνη μακρή, ὁ δὲ καιρὸς ὀξύς, ἡ δὲ πεῖρα σφαλερή, ἡ δὲ κρίσις χαλεπή [1]. He also stated that a physician should consider the place, the time and the age and other diseases for which treatment is needed or not. He anticipated the difficulties we now face in applying the findings of clinical trials to individual patients. Clinical trials are essential in establishing the efficacy of pharmacologic and other interventions, but it may be difficult to make decisions on individual patients since the trials include large numbers of participants. In Hippocratic terms the "experience" derived from clinical trials may be "misleading" in the care of some patients. The principles of clinical trials and the statistical procedures used currently were initially developed in 1923 [2] by R. R. Fisher and W. A. Mackenzie studying the manurial response of different potato varieties to different types of manure. Fields of the same size were assigned to use different kinds of manure or no manure at all. They observed a significant variation in weight of potato yield measured in pounds per field. The unit of measurement was the total weight of the potatoes rather than the number and size of the potatoes [3]. Thus, the weight of potatoes per field, the primary endpoint in today's language, included very small potatoes where the manurial treatment was not beneficial, analogous to patients who suffer a serious adverse event from a treatment proven beneficial by the clinical trial. This difficulty in applying the results of clinical trials to individual patients is emphasized by the statement of a experienced clinician who stated "my patients do not walk into my office 3,000 at a time".

W. J. Kostis
Cardiovascular Institute, Rutgers Robert Wood Johnson Medical School, New Brunswick, NJ, USA

Medicine at Massachusetts General Hospital, Boston, MA, USA

J. M. Dobrzynski · J. B. Kostis (✉)
Cardiovascular Institute, Rutgers Robert Wood Johnson Medical School, New Brunswick, NJ, USA
e-mail: kostis@rwjms.rutgers.edu

V. Papademetriou et al. (eds.), *Management of Hypertension*,
https://doi.org/10.1007/978-3-319-92946-0_12

Dr. Arun Bhatt has described the evolution of clinical research from biblical times to 2010 [4]. It appears that the first recorded clinical trial is in the Book of Daniel of the old testament, in which King Nebuchadnezzar ordered his citizens to eat only meat and drink only wine because he believed that such a diet would make his people stronger. However, several persons of his retinue ate vegetables, legumes and drank water. At the end, the vegetarians appeared better nourished than the meat eaters [5]. The first controlled clinical trial was performed by James Lind in 1747, who while working on a ship, performed a comparative trial where eating two oranges and one lemon every day showed an improvement in the manifestations of scurvy compared to several types of control. The first use of placebo, "an epithet given to any medicine more to please than benefit the patient" was reported in 1963 by Austin Flint, of Austin Flint murmur fame. The first double blind, controlled clinical trial was performed in 1943 by the Medical Research Council (MRC) of the UK chaired by Sir Harold Himsworth, in over 1000 workers suffering from colds. Both the physicians and the patients were blinded as to the nature of the allocation. They proved that the active agent (patulin) was not effective in alleviating the cold. The first randomized clinical trial was performed by the MRC in evaluating streptomycin for pulmonary tuberculosis in 1946. The committee was chaired by Sir Geoffrey Marshall with statistical advice by Sir Austin Bradford Hill and Philip Hart [6, 7].

Methods of Establishing Scientific Truth

Medical inference is the derivation of conclusions from given information or premises by an acceptable form of reasoning. It is based on the fact that there are patterns in nature and that the past predicts the future. As implied by many philosophers beginning with Aristotle (e.g. Carneades, Francis Bacon, Charles Sanders Peirce, Carnap, Poper, Levi-Strauss, Derrida, John Locke, William James, Avicena, Richard Rorty, etc.), we can make inferences using deductive logic. The statistical techniques were formulated by Fermat, Pascal, Bernoulli, Galton, RA Fisher, Tukey, Bradley Efron, Pearson, Chalmers, Benjamini and others.

Carneades, a leader of the Athenian Academy in the second century B.C., should be given credit for developing the notion of probability now used widely in science. He was considered a leader in thinking about probabilities since he understood that "the true and the false may coexist, and by weighing the strength of the probability (την του πιθανού ροπήν) of each, he considered neither of them certain". He considered that statements may be: (1) probable by themselves, (2) probable and un-contradicted, or (3) probable, un-contradicted and confirmed. This is in agreement with the Aristotelian phrase "Ως επι το πολύ", most of the time, about 150 years earlier. An example of a finding that was probable and un-contradicted, but not confirmed, was the effect of estrogen replacement therapy on health outcomes in post-menopausal women. Observational studies reported that estrogen replacement therapy markedly decreased the rate of acute myocardial infarction [8]. An increase in cardiovascular disease, rather than the benefit suggested by observational studies, was proven by the randomized, double-blind, placebo-controlled Women's Health Initiative, that showed an increase in coronary heart disease and stroke [9]. This example highlights the difficulty in assigning causality and in understanding the relationship between intervention and outcome.

The following four types of relationship between two entities can be defined: (1) none (each entity is independent of the other); (2) artefactual association (spurious or false association) that could be classified into two subcategories i.e. chance (stochastic, that is unsystematic variation or noise) and bias (systematic variation i.e. variation in one direction); (3) indirect association (confounding) where the two entities are both related to another entity. Confounding gives the false impression that the two entities in question are directly related, and finally; (4) causal or direct association where one entity causes the other. An experiment (e.g. a clinical trial) is usually needed to determine the presence of direct (causal) association. The many types of bias that have been described include popularity bias, centripetal bias, referral filter bias, diagnostic access bias, diagnostic suspicion bias, unmasking (detection signal) bias, mimicry bias, previous opinion bias, wrong sample size bias, admission rate (Berkson) bias, prevalence-incidence (Neyman) bias, diagnostic vogue bias, diagnostic purity bias, procedure selection bias, missing clinical data bias, starting time bias, unacceptable disease bias, migrator bias, membership bias, nonrespondent bias, volunteer bias, contamination bias, withdrawal bias, compliance bias, therapeutic personality bias, bogus control bias, unacceptability bias, obsequiousness bias, expectation bias, substitution game, family information bias, exposure suspicion bias, recall bias, Hawthorne attention bias, instrument bias, post-hoc significance bias, data dredging bias ("looking for the pony"), scale degradation bias, tidying-up bias, repeated peeks bias, the biases of rhetoric, all's well literature bias, one-sided reference bias, positive results bias, hot stuff bias, mistaken identity bias, cognitive dissonance bias, magnitude bias, significance bias, correlation bias, under-exhaustion bias, insensitive measure bias, rumination (underlying cause) bias, and last-digit preference bias, etc.

One would expect that random variation (error) would result in a decrease of the likelihood of finding an effect. However, the assumption that measurement error always reduces the effect size is false, and is observed primarily in studies with small (less than 1000 participants) sample size. [10].

The first hypertension randomized clinical trial, the Veterans Administration Cooperative Study Group on Anti-hypertensive Agents, was published in JAMA in 1967 [11]. It included only 143 patients with a diastolic blood pressure between 115 and 129 mm Hg and proved overwhelmingly that treatment was superior to placebo. Since that time, a plethora of clinical trials on hundreds of thousands of patients has proven the benefits of pharmacologic therapy in treating hypertension. These trials answer different questions at different time periods in the evolution of pharmacologic therapy for hypertension (Fig. 12.1). After the first VA study, the first MRC trial and the first Australian Blood Pressure trial proved that control of hypertension at lower levels than the VA study was beneficial. The EWPHE trial, the second MRC trial,

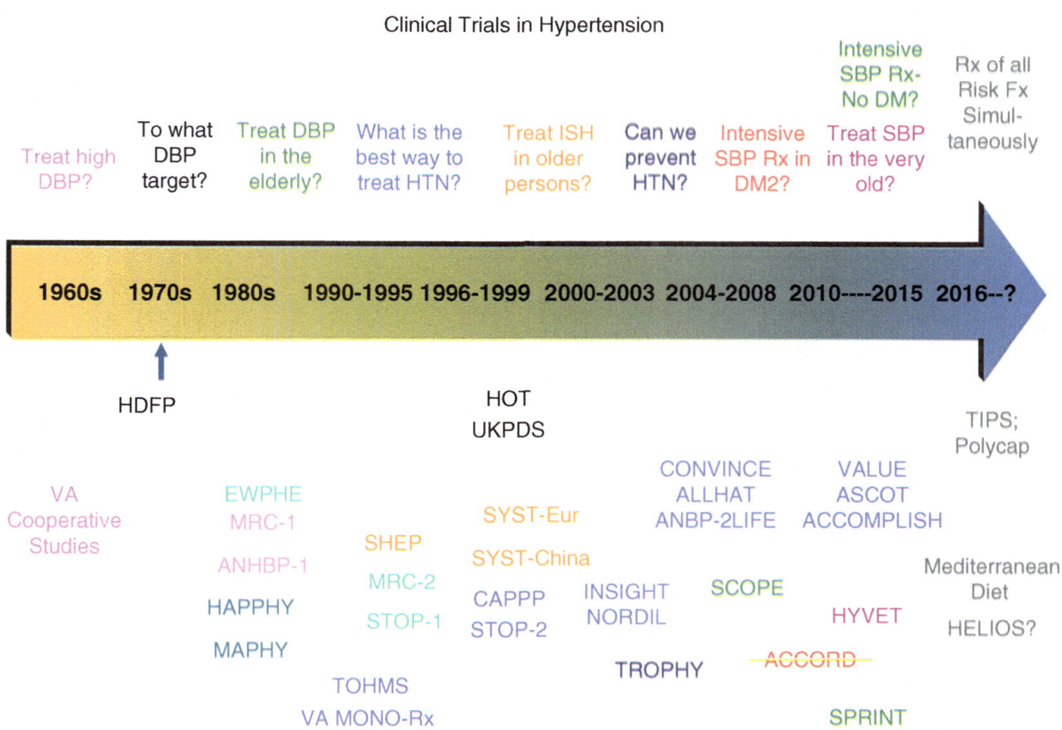

Fig. 12.1 Timeline of clinical trials in hypertension color-coded to correspond to the questions on the top of the figure. The answer is always yes with the exception of "What is the best way to treat hypertension?" where different pharmacologic approaches have been used

and the STOP Hypertension trial reported a benefit of treatment in older patients with hypertension. In the 1990s, SHEP, SYST-EUR and SYST-China demonstrated the benefit of treating isolated systolic hypertension in older adults. HYVET extended the benefit of antihypertensive therapy to the very old, while TROPHY indicated that hypertension may be prevented or postponed. Current studies are examining the benefit of multifactorial intervention in treating hypertension and other risk factors (TIPS, polypill), the benefit of lower systolic blood pressure targets [12], and the use of the Mediterranean diet (HELIOS). In addition, SPRINT, and to a lesser extent ACCORD, as well as a meta-analysis by the BPLTTC indicate that lower targets result in better outcomes [13].

The Bradford Hill Criteria

The Bradford Hill Criteria that are commonly used in accepting causal associations were proposed by Bradford Hill in 1937 [14]. The criteria included coherence with existing information, time sequence, specificity, consistency (reproducibility), strength i.e. quantitative strength (effect size), dose-response relationship (biological gradient), biological plausibility and quality of study design [15]. These criteria do not guarantee reproducibility as he has stated. “At its best such a trial shows what can be accomplished with a medicine under careful observation and certain restrictive conditions. The same results will not invariably or necessarily be observed when the medicine passes into general use.” The criteria have been modified from time to time to include consistency of the effect, association with other studies, analogy (other similar associations) and randomized controlled trials [16, 17].

Types of Studies in Clinical Medicine

Case Reports and Case Series

These are useful in bringing to the attention of the scientific community unusual or interesting clinical scenaria. Case reports are inexpensive, include detailed data, are useful for rare diseases, and may be used for comparison of different interventions. In some instances, case reports and case series open new avenues for research. For example, early papers about PCSK9 mutations resulted in the growing volume of research and publications, as well as the marketing of new pharmacologic agents [18].

Cross Sectional Studies

These studies provide information on a cross section of a population at a given time. They may be very large, and are useful especially in epidemiology. They include information on exposure and outcome, and can be conducted rapidly. However, since it is difficult to examine causal relationships and evaluate confounding, these studies are frequently used to generate rather than confirm hypotheses.

Cohort Studies

Cohort studies compare groups of individuals who are exposed or not exposed to a risk factor. They measure what percentage of those exposed and those not exposed who will develop the disease during follow-up (Fig. 12.2). Cohort studies can be used to study multiple outcomes with one exposure. They may be used for hypothesis confirmation when the hypothesis is pre-stated

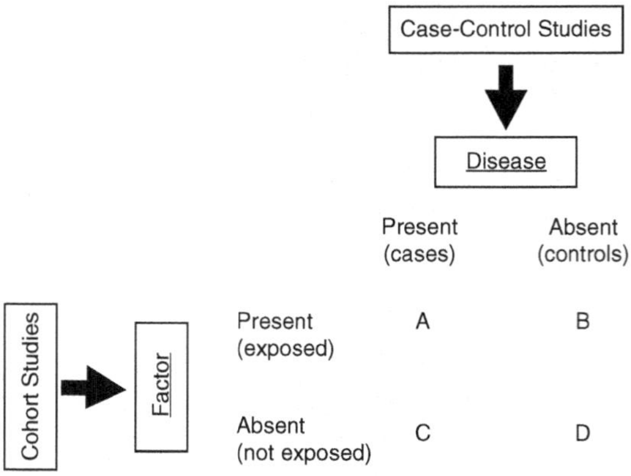

Fig. 12.2 Cohort studies and case control studies. Both types of studies examine exposed or cases (A) and unexposed controls (B, C) patients. Case control studies are uniquely suited for rare conditions (comparing A to B). In that situation cohort studies would be very large and impractical. On the other hand, cohort studies (comparing A to C) provide data on incidence of events at different points of time

or hypothesis generation when a significant finding is observed that was not in a pre-stated hypothesis. Cohort studies may be prospective or retrospective. Both report on temporal relationships, can evaluate several outcomes simultaneously, are useful in examining uncommon risk factors, and allow for nested studies. A significant advantage of retrospective cohort studies is that they can be conducted rapidly. Limitations are that they are not efficient in studying rare diseases and that prospective cohort studies may be expensive. Retrospective cohort studies have the additional problem of incomplete recall. Cohort studies provide information on the incidence of the disease in the exposed and unexposed groups. This information cannot be obtained from case control studies.

Case Control Studies

Case controlled studies are similar to cohort studies with respect to having exposed and unexposed groups and the occurrence or nonoccurrence of the disease. Unlike cohort studies, cases are matched to controls and then the occurrence of disease in cases and controls is evaluated either prospectively or retrospectively. Case control studies are uniquely suitable for rare conditions, where cohort studies require a very large number of participants. However, case studies do not provide information of the incidence of the disease in the exposed and unexposed groups (Fig. 12.2).

Randomized Clinical Trials

In discussing the significance of clinical trials we need to distinguish several types of significance: (1) stochastic significance, described by the p value (related to alpha error), the point estimate and confidence interval as well as the statistical power (related to beta error) (2) the scientific inference (Bayesian), determined by the findings of the trial in conjunction with plausibility from basic science, epidemiology, prior trials, and other information and (3) clinical (quantitative) significance.

Variables used in describing clinical trials from the quantitative point of view include the rate difference, risk ratio and odds ratio as defined by a two-way contingency table as shown in Fig. 12.3.

The risk of an event in the active group is the number of events divided by events plus non-events i.e. the probability of an event among all subjects randomized to active.

The risk of an event in the control group is the number of events in the control group divided by events plus non-events i.e. the probability of an event among all subjects randomized to control.

The risk ratio is the event rate in the active group divided by the event rate in the control group.

The risk difference (absolute risk reduction) is the event rate in the control group minus the event rate in the active group. The number needed to treat (NNT) is the number needed to treat to prevent one event and it is the reciprocal of the risk difference. The number needed to harm (NNH) is the number needed to cause one (adverse) event and it is the reciprocal of the event difference or risk difference (increase risk of adverse event).

The odds in the active group are the risk of an event divided by the number of non-events. This is equal to risk of an event in the active group divided by one minus risk of an event in the active group.

The odds in the control group are the risk of an event divided by the number of non-events. This is equal to risk of an event in the control group divided by one minus risk of an event in the control group.

The odds ratio is the ratio of the odds in the active group divided by the odds in the control group.

The relationships among these variables are not linear and they depend on the risk difference or risk ratio of an event as described above. A statistically significant quantitative clinical effect is not necessarily a clinical relevant effect. The latter depends on the clinical scenario and the individual patient.

Clinical trials are also analyzed from a Bayesian perspective. Here, each trial adds to previous knowledge suggesting that a hypothesis is true (prior probability). In this type of analysis,

Risk Difference, Risk Ratio, Odds Ratio from 2 by 2 Table

- A 2-way contingency table

	Event	Non-event	Total
Active	a	b	a+b
Control	c	d	c+d

- Risk of event in active: $p_1 = \frac{a}{a+b}$; risk of event in control: $p_2 = \frac{c}{c+d}$
- Risk ratio = $\frac{p_1}{p_2} = \frac{\frac{a}{a+b}}{\frac{c}{c+d}} = \frac{a(c+d)}{c(a+b)}$
- Risk difference = $p_1 - p_2 = \frac{a}{a+b} - \frac{c}{c+d}$
- Odds in active: $odds_1 = \frac{p_1}{1-p1}$; odds in control: $\text{odds}_2 = \frac{p_2}{1-p2}$
- Odds ratio = $\frac{odds_1}{\text{odds}_2} = \frac{\frac{p_1}{1-p_1}}{\frac{p_2}{1-p_2}} = \frac{p_1(1-p_2)}{p_2(1-p)} = \frac{a/(a+b)\times d/(c+d)}{b/(a+b)\times c/(c+d)} = \frac{ad}{bc}$

Risk Difference, Risk Ratio, and Odds Ratio April 6, 2017 2 / 6

Kostis 2017

Fig. 12.3 Data used in meta-analyses are in 2-way contingency tables (top of the figure). The definitions of risk of an event in the active and control groups, the risk ratio (also called relative risk reduction), the risk difference (also called absolute risk reduction), the odds in the active an control groups and the odds ratio are explained in the respective formulas

each new study refines the prior probability using the findings of the new trial. In this analysis, the "Bayes factor" or the likelihood ratio (LR) is the probability of the new study finding its set of data given (assuming) the null hypothesis divided by probability of finding the data given (assuming) the alternate hypothesis.

The LR is either positive LR+ = sensitivity/(1-specificity) or negative LR- = (1-sensitivity)/specificity. The posterior odds after the new trial are equal to the prior odds multiplied by the Bayes factor (LR). The simple Bayes factor is also called likelihood ratio. The "weight of evidence" is equal to the log Bayes factor (LR). The likelihood ratio is easy to use because it is additive.

Mendelian Randomization

Mendelian randomization studies combine elements of epidemiology and randomized clinical trials and are used in many fields including cardiovascular medicine. These studies address the issue of causal relationships in a way that was not predicted by Bradford Hill. Mendelian randomization studies can be classified as experiments of nature on the relationship of risk factor and a disease. They decrease the risk of confounding and reverse causality that are significant problems of observational studies but have other drawbacks as shown in Fig. 12.4. In Mendelian studies, the risk (exposure) is the presence or absence of a specific allele or group of alleles. Such studies have indicated a causal

Box 1: Strengths and limitations of study types

Although none of the following study types are infallible, all are able to provide useful information about causal inference and can complement each other to achieve increasing certainty about causality

Observational studies

- Aim to examine the association between an exposure and an outcome and to test whether the association is caused by chance, bias, or confounding
- Typically are affected by residual confounding, undetected bias, or reverse causality, which may generate associations that are not reliable indicators of causality

Randomised controlled trials

- An approach to obtain evidence of a causal effect of a treatment or intervention on a disease process
- Eliminates many of the biases and confounding factors that are present in observational studies
- Limitations include non-adherence to the assigned intervention, limited external validity, short term intervention effects, and non-retention, which can all render the results invalid or questionable
- High costs and ethical concerns can also limit the application of the trials in scientific research

Mendelian randomisation studies

- Provide a cost effective analogy to a randomised controlled trial by using genetic variants as proxies to test the causality of an association between exposure and outcome
- Is not influenced by the confounding inherent in observational studies and not seriously affected by reverse causality, but does rely on several assumptions (the genetic instruments should be associated with the exposure of interest, they should not be associated with known confounders, and they should affect the outcome solely through the exposure) that can be hard to identify and control
- May lack power when the proportion of trait variance explained by the genetic instruments is small

BMJ. 2017; 357: j2376.
PMCID: PMC5461476
Published online 2017 Jun 7. doi: 10.1136/bmj.j2376
Serum uric acid levels and multiple health outcomes: umbrella review of evidence from observational studies, randomised controlled trials, and Mendelian randomisation studies
Xue Li, PhD student,1 Xiangrui Meng, PhD student,1 Maria Timofeeva, statistical geneticist,2 Ioanna Tzoulaki, senior lecturer,3 Konstantinos K Tsilidis, assistant professor,3 ,4 P A Ioannidis, professor,5 ,6 ,7 Harry Campbell, professor, 1 and Evropi Theodoratou, chancellor's fellow1 ,2

Fig. 12.4 Box 1 describes the strengths and limitations of observational studies, randomized controlled trials and Mendelian randomization studies (from BMJ 2017;357:j2376)

relationship between specific alleles affecting cholesterol metabolism with coronary heart disease. The same was observed for Lp(a) while no definite relationship was observed for high sensitivity C-reactive protein. In the field of hypertension, a relationship using the GLUT9 gene that codes for an important urate transporter, indicates that a decrease in serum uric acid is causally related to blood pressure lowering. Mendelian randomization addresses three specific associations: (1) the association between the risk allele or gene (genetic risk) and the risk factor (clinical risk factor); (2) the association between the genetic risk and the outcome of interest (hypertension); and (3) the association between the clinical risk factor (uric acid) and the outcome (hypertension). The authors identified four non-synonymous SNPs within GLUT9 with one missense SNP (rs16890979) showing the best association. This genetic risk was strongly associated with uric acid levels ($p = 10e-11$). They also found that the uric acid levels were correlated with blood pressure. When patients were on a standardized high salt diet, the effect was more pronounced than when the patients were on a regular diet (0.44 mm reduction in serum uric acid, mean decrease in SBP was 2.2 vs. 1.5 mm hg) [19]. Limitations of the approach of Mendelian randomization include that there may be variation in the association of the clinical risk (uric acid), but not with other factors that affect the outcome since there may be many false positive associations between the genetic risk and the clinical risk factor (uric acid). Although Mendelian randomization studies may provide strong support that the clinical factor e.g. urate level is causally related to the outcome (hypertension), this type of study does not provide proof that the genetic risk should be used as a predictor in managing patients. Also, Mendelian randomization studies, including the one discussed above, may have low statistical power (Fig. 12.4). Thus, most Mendelian studies require careful study and validation in other cohorts [20].

Pragmatic Trials

The limitations of randomized controlled clinical trials that are described below in a specific section of this review, have provided the impetus to develop newer methods to obtain information including pragmatic trials [21]. Pragmatic trials aim to emulate real world situations by comparing two or more interventions [22]. Because of their nature pragmatic trials help patients, physicians and regulators in making clinical decisions. In contrast, randomized trials focusing on a specific hypothesis and carried out by trial specialists on volunteers who fulfill specific inclusion and exclusion criteria are difficult to apply to the usual patient in the community (Fig. 12.5). By using randomization and allocation concealment, randomized trials optimize internal validity at the expense of external validity. Pragmatic trials have high generalizability and external validity, can be conducted at a relatively low cost and report on practices used in the community. Weaknesses could include potential variability of the quality of the data, cross over, lack of standardization and possibly loss of follow up.

Ecologic Studies

Similar to pragmatic trials are ecologic studies. These studies provide population level data and can describe outcomes of natural experiments as mentioned above. They can be conducted very rapidly, but suffer from the potential of non-causal associations because of residual confounding (ecological fallacy). Also, the data are usually not standardized and not comparable from one study to another.

Analyses of Secular Trends

Secular trends of ecologic studies, pragmatic trials, cohort studies, and cross-sectional studies provide useful information on changing patterns

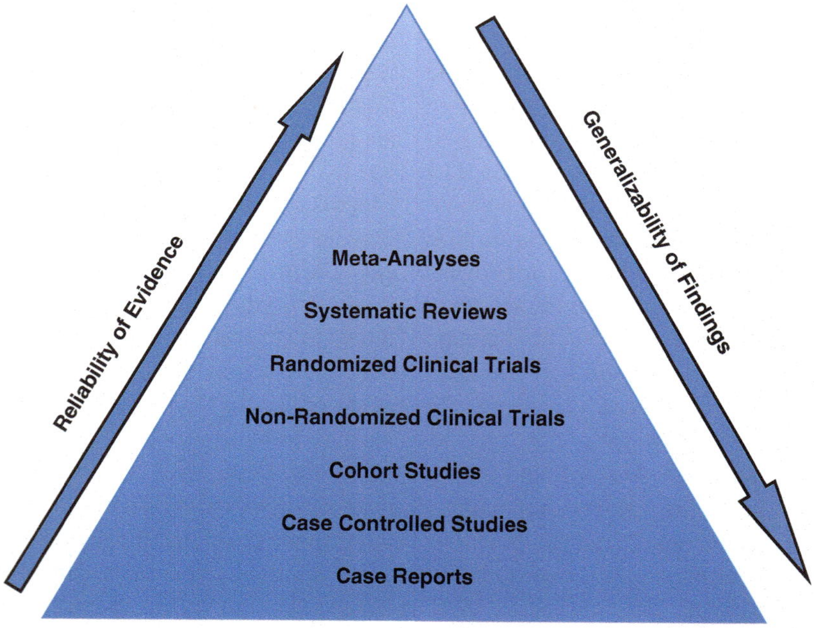

Fig. 12.5 The reliability of the evidence of the different types of studies is inversely related to the generalizability of the findings. On the top, meta-analyses provide the most reliable evidence, but their applicability to an individual patient may be limited. On the other hand, case reports and case controlled studies are specifically applicable to the individual study, but they do not provide reliable generalizable evidence

of disease as affected by environmental, political, new preventive and therapeutic modalities and other factors. It is important to consider methodology drift in performing and interpreting studies analyzing secular strengths, since with the passage of time, new diagnostic modalities and interventions are developed.

Non-inferiority Trials

In non-inferiority trials the null hypothesis is that the result of the new intervention is worse than the control (current intervention) by a non-interiority margin that is stated *a priori*. If this null hypothesis is rejected at a pre-specified level of statistical significance, a conclusion can be reached that the new intervention is non-inferior to the old one. If the upper confidence interval of the study is less than 1, the odds ratio value of no difference between the old and new trial, superiority of the new treatment can be inferred. If the upper value of the confidence interval of the new study does not exceed the pre-specified non-inferiority margin, non-inferiority is demonstrated. If non-inferiority is present but the lower confidence interval is above 1, both non-inferiority and inferiority are proven. The study is inconclusive when the confidence interval of the new study extends above the non-inferiority margin and below 1 (the no difference point). The careful selection of the control intervention using well performed randomized clinical trials is an important consideration in conducting non-inferiority trials. A problem with this could be that placebo controlled clinical trials may not have been performed. In designing non-inferiority trials, caution should be exercised in selecting large well controlled placebo controlled trials where superiority of the active intervention is evident and there is no significant change from the time the clinical trials were done and the testing time and that represent the standard of care. Attention to the selection of the endpoint and to possible changes in the metrics used are very important, as are high rates of adherence to the protocol and avoidance of cross over [23].

Digital (Internet) Trials

The nearly exponential increase in computing power and mobile connectivity has fostered the development of mobile health technologies that are transforming the form and quality of clinical research and healthcare on a global scale [24].

The face of clinical trials is undergoing a huge transformation because of these advances combined with the increased use of wearable devices such as smart phones and the nearly ubiquitous availability of WiFi wireless access points. Sixty-four percent of the worldwide population uses mobile devices, including 91% of US adults. Wearable biometric sensors including Fitbits, watches, ear phones, head bands and skin patches have been developed. These devices continuously record physiological functions without being prompted and the connectivity allows seamless transmission to "cloud" computers. The devices have computational power that would cost millions of dollars a few decades ago. The emergence of machine learning and of artificial intelligence has caused great strides as exemplified by their ability to beat worldwide champions in Chess and Go. Cloud computing may include individual data on the usual history, family history, risk factors, habits as well as genomic data that are becoming widely available. The data will be much more precise and much more inclusive than what can be obtained today even in the most advanced electronic health records. Blood pressure monitoring without the use of inflatable devices using photopletysmography and pulse wave transmission allow almost continuous monitoring of blood pressure. Single lead and 12 lead EKG monitoring simultaneous with activity level and respiratory rate can be recorded and microfluidics and microelectronics allow examination of blood, sweat, saliva, tears, urine and breath. Also, increased resolution of smartphone cameras that can evaluate our eyes for refractive errors and help in dermatologic diagnosis [25]. Michael Lauer and associates have recommended that literature search and retrieval of publications can be improved by peer review comparing the findings of other similar publications, meta-analyses and guidelines. In this proposal, the published paper will not be the final word on the matter as described above and will allow continuing post publication dialogue [26].

New medical specialists, the Medical Virtualists, are becoming important in the new healthcare and research operations. This term could be used to describe physicians who will spend the majority or all of their time caring for patients using a virtual medium. A professional consensus will be needed on a set of core competencies to be further developed over time. It is possible that there could be a need for physicians across multiple disciplines to become full-time medical virtualists with subspecialty differentiation. Medical virtualists will need specific core competencies and curricula that are being developed at some institutions. In addition to the medical training for a specific discipline, the curriculum for certification should include knowledge of legal and clinical limitations of virtual care, competencies in virtual examination using the patient or families, "virtual visit presence training," inclusion of on-site clinical measurements, as well as continuing education [27].

An essential part of clinical trials is a written informed consent that has recently become increasingly regulated and standardized [28]. The opportunity to answer important clinical questions using internet data and "big data" and the nearly exponential increase in computer power and connectivity would require novel approaches to obtaining informed consent. Big data that are voluminous, vary in content, possess veracity, change with time (velocity) and are valuable (The 5 Vs). Traditionally, the informed consent is written on a paper after fact to face discussion with the investigator and after all questions have been satisfactorily answered by the investigator. An electronic and digital informed consent can include electronic information including multimedia, videos and interactive computer interface. The consent must incorporate full disclosure, discussion, responding to questions and evaluating patient understanding by the investigator. Also, the investigator must be assured that the consent is voluntary and that it is signed. Decisions on the amount, style and complexity of the information that is provided to potential research volunteers need careful consideration. Internet based (digital) research studies involve the introduction, determination of eligibility, signing an informed consent and permission to access the information concurrently or in the future. The investigator does not have to be present during the consent process but development of user-friendly platforms is essential. This may be accomplished with the ResearchKit on the Apple iOS platform [29]. For research cases that require specialized assessment or treatments that cannot be performed through the internet, treatments can be made by research nurses who can make home visits. Medications may be delivered, and unused medications returned, by the patient through secure over night delivery with signature confirmation of receipt. The problem of clinically important heterogeneity in assigning intensive blood pressure treatment effects that may be undetectable in digital trials can be diminished using sequential randomization trial designs [30].

Meta-analyses of Clinical Trials

Meta-analyses allow pooling of results to prove more robust effects, can adjust for quality of included studies and, most important, do not require new data collection. Because of this, many meta-analyses testing different hypotheses are published. However, there is a possibility of publication bias if only meta-analyses with positive results are reported. Use of appropriate statistical models (random effects) and using more stringent values for signifcant repeated meta-analyses are important.

Meta-analyses are at the top of evidence-based medicine (Fig. 12.5). However, they have many limitations including publication bias, heterogeneity in effects, variability in the quality of the studies included, heterogeneity in inclusion criteria, exclusion criteria, duration of follow-up, end points of interest, etc. A commentary entitled Meta-Analysis, Meta-Regression, and Meta-Physics implies the similarity in the underlying methodology of the three entities [31]. In the first sentence of meta-physics, Aristotle stated that by nature humans thirst for knowledge. Reading only the first sentence would encourage persons to learn including performing meta-analyses. The second sentence, however, states that a sign (of the thirst for knowledge) is our love of the senses, especially the eye sight. This is consonant with a preference of many of us of looking at each clinical trial in itself rather than performing a meta-analysis [31]. On the other hand, well performed meta-analyses employing good quality studies and appropriate statistical techniques may be useful especially in analyzing effects of medications or other interventions among patient subsets that are under represented in existing studies. For example, since women were under-represented in trials of statins, some health care providers assumed that absence of a significant effect in women was proof of lack of an effect, a classical type 2 error. A meta-analysis proved that women and men benefited to a similar degree in primary prevention and secondary prevention [32]. Readers of meta-analyses must understand and scrutinize the following terms: confounding where a variable (confounder) is related to exposure and outcome and may account for an association or lack of an association between exposure and outcome. Confounding may be ameliorated using matching to produce similar distribution of the confounder across the two groups examined. This may be done using propensity scores. I^2 is a quantitative measure of the consistency of treatment effects across the studies that were included in the meta-analysis and of statistical heterogeneity in the effects observed from every study in the meta-analysis [33]. Most meta-analyses are performed according to the Preferred Reporting Items for Systematic Reviews and Meta-Analyses (PRISMA) statement that includes developing a protocol, formulating the research question(s), searching for the evidence, assessing the quality of studies displaying the results, evaluating publication bias, exploring heterogeneity describing the reliability of the statistical methods performing metaregression to examine the influence of the level of a baseline on the magnitude of the observed effect and reporting on the stability of the results. Random effects models are more conservative and should be employed in all meta-analyses unless there is very small heterogeneity.

There is an inverse relationship between the reliability of the conclusions and the applicability of the results in individual patients. Large clinical trials and meta-analyses provide precise effect measures but are difficult to apply to individual patients. The opposite is true of case reports and case series where the findings pertain to one or a small number of patients but the findings cannot be generalized to the patients at large (Fig. 12.5).

Strengths of Randomized Clinical Trials

Randomization, Blinding and Allocation Concealment

Randomization and allocation concealment assure accounting for known and unknown confounders and is a *sine qua non* for determining efficacy of interventions.

Effect Size

As stated above and shown in Fig. 12.3 there are important differences among the ways that the findings of randomized clinical trials are presented. Figure 12.6 shows the effect of placebo and active chlorthalidone based therapy among patients with isolated systolic hypertension. In the inset, one may observe that the relative risk reduction (approximately 50%, in red) is much higher than the absolute risk reduction (about 2%, in light blue) [34]. The effect of clinical trials in cardiovascular medicine is affected markedly by the duration of follow up. With the passage of time, all patients in a randomized clinical trial die (when the endpoint is death) or are censored or develop another non-fatal event. The differences between active and placebo depends on the time of observation and it increases with the passage of time, until approximately 17 years with SHEP, and the placebo and control groups survival curves converge until everyone is either dead or has developed the non-fatal endpoint. The idealized diagram included in Fig. 12.7, the gain in survival

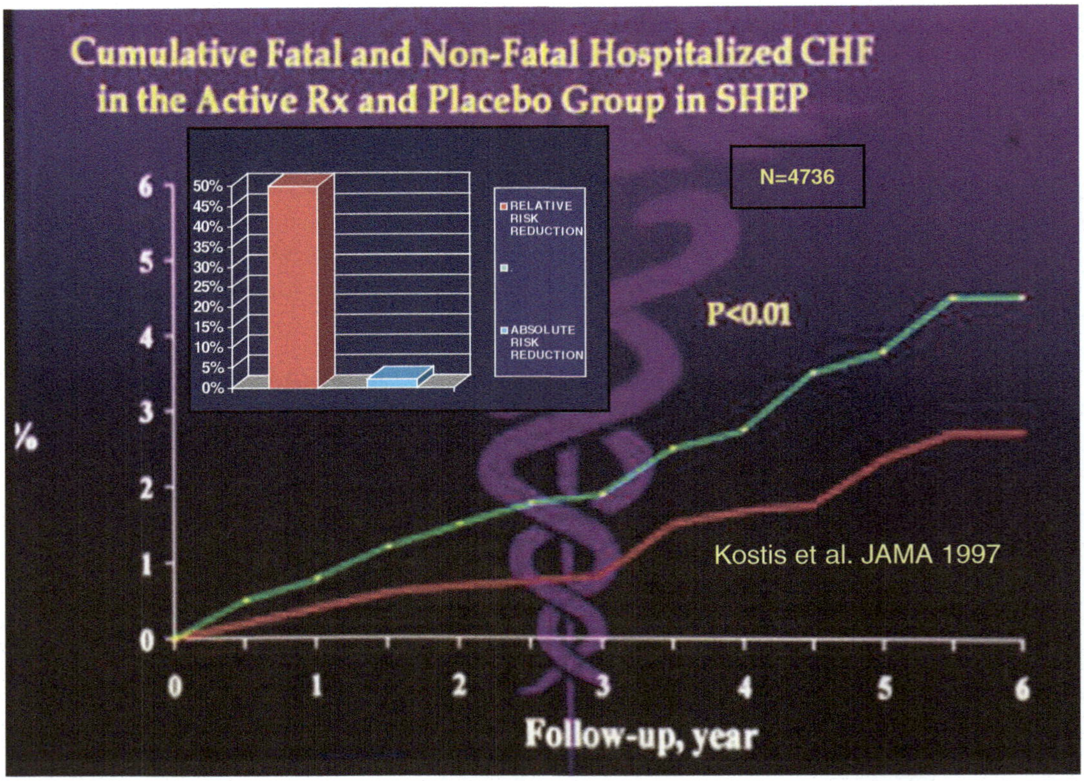

Fig. 12.6 An example of the importance of risk ratio or relative risk reduction as compared to risk difference or absolute risk reduction is shown in the figure. In SHEP the relative risk reduction of heart failure is about 50%, but this corresponds to only a 2% absolute risk reduction. Both notions must be used in examining the efficacy of clinical trials (Kostis et al. JAMA 1997;278:212–6)

associated with active treatment, is shown as the difference between the two curves at any given probability of survival. Using the 50% probability of survival, one may estimate the gain in median survival time. Using the horizontal axis, one may examine the gain in survival at any given time interval (5 years) (Fig. 12.7). The overall effect between treatment and control group, is the difference between the two survival curves. Figure 12.8 presents the difference in survival between the active and placebo groups in the SHEP clinical trial. An increase in survival free of cardiovascular death is observed in the active treatment group.

Blinding

A blind study that involved historical figures was performed in 1785 [35] by a committee convened by Louis XVI, the King of France, to report on the existence of animal magnetism. The panel included Benjamin Franklin of Philadelphia, and the equally famous chemist Lavoisier. They reported that when there was visual contact between the subject and the experimenter, the magnetism was present, while when visual contact became impossible because of intervening screen, there was no animal magnetism [35].

There are several levels of blinding including un-blinded studies, where no one in the investigative team is blinded. In a single blind study, only the patients are blinded on the treatment allocation. A more common design is a double-blind study where both the experimenters and the research subjects are blind. Blinding per-se is not useful if the allocation to active or placebo or to different treatments is not maintained. It is possible that after the patients have been

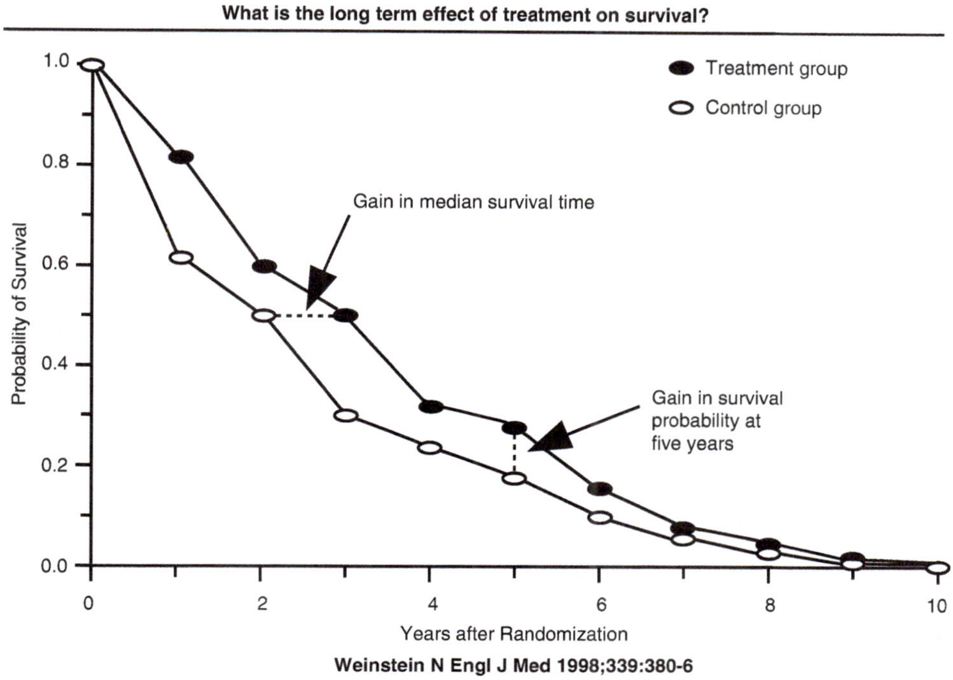

Fig. 12.7 A hypothetical description of the long-term effect of an intervention compared to control on survival. It is assumed that at the end of the follow-up (in this case 10 years) all patients in both the intervention and control groups are dead. This allows the evaluation of differences between intervention and control groups at any survival probability level e.g. median survival on the horizontal axis as well as the differences between the two conditions at any given time (5 years in this figure) (Weinstein N Engl J Med 1998;339:380-6). The area between the two curves corresponds to the net benefit of the intervention throughout the follow-up

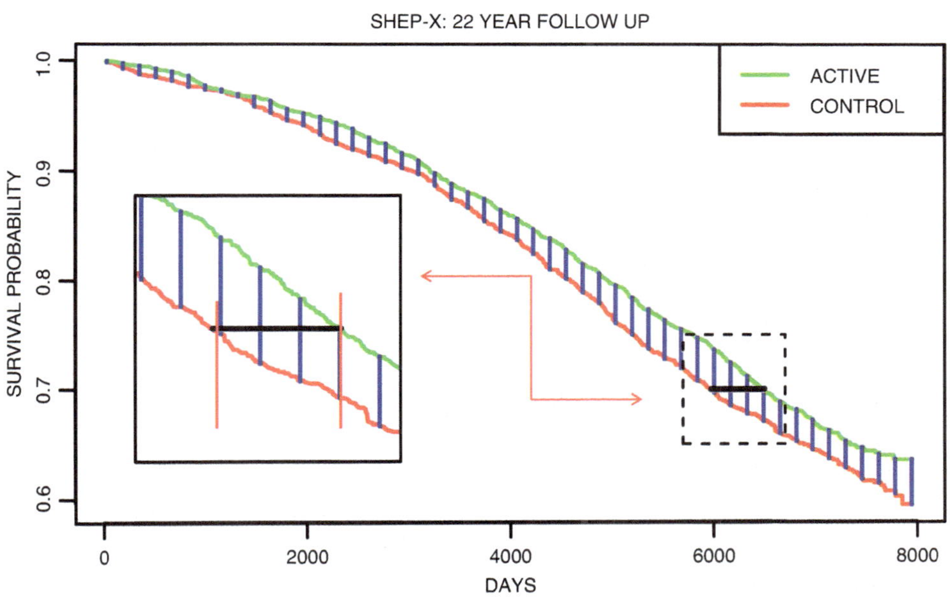

Fig. 12.8 The survival at the 22-year follow-up of SHEP was examined using the concept described in Figure 12.7. Life expectancy gain, expressed as the area between the active and placebo groups, was 158 days (95% CI, 36-287; P = .009) for cardiovascular death (Kostis et al. 2011;306:25888–93)

randomized and received the allocated therapy, the allocation assignment may be revealed to the subject and/or the investigator. This may be done unwittingly or because of obvious differences in physical or laboratory findings during the conduct of the study. For example, a common side effect (unrelated to the outcome of the study) occurring among individuals in one of the randomized groups may occur, in which case the patients or investigators may be unblinded. In other studies, the patients, the data collectors, and the investigators may be blinded. Although the function of the DSMB is to protect human subjects from harm, and members of the DSMB see summary and individual data on all patients, blinding may be maintained by naming the groups with a code (A, B, C). Unblinding is performed when the outcomes are unbalanced as determined by the Lan-DeMets stopping boundaries. In some instances, two sequential crossings of the boundaries, in the same direction, may be used to stop the study. This decreases the stochastic (chance, noise) variability. It takes careful consideration of the ethics to decide to stop or continue the study. Continuing the study when there are more serious adverse events in the active treatment group, exposes the participants to unnecessary harm. On the other hand, stopping the study prematurely may make the study uninterpretable and the effort and expense could be for naught. Studies may be stopped for three reasons: therapeutic triumph (where the active treatment is clearly worse than control), toxic catastrophe (where the active is clearly better than the intervention), and futility (when continuation of the study to it's conclusion would not yield significant differences among the randomized groups). It has been proposed, and usually accepted, that analysts be blinded as well. Since many of the decisions to stop, as well as other aspects of the analysis are to a certain degree arbitrary, caution should be exercised to protect "our obsession with eminence warps research" [36]. This tendency to assign more weight to studies with well-known researchers could be decreased by performing the initial work with blinded authors and institutions where the research was done.

Intention to Treat (ITT) Analysis

Clinical trials should be analyzed using the intention to treat (ITT) rule. This, in addition to blinding, allocation concealment, completeness of follow up and adherence to medication assures unbiased findings. ITT analysis of longitudinal studies rests on two principles i.e. all patients who are randomized to the study groups (active and control) should be included in the analysis, and this analysis would determine the size of the treatment effect. ITT analysis suffers from drop-outs, especially when the duration of follow-up is long. This could decrease statistical power, because the reason for dropping out is not known. If the reason for the drop out is the occurrence of side effects or decreased tolerability related to the primary end-point of the trial, ITT analysis could be overly optimistic. The alternative is to do as-treated or per protocol analysis, where the subjects randomized to either the control or the active groups would be compared according to whether they took the assigned randomized treatment. In large, well-controlled clinical trials such as the Women's Health Initiative, the two analyses yield similar results both directionally and with similar effect size and confidence intervals. A problem occurs when the two analyses diverge, a situation that may occur especially when the rate of drop-outs is high. When the event is not fatal, and other variables are examined, the LOCF (last observation carried forward) may be used although it suffers from the bias that the drop-outs may be different than those who continued. Methods of multiple imputations of the missing values, following drop-out, have been described and yield less biased results [37].

The Placebo and Nocebo Effects

The placebo and nocebo effects are very powerful, especially when subjective effects are evaluated. In a study we performed several years ago, patients with angina who were on placebo improved almost to the same extent as those who were treated with beta-blockers, and both of those improvements in time on the treadmill were lower than those obtained by exercise conditioning. However, the double-product (SBPxHR) that quantifies the work of the heart, was lower after beta-blockade, unchanged after conditioning, and higher with placebo. The results of this study imply that placebo allowed the patients to exercise to a higher cardiac workload before the occurrence of angina. The importance of the placebo effect was demonstrated in the ORBITA randomized trial of the effect of PCI and a placebo procedure on angina relief [38]. Symptomatic and exercise improvement from baseline was similar in the PCI and placebo groups.

The presence and magnitude of the placebo effect depend on the context including characteristics of the treatment (such as color, size and shape of the medication), characteristics of the patient (specific illness, adherence to medication and anxiety), the characteristics of the physician (e.g. gender, status, treatment and illness beliefs), on the physician-patient relationship (e.g. compassion, reassurance and suggestion of potency of the medication), and the health-care setting (e.g. home, hospital, office, room layout). The placebo effect is more pronounced when continuous and subjective, rather than objective or binary, variables are considered.

Adherence to placebo is also related to mortality. This was made clear in a report from the Coronary Drug Project where the effect of good adherence (>80%) to placebo and to active medication (clofibrate) was associated with lower all-cause death. Although there was no difference between placebo and clofibrate at 5-year adjusted mortality, patients with good adherence to placebo (or clofibrate) had 40% lower mortality than patients with low adherence [39]. This lower mortality of patients who adhere to placebo may be attributed to the higher attention to other risk factors and better attention to their health. After logistic regression analysis, where adherence and the percentage of persons lost-to-follow up, were accounted for separately, the difference attributed to the placebo effect decreased markedly but remained statistically significant [40].

Nocebo, describes a situation where unwelcome adverse effects are attributed to placebo. These effects are not explained by known pathophysiologic mechanisms, increase the burden and cost of illness and decreases adherence. In addition, the nocebo effect may lead to additional unnecessary therapy used to treat the "imaginary" adverse effects of nocebo. A current example is the rate of adverse joint, muscle and CNS effects attributed to statins. While such differences are not observed in randomized, double-blind studies, they are observed in unblinded studies. In the ASCOT trial, these adverse effects of statin therapy were observed only in the unblinded phase of the study but not in the placebo controlled blinded phase [41].

Methods of Evaluation of Clinical Trials

Items that are commonly examined in evaluating clinical trials include the type of patients included or excluded by the protocol, the pool from where the patients are recruited, and the percentage of participants who were recruited from the pool. These items evaluate the external validity of a study, i.e. to the applicability to the population of patients with the disease in question. The internal validity is determined by drop-outs, crossover, contamination and cointervention [42].

A one-to-one randomization ratio is more efficient from the statistical point of view, while higher ratios, e.g. 2-1 or 3-1, in favor of the active medication, are frequently used when long-term follow-up of patients is planned in order to evaluate adverse effects and long-term efficacy. Balance of baseline characteristics and allocation concealment are important. Contamination, crossover, compliance, co-intervention, and count, the five "Cs", are easy to remember items to use in evaluating the quality of clinical trials. Choice of a well-defined clinically relevant outcome is important in assuring the implementation of the findings of a trial. Analyses, it could be ITT (as discussed above) or per protocol, subgroup analyses, are more reliable if pre-specified, and the precision should be reported with confidence intervals rather than p-values. In addition to the statistical quantification of the effect (RRR vs ARR), the clinical importance of the effect should be described, and the findings of the trial should be put in broader perspective using Bayesian analysis and the Bradford Hill criteria.

Many issues and stakeholders affect the complexity and influence the design and conduct of multi-center clinical trials. They are (1) geography (including multiple sites, multiple investigators, multiple IRBs, differences in care, variation in ethnic background, variation in diet, and tobacco use, (2) regulatory agencies (multiple requirements, variety of approval tracks, variety of documentation) (3) payers (including health insurers, national health agencies, patients), (4) clinical operations (pertaining to protocol implementation, collection and security of data, patient selection, recruitment and retention, end point adjudication, and use of placebo), (5) personnel (investigators, monitors, statisticians, managers, DSMB, consultants, academic collaboration), (6) design (endpoints, composite endpoints, surrogate markers, and biomarkers) and (7) advocacy organizations and professional societies and medical journals [43]. Xue and associates have tabulated the strengths and limitations of observational studies, randomized controlled trials and Mendelian randomization studies (Fig. 12.4, [44]).

The Hawthorne Effect in Research

The Hawthorne effect was publicized by Henry A. Landsberger in 1958 when he analyzed earlier experiments from 1924–32 at the Hawthorne Works (a Western Electric factory outside Chicago) (Wikipedia accessed December 18, 2017). The Hawthorne Works had commissioned a study to see if their workers would become more productive in higher or lower levels of light. The productivity appeared to improve when changes were made, and slumped when the study ended. Other changes such as maintaining clean work stations, clearing floors of obstacles, and even relocating workstations resulted in increased productivity for short periods.

The Hawthorne effect describes a change in behavior where individuals modify or improve an aspect of their behavior in response to their awareness of being observed.

The Hawthorne effect may affect the behavior and behavior related outcomes in research studies where some or all research subjects know that their behavior is observed by data collection.

The "Secondary Hawthorne Effect"

The Hawthorne effect may also influence the investigators. This "secondary Hawthorne effect" was described by Nat Breslau who observed that researchers arrived at different results when analyzing the same secondary data using the same methods [45]. The Secondary Observer Effect where researchers working with secondary data such as survey data or various indicators may impact the results of their scientific research. The researchers may choose different seemingly innocuous steps in their analyses that end up causing significantly different results using the same data [46].

The Trial Effect

Similar to Hawthorne effect is the trial effect. Various medical scientists postulate that, beyond the attention and observation of trial participants, other factors such as better care, better compliance/adherence and selection bias may explain the effect. It may be due to the recruitment of patients with better adherence potential and lesser likelihood of drop out. Also, the inclusion/exclusion criteria of trials often exclude at least some patients with comorbidities; although this is often necessary to prevent confounding, it also means that trials may tend to work with healthier patient subpopulations [47, 48].

Specific Limitations of Clinical Trials

No Inclusion of all Available Information

By design, clinical trials address an important but limited aspect of a clinical problem and do not explore the entire spectrum of severity, comorbidities and co-interventions aspects of the clinical question. As a result, clinical trials apply to a limited proportion of the patients with the clinical problem under study and may lead to recommendations that are not supported by the totality of evidence on each issue. Putting the findings of the trials in better perspective needs additional information including epidemiologic facts pertaining to the same or similar problem, and integration with pathophysiology and all other available information. The Bradford Hill criteria are helpful when applied correctly with respect to the type and size of prior information that is considered.

Imbalance Between Errors of Commission Versus Errors of Omission

Application of the results of clinical trials may lead to two types of adverse consequences or errors: (a) errors of commission, e.g. the occurrence of an adverse event after prescribing a medication that was proven by the trial to be beneficial overall (e.g. rhabdomyolysis after statin treatment) and, (b) errors of omission, the occurrence of an serious adverse event that could have been avoided if a patient was not prescribed a medication proven to prevent such events (e.g. a fatal myocardial infarction in patients eligible for secondary prevention). The practice of assigning more blame to the first error (of commission) than to the second error (of omission) in other words, aiming to avoid errors of commission while increasing the probability of errors of omission is not justified. It is not supported by utilitarian ethics (biggest good for the highest number of persons).

False Positive or False Negative Clinical Trials

Single or very small number of clinical trials may lead to erroneous recommendations similar to those of diagnostic tests where false positive and false negative results are considered. False positive clinical trials may lead to the use of unnecessary or harmful interventions while false negative trials may result in not using beneficial medications. An instructive example is the Aspirin Myocardial Infarction Study (AMIS), an NIH sponsored double blind trial with good adherence that arrived at the conclusion "Based on AMIS results, aspirin is not recommended for routine use in patients who have survived an MI.", a statement that has been proven wrong by studies in over 100,000 patients [49]. Although some have raised the issue of the high dose of aspirin used in this trial, the probable explanation for the inconsistency is that AMIS was a false negative trial, in a fashion similar to a false negative stress test in an older man who smokes, has typical angina on effort, an LDL-c of 220 mg/dl an SBP of 190 mm Hg and a strong family history. Over a period of 50 years, more than 50% of the conclusions on medical publications became obsolete, and interestingly, reports of studies using good methodology did not have much longer survival than others [50].

Undue Emphasis on Statistics and p Values

The p-value is defined as the probability, under "the null hypothesis", that there is no difference between the two drugs or interventions that are tested, of obtaining a result equal to or more extreme than what was actually observed. The p-value is not the probability of accepting the null hypothesis. It is not the false positive error rate, not the probability that drug A and drug B are the same. The p-value is the probability of finding a result equal or more extreme than that observed in the study under the assumption of no difference, the null hypothesis. The p-value measures discrepancy of the data of a given study from the hypothesis and thus describes the study not the hypothesis.

Mark and associates have recently stated "P values and hypothesis testing methods are frequently misused in clinical research. Much of this misuse appears to be owing to the widespread, mistaken belief that they (p-values) provide simple, reliable, and objective triage tools for separating the true and important from the untrue or unimportant [51]. The p-value reflects the degree to which the observed data are incompatible with the null hypothesis. R. A. Fisher, the proponent of the p value, acknowledged the arbitrariness of this number stating that it is convenient to take P = .05, or 1 in 20 as a limit in judging whether a deviation is to be considered significant or not [2].

On March 7, 2016, the American Statistical Association released a statement on statistical significance and p-values [52] and enunciated with six principles underlying the proper use and interpretation of the p-value as follows.

1. P-values can indicate how incompatible the data are with a specified statistical model.
2. P-values do not measure the probability that the studied hypothesis is true, or the probability that the data were produced by random chance alone.
3. Scientific conclusions and business or policy decisions should not be based only on whether a p-value passes a specific threshold.
4. Proper inference requires full reporting and transparency.
5. A p-value, or statistical significance, does not measure the size of an effect or the importance of a result.
6. By itself, a p-value does not provide a good measure of evidence regarding a model or hypothesis.

Similarly, Nature published an article written by five influential statisticians who recommended the following [53]. (1) Consider and make adjustments for human cognition in the era of big data and newer statistical techniques. Methods that were developed in an era of rare and hard to collect information are not appropriate to handle the more diverse, more complex and much bigger data sets available now. Use of outdated statistics (e.g. p-value), misapplication of the tests and misinterpretation of results are not uncommon. The p value is one of them. (2) Abandon statistical significance altogether. Unlike prior effects that were rather large, nowadays scientists are required to make strong claims from noisy data in situations where the effects are small. The current approach of null hypothesis significance testing i.e. deciding between two inverse claims ("uncertainty laundering"), prevents investigators from using many additional ways of analyzing data. It is proposed to move beyond binary statements and accept variation under different circumstances rather than tightening the thresholds for statistical significance in multiple comparisons or using the false discoveries methods. (3) Report on the false positive risk in hypothesis testing to complement the p-value. The false positive risk is easy to calculate by online available programs (http://fpr-calc.ucl.ac.uk). (4) Share the analytic plan, the results and the entire data set and preregister all analyses. This will go a long way in reducing the reproducibility problem and allow description of the distribution of outcomes in different circumstances rather than relying on a categorical yes or no. (5) Change should be done from within, with explanations and adoption of different norms for different types of results and hypotheses.

Inclusion of Participants Who Do Not Represent the Average Patient

The findings of RCTs pertain only to the patients that participated in the respective trials or to patients very similar to those included in the randomized clinical trials. However, frequently this is not the case. At 22 years of follow up the Systolic Hypertension in the Elderly Program (SHEP) participants had much lower all-cause mortality compared to actuarial controls who fulfilled the following criteria: (1) Each one of them was born on the same day as a SHEP participant, (2) They were of the same gender and race of the SHEP participant, and (3) They were alive on the day the relevant SHEP participant was randomized (Fig. 12.9). The better outcome in RCTs is the exclusion of sicker and unreliable subjects by the protocol, the tendency of the investigating team to recruit healthier patients who fulfill the

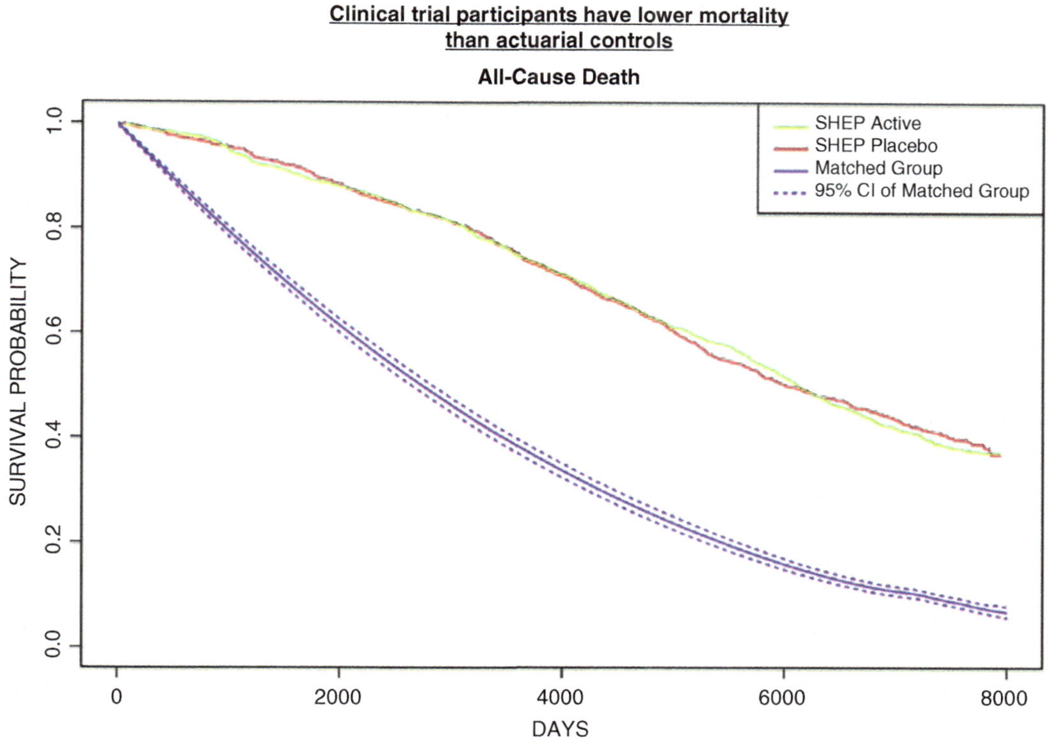

Fig. 12.9 Survival probability of patients in the active and placebo groups in SHEP compared to controls. The control group was constructed from actuarial tables where each SHEP participants was matched to an actuarial control of the same gender and race who was born on the day of the SHEP participant and was alive on the day of randomization of each SHEP participant (Kostis et al. 2011;306:25888–93)

inclusion and exclusion criteria, to self-selection of healthier, health conscious volunteers with better lifestyle, the placebo effect as described above, and discovery and management of abnormal findings (incidentalomas") that when treated do not lead to adverse outcomes [48].

Also, there may be a big difference between the efficacy observed in clinical trials and the effectiveness when a successful therapy is implemented in the community. Juurlink and associates reported that after the Randomized Aldactone Evaulation Study (RALES), demonstrating decreased all cause mortality with spironolactone, there was an abrupt increase in the rate of prescriptions for spironolactone and in hyperkalemia-associated morbidity and mortality. Also, there were significant increases in the rate of readmission for heart failure or death from all causes. Possible explanations are the use of higher doses of spironolactone, less careful monitoring of serum potassium, and treatment of patients who did not fulfill the criteria for inclusion in RALES [54].

Short Duration

The duration of clinical trials is rather short (4 or 5 years), while the life-expectancy of the persons included in the trials is usually much longer (both in truth and in patient expectations). Methods of examining the effects of different durations of follow up on the difference on survival between intervention and control at specific time intervals and determination of the time when a given percentage of participants in the two groups have died, are presented in the effect size section above (Fig. 12.7).

The Legacy Effect

Randomized clinical trials do not consider the legacy effect where treatment at an early stage results in better outcomes. An instructive example of the legacy effect is the follow up of the Anglo-Scandinavian Cardiac Outcomes Trial (ASCOT) [55]. The ASCOT trial compared two different antihypertensive treatment strategies on cardiovascular outcomes i.e. combined fatal coronary heart disease (CHD) or non-fatal myocardial infarction). The lipid lowering arm was a double-blind placebo-controlled trial of atorvastatin in participants with high total cholesterol concentrations at baseline. The lipid arm was stopped prematurely after a median 3.3 years follow-up because of substantial cardiovascular benefits in those assigned to atorvastatin. However, the patients in this arm continued to be followed to the end of the blood pressure arm. At that time, 2.2 years later, the relative risk reduction in primary events among those originally assigned to statin (10 mg atorvastatin) treatment remained unchanged although all patients received atorvastatin and LDL was similar. Carry-over benefits from those originally assigned atorvastatin, but no longer taking the drug, may account for unchanged relative risk reductions in most cardiovascular endpoints.

Our group published a meta-analysis of all randomized lipid lowering trials in which the patients were followed after discontinuation of the lipid lowering treatment. This analysis showed a legacy effect where at long term follow-up a statistically significant benefit in all-cause mortality was observed years after discontinuation of lipid therapy. The Legacy effect may be attributed to delay of progression (or regression) of atherosclerotic disease and to the prevention of non-fatal events that damage the heart to increase the risk of future mortality [56]. In the niacin arm of the Coronary Drug Project trial a decrease in non-fatal myocardial infarction by niacin during the randomized phase of the trial resulted in a decrease of all-cause mortality 11 years later. A similar legacy effect has been shown with blood pressure lowering agents [56].

Delay Between Hypothesis and Publication

A less publicized limitation of clinical trials is the long time between the design of the study (presumably after consideration of the majority of relevant information and establishing equipoise) and the publication and dissemination of the results (the shifting target problem). New knowledge from biology and epidemiology, lower than projected event rates, delays between the completion of the trial, analysis and publication, and the development of newer pharmacological interventions detract from the usefulness of the trials.

The Statistical Power of Clinical Trials

Estimating the statistical power of clinical trials is important because underpowered trials do not arrive at firm conclusions in spite of great expense and effort on the part of the organizers, the sponsors, the investigators, and the patients who volunteer their time and take clinical risks. For these reasons, designing a clinical trial without explicit estimation of statistical power for an important relevant endpoint verges on the unethical. Clinical trials that are discontinued because of futility frequently have overestimated the event rate in the control group, the size of the projected effect, or the efficiency of recruitment. Usually a fixed sample size is calculated using standard 5% level of significance and 80% power to detect a given (usually 15–25%) difference in the primary outcome between interventions. Design of event driven clinical trials with competitive recruitment mitigates this problem. Another approach is to design adaptable clinical trials where the conduct of the study is adapted based on information collected in the early phases of the trial. For example, in trials examining different doses or aspects of an intervention, randomization groups that appear unlikely to be optimal are discontinued allowing more resources, including the number of patients, to be allocated to more promising randomization branches. Sequential designs including group sequential designs, and adaptive designs evaluate accumulating information from a clinical trial and may reduce the size of a trial with savings in time, effort, risk and funding. The sample size attained at the end of the trial is unknown at the start. The sample size for a given set of alpha, beta, and effect size may turn out to be larger than with a classical fixed sample size approach [57].

A group sequential, response-adaptive design partially addresses the underpowering issue while at the same time allowing for early stopping [58].

Ethics of Clinical Trials

In the Epidemics and the oath Hippocrates states that the duty of the physician is to help or not to harm accepting the possibility that unintentional harm can occur while treating a patient and that the paramount ethical duty of the physician is to take care of patients without harming them. The ethics of clinical trials have been codified in the Nuremberg code in 1947 (international guidance on the ethics of medical research involving patients). In 1948 the Universal Declaration of Human Rights was adopted and in 1964 the World Medical Association formalized general and specific guidelines for human subjects in medical research (the Helsinki Declaration). The National Research Act of 1974, the Belmont Report of 1979, and the 1996 International Conference on Harmonization Good Clinical Practice as well as the Food and Drugs Act have helped protect human subjects participating in research.

Clinical trials have also been accused of being deceitful with false signatures and misconduct; of being disputable since they emphasize the positive with primary reports of relative risk reduction. Even when applying the CONSORT guidelines, clinical trials may be unreliable with imperfect peer review and conflicts. They are not always helpful because they only provide a binary answer to complex clinical problems and do not include all information as suggested by Bradford Hill. They do not address appreciation of the subjectivity of interpretation of their statements by the reader. They may be shameful since they may include results from poor countries where investigators have financial gain to fabricate data and may exploit vulnerable persons who seek participation in a trial for monetary reasons [59]. Although this paper on limitations of clinical trials was published more than 15 years ago, most of these issues seem to persist today. Misinformation should be nipped in the bud since frequently fact checking is often too little and too late [60]. An important problem in studying the effects of new medications or interventions is the use of placebo. Lewis and associates, quoting a strict interpretation of the 2000 Declaration of Helsinki, have proposed a limited use of placebo in clinical trials preferring the use of active controls. Since the efficacy of new medications can be satisfactorily established by comparison to active controls, the judicious use of placebo may be justifiable if it is essential to establish their effectiveness [61].

Summary, Conclusion and Future Prospects

Clinical trials in their great variety are necessary for progress of clinical medicine. Because of the complexity of the issues involved and the great demand for time, effort and expense and because they may expose participants to discomfort and risk clinical trials, they should be conducted and executed with great care. They should be thoughtfully designed and executed in a disciplined fashion with attention to detail, adherence to the protocol, encouragement to participants to adhere to visits, medication and other aspects of the protocol, and in agreement to good clinical practice rules, as well as federal and local regulations. Accurate interpretation of the results requires understanding of their limitations, including the transience of their findings. Their application to individual patients should be done after consideration of the totality of the clinical situation including demographics, comorbidities and co-interventions. Also, there is need to shift emphasis of the trials from primary and secondary prevention with lifestyle change, devices and medications to primordial prevention i.e. preventing the atherosclerotic disease at the earliest stage rather than focusing on complications of atherosclerotic disease such as myocardial infarction, stroke and heart failure. We have come a long way from Providence Based Medicine (based on religious beliefs), to Eminence Based Medicine (based on the opinions and practices of eminent physicians an academicians), to Evidence Based Medicine (based on the finding of randomized trials as well as observational and epidemiologic data), to Evidence Biased Medicine (where trials are designed and question addressed are influenced by profit considerations), to Evidence Bayesed. Medicine (both frequentist and Bayesian statistics are used in conjunction with the Bradford Hill criteria to make decisions). We also need to understand, accept and embrace the rapidly evolving computer power, wearable devices and wireless connectivity and to evolve toward Internet and Cloud-based medicine.

Repeated experiments, as Fisher recognized years ago, may be the best way to tame much of the messiness of nature. If that is not feasible, and it often is not, medicine can still accomplish much by making pragmatic, well-reasoned use of the evidence that is available [51].

References

1. Hippocrates. In: Adams CD, editor. The genuine works of Hippocrates. New York: Dover; 1868.
2. Fisher RA, Mackenzie WA. Studies in crop variation. II. The manorial response of different potato varieties. J Agric Sci. 1923;13:311–20.
3. Fisher RA. On the "probable error" of a coefficient of correlation deduced from a small sample. Metro. 1921;1:3–32.
4. Bhatt A. Evolution of clinical research: a history before and beyond James Lind. PICR. 2010;1(1):6–10.
5. Collier R. Legumes, lemons and streptomycin: a short history of the clinical trial. CMAJ. 2009;180:23–4.
6. MRC Streptomycin in Tuberculosis Trials Committee. Streptomycin treatment of pulmonary tuberculosis. BMJ. 1948;2:769–83.
7. Hart PD. A change in scientific approach: from alternation to randomised allocation in clinical trials in the 1940s. BMJ. 1999;319(7209):572–3.
8. Stampfer MJ, Colditz GA, Willett WC, et al. Postmenopausal estrogen and cardiovascular disease. Ten-year follow-up from the nurses' health study. N Engl J Med. 1991;325(11):756–62.
9. Writing Group for the Women's Health Initiative Investigators. Risks and benefits of estrogen plus progestin in healthy post-menopausal women. Principal results from the Women's Health Initiative Randomized Controlled Trial. JAMA. 2002;288(3):321–33.
10. Loken E, Gelman A. Measurement error and the replication crisis. Science. 2017;355(6325):584–5.
11. Veterans Administration Cooperative Study Group on Anti-hypertensive Agents. Effects of treatment on morbidity and mortality in hypertension: I. Results in patients with diastolic blood pressure averaging 115–129 mm Hg. JAMA. 1967;202:116–22.
12. Whelton PK, Carey RM, Aronow WS, et al. ACC/AHA/AAPA/ACPM/AphA/ASH/NMA/PCNA Guideline for the prevention, detection, evaluation, and management of high blood pressure in adults: A report of the American College of Cardiology/American Heart Association Task Force on Clinical Practice Guidelines. Hypertension. 2018;71(6):e13–e115.
13. Blood Pressure Lowering Treatment Trialists' Collaboration, Turnbull F, Neal B, Pfeffer M, et al. Blood pressure-dependent and independent effects of agents that inhibit the renin-angiotensin system. J Hypertens. 2007;25(5):951–8. Erratum in: J Hypertens. 2007;25(7):1524.
14. Hill AB. Principles of medical statistics. Lancet. 1937;229:706–8.
15. Hill AB. The environment and disease: association or causation? Proc R Soc Med. 1965;58(5):295–300.
16. Bothwell LE, Podolsky SH. The emergence of the randomized, controlled trial. N Engl J Med. 2016;375:501–4.
17. Grimes DA, Schulz KF. Bias and causal associations in observational research. Lancet. 2002;359(9302):248–52.
18. Abifadel M, Varret M, Rabès JP, et al. Mutations in PCSK9 cause autosomal dominant hypercholesterolemia. Nat Genet. 2003;34(2):154–6.
19. Parsa A, Brown E, Weir MR, et al. Genotype-based changes in serum uric acid affect blood pressure. Kidney Int. 2012;81:502–7.
20. Thanassoulis G, Campbell CY, Owens DS, et al. Genetic associations with valvular calcification and aortic stenosis. N Engl J Med. 2013;368:503–12.
21. Frieden TR. Evidence for health decision-making – beyond randomized, controlled trials. N Engl J Med. 2017;377:465–75.
22. Treweek S, Zwarenstein M. Making trials matter: pragmatic and explanatory trials and the problem of applicability. Trials. 2009;10:37. https://doi.org/10.1186/1745-6215-10-37.
23. Mauri L, D'Agostino RB Sr. Challenges in the design and interpretation of noninferiority trials. N Engl J Med. 2017;377:1357–67.
24. Steinhubl SR, McGovern P, Dylan J, Topol EJ. The digitised clinical trial. Lancet. 2017;390(10108):2135.

https://doi.org/10.1016/S0140-6736(17)32741-1. Epub 2017 Nov 9.
25. Steinhubl SR, Muse ED, Topol EJ. The emerging field of mobile health. Sci Transl Med. 2015;7(283):283rv3. https://doi.org/10.1126/scitranslmed.aaa3487.
26. Lauer MS, Krumholz HM, Topol EJ. Time for a prepublication culture in clinical research? Lancet. 2015;386(10012):2447–9.
27. Nochomovitz M, Sharma R. Is it time for a new medical specialty?: The medical virtualist. JAMA. 2018;319(5):437–8.
28. Grady C. Enduring and emerging challenges of informed consent. N Engl J Med. 2015;372:855–62.
29. Grady C, Cummings SR, Rowbotham MC, McConnell MV, Ashley EA, Kang G. Informed consent. N Engl J Med. 2017;376:856–67.
30. Basu S, Sussman JB, Hayward RA. Detecting heterogeneous treatment effects to guide personalized blood pressure treatment: a modeling study of randomized clinical trials. Ann Intern Med. 2017;166(16695):354–60.
31. Kostis JB. Meta-analysis, meta-regression, and meta-physics. JCH. 2003;1:64–5.
32. Kostis WJ, Cheng JQ, Dobrzynski JM, Cabrera J, Kostis JB. Meta-analysis of statin effects in women versus men. JACC. 2012;59:572–82.
33. Cornell JE, Liao JM, Stack CB, Mulrow CD. Annals understanding clinical research: evaluating the meaning of a summary estimate in a meta-analysis. Ann Intern Med. 2017;167(4):275–7.
34. Kostis JB, Davis BR, Cutler J, for the SHEP Cooperative Research Group, et al. Prevention of heart failure by antihypertensive drug treatment in older persons with isolated systolic hypertension. JAMA. 1997;278:212–6.
35. Franklin B, Bailly JS, Lavoisier A. Chez Gabliel Floteron, Nice. Papport des commissaires decharges par le Roi a l'examen du magnetisme animal 1785.
36. Vazire S. Our obsession with eminence warps research. Nature. 2017;547(7661):7.
37. Little R, Yau L. Intent-to-treat analysis for longitudinal studies with drop-outs. Biometrics. 1996;52(4):1324–33.
38. Al-Lemee R, Thompson DHM, et al. Percutaneous coronary intervention in stable angina (ORBITA): a double-blind, randomized controlled trial. Lancet. 2018;391:31–40.
39. Coronary Drug Project Research Group. Influence of adherence to treatment and response of cholesterol on mortality in the coronary drug project. N Engl J Med. 1980;303(18):1038–41.
40. Murray EJ, Herman MA. Adherence adjustment in the Coronary Drug Project: a call for better per-protocol effect estimates in randomized trials. Clin Trials. 2016;13:372–8.
41. Gupta A, Thompson D, Whitehouse A, Collier T, ASCOT Investigators, et al. Adverse events associated with unblended, but not with blinded, statin therapy in the Anglo-Scandinavian Cardiac Outcomes Trial-Lipid-Lowering Arm (ASCOT-LLA): a randomized double-blind placebo-controlled trial and its non-randomised non-blind extension phase. Lancet. 2017;389(10088):2473–81.
42. Attia J, Page J. A graphic framework for teaching critical appraisal of randomized controlled trials. ACP J Club. 2001;134(4):A11–2.
43. Rosenblatt M. The large pharmaceutical company perspective. N Engl J Med. 2017;376(1):52–60.
44. Xue L, Meng X, Timofeeva M, et al. Serum uric acid levels and multiple health outcomes: umbrella review of evidence from observational studies, randomised controlled trials, and Mendelian randomisation studies. BMJ. 2017;357:j2376.
45. Breznau N. Secondary observer effects: idiosyncratic errors in small-N secondary data analysis. Int J Soc Res Methodol. 2016;19:301–18.
46. Hawthorne Effect. Wikipedia accessed January 15, 2017.
47. Braunholtz DA, Edwards SJ, Lilford RJ. Are randomized clinical trials good for us (in the short term)? Evidence for a "trial effect". J Clin Epidemiol. 2001;54(3):217–24.
48. Kostis WJ, Cabrera J, Messerli FH, Cheng JQ, Sedjro JE, Cosgrove NM, et al. Competing cardiovascular and noncardiovascular risks and longevity in the Systolic Hypertension in the Elderly Program. Am J Cardiol. 2014;113(4):676–81.
49. Aspirin Myocardial Infarction Study Research Group. A randomized, controlled trial of aspirin in persons recovered from myocardial infarction. JAMA. 1980;243:661–9.
50. Poynard T, Munteanu M, Ratziu V. Truth survival in clinical research: an evidence-based requiem? Ann Intern Med. 2002;136:888–95.
51. Mark DB, Lee KL, Harrell FE Jr. Understand the role of p values and hypothesis tests in clinical research. JAMA Cardiol. 2016;1(9):1048–54.
52. Wasserstein RL, Lazar NA. The ASA's statement on p-values: context, process, and purpose. Am Stat. 2016;70:129–33.
53. Lee J, McShane BB, Gelman A, Colquhoun D, Nuijten MB, Goodman SN. Five ways to fix statistics. Nature. 2017;551:557–9.
54. Juurlink DN, Mamdani MM, Lee DS, et al. Rates of hyperkalemia after publication of the randomized aldactone evaluation study. N Engl J Med. 2004;351(6):543–51.
55. Sever PS, Poulter NR, Dahlof B, ASCOT Investigators, et al. The Anglo-Scandinavian Cardiac Outcomes Trial lipid lowering arm: extended observations 2 years after trial closure. Eur. Heart. 2008;29(4):499–508.
56. Kostis WJ, Thijs L, Richart T, Kostis JB, Staessen JA. Persistence of mortality reduction after the end of randomized therapy in clinical trials of blood pressure lowering medications. Hypertension. 2010;56:1060–8.
57. van der Lee JH, Wesseling J, Tanck MW, Offringa M. Efficient ways exist to obtain the optimal sample size in clinical trials in rare diseases. J Clin Epidemiol. 2008;61(4):324–30.

58. Karrison TG, Huo D, Chappell R. A group sequential, response-adaptive design for randomized clinical trials. Control Clin Trials. 2003;24(5):506–22.
59. Horton R. The clinical trial: deceitful, disputable, unbelievable, unhelpful, and shameful-what next? Control Clin Trials. 2001;22:593–604.
60. Weiss R. Nip misinformation in the bud. Science. 2017;358(6362):427.
61. Lewis JA, Jonsson B, Kreutz G, Sampaio C, van Zwieten-Boot B. Placebo-controlled trials and the declaration of Helsinki. Lancet. 2002;359(9314):1337–40.

Arterial Hypertension: What Is the Optimal Goal of Treatment?

13

Emmanuel A. Andreadis
and Charalampia V. Geladari

A Historical Perspective

It was in 1896 when the Italian Internist Scipione Riva-Rocci first introduced the mercury sphygmomanometer for the measurement of blood pressure (BP) [1]. Since then, and for decades, arterial hypertension (HTN) was considered to be essential for the perfusion of vital organs, such as the brain, heart, and the kidneys. The term essential hypertension ("essentiellehypertonie") was coined by the German Eberhard Frank in 1911 to describe elevated BP for which no cause could be found [2, 3]. At that time, BP was meant to be the essence of life, and it was indeed widely believed that there could be no life without BP [4].Interestingly, Paul Dudley White, a top American physician and cardiologist in Harvard Medical School and one of the founders of the American Heart Association, the American Red Cross, and the National Institute of Health, and who served as the President's Dwight D. Eisenhower personal physician following his heart attack in 1955, stated that: "*Hypertension may be an important compensatory mechanism, which should not be tampered with, even were it certain we could control it.*" [5]. It is widely known that a prominent individual with essential HTN was Franklin D. Roosevelt, the 32nd President of the USA, from 1933 till his death in 1945. It is certain that the understanding of the medical community regarding HTN during the Great Depression and World War II was still in a "medieval" state and this greatly contributed to the deterioration of Roosevelt's health, whose BP rose steadily during his presidency [6]. According to existing historical data, it was on the afternoon of April 12, 1945, when Roosevelt, while sitting for a portrait being painted by the artist Elizabeth Shoumatoff, complained of a terrible headache (Fig. 13.1). Fifteen minutes later, the president was dead of a massive cerebral hemorrhage [7–9]. His successor, the President Harry S. Truman, signed into lawthe pivotal National Heart Act, 3 years following his death [10]. This served as the trigger for the study of HTN and associated heart diseases, and led to the significant results of the VA Co-operative Studies and the Framingham Heart Study. Until then, research grants were rewarded almost exclusively to those who sought the causes of hypertension. The question on whether hypertension should be treated by antihypertensive drugs was hotly

E. A. Andreadis (✉)
Hypertension and Cardiovascular Disease Prevention Center, Evangelismos General Hospital, Athens, Greece

Fourth Internal Medicine Department, Evangelismos State General Hospital, Athens, Greece

C. V. Geladari
Fourth Internal Medicine Department, Evangelismos State General Hospital, Athens, Greece

Department of Medicine, Division of Cardiology, Beth Israel Deaconess Medical Center, Harvard Medical School, Boston, MA, USA

V. Papademetriou et al. (eds.), *Management of Hypertension*,
https://doi.org/10.1007/978-3-319-92946-0_13

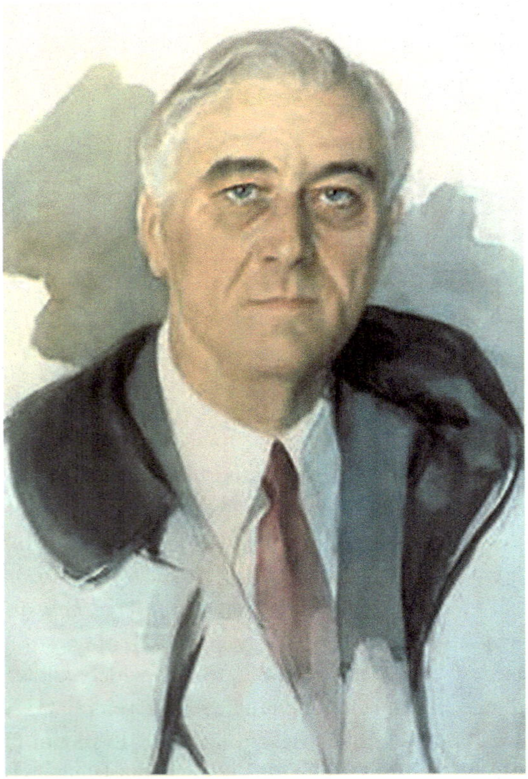

Fig. 13.1 Used with permission from the Georgia Department of Natural Resources Roosevelt's Little White House State Historic Site

debated during the 1950s and the 1960s. Edward D. Freis, an American farsighted physician, was the first to answer this question by carrying out the famous VA-Co-operative studies. As he stated: "*The VA Co-Operative study will be remembered for changing the management of hypertension. It altered the emphasis from secondary forms of hypertension, which while still important, applied only to a small percentage of the hypertension population. It convinced physicians that the numerically much more prevalent essential or primary hypertension could be benefited by antihypertensive drug treatment. Our study demonstrated that by controlling the blood pressure, we could prevent most of the complications of the disorder, and equally important, its progression to a more severe state could be arrested.*" [11] In addition, scientists from the Framingham Heart Study proved that HTN and hyperlipidemia, were associated with many cardiovascular morbidities such as cerebral stroke, heart failure, and myocardial infarctions leading to premature deaths and the risk was clearly higher with higher BP (systolic and diastolic) [12, 13]. Nowadays, that HTN has been showed clearly to be a significant risk factor for cardiovascular morbidity and mortality, this question has shifted to whether the optimal BP goal should be lowered to levels below 140/90 mmHg for systolic and diastolic BP, respectively, and will be the main focus of this chapter.

Epidemiologic Data

Arterial hypertension (HTN) remains a growing-threat in modern societies despite the implementation of new clinical guidelines and the broad availability of effective pharmaceutical agents [14]. According to the World Health Organization (WHO), the prevalence of HTN in the United States of America, in 2015 was estimated to be about 15.3% and 10.5% among males and females, respectively [15]. Pooled worldwide data analyses have reported that the prevalence of HTN was 26.4% in the beginning of the twenty-first century, and it is expected to rise by 60% by the year 2025 [16, 17]. Arterial HTN is associated with all forms of stroke, cardiac, kidney and peripheral artery disease [18–21], and it is considered to kill 9.4 million people every year [22]. More recently, Forouzanfar et al., reported in the JAMA that both the rate of raised systolic blood pressure (BP) ($\geq$110–115 and $\geq$140 mmHg), and disability-adjusted life-years (DALYs) and deaths associated with elevated systolic BP, increased substantially between 1990 and 2015 [23]. Therefore, setting optimal BP goals is central to prevent fatal complications among hypertensive subjects. However, the optimal BP target that is protective against cardio-cerebrovascular disease risk remains controversial and the ongoing scientific debate is of substantial public health importance.

In this chapter, we will examine which is the ideal BP goal for the general hypertensive population, by focusingprimarily on available milestone studies and on updated evidence-based clinical HTN guidelines. More specifically, we will review the MRC trial published before 1995, the HDFP, and the HOT, the SPRINT, the ACCORD and the HOPE-3 studies, published after this year. We will also focus on interesting meta-analyses stratifying the different trials according to the BP levels achieved by active treatment. It is under no question that different BP goals should be achieved for special population groups (ie. the elderly, diabetics, patients with chronic kidney disease, etc). However, we will not discuss BP goals for these hypertensive populations in depth, since those are described thoroughly in other chapters of this book.

Landmark Trials in Hypertension Research – The Optimal Goal of Blood Pressure

It has been shown that antihypertensive therapy is helpful in protecting against cardiovascular disease (CVD) progression and death, as demonstrated by several studies conducted before 1995 and including a considerable number of patients. In all these trials, the primary drugs used were either beta-blockers, or diuretics, in low or higher doses. Subsequently, the 1995 trials determined the effects of the newer antihypertensive drugs such as angiotensin-converting enzyme inhibitors (ACEIs), angiotensin receptor blockers (ABRs) and calcium channel blockers (CCBs), in the prevention of CVD [24]. Meanwhile, a series of trials were designed to assess the reduction of cardiovascular (CV) events according to different BP levels as optimal targets. It should be noted that in these trials, the entry BP criterion was the diastolic BP, and not the systolic BP as it is observed in more recent trials, because diastolic BP was considered as the major determinant of risk [25].

The first randomized controlled trial (RCT) to provide evidence of benefits in treating mild HTN in younger cohort was theMedical Research Council (MRC) trial conducted by the Medical Research Council Working Party in 1985. The study included a population of 17,354 men and women, aged 35–64 years, followed up for an average of 4.9 years. Mean patient BP level systolic/diastolic was 158/98 mmHg at entry. The primary objective of the study was to examine the effect of the drug treatment of mild HTN on the rates of stroke, of death due to HTN, and of coronary events in the studied population, whereas, the secondary objectives of the trial were to compare the effectiveness and adverse effects of the two antihypertensive drugs used, bendrofluzide and propranolol. The mean attained BP was approximately 137/86 mmHg in the two treated groups and 150/92 mmHg in the placebo group. The treatment was found to be effective in preventing complications in patients with mild HTN. Baseline patient data at entry showed that the level of systolic blood pressure(SBP) was significantly associated with the risk of stroke, coronary events, all cardiovascular events, and all cause mortality whereas it was not significantly related to the percentage benefit associated with active treatment. The level of diastolic pressure at entry was less clearly associated with the risk of subsequent events [26]. In general, patients in the MRC trial had a significant reduction only for the primary endpoint of stroke and all CV events but not for coronary events and mortality from all causes suggesting a goal BPof less than 140 mmHg systolic and/or less than 90 mmHg diastolic [27]. Interestingly, both bendrofluzide and propranolol were associated with reduced rates of stroke as well as with reduced rates of all CV events. In contrast, for coronary events and for all cause mortality there were no statistically significant differences between the effects associated with the two drugs (p = 0,24 for bendrofluzide and 0,71 for propranolol, respectively) [26] (Table 13.1).

The Hypertension Detection and Follow-up Program (HDFP) study published in 1979,was the first study to demonstrate a mortality benefit of goal-directed, stepped care BP treatment compared to usual care. This study established the practice of stepped care approach to achieve BP goal which became the norm of HTN treatment strategy ever since. High or lower doses of diuretics, and b-blockers, were used as primary drugs. A total of 10,940 subjects were recruited by population-based screening of 158,906 people aged 30–69 years in 14 communities throughout the United States and were randomly assigned to stepped-care or referred-care groups within each center and by entry diastolic blood pressure (DBP) above 90 mmHg (90 to 104, 105 to 114, and 115+ mmHg). The studied population was followed-up for a mean period of 5 years. Half of the patients were more intensively treated (equivalent to 50 mg or more of

Table 13.1 Brief description of the MRC trial

Year of publication	1985
Journal	British medical journal
No of patients recruited	17,354
Sex studied	Both sexes, men and women
Mean patient age	35–64 years
Start of patient recruitment	1973
End of patient recruitment	1982
Study design	Single-blinded RCT
Main objective	To determine any treatment benefit of mild HTN in a younger cohort
Secondary objective	1. To compare the course of BP in the two treatment groups 2. To examine the adverse effects caused by these drugs
Drugs used in the study	1. Bendrofluazide, 10 mg daily (or matching placebo) 2. Propranolol,could be titrated up to 240 mg daily (or matching placebo)
Eligibility criterion for entry in the study	Mean DBP 90-109 mmHg *and* SBP <200 mmHg
Exclusion criteria	1. Secondary HTN 2. Taking antihypertensive treatment 3. Normally accepted indications for antihypertensive treatment (such as CHF) present 4. MI or stroke within the previous 3 months 5. Presence of angina, intermittent claudication, diabetes, gout, bronchial asthma, serious intercurrentdisease 6. Pregnancy
Definition of entry pressure	Screening pressure was defined as the mean of four readings taken on two separate occasions and confirmed by the mean of two later readings still in this range
Target BP	DBP <90 mmHg (for those randomized to active treatment)
Primary endpoint	1. Fatal or non-fatal stroke 2. Coronary events, including both fatal and non-fatal MI 3. Sudden death thought to be a result ofCAD 4. Death due to hypertensivecardiac or renal disease or to rupture or dissection of aortic aneurysm 5. Death from any other cause
Mean BP in the treated groups	**137/86 mmHg**
Mean BP in the placebo group	150/92 mmHg
Main result	Drug treatment was effective in preventing complications in patients with mild HTN; Total no of CV events in the active treatment group: 286 Total no of CV events in the placebo group: 352 ($p < 0.05$)

MRC indicates medical research council, *No* number, *RCT* randomized controlled trial, *HTN* hypertension, *BP* blood pressure, *DBP* diastolic blood pressure, *SBP* systolic blood pressure, *CHF* congestive heart failure, *MI* myocardial infarction, *CAD* coronary artery disease and *CV* cardiovascular

hydrochlorothiazide-stepped care) while the other half received less intensive treatment (equivalent to 12.5–25.0 mg hydrochlorothiazide-referred care). The separation of the data by doses revealed a beneficial effect both on patients treated with diuretic in low doses and those receiving b-blockers. No protection was observed against coronary heart disease by high doses of diuretics. On the other hand, all therapies had a significant impact on stroke. The average attained diastolic BP was 85 and 90 mmHg in the stepped care; systolic BPswere not given. Researchers concluded that the systematic effective management of HTN has a great potential for reducing mortality for the large numbers of people with high BP in the population, including those with "mild" HTN [28].Both the MRC and the HDFP trials supported that the optimalBP goal the general hypertensive population should be <140/90 mmHg for systolic and diastolic BP, respectively. Importantly, these trials did not include patients at increased risk for CV disease occurrence, such as patients with atherosclerotic CV disease and/or dia-

Table 13.2 Brief description of the HDFP trial

Year of publication	1979
Journal	Journal of the American Medical Association
No of patients recruited	10,940
Sex studied	Both sexes, men and women
Race	White and blacks
Mean patient age	30–69 years
Start of patient recruitment	February, 1973
End of patient recruitment	May, 1974
End of therapeutic intervention	June, 1979
Main objective	To determine whether a systematic and effective management of HTN could yield a mortality benefit for all patients with high BP
Intervention used	Stepped-care (patients received antihypertensive drug therapyaccording to a predetermined protocol in hospital-based clinics) versus usual-care (referred back to their usual medical practitionerto receive whatever therapy he or she might deem appropriate)
Drugs used in the study	1. Chlorthalidone 2. Reserpine 3. Potassium-sparing diuretics 4. Methyldopa 5. Hydralazine 6. Guanethidine
Eligibility criterion for entry in the study	DBP >90 mmHg
Entry BP	Stepped-care group: 159/101 mmHg Referred-care group: 159/101 mmHg
Primary endpoint	To determine the mortality rate in the two-groups (stepped-care versus usual-care)
Mean BP in the stepped-care groups	DBP: **85–90 mmHg**
Main result	Five-year mortality from all causes was 17% lower for the stepped-care group compared to the referred-care group

HDFP indicates Hypertension Detection and Follow-up trial, *No* number, *HTN* hypertension, *BP* blood pressure, *DBP* diastolic blood pressure

betes mellitus or patients with proteinuric chronic kidney disease (CKD) (Table 13.2).

It is well known that the VA-Cooperative studies were the first randomized trials of HTN anywhere in the world. Edward Freis et al., addressed HTN at the severe level of DBP 115–129, and demonstrated a clear treatment effect. In the late 1960s another trialdemonstrated the significant CV benefits of treatingpatients with "mild to moderate HTN" and DBP levels averaging 90–114 mmHg. Since then, DBP target had been 90 mmHg, and no other trial was conducted to determine if lowering target DBP below 90 mmHg reduces CV events further [29, 30]. The VA Co-operative studies are discussed in detail in a separate chapter of this book. There is no doubt however that after the publication of the VA Co-operative studies, the antihypertensive treatment was deemed beneficial for CV disease prevention. At the same time the observed side effects of treatment were generally tolerable.

The Hypertension Optimal Treatment (HOT) study, published in the Lancet in 1998 was the first large RCT to investigate the appropriate goal for DBP in order to protect hypertensives against CVD. A total of 18 790 men and women, aged 50–80 years, were recruited for the study, across 26 countries. All subjects were diagnosed with HTN and had a DBP between 100 and 115 mmHg. Subsequently, all participants were randomly assigned a target DBP. Researchers evaluated the intensity of treatment using a calcium antagonist as baseline therapy in hypertensives with an average BP of 170/105 mmHg, 1501 of whom had type 2 diabetes. The study showed a significant reduction in stroke incidence rates in patients with lower target BP, especially in hypertensives with a history of ischemic heart disease. They also found no significant difference in coronary

Table 13.3 Brief description of the HOT trial

Year of publication	1998
Journal	The lancet
No of patients recruited	18,790
Sex studied	Both sexes, men and women
Mean patient age	61.5 years
Study design	Prospective, randomized, multicenter
Main objective	To determine what is the optimal target DBP during antihypertensive treatment with regard to the reduction in cardiovascular morbidity and mortality.
Secondary objective	To examine the effect of low dose aspirin in preventing stroke further in treated hypertensives
Drugs used in the study	1. Felodipine 5–10 mg daily 2. Addition of an ace inhibitor or beta blocker if BP target not achieved, and 3. Addition of thiazide diuretic if still BP target not achieved Also, 75 mg daily of acetylsalicylic acid (9399 patients) versus placebo (9391 patients)
Eligibility criterion for entry in the study	DBP 100–115 mmHg
Definition of entry pressure	170/105 mmHg
Target BP	Patients were randomized to three different therapeutic goals: 1. DBP ≤90 mmHg (group 1) 2. DBP ≤85 mmHg (group 2), or 3. DBP ≤80 mmHg (group 3)
Primary endpoint	CV event occurrence or mortality
Mean BP in the treated groups	**1. DBP = 85 mmHg** in group 1 **2. DBP = 83 mmHg** in group 2, and **3. DBP = 81 mmHg** in group 3
Main result	No significant differencein outcome between all three groups was observed

HOT indicates Hypertension Optimal Treatment trial, *No* number, *DBP* diastolic blood pressure, *BP* blood pressure, *CV* cardiovascular

heart disease at low DBP. It is worthy of note that a goal below 80 mmHg in diabetic patients proved protective. Therefore, an appropriate DBP goal below 80–85 mmHg was supported by the results of the study, especially in patients with diabetes who exhibit the greatest risk of CV death. Levels lower than 70 mmHg were associated with elevated CVD risk and as such should be avoided [31] (Table 13.3).

The existing European and previous American guidelines, ESH/ESC and JNC 8 published in 2013 and 2014, respectively, suggest that most patients should have their BP brought down to 140/90 mmHg. Specifically, the ESH/ESC Guideline recommendations suggest a systolic BP goal of <140 mmHg. The only exception seems to concern elderly patients where a value of up to 150 mmHg might be appropriate. As far as DBP is concerned, it is recommended that <90 mmHg should be the target for all patients, with the possible exception of those with diabetes where <85 mmHg might be preferable. However, it remains unanswered which is the optimal BP target for young hypertensive patients; if well tolerated, more aggressive BP goals could be considered [32].

More specifically, the 2013 European guidelines for the management of arterial HTN included simplified BP targets across patient groups, evaluation of the benefit of monotherapy vs. combination therapy, as well as assessment of the importance of out-of-office BP measurements. Given the fact that evidence for an aggressive BP treatment approach was lacking, more relaxed BP targets for high-risk hypertensive patients in the 2013 ESH/ESC guidelines were suggested. However, substantial evidence demonstrates cardiovascular benefits from more intensive BP lowering across patient groups. Individualized treatment of high-risk patients may be prudent until more solid evidence is available. Individual patient profiles and preferences and evidence for preferential therapy benefits should be considered when deciding upon the optimal antihypertensive regimen. CCBs appear to be a positive choice for monotherapy, and in combination with other agent classes, and may provide specific benefits beyond BP lowering. Ambulatory and home BP monitoring have an increasing role in defining the diagnosis and prognosis of HTN (especially non-sustained); however, their value for comprehensive diagnosis and appropriate treatment selection should be more widely acknowledged. In conclusion, further evidence may be required on BP targets in high-risk patients, and optimal treatment selection based upon individual patient profiles and comprehensive diagnosis using out-of-office BP measurements may improve patient management.

JNC 8 committee suggests commencement of treatment when BP is ≥140/90 mmHg in the general population, with or without risk factors or organ damage, and in those with diabetes and chronic kidney disease. JNC8 highlighted that the previous recommendations to lower BP to <130/80 mmHg in patients with diabetes are not supported by the extensive review of randomised controlled trials. Only in persons aged 60 years or over does the treatment target range from 140 to 149 mmHg, increasing the treatment threshold to150 mmHg systolic BP [33].

One year later, in November 2015, the publication of the Systolic Blood Pressure Intervention Trial (SPRINT) in the NEJM, and its remarkable results would change the approach to diagnosing and treating HTN. This study involved a large, well-designed, randomized, controlled, open label clinical trial funded by the NIH and conducted at 102 clinical sites in the United States (organized into 5 clinical center networks), including Puerto Rico. SPRINT compared the effect of lowering SBP to either less than 120 mmHg or less than 140 mmHg, intensive vs. standard care, in 9361 hypertensive subjects without diabetes or a history of stroke. The study included individuals aged 50 years or older, either with a history of CVD or at high risk. The results showed that in the intensively treated group, cardiovascular incidence fell significantlyby 25% and mortality rates dropped by 27% compared to subjects receiving standard treatment (absolute rates 5.2% vs. 6.8% and 3.3% vs. 4.5%, respectively). However, in the intensively treated group, an increased number of episodes of hypotension, syncope or acute renal failure were recorded [34].SPRINT results suggest that treatment should be continued even when treated SBP is <130 mmHg, especially for the SPRINT-like hypertensive population. As expected, SPRINT raised several controversies since its publication. The debate concerned mainly the question whether the SPRINT results should be applied safely to the general hypertensive population, seen in daily clinics, and whether they should be embedded into the future HTN guidelines. The methodological way of obtaining the BP measurements in SPRINT trial has contributed highly to the dispute of the generalization of its results to the general population [35].The automated office blood pressure (AOBP) technique, methodology adopted in SPRINT, used a fully automated oscillometric device with the patient sitting alone in the examination room for 5 min after which three readings were taken automatically at one-minute intervals with all three values averaged. In so doing, human involvement was reduced to the minimum, eliminating the white coat effect, and AOBP readings correlated more closely with those of ABPM than conventional office recordings [36]. Thus, seasoned European researchers claimed that BPs taken in SPRINT cannot be directly compared with BPs in other trials which utilized the conventional oscillometric office BP technique for BP characterization levels, and strongly support that the treatment arm of<120 mmHg in SPRINT compares with a higher SBP value close to 140 mmHg in other trials [35]. Thus, they conclude that SBP target in the treatment of hypertension should remain unchanged at <140 mmHg (Table 13.4).

Soon after the publication of the SPRINT trial, a large systematic review and meta-analysis which identified 123 studies with 613,815 participants, was published in the Lancet. The analysis indicated that a 10 mmHg reduction in SBP achieved an overall 13% reduction in all-cause mortality (95% CI, relative risk 0.84–0.91) but had no significant impact on the risk of renal failure events. These effects remained similar even when the effects were compared between trials including patients with higher mean baseline

SBP, and positive history of coronary heart disease, or other cardiovascular disease [37]. Bangalore et al., conducted a meta-analysis of 17 trials that enrolled 55,163 patients with 204,103 patient-years of follow-up. Results indicated that lower SBP levels were associated with a significant decrease in stroke incidence and myocardial infarction, whereas there was no difference in death, cardiovascular death, or heart failure when comparing any of the study BP targets. More specifi-

Table 13.4 Brief description of the SPRINT trial

Year of publication	2015
Journal	New England journal of medicine
No of patients recruited	9361
Sex studied	Both sexes, men and women
Mean patient age	67.9 years
Start of patient recruitment	November, 2010
End of patient recruitment	March, 2013
Study design	RCT, open-label
Main objective	To determine the most appropriate targets for SBP to reduce CV morbidity and mortality among persons without diabetes To answer this question patients were assigned to two treatment groups: 1. Intensive treatment group 2. Standard treatment group
Drugs used in the study	1. Thiazide-type diuretics 2. Calcium channels blockers, and 3. Angiotensin-converting enzymeinhibitors or angiotensin receptor blockers Other agents, including: 1. Spironolactone 2. Amiloride 3. β-blockers 4. Vasodilators, or 5. α-receptor blockers, could be added if necessary
Eligibility criterion for entry in the study	1. Age ≥50 years 2. SBP 130-180 mmHg (treated or untreated) 3. Additional CV disease risk
Exclusion criteria	1. Stroke 2. Diabetes mellitus 3. Polycystic kidney disease 4. Congestive heart failure (symptoms or EF <35%) 5. Proteinuria >1 g/d 6. CKD with eGFR<20 mL/min/1.73 m2 (MDRD) 7. Adherence concerns
Target BP	Intensive treatment group: SBP ≤120 mmHg Standard treatment group: SBP ≤140 mmHg
Median follow-up period	3.26 years
Primary endpoint	CVD composite – first occurrence of: 1. MI 2. Non-MI ACS 3. Stroke 4. Acute decompensated HF 5. CVD death
Mean BP in the treated groups	Intensive treatment group:**122 mmHg** Standard treatment group:**135 mmHg**
Main result	Incidence of primary outcome (composite of CVD events) 25% lower in the intensive compared to standard treatment group and all-cause mortality reduced by 27%

SPRINT indicates Systolic Blood Pressure Intervention Trial, *No* number, *RCT* randomized controlled trial, *SBP* systolic blood pressure, *CV* cardiovascular, *EF* ejection fraction, *CKD* chronic kidney disease, *eGFR* estimated glomerular filtration rate, *BP* blood pressure, *CVD* cardiovascular disease, *MI* myocardial disease, *ACS* acute coronary syndrome, *HF* heart failure cally, BP targets of <120 mmHg and <130 mmHg were ranked as the two most efficacious targets, whereas BP targets <140 mmHg and <150 mmHg were ranked as the two safest targets for the outcome of serious adverse effects. An optimal balance between efficacy and safety was achieved with a target SBP of <130 mmHg [38]. It should be noted that SPRINT patients aged ≥75 years benefited to a similar extent as younger individuals. Despite, concerns of excessive lowering of diastolic BP provide complementary and additional data to clarify the impelling question of the optimal level to which BP should be brought by treatment [39, 40].

At the same time as SPRINT, another randomized, controlled study was conducted, namely the Action to Control Cardiovascular Risk in Diabetes (ACCORD) trial that included patients with both HTN and diabetes. The ACCORD trial was a double-blinded RCT that mainly tested the effect of lowering the SBP to <120 mmHg on CV events in diabetic patients compared to the usual systolic 140. Like SPRINT, ACCORD was designed to compare the effects of lowering SBP to either less than 140 mmHg or less than 120 mmHg. A total of 4733 participants were followed for a mean follow-up period of 4.7 years. The primary outcomes included non-fatal myocardial infarctions, non-fatal strokes, or death from any cardiovascular causes. No significant decrease in CVD was observed between the two groups, other than the stroke incidence that was significantly reduced in the intensively treated group, but this was one of the eight secondary outcomes of the study [41].Thus, the authors concluded that compared to usual BP control intensive BP control in diabetics does not confer any significant benefit. Another concern that emerged was that the results of SPRINT would not be applicable to individuals at low or medium

Table 13.5 Brief description of the ACCORD trial

Year of publication	2010
Journal	New England journal of medicine
No of patients recruited	4733
Sex studied	Both sexes, men and women
Mean patient age	62.2 years
Study design	Double-blinded RCT
Main objective	To determine whether therapy targeting normal SBP (i.e., <120 mmHg) reduces major CV events in patients with type 2 diabetesat high risk for CV events
Eligibility criterion for entry in the study	1. Type 2 diabetes 2. HbA1C ≥7.5% 3. ≥40 years of age with CVD or 4. ≥55 years of age withanatomical evidence of risk 5. Individuals with SBP 130–180 mmHg takingthree or fewer antihypertensivemedications, and 6. a 24protein of less than 1 gm
Exclusion criteria	1. BMI more than 45 2. Serum creatinine more than 1.5 mg/dl 3. Other serious illness
Definition of entry pressure	139/76 mmHg in both the intensive and the standard treatment group
Primary endpoint	First occurrence of a major CV event: 1. The composite of nonfatal MI 2. Nonfatal stroke, or 3. Cardiovascular death
Mean follow-up period	4.7 years
Mean BP in the treated groups	**Mean SBP = 119.3 mmHg** in the intensive treatment group **Mean SBP = 133.5 mmHg** in the standard treatment group
Main result	No significant differencein primary outcomes of death from CVD or nonfatal MI or stroke (P = 0.20)

ACCORD indicates Action to Control Cardiovascular Risk in Diabetes Trial, *No* number, *RCT* randomized controlled trial, *SBP* systolic blood pressure, *CV* cardiovascular, *HbA1C* glycosylated hemoglobin, *CVD* cardiovascular disease, *BMI* body mass index, *MI* myocardial infarction, *BP* blood pressure

Table 13.6 Brief description of the HOPE trial

Year of publication	2016
Journal	New England journal of medicine
No of patients recruited	12,705
Sex studied	Both sexes, men and women
Mean patient age	65.8 years
Start of patient recruitment	April, 2007
End of patient recruitment	November, 2010
Study design	Multicenter, long-term,international, double-blind, RCT
Main objective	To determine whether the benefits of statins in reducing CVD risk among patients without CVD, can be extended toan intermediate-risk, ethnically diverse population without CVD
Drugs used in the study	1. Daily rosuvastatin (10 mg) or placebo, plus 2. Daily candesartan/hydrochlorothiazide (16 mg/12.5 mg) or placebo
Eligibility criterion for entry in the study	Men ≥55 years of age and women ≥65 years of age, who had atleast one of the following CV risk factors: 1. Elevated waist-to-hip ratio 2. History of alow level of high-density lipoprotein cholesterol 3. Current or recent tobacco use 4. Dysglycemia 5. Familyhistory of premature coronary disease, and 6. Mild renal dysfunction Women ≥60 years of age who had at least twosuch risk factors.
Exclusion criteria	Participants with CVD and those with an indication for or contraindicationto statins, angiotensin-receptor blockers, Angiotensin-converting–enzyme inhibitors,or thiazide diuretics
Definition of entry pressure	138/82 mmHg in both the treatment and the placebo group
Primary endpoint	Thefirst co-primary outcome was the composite of Death from CV causes, nonfatal MI, or nonfatal stroke, and thesecond co-primary outcome additionally included Resuscitated cardiac arrest, HF, and revascularization
Median follow-up period	5.6 years
Mean BP reduction in the treated groups	6.0/3.0 mmHg greater in the active-treatmentgroup than in the placebo group
Main result	Treatment with rosuvastatin at a dose of 10 mg per day resulted in a significantlylower risk of CV events than placebo in an intermediate-risk, ethnicallydiverse population without CVD. Therapy with candesartan at a dose of 16 mg per day plus hydrochlorothiazide ata dose of 12.5 mg per day was not associated with a lower rate of major CV events than placebo among persons at intermediate risk who did not have CVD.

HOPE-3 indicates Heart OutcomesPrevention Evaluation trial, *No* number, *RCT* randomized-controlled trial, *CVD* cardiovascular disease, *CV* cardiovascular, *MI* myocardial infarction, *BP* blood pressure, *HF* heart failure

risk of CVD given that such patients were excluded from the study (Table 13.5).

The Heart Outcomes Prevention Evaluation (HOPE-3) study, published in sought to address this concern [42]. This multicenter, long-term, international, double-blind, randomized, placebo-controlled trial included men aged 55 years or older or women 65 years or older, at low or medium risk of CVD, all of whom were under treatment with BP and cholesterol-lowering drugs, irrespective of pretreatment levels of BP or low-density lipoprotein cholesterol levels (Table 13.6). The study results revealed that triple combination vs. double placebo treatment achieved a significant decrease in the incidence of CVD. According to Chobanian a key caveat of the HOPE-3 trial is that “the findings are not relevant to making practical recommendations about BP goals” [43].It is generally accepted that the ultimate goal in all patients with HTN is to lower BP to specific BP levels in order to reduce CV complications. SPRINT considered a target of systolic BP lower than 120 mmHg in high risk patients older than 50 years of age. Evidence is lacking for adults younger than 50 years of age and for those for whom SPRINT results would not be applicable, such as individuals with type 2 diabetes, a history of stroke, non-ambulatory elderly persons and those residing in institutions. Consequently, the currently available evidence is based on meta-analyses stratifying the different trials according to the BP levels achieved by active treatment. In a meta-analysis of 34 trials including SPRINT results, a target between 130 and 140 mmHg might be considered in view of the observed benefit of reducing all major CV events and mortality [44]. In addition, a somewhat lower target below 130 mmHg might also be contemplated given the benefit seen in reducing CV risk [41] but patients should be monitored for permanent discontinuation of treatment due to adverse events.

The initiation of antihypertensive therapy should continue to be guided by elevated office BP above 140 mmHg or 90 mmHg for systolic or diastolic BP, respectively, confirmed either by ambulatory or home monitoring. Clinicians in their practice should take into account not only the BP level but also the overall CV risk in order to decide on the course of treatment. The 2013 European Guidelines use risk factors, target organ damage and the presence of overt CV or renal disease. In contrast, no mention is made of the overall risk in the JNC 8 recommendations, neither in those submitted by the American Society of Hypertension (ASH)/International Society of Hypertension (ISH) or the ACC/AHA/CDC guidelines. Based on the available evidence, Chobanian in his monography in the JAMA [43] suggests a reasonable approach regarding the goal for treatment of hypertension in the general population and in high-risk populations. Control of other CVD risk factors, such as appropriate lifestyle modifications (ie. body weight reduction, lipid lowering, avoidance of smoking and alcohol, etc) is crucial to prevent CV complications in hypertensive subjects. Moreover, the use of statins seems necessary for an integrated management approach for high-risk patients.

More recently, the new American 2017 ACC/AHA Hypertension guidelines were published in JACC. The writing committee recommends BP-lowering medication for those with stage 1 HTN (130-139 mmHg and/or 80-89 mmHg, for systolic and DBP, respectively) with clinical CV disease or a 10-year risk of ASCVD 10% or greater, as well as for those with stage 2 hypertension (≥140 mmHg and/or ≥90 mmHg, for systolic and DBP, respectively). For stage 2 HTN, the updated guidelines recommend using 2 BP-lowering medications in addition to healthy lifestyle changes, which is a more aggressive treatment standard. In contrast, previous guidelines recommended starting patients on only 1 BPlowering medication [45]. Moreover, the new BP guidelines are focusing on the importance of ensuring that BP measurements are accurate and underline the need for using calibrated BP monitors, stressing in parallel the need for utilizing the proper cuff size. In addition they make clear that failure to position patients and their arms appropriately, or failure to allow time to rest before performing three blood-pressure readings can result in falsely elevated BP levels [46]. Furthermore, they emphasize the significance of frequent self-measurement of BP at home, since conventional office BPs are often higher than ambulatory or home BPs, and recording them appropriately and bringing them to all clinic appointments to help physicians in accurate clinical decision-making [47]. Undoubtedly, the updated 2017 ACC/AHA Guidelines on High Blood Pressure greatly expand the number of adults who will qualify for the diagnosis of HTN and millions more Americans will need to lower blood pressure. (In Tables 13.7 and 13.8 the major HTN Guidelines are summarized).

As anticipated, the release of the 2017 American HypertensionGuidelines gave rise to a heated discussion regarding which is the optimal BP goal. Americans, for the first time, as described above, are focusing on calculating the 10-year ASCVD risk in all patients with stage 1 HTN, whereas antihypertensive drugs are not warranted unless there is a greater than 10% ASCVD risk [45].At the same time, they define systolic/diastolic BP levels of 120-129 mmHg/<80 mmHg,

Table 13.7 Comparison between hypertension guidelines in the adult general population without comorbidities

	JNC 7 2003	JNC 8 2014	CHEP 2015	ESH/ ESC 2013	ASH/ ISH 2014	Australian 2008 (updated 2010)	BHS/ NICE 2011	ACC/AHA 2017
BP target in the adult general population (mmHg)	<140/90	<140/90	<140/90	<140/90	<140/90	<140/90 or lower if well-tolerated	<140/90 (OBP) <135/85 (ABP/HBP)	<130/80 mmHg The New Guidelines give emphasis on the following: 1. 10-year ASCVD risk assessment 2. Eliminate the term prehypertension and instead use the term elevated BP for SBP 120–129 and DBP<80 mmHg 3. Accurate BP measurement 4. Accurate self BP monitoring 5. Lifestyle changes

BP blood pressure, *JNC-7* Seventh Joint National Committee, *JNC-8* Eighth Joint National Committee, *CHEP* Canadian Hypertension Education Program, *ESH/ESC* European Society of Hypertension/European Society of Cardiology, *ASH/ISH* American Society of Hypertension/International Society of Hypertension, *BHS/NICE* British Hypertension Society/National Institute for Health and Care Excellence, *SBP* Systolic blood pressure, *OBP* office blood pressure, *ABP* ambulatory blood pressure, *HBP* home blood pressure, *ACC/AHA* American College of Cardiology/American Heart Association, *ASCVD* atherosclerotic cardiovascular disease, *SBP* systolic blood pressure, *DBP* diastolic blood pressure

Table 13.8 Comparison between hypertension guidelines in patients with comorbidities

	JNC 7 2003	JNC 8 2014	CHEP 2015	ESH/ESC 2013	ASH/ISH 2014	Australian 2008 (updated 2010)	BHS/ NICE 2011	ACC/AHA 2017
Goal BP in patients with DM	<130/80	<140/90	<130/80	<140/85	<140/90	<130/80	<140/90	<130/80 mmHg If goal is met after 1 month, reassess in 3–6 months If goal is not met after 1 month, consider different medication or titration Continue monthly follow-up until control is achieved
Goal BP in patients with CKD	<130/80	<140/90	<140/90	SBP of < than 140 SBP of < than 130, if proteinuria is present	<140/90 <130/80, if proteinuria is present	<130/80, if proteinuria exceeds 300mg/day <125/75, if proteinuria exceeds 1gr/day (+/- DM)	<140/90	<130/80 mmHg If goal is met after 1 month, reassess in 3–6 months If goal is not met after 1 month, consider different medication or titration Continue monthly follow-up until control is achieved

BP blood pressure, *DM* diabetes mellitus, *CKD* chronic kidney disease, *JNC-7* Seventh Joint National Committee, *JNC-8* Eighth Joint National Committee, *CHEP* Canadian Hypertension Education Program, *ESH/ESC* European Society of Hypertension/European Society of Cardiology, *ASH/ISH* American Society of Hypertension/International Society of Hypertension, *BHS/NICE* British Hypertension Society/National Institute for Health and Care Excellence, *SBP* Systolic blood pressure respectively, as "elevated blood pressure", eliminating the term "prehypertension" [45].Moreover, recent estimates calculated that among patients aged 35–74 years, adding intensive BP goals for high-risk groups to JNC7 and JNC8 HTN treatment guidelines prevents additional CV disease deaths while saving costs provided that medication costs are controlled [48].Beyond doubt, every life counts. It should be made clear, however, that intensive treatment of BP should not apply to all with HTN. It remains to be known what the European HTN specialists will recommend as the appropriate treatment target for the general hypertensive population, as well as for the highrisk groups. Will they take into account the results of the SPRINT trial, which is considered from many in the field a landmark study? Perhaps, one could find the answer about which should be the optimal BP target in the past. The HTN pioneer Edward Freis had stated: "*Some of you may be curious if I take antihypertensive drugs. I do, and at age 91 years, my blood pressure is maintained between 110/60mm Hg and 125/70 mmHg. I have never felt weak or faint at these levels*" [49].

References

1. Roguin A. Scipione Riva-Rocci and the men behind the mercury sphygmomanometer. Int J Clin Pract. 2006;60:73–9.
2. Korner PI. Essential hypertension and its causes: neural and non-neural mechanisms. Oxford/New York: Oxford University Press. ISBN 978-0-19-535740-0.
3. Rossi GP. The challenges of arterial hypertension. Front Cardiovasc Med. 2015;2:2.
4. Chrysant SG. Current status of aggressive blood pressure control. World J Cardiol. 2011;3:65–71.
5. White PD. Heart disease. 3rd ed. New York: MacMillan; 1944. Zanchetti A. Hypertension: past, present, and future. Rev Fed Arg Cardiol. 2015;44.
6. Bishop T, Figueredo VM. Hypertensive therapy: attacking the renin-angiotensin system. West J Med. 2001;2:119–24.
7. Bumgarner J. The health of the presidents: the 41 United States presidents through 1993 from a physician's point of view. Jefferson: McFarland & Company, Inc.; 1994.
8. Deppisch LM. The White House physician: a history from Washington to George W. Bush. Jefferson: McFarland & Company; 2007.
9. Evans H. The hidden campaign: FDR's health and the 1944 election. Armonk: M.E. Sharpe; 2002.
10. Fye WB. Caring for the heart: Mayo Clinic and the rise of specialization. Oxford: Oxford University Press; 2015.
11. Freis ED. Reminiscences of the Veterans Administration trial of the treatment of hypertension. Hypertension. 1990;16(4):472–5.
12. Kannel WB, Wolf PA, Veter J, McNamara PM. Epidemiologic assessment of the role of blood pressure in stroke. JAMA. 1970;214:301–10.
13. Kannel WB, Schwartz MJ, McNamara PM. Blood pressure and risk of coronary heart disease: the Framingham study. Dis Chest. 1969;56:43–52.
14. Andreadis EA. Hypertension: a growing threat. In: Andreadis EA, editor. Hypertension and cardiovascular disease. Cham: Springer Nature; 2016. p. 1–17.
15. WHO. Global status report on noncommunicable diseases 2014. World Health Organization, Geneva; 2015.
16. Chockalingam A, Campbell NR, Fodor JG. Worldwide epidemic of hypertension. Can J Cardiol. 2006;22:553–5.
17. Kearney PM, Whelton M, Reynolds K, Muntner P, Whelton PK, He J. Global burden of hypertension: analysis of worldwide data. Lancet. 2005;365: 217–23.
18. O'Donnell MJ, Xavier D, Lio L, Zhang H, Chin SL, Rao-Melacin P, et al. Risk factors for ischemic and intracerebral hemorrhage stroke in 22 countries (the INTERSTROKE study): a case-control study. Lancet. 2010;376:112–23.
19. Yusuf S, Hawken S, Ounpuu S, Dans T, Avezum A, Lanas F, et al. Effect of potentially modifiable risk factors associated with myocardial infarction in 52 countries (the INTERHEART study); case-control study. Lancet. 2004;364:937–52.
20. Botdorf J, Chaudhary K, Whaley-Connell A. Hypertension in cardiovascular and kidney disease. Cardiorenal Med. 2011;1:183–92.
21. Murabito JM, D'Agostino RB, Silbershtz H, Wilson WF. Intermittent claudication: a risk profile from the Framingham Heart Study. Circulation. 1997;96: 44–9.
22. World Health Organization. A global brief on hypertension: silent killer, global public health crisis 2013. http://www.who.int/cardiovascular_diseases/publications/global_brief_hypertension/en/. Accessed 31 Aug 2014.
23. Forouzanfar MH, Liu P, Roth GA, et al. Global burden of hypertension and systolic blood pressure of at least 110 to 115 mm Hg, 1990–2015. JAMA. 2017;317:165–82.
24. Bakris GL, Frohlich ED. An overview of four decades of experience. JACC. 1989;7:1595–608.
25. Rutan GH, McDonald RH, Kuller LH. A historical perspective of elevated systolic vs diastolic blood pressure from an epidemiological and clinical trial viewpoint. J Clin Epidemiol. 1989;7:663–73.
26. MRC Trial of treatment of mild Hypertension: principal results. Medical Research Council Working Party. Br Med J. 1985;291:97–104.

27. Zhang X, Fan F, Huo Y, Xu X. Identifying the optimal blood pressure target for ideal health. J Transl Intern Med. 2016;4:1–6.
28. Hypertension Detection and Follow-Up Program Cooperative Group. Five-year findings of the hypertension detection and follow-up program. I. Reduction in mortality of persons with high blood pressure, including mild hypertension. JAMA. 1979;242:2562–71.
29. Veterans Administration Cooperative Study Group on Antihypertensive Agents. Effects of treatment on morbidity and hypertension: results in patients with diastolic pressures averaging 115 through 129 millimeters of mercury. JAMA. 1967;202:1028–34.
30. Veterans Administration Cooperative Study Group on Antihypertensive Agents. Effects of treatment on morbidity and hypertension. II. Results in patients with diastolic blood pressure averaging 90 through 114 millimeters of mercury. JAMA. 1970;213:1143–52.
31. Hansson L, Zanchetti A, Carruthers SG, Dahlof B, Elmfeldt D, Julius S, et al. Effects of intensive blood-pressure lowering and low-dose aspirin in patients with hypertension: principal results of the Hypertension Optimal Treatment (HOT) randomised trial. Lancet. 1998;351:1755–62.
32. Mancia G, Fagard R, Narkiewicz K, et al. 2013 ESH/ESC guidelines for the management of arterial hypertension. J Hypertens. 2013;31:1281–357.
33. James PA, Oparil S, Carter BL, et al. 2014 evidence-based guideline for the management of high blood pressure in adults: report from the panel members appointed to the Eight Joint National Committee (JNC 8). JAMA. 2014;311:507–20.
34. Wright JT Jr, Williamson JD, Whelton PK, Snyder JK, Sink KM, Rocco MV, et al. A randomized trial of intensive versus standard blood-pressure control. N Engl J Med. 2015;373:2103–16.
35. Kjeldsen SE, Mancia G. Unobserved automated office blood pressure measurement in the systolic blood pressure intervention trial (SPRINT): systolic blood pressure treatment target remains below 140 mmHg. Eur Heart J Cardiovasc Pharmacother. 2016;2:79–80.
36. Parati G, Ochoa JE, Bilo G, Zanchetti A. SPRINT blood pressure: sprinting back to Smirk's basal blood pressure? Hypertension. 2017;69:15–9.
37. Ettehad D, Emdin CA, Kiran A, et al. Blood pressure lowering for prevention of cardiovascular disease and death: a systematic review and meta-analysis. Lancet. 2016;387:957–67.
38. Bangalore S, Toklu B, Gianos E, Schwartzbard A, Weintraub H, Ogedegbe G, et al. Optimal systolic blood pressure target after SPRINT: insights from a network meta-analysis of randomized trials. Am J Med. 2017;130(6):707–719 e8.
39. Zanchetti A, Liu L, Mancia G, Parati G, Grassia G, MarcoStramba-Badialea M, et al. Continuation of the ESH-CHL-SHOT trial after publication of the SPRINT: rationale for further study on blood pressure targets of antihypertensive treatment after stroke. J Hypertens. 2016;34:393–5.
40. Williamson JD, Supiano MA, Applegate WB, Berlowitz DR, Campbell RC, Chertow GM, et al. Intensive vs standard blood pressure control and cardiovascular disease outcomes in adults aged ≥75 years. JAMA. 2016;315:2673–82.
41. Cushman WC, Evans GW, Byington RP, Goff DC, Grimm RH, Cutler JA. Effects of intensive blood-pressure control in type 2 diabetes mellitus. N Engl J Med. 2010;362:1575–85.
42. Yusuf S, Lonn E, Pais P, Bosch J, Lopez-Jaramillo P, Zhu J, et al. Blood-pressure and cholesterol lowering in persons without cardiovascular disease. N Engl J Med. 2016;374:2032–43.
43. Chobanian AV. Hypertension in 2017-what is the right target? JAMA. 2017;317:579–80.
44. Thomopoulos C, Parati G, Zanchetti A. Effects of blood pressure lowering on outcome incidence in hypertension. 7. Effects of more versus less intensive blood pressure lowering and different achieved blood pressure levels-updated overview and meta-analyses of randomized trials. J Hypertens. 2016;34:613–22.
45. Whelton PK, et al. 2017 ACC/AHA/AAPA/ABC/ACPM/AGS/APhA/ASH/ASPC/NMA/PCNA guideline for the prevention, detection, evaluation, and Management of High Blood Pressure in adults. JACC. 2018;71:e127–248. https://doi.org/10.1016/j.jacc.2017.11.006.
46. Handler J. The importance of accurate blood pressure measurement. Perm J. 2009;13:51–4.
47. Bakris G, Sorrentino M. Redefining hypertension — assessing the new blood-pressure guidelines. NEJM. 378:497–9. https://doi.org/10.1056/NEJMp1716193.
48. Moise N, Huang C, Rodgers A, Kohli-Lynch CN, Tzong KY, Coxson PG, et al. Comparative cost-effectiveness of conservative or intensive blood pressure treatment guidelines in adults aged 35–74 years the cardiovascular disease policy model. Hypertension. 2016;68:88–96.
49. Freis ED. Hypertension treatment: contributions and comments on challenges. J Clin Hypertens. 2004;1:45–6.

Part III

Blood Pressure Assessment Methods Used in Landmark Trials

Methods of Blood Pressure Assessment Used in Milestone Hypertension Trials

14

Yi Chen, Lei Lei, and Ji-Guang Wang

Introduction

Accurate blood pressure measurement is critical for the clinical management of hypertension and for clinical trial research in hypertension as well. The methodology of blood pressure measurement therefore has to be carefully chosen to assure the accuracy of blood pressure measurement in a hypertension trial. Indeed, small discrepancies in blood pressure measuring protocols may have substantial impact on the recorded blood pressure levels and subsequent therapeutic decisions during a trial, and sometimes on the results of the whole trial.

In principle, the methods of blood pressure measurement used in a hypertension trial should stringently follow most recent guideline recommendations [1–3]. If the results of such a trial would be clinically relevant for clinical practice and used for guideline recommendations, the corresponding methods of blood pressure measurement may also be used to formulate recommendations on blood pressure measurement in clinical practice.

Over the years, dozens of clinical trials in hypertension had been conducted with various blood pressure measuring techniques and protocols. Because the technology and knowledge for blood pressure measurement have been advancing rapidly, the blood pressure measuring techniques and protocols changed from the early to the most recent trials in hypertension. In this chapter, we will summarize the blood pressure measurement protocols used in the milestone hypertension trials [4–82], and explore the clinical relevance and implications for the management of hypertension.

Y. Chen · L. Lei · J.-G. Wang (✉)
Centre for Epidemiological Studies and Clinical Trials, The Shanghai Institute of Hypertension, Ruijin Hospital, Shanghai Jiaotong University School of Medicine, Shanghai, China

Methodological Issues of Blood Pressure Assessment in Milestone Hypertension Trials

A literature search limited to clinical trials published in English between 1 January 1990 and 1 April 2017 was performed using the PubMed with the keywords "hypertension" or "blood pressure", "randomized controlled trial" and "cardiovascular event". Additional relevant trials were included from the references of the identified studies. Selected studies were randomized controlled outcome trials with a blinded or open design. We excluded studies of a surrogate outcome measure or in patients with congestive heart failure, end-stage renal disease on dialysis, or acute stroke (<30 days of onset). Relevant information was also obtained from prior publications related to the trial design of the individual studies.

V. Papademetriou et al. (eds.), *Management of Hypertension*,
https://doi.org/10.1007/978-3-319-92946-0_14

We selected 37 milestone hypertension trials that formed the basis for the past and current hypertension management guidelines. Although ambulatory blood pressure monitoring was performed in a subset of randomized patients in some of these trials, such as the Hypertension Optimal Treatment (HOT) trial [22] and Systolic Blood Pressure Intervention Trial (SPRINT) [80], clinic or office blood pressure measurement was used in all these milestone hypertension trials. We evaluated nine different aspects of blood pressure measurement (Table 14.1), in terms of the accordance with recent blood pressure measurement guidelines [1–3].

Observers

Physicians measured blood pressure in most of the earlier trials [10, 11]. However, non-physician health professionals, such as nurses, were increasingly involved in many of the recent trials [42, 46]. In addition to the increased use of automated blood pressure monitors in clinical practice and research, several other reasons drove this shift. Although physicians are usually adequately trained to measure blood pressure, they do not often measure blood pressure in complete compliance with the standards of blood pressure measurement guidelines [83, 84]. When an auscultatory device (mercury, aneroid, or hybrid) is used, they often have reading bias, in other words, digit preference and commonly round blood pressure readings to zero or five. In addition, the white-coat effect may also dilute the validity and usefulness of blood pressure measured by physicians. Therefore, some experts recommended that physicians should not measure blood pressure themselves but should rely on blood pressures measured by trained observers using validated automated devices to improve the quality of care of hypertensive patients in general and the accuracy of blood pressure assessment in clinical research in particular [83].

However, people believe that even though blood pressure is measured by nurses, other "trained observers," or automated devices, the white-coat effect is still possible in clinic blood pressure measurement. Many patients still become anxious in the clinical setting even in the absence of physicians. And the presence of a nurse or other trained observers may lead to conversation and therefore increase blood pressure. That is actually the rationale for establishing unattended blood pressure measurement facilities. Such an unattended blood pressure measurement was used in the recent SPRINT study [78, 79]. In SPRINT, clinic blood pressure was measured automatically three times with a validated oscillometric device, with the patient being quiet and isolated in a room [79]. This methodology has been labelled as automated office blood pressure measurement (AOBP). This so-called AOBP used in the SPRINT trial had two key elements. First, everybody except the patient him/herself was out of the room during measurements and the resting period prior to measurements. Second, the blood pressure measurement device (HEM-907, OMRON Healthcare, Kyoto, Japan) was preset to wait for 5 min before measurements were started. Blood pressure was measured three times at 1 min interval.

This unattended blood pressure measurement is considered to be superior to conventional office blood pressure measurement because it reduces the white-coat effect and shows a better correlation with ambulatory blood pressure and target organ damage than conventional office blood pressure [85, 86]. This approach to measuring blood pressure is, in some researchers' opinion, probably better than conventional office blood pressure measurement methods. However, systolic blood pressure, assessed by unattended measurements, is lower than measurements in the presence of a physician or a nurse [87, 88]. According to some researchers, the blood-pressure levels attained in the SPRINT intensive treatment group (systolic blood pressure < 120 mmHg) might correspond to a conventional office systolic blood pressure < 136 mmHg, which is more or less the same as the currently recommended therapeutic target of adequate blood pressure control (systolic blood pressure <140 mmHg) [87].

The 2005 recommendations on blood pressure measurement do not mandate who should measure blood pressure, but do require that the

Table 14.1 Methodology of blood pressure measurement in major hypertension trials

Study acronym, year of publication (reference)	Observer	Device description	Number of measurements	Time interval between measurements	Resting period	Position(s)	Arm	Cuff	Drug timing[a]
SHEP, 1991 [4–6]	Trained, certified technician	Random zero sphygmomanometer	Average of 4 readings (twice at 2 visits)	30 s	After 5 min of seated rest, and 1 to 3 min of standing	Seated and standing	Right arm	Appropriate size	–
STOP-H, 1991 [7–10]	Nurse or doctor	Mercury sphygmomanometer	Average of 2 readings	–	After 5 min supine, and after 1 and 3 min of standing	Supine and standing	–	Appropriate size	–
MRC old, 1992 [11]	Nurse and/or doctor	Random zero sphygmomanometer	Average of the 2nd and the 3rd of 3 readings	–	–	Seated	–	–	–
TOMHS, 1993 [12, 13]	Trained, certified, and monitored observer	Random zero sphygmomanometer	Average of 2 readings	30 s	After 5 min of rest	Seated	Right arm	Appropriate size	Morning BP 1–4 h after medication
SYST-EUR, 1997 [14–17]	–	Mercury sphygmomanometer	Average of 6 sitting and 6 standing readings—2 in each position at 3 visits	–	After 2, 5, 2 min of rest in supine, seated & standing, respectively	Seated, supine and standing	–	–	–
Syst-China, 1998 [18, 19]	Physician	Mercury sphygmomanometer	Average of 6 readings (twice at 3 visits)	1 min	After 5 and 2 min of seated and standing rest, respectively	Seated	–	–	At trough
HOT, 1998 [20–22]	–	Oscillometric semiautomatic device	3 readings	–	After 5 min of rest	Seated	–	–	–
NICS-EH, 1999 [23]	–	–	–	–	–	–	–	–	–

(continued)

Table 14.1 (continued)

Study acronym, year of publication (reference)	Observer	Device description	Number of measurements	Time interval between measurements	Resting period	Position(s)	Arm	Cuff	Drug timing[a]
CAPPP, 1999 [24]	–	Mercury sphygmomanometer	Average of 3 readings	–	–	Supine	–	Appropriate size	–
NORDIL 2000 [25, 26]	–	–	Single readings in at least 2 visits	–	After 10 min of rest	Seated	–	–	–
INSIGHT, 2000 and Substudy [27, 28]	–	Mercury sphygmomanometer	3 readings	–	After 5 min of rest	–	–	–	At trough
PROGRESS, 2001 [29–32]	Trained observer	Mercury sphygmomanometer	Average of 2 readings	2 min	After 5 min of rest	Seated	–	–	–
IDNT, 2001 [33–35]	–	–	–	–	–	Seated	–	–	–
HOPE, 2001 and substudy [36, 37]	–	Mercury sphygmomanometer	Average of 2 readings in each arm	–	–	–	Arm with higher BP	–	–
LIFE, 2002 [38–41]	–	Validated, calibrated manual manometer	Average of 2 readings	1 min	After 5 min of rest	Seated and standing	Right or left arm	Appropriate size	At trough (22–26 h)
ALLHAT, 2002 [42–45]	Trained observer	–	Average of 2 readings	30 s	–	Seated	–	–	–
ANBP 2, 2003 [46, 47]	Trained study nurse	Mercury sphygmomanometer	The average of the 2nd and 3rd of 3 readings if BP differences <10/6 mm Hg between readings	–	After 5 min of rest	Seated	–	Appropriate size	–
SCOPE, 2003 [48, 49]	–	–	Average of the 2nd and the 3rd of 3 readings	1 min	After 10 min of rest	Seated and standing	–	Appropriate size	–
INVEST, 2003 [50, 51]	–	Mercury sphygmomanometer, calibrated aneroid manometer or an electronic device	Average of 2 readings. Additional readings if difference > 5 mmHg between readings	2 min	After 5 min of rest	Seated	Right or left arm	Appropriate size	–

Study acronym, year of publication (reference)	Observer	Device description	Number of measurements	Time interval between measurements	Resting period	Position(s)	Arm	Cuff	Drug timing[a]
WHI-OS, 2004 [52, 53]	Certified staff	Mercury sphygmomanometer	Average of 2 readings	30 s	After 5 min of rest	Seated	Right arm	Appropriate size	–
VALUE, 2004 [54]	–	–	–	–	After 5 min of rest	Seated	–	–	At trough (24 h post-dose)
ASCOT-BPLA, 2005 [55, 56]	–	Semiautomated device (Omron HEM 705-CP)	Average of the 2nd and the 3rd of 3 readings	–	After 5 min of rest	Seated	–	–	All drugs taken no more than 24 h before study visits
FEVER, 2005 [57]	–	Mercury sphygmomanometer	Average of 3 readings	1 min	After 5 and 2 min of seated and standing rest, respectively	Seated and standing	–	Appropriate size	–
E-COST, 2005 [58]	–	–	Average of readings	–	–	Seated	–	–	At trough
ADVANCE, 2007 [59]	–	Automatic (Omron HEM-705CP)	Average of 2 readings	–	After 5 min of rest	Seated	–	–	–
AVOID, 2008 [60]	–	Mercury sphygmomanometer	Average of 3 readings	2 min	After 5 min of rest	–	–	Appropriate size	At trough
ONTARGET 2008, and sub-study [61–63]	–	Semiautomatic device (OMRON HEM-757)	Duplicate readings	–	After 3 min of rest	Seated	–	–	–
ACCOMPLISH, 2008 [64–66]	–	–	Average of 3 readings	2 min	After 5 min of rest	Seated	–	–	–
JATOS, 2008 [67, 68]	–	Sphygmomanometer	Average of at least 2 readings per visit	–	After 10 min of rest	Seated	–	–	–
CASE J, 2008 [69]	–	–	2 readings	–	–	Seated	–	–	–
HIJ CREATE, 2009 [70]	–	Mercury sphygmomanometer	–	–	After 5 min of rest	Seated	–	–	–

(continued)

Table 14.1 (continued)

Study acronym, year of publication (reference)	Observer	Device description	Number of measurements	Time interval between measurements	Resting period	Position(s)	Arm	Cuff	Drug timing[a]
ACCORD BP, 2010 [71, 72]	–	Automatic sphygmomanometer (Omron HEM-907)	Average of 3 readings	–	–	Seated	–	–	–
COPE, 2011 [73]	Physician	–	Average of 2 stable readings	2 min	After 5 min of rest	Seated	–	–	–
OSCAR, 2012 [74, 75]	–	Mercury or automatic sphygmomanometer	Single readings in 2 different visits	–	–	Seated	–	–	–
NAGOYA-HEART, 2012 [76, 77]	–	–	Single readings in at least 2 visits	–	–	–	–	–	–
SPRINT,2015 [78–80]	Unattended	Automatic sphygmomanometer (Omron HEM-907)	Average of 3 measurements	1 min	After 5 min of rest	Seated	–	Proper cuff size	–
HOPE-3, 2016 [81, 82]	–	Automatic (Omron HEM-711DLXCAN) or mercury sphygmomanometer	Average of 2 measurements	At least 1 min	After 5 min of rest	Seated	Right arm	Evenly tight	–

– not reported
[a]Timing of the blood pressure measurement in relation to the last medication dosage. For instance, "trough" usually refers to a blood pressure measured 20–26 h after the last study medication was taken

observer be properly trained [1, 2]. AOBP was recommended in the 2013 European Society of Hypertension guidelines for the management of hypertension as a superior method to improve reproducibility and to make office blood pressure values closer to daytime ambulatory and home blood pressure [89].

Devices

Before electronic blood pressure monitors became readily available in clinical practice a few decades ago, mercury sphygmomanometers were the major instrument for blood pressure measurement in earlier clinical trials, including Hawksley random-zero sphygmomanometer [4, 11]. However, even in the era of electronic blood pressure measuring devices, both aneroid and mercury sphygmomanometers had been used in parallel with automated and semi-automated electronic devices in the International Verapamil SR-Trandolapril Study (INVEST) [50, 51]. In fact, this multiple-device approach was also seen in several other multicentre clinical trials, such as the recent Heart Outcomes Prevention Evaluation-3 (HOPE-3) trial [81, 82], and even in the single-centre Olmesartan and Calcium Antagonists Randomized trial (OSCAR) [74, 75].

The standard sphygmomanometry has been the mainstay of clinic blood pressure measurement since blood pressure could be measured non-invasively. This technique usually requires a mercury manometer. It has been removed from clinical practice in several countries and will eventually be eliminated from blood pressure measurement in all countries not before long, because of serious environmental concerns about mercury pollution. In addition, manual auscultatory blood pressure measurement is prone to observers' error or bias. For these reasons, manual blood pressure measurement is gradually being supplanted by automated techniques.

Currently, the most widely used mercury-free devices are automated oscillometric blood pressure monitors [90]. Some professional oscillometric devices allow consecutive repeated automated measuring and averaging and simultaneous two-arm measurements, with some optional functions, such as, associated auscultatory blood pressure measurement mode, detection of irregular heart beat or specifically atrial fibrillation, automated memory, and computer link or blue-tooth transfer of readings [91]. The use of oscillometric devices for office blood pressure measurement is still debatable in the presence of atrial fibrillation [92]. However, the results of recent studies suggested that in atrial fibrillation, oscillometric blood pressure monitors had similar accuracy in both systolic and diastolic blood pressure measurements as the repeated auscultatory method [92].

Whatever devices are used, they should be regularly calibrated. When automated blood pressure monitors are used, they should be validated. In the latter case, mercury column-based sphygmomanometers, although being phasing out in office blood pressure measurement, are still critical for evaluating the accuracy of algorithm-based electronic devices [1].

Body Position; Resting Period

Most studies reported seated blood pressure levels, and the resting time before the initial measurement varied from 3–10 min, with the most frequent resting period being 5 min. In several early studies (before 2000), blood pressure was measured at supine position [24] or both supine and standing positions [7], usually after 5 min rest in the supine position. In some other studies, blood pressure was measured at both seated and standing positions [38, 48, 57]. Standing blood pressure was measured usually after 1–3 min standing.

Number of Blood Pressure Readings; Time of Interval

In most trials, multiple (2 to 6) blood pressure readings were obtained. However, the ultimately recorded value varied from the lowest to an average of two or three readings or the last two of three readings. The time interval between consecutive readings ranged from 30–120 s (Table 14.1).

Arm Side and Cuff

Blood pressure was measured on the upper arm in almost all trials, although this was rarely acknowledged explicitly. The arm side for blood pressure measurement was also infrequently noted. However, most commonly it was the right arm or the arm with the higher blood pressure value. The actual protocol used to determine the correct cuff size was rarely stated. However, an "appropriate size" was frequently delineated. Other aspects, such as whether the brachial artery was positioned at the "heart level" as per guideline, could not be assessed in most trials.

Timing of Blood Pressure Measurement

"Trough" blood pressure levels were most commonly obtained although indicated in only a minority of trials, and the trough time is usually at 20–26 h after the last antihypertensive medication dosage.

The blood pressure measurement guidelines do not mandate timing of blood pressure measurement. However, for the purpose of comparability between trial groups and over time, blood pressure should be measured at "trough" effect hours in all comparison studies. This is indeed mandatory for the approval of any medication by the Food and Drug Administration [93]. For a claimed once daily medication, the trough efficacy of blood pressure lowering has to be at least 50% of the peak effect [93]. However, the timing in relation to the last medication dosage is rarely discussed in the guidelines [1–3].

Clinical Implications

Office blood pressure measurement has been used for the diagnosis and therapeutic monitoring of hypertension for more than a century. Office blood pressure still has a role in the screening, diagnosis, and follow-up of hypertension, but has apparent drawback of over-diagnosis and under-diagnosis of hypertension because of the white-coat and masked hypertension, respectively [92].

AOBP seems to be a superior office blood pressure measurement method. However, it should be recognized that although the blood pressure values of AOBP may be more strongly associated with hypertension-related target organ damage, there is no evidence to date that treatment decisions on the basis of AOBP yield better cardiovascular outcomes than the conventional office blood pressure measurement [94]. More research, especially outcome trial research, is needed before a universal recommendation can be made on the use of automated office blood pressure in clinical practice. A lower cut-off value of 135/85 mmHg has been proposed when AOBP is used for the diagnosis of hypertension, as compared with the conventional office blood pressure measurement [95, 96]. The results of a recent study in 3627 participants also suggested that 135/85 mmHg may be an appropriate threshold for the diagnosis of hypertension in older subjects using AOBP [97].

As compared with any office blood pressure measurement, out-of-office blood pressure measurement, such as ambulatory and home blood pressure monitoring, has apparent advantages. It is devoid of white-coat effect, and by comparing with office blood pressure may identify white-coat hypertension. It may help in the diagnosis of masked hypertension, including nocturnal hypertension [98]. It may also improve cardiovascular prediction by measuring nocturnal dipping, morning blood pressure surge, and reading-to-reading blood pressure variability [99]. Nonetheless, the superiority of ambulatory and home blood pressure monitoring over office blood pressure in guiding antihypertensive therapy, in terms of cardiovascular disease prevention, has not yet been fully proven by randomized controlled trials [100], needless to say its limited availability in both high and low-income settings.

Future randomized clinical trials should consider the use of these novel office or out-of-office blood pressure measurements in the guidance of antihypertensive therapy and prevention of cardiovascular events.

References

1. Pickering TG, Hall JE, Appel LJ, Falkner BE, Graves J, Hill MN, et al. Recommendations for blood pressure measurement in humans and experimental animals: part 1: blood pressure measurement in humans: a statement for professionals from the Subcommittee of Professional and Public Education of the American Heart Association Council on High Blood Pressure Research. Circulation. 2005;111:697–716.
2. O'Brien E, Asmar R, Beilin L, Imai Y, Mancia G, Mengden T, et al. Practice guidelines of the European Society of Hypertension for clinic, ambulatory and self blood pressure measurement. J Hypertens. 2005;23:697–701.
3. O'Brien E, Asmar R, Beilin L, Imai Y, Mallion JM, Mancia G, et al. European Society of Hypertension recommendations for conventional, ambulatory and home blood pressure measurement. J Hypertens. 2003;21:821–48.
4. The Systolic Hypertension in the Elderly Program (SHEP) Cooperative Research Group. Prevention of stroke by antihypertensive drug treatment in older persons with isolated systolic hypertension. Final results of the SHEP. JAMA. 1991;265:3255–64.
5. The Systolic Hypertension in the Elderly Program (SHEP) Cooperative Research Group. Rationale and design of a randomized clinical trial on prevention of stroke in isolated systolic hypertension. J Clin Epidemiol. 1988;41:1197–208.
6. Labarthe DR, Blaufox MD, Smith WM, Lacy CR, Schnaper H, LaBaw F, et al. Systolic Hypertension in the Elderly Program (SHEP). Part 5: baseline blood pressure and pulse rate measurements. Hypertension. 1991;17(3 Suppl):II62–76.
7. Dahlof B, Lindholm LH, Hansson L, Schersten B, Ekbom T, Wester PO. Morbidity and mortality in the Swedish Trial in Old Patients with Hypertension (STOP-Hypertension). Lancet. 1991;338:1281–5.
8. Dahlöf B, Hansson L, Lindholm L, Råstam L, Scherstén B, Wester PO. STOP-Hypertension: Swedish trial in old patients with hypertension. J Hypertens. 1986;4:511–3.
9. Dahlöf B, Hansson L, Lindholm L, Schersten B, Wester PO. STOP-Hypertension-preliminary communication from the pilot study of the Swedish Trial in Old Patients with Hypertension. J Hypertens. 1987;5(Suppl. 5):S607–10.
10. Hansson L, Dahlöf B, Ekbom T, Lindholm L, Scherstén B, Wester PO. Key learnings from the STOP-Hypertension study: an update on the progress of the ongoing Swedish study of antihypertensive treatment in the elderly. Cardiovasc Drugs Ther. 1991;4(Suppl 6):1253–5.
11. MRC Working Party. Medical Research Council trial of treatment of hypertension in older adults: principal results. BMJ. 1992;304:405–12.
12. Neaton JD, Grimm RH Jr, Prineas RJ, Stamler J, Grandits GA, Elmer PJ, et al. Treatment of Mild Hypertension Study Research Group. Treatment of Mild Hypertension Study. Final results. JAMA. 1993;270:713–24.
13. Treatment of Mild Hypertension Research Group. A randomized, placebo-controlled trial of a nutritional-hygienic regimen along with various drug monotherapies. Arch Intern Med. 1991;151:1413–23.
14. Staessen JA, Fagard R, Thijs L, Celis H, Arabidze GG, Birkenhäger WH, et al. The Systolic Hypertension in Europe (Syst-Eur) Trial Investigators. Randomised double-blind comparison of placebo and active treatment for older patients with isolated systolic hypertension. Lancet. 1997;350:757–64.
15. Amery A, Birkenhäger W, Bulpitt CJ, Clément D, De Leeuw P, Dollery CT, et al. Syst-Eur: a multicentre trial on the treatment of isolated systolic hypertension in the elderly: objectives, protocol, and organization. Aging Clin Exp Res. 1991;3:287–302.
16. Slovick DI, Amery A, Birkenhager W, Bulpitt CJ, Cox J, de Leeuw P, et al. SYST-EUR multicentre trial on the treatment of isolated systolic hypertension in the elderly: first interim report. J Hum Hypertens. 1993;7:201–3.
17. Staessen J, Bert P, Bulpitt C, De Cort P, Fagard R, Fletcher A, et al. Nitrendipine in older patients with isolated systolic hypertension: second progress report on the SYST-EUR trial. J Hum Hypertens. 1993;7:265–71.
18. Liu L, Wang JG, Gong L, Liu G, Staessen JA. Systolic Hypertension in China (Syst-China) Collaborative Group. Comparison of active treatment and placebo in older Chinese patients with isolated systolic hypertension. J Hypertens. 1998;16:1823–9.
19. Wang JG, Liu G, Wang X, Zhang S, Sun M, Pan X, et al. Long-term blood pressure control in older Chinese patients with isolated systolic hypertension: a progress report on the Syst-China trial. J Hum Hypertens. 1996;10:735–42.
20. Hansson L, Zanchetti A, Carruthers SG, Dahlof B, Elmfeldt D, Julius S, et al. Effects of intensive blood-pressure lowering and low-dose aspirin in patients with hypertension: principal results of the Hypertension Optimal Treatment (HOT) randomised trial. HOT Study Group. Lancet. 1998;351:1755–62.
21. Kjeldsen SE, Hedner T, Jamerson K, Julius S, Haley WE, Zabalgoitia M, et al. Hypertension Optimal Treatment (HOT) study home blood pressure in treated hypertensive subjects. Hypertension. 1998;31:1014–20.
22. Mancia G, Omboni S, Parati G, Clement DL, Haley WE, Rahman SN, et al. Twenty-four hour ambulatory blood pressure in the Hypertension

Optimal Treatment (HOT) study. J Hypertens. 2001;19:1755–63.
23. National Intervention Cooperative Study in Elderly Hypertensives Study Group. Randomized double-blind comparison of a calcium antagonist and a diuretic in elderly hypertensives. Hypertension. 1999;34:1129–33.
24. Hansson L, Lindholm LH, Niskanen L, Lanke J, Hedner T, Niklason A, et al. Effect of angiotensin converting enzyme inhibition compared with conventional therapy on cardiovascular morbidity and mortality in hypertension: the Captopril Prevention Project (CAPPP) randomised trial. Lancet. 1999;353:611–6.
25. Hansson L, Hedner T, Lund-Johansen P, Kjeldsen SE, Lindholm LH, Syvertsen JO, et al. Randomised trial of effects of calcium antagonists compared with diuretics and beta-blockers on cardiovascular morbidity and mortality in hypertension: the Nordic Diltiazem (NORDIL) study. Lancet. 2000;356:359–65.
26. Lund-Johansen P, Omvik P. Effect of long-term diltiazem treatment on central haemodynamics and exercise endurance in essential hypertension. Eur Heart J. 1990;11:543–51.
27. Brown MJ, Palmer CR, Castaigne A, de Leeuw PW, Mancia G, Rosenthal T, et al. Morbidity and mortality in patients randomised to double-blind treatment with a long-acting calcium-channel blocker or diuretic in the International Nifedipine GITS study: Intervention as a Goal in Hypertension Treatment (INSIGHT). Lancet. 2000;356:366–72.
28. Mancia G, Omboni S, Parati G. Investigators of the INSIGHT ABPM substudy. Twenty-four hour ambulatory blood pressure in the International Nifedipine GITS study Intervention as a Goal in Hypertension Treatment (INSIGHT). J Hypertens. 2002;20:545–53.
29. PROGRESS Collaborative Group. Randomised trial of a perindopril-based blood-pressure-lowering regimen among 6,105 individuals with previous stroke or transient ischaemic attack. Lancet. 2001;358:1033–41.
30. PROGRESS Management Committee. Blood pressure lowering for the secondary prevention of stroke: rationale and design for PROGRESS. J Hypertens Suppl. 1996;14:S41–5; discussion S45–6
31. PROGRESS Management Committee. PROGRESS – perindopril protection against recurrent stroke study: characteristics of the study population at baseline. J Hypertens. 1999;17:1647–55.
32. Arima H, Anderson C, Omae T, Woodward M, Hata J, Murakami Y, et al. Effects of blood pressure lowering on major vascular events among patients with isolated diastolic hypertension: the perindopril protection against recurrent stroke study (PROGRESS) trial. Stroke. 2011;42:2339–41.
33. Lewis EJ, Hunsicker LG, Clarke WR, Berl T, Pohl MA, Lewis JB, Collaborative Study et al. Group. Renoprotective effect of the angiotensin-receptor antagonist irbesartan in patients with nephropathy due to type 2 diabetes. N Engl J Med. 2001;345:851–60.
34. Berl T, Hunsicker LG, Lewis JB, Pfeffer MA, Porush JG, Rouleau JL, et al. Cardiovascular outcomes in the Irbesartan Diabetic Nephropathy Trial of patients with type 2 diabetes and overt nephropathy. Ann Intern Med. 2003;138:542–9.
35. Rodby RA, Rohde RD, Clarke WR, Hunsicker LG, Anzalone DA, Atkins RC, et al. For the Collaborative Study Group. The Irbesartan type II diabetic nephropathy trial: study design and baseline patient characteristics. Nephrol Dial Transplant. 2000;15:487–97.
36. Svensson P, de Faire U, Sleight P, Yusuf S, Ostergren J. Comparative effects of Ramipril on ambulatory and office blood pressures a HOPE substudy. Hypertension. 2001;38:e28–32.
37. Yusuf S, Sleight P, Pogue J, Bosch J, Davies R, Dagenais G. Effects of an angiotensin-converting-enzyme inhibitor, ramipril, on cardiovascular events in high-risk patients. The Heart Outcomes Prevention Evaluation Study Investigators. N Engl J Med. 2000;342:145–53.
38. Dahlof B, Devereux RB, Kjeldsen SE, Julius S, Beevers G, de Faire U, et al. Cardiovascular morbidity and mortality in the Losartan Intervention for Endpoint reduction in hypertension study (LIFE): a randomized trial against atenolol. Lancet. 2002;359:995–1003.
39. Dahlöf B, Devereux RB, de Faire U, Fyhrquist F, Hedner T, Ibsen H, et al. The Losartan Intervention for Endpoint reduction (LIFE) in hypertension study: rationale, design, and methods. Am J Hypertens. 1997;10:705–13.
40. Dahlöf B, Devereux RB, Julius S, Kjeldsen SE, Beevers G, de Faire U, et al. Characteristics of 9,194 patients with left ventricular hypertrophy: the LIFE study. Hypertension. 1998;32:989–97.
41. Kjeldsen SE, Dahlöf B, Devereux RB, Julius S, de Faire U, Fyhrquist F, et al. Lowering of blood pressure and predictors of response in patients with left ventricular hypertrophy: the LIFE study. Am J Hypertens. 2000;13:899–906.
42. The ALLHAT Officers and Coordinators for the ALLHAT Collaborative Research Group. Major outcomes in high-risk hypertensive patients randomized to angiotensin-converting enzyme inhibitor or calcium channel blocker vs diuretic: The Antihypertensive and Lipid-Lowering Treatment to Prevent Heart Attack Trial (ALLHAT). JAMA. 2002;288:2981–97.
43. Davis BR, Cutler JA, Furberg CD, Wright JT, Farber MA, Felicetta JV, et al. Relationship of antihypertensive treatment regimens and change in blood pressure to risk for heart failure in hypertensive patients randomly assigned to doxazosin or chlorthalidone: further analyses from the Antihypertensive and Lipid-Lowering treatment to prevent Heart Attack Trial. Ann Intern Med. 2002;137(5 Part 1):313–20.

44. ALLHAT Collaborative Research Group. Major cardiovascular events in hypertensive patients randomized to doxazosin vs chlorthalidone: the antihypertensive and lipid-lowering treatment to prevent heart attack trial (ALLHAT). JAMA. 2000;283:1967–75.
45. Grimm RH Jr, Margolis KL, Papademetriou V, Cushman WC, Ford CE, Bettencourt J, et al. Baseline characteristics of participants in the Antihypertensive and Lipid Lowering Treatment to Prevent Heart Attack Trial (ALLHAT). Hypertension. 2001;37:19–27.
46. Wing LM, Reid CM, Ryan P, Beilin LJ, Brown MA, Jennings GL, et al. A comparison of outcomes with angiotensin-converting–enzyme inhibitors and diuretics for hypertension in the elderly. N Engl J Med. 2003;348:583–92.
47. Management Committee on behalf of the High Blood Pressure Research Council of Australia. Australian comparative outcome trial of angiotensin-converting enzyme inhibitor and diuretic based treatment of hypertension in the elderly (ANBP2): objective and protocol. Clin Exp Pharmacol Physiol. 1997;24:188–92.
48. Lithell H, Hansson L, Skoog I, Elmfeldt D, Hofman A, Olofsson B, et al. The Study on Cognition and Prognosis in the Elderly (SCOPE): principal results of a randomized double-blind intervention trial. J Hypertens. 2003;21:875–86.
49. Hansson L, Lithell H, Skoog I, Baro F, Bánki CM, Breteler M, et al. Study on cognition and prognosis in the elderly (SCOPE). Blood Press. 1999;8:177–83.
50. Pepine CJ, Handberg EM, Cooper-DeHoff RM, Marks RG, Kowey P, Messerli FH, et al. Acalcium antagonist vs a non-calcium antagonist hypertension treatment strategy for patients with coronary artery disease. The International Verapamil-Trandolapril Study (INVEST): a randomized controlled trial. JAMA. 2003;290:2805–16.
51. Pepine CJ, Handberg-Thurmond E, Marks RG, Conlon M, Cooper-DeHoff R, Volkers P, et al. Rationale and design of the International Verapamil SR/Trandolapril Study (INVEST): an Internet-based randomized trial in coronary artery disease patients with hypertension. J Am Coll Cardiol. 1998;32:1228–37.
52. Wassertheil-Smoller S, Psaty B, Greenland P, Oberman A, Kotchen T, Mouton C, et al. Association between cardiovascular outcomes and antihypertensive drug treatment in older women. JAMA. 2004;292:2849–59.
53. WHI Study Group. Design of the Women's Healthi nitiative clinical trial and observational study. Control Clin Trials. 1988;19:61–109.
54. Julius S, Kjeldsen SE, Weber M, Brunner HR, Ekman S, Hansson L, et al. Outcomes in hypertensive patients at high cardiovascular risk treated with regimens based on valsartan or amlodipine: the VALUE randomised trial. Lancet. 2004;363:2022–31.
55. Dahlof B, Sever PS, Poulter NR, Wedel H, Beevers DG, Caulfield M, et al. Prevention of cardiovascular events with an antihypertensive regimen of amlodipine adding perindopril as required versus atenolol adding bendroflumethiazide as required, in the Anglo-Scandinavian Cardiac Outcomes Trial-Blood Pressure Lowering Arm (ASCOT-BPLA): a multicenter randomized controlled trial. Lancet. 2005;366:895–906.
56. Sever PS, Dahlöf B, Poulter NR, Wedel H, Beevers G, Caulfield M, et al. Rationale, design, methods and baseline demography of participants of the Anglo-Scandinavian Cardiac Outcomes Trial. J Hypertens. 2001;19:1139–47.
57. Liu L, Zhang Y, Liu G, Li W, Zhang X, Zanchetti A. The Felodipine Event Reduction (FEVER) study: a randomized long-term placebocontrolled trial in Chinese hypertensive patients. J Hypertens. 2005;23:2157–72.
58. Suzuki H, Kanno Y. Effects of candesartan on cardiovascular outcomes in Japanese hypertensive patients. Hypertens Res. 2005;28:307–14.
59. ADVANCE Collaborative Group. Effects of a fixed combination of perindopriland indapamide on macrovascular and microvascular outcomes in patients with type 2 diabetes mellitus (the ADVANCE trial): a randomised controlled trial. Lancet. 2007;370:829–40.
60. Parving HH, Persson F, Lewis JB, Lewis EJ, Hollenberg NK, AVOID Study Investigators. Aliskiren combined with losartan in type 2 diabetes and nephropathy. N Engl J Med. 2008;358:2433–46.
61. ONTARGET Investigators. Telmisartan, ramipril, or both in patients at high risk for vascular events. N Engl J Med. 2008;358:1547–59.
62. Redon J, Mancia G, Sleight P, Schumacher H, Gao P, Pogue J, et al. Safety and efficacy of low blood pressures among patients with diabetes: subgroup analyses from the ONTARGET (ONgoing Telmisartan Alone and in combination with Ramipril Global Endpoint Trial). J Am Coll Cardiol. 2012;59:74–83.
63. Teo K, Yusuf S, Sleight P, Anderson C, Mookadam F, Ramos B, et al. Rationale, design, and baseline characteristics of 2 large, simple, randomized trials evaluating telmisartan, ramipril, and their combination in high-risk patients: the Ongoing Telmisartan Alone and in Combination with Ramipril Global Endpoint Trial/Telmisartan randomized assessment study in ACE intolerant subjects with cardiovascular disease (ONTARGET/TRANSCEND) trials. Am Heart J. 2004;148:52–61.
64. Jamerson K, Weber MA, Bakris GL, Dahlof B, Pitt B, Shi V, et al. Benazepril plus amlodipine or hydrochlorothiazide for hypertension in high-risk patients. N Engl J Med. 2008;359:2417–28.
65. Jamerson KA, Bakris GL, Wun CC, Dahlöf B, Lefkowitz M, Manfreda S, et al. Rationale and design of the Avoiding Cardiovascular events through COMbination therapy in Patients LIving with Systolic Hypertension (ACCOMPLISH) trial:

the first randomized controlled trial to compare the clinical outcome effects of first-line combination therapies in hypertension. Am J Hypertens. 2004;17:793–801.
66. Weber MA, Bakris GL, Dahlöf B, Pitt B, Velazquez E, Gupte J, et al. Baseline characteristics in the Avoiding Cardiovascular events through Combination therapy in Patients Living with Systolic Hypertension (ACCOMPLISH) trial: a hypertensive population at high cardiovascular risk. Blood Press. 2007;16:13–9.
67. JATOS Study Group. Principal results of the Japanese trial to assess optimal systolic blood pressure in elderly hypertensive patients (JATOS). Hypertens Res. 2008;31:2115–27.
68. JATOS Study Group. The Japanese Trial to Assess Optimal Systolic Blood Pressure in Elderly Hypertensive patients (JATOS): protocol, patient characteristics, and blood pressure during the first 12 months. Hypertens Res. 2005;28:513–20.
69. Ogihara T, Nakao K, Fukui T, Fukiyama K, Ueshima K, Oba K, et al. Effects of candesartan compared with amlodipine in hypertensive patients with high cardiovascular risks: candesartan antihypertensive survival evaluation in Japan trial. Hypertension. 2008;51:393–8.
70. Kasanuki H, Hagiwara N, Hosoda S, Sumiyoshi T, Honda T, Haze K, et al. Angiotensin II receptor blocker-based vs. non-angiotensin II receptor blocker based therapy in patients with angiographically documented coronary artery disease and hypertension: the Heart Institute of Japan Candesartan Randomized Trial for Evaluation in Coronary Artery Disease (HIJCREATE). Eur Heart J. 2009;30:1203–12.
71. The ACCORD Study Group. Effects of intensive blood-pressure control in type 2 diabetes mellitus. N Engl J Med. 2010;362:1575–85.
72. Cushman WC, Grimm RH Jr, Cutler JA, Evans GW, Capes S, Corson MA, et al. Rationale and design for the blood pressure intervention of the Action to Control Cardiovascular Risk in Diabetes (ACCORD) trial. Am J Cardiol. 2007;99(Suppl 12A):44i–55i.
73. Matsuzaki M, Ogihara T, Umemoto S, Rakugi H, Matsuoka H, Shimada K, et al. Prevention of cardiovascular events with calcium channel blocker-based combination therapies in patients with hypertension: a randomized controlled trial. J Hypertens. 2011;29:1649–59.
74. Ogawa H, Kim-Mitsuyama S, Matsui K, Jinnouchi T, Jinnouchi H, Arakawa K. Angiotensin II receptor blocker-based therapy in Japanese elderly, high-risk, hypertensive patients. Am J Med. 2012;125:981–90.
75. Ogawa H, Kim-Mitsuyama S, Jinnouchi T, Matsui K, Arakawa K. Rationale, design and patient baseline characteristics of OlmeSartan and calcium antagonists randomized (OSCAR) study: a study comparing the incidence of cardiovascular events between high-dose angiotensin II receptor blocker (ARB) monotherapy and combination therapy of ARB with calcium channel blocker in Japanese elderly high-risk hypertensive patients. Hypertens Res. 2009;32:575–80.
76. Muramatsu T, Matsushita K, Yamashita K, Kondo T, Maeda K, Shintani S, et al. Comparison between valsartan and amlodipine regarding cardiovascular morbidity and mortality in hypertensive patients with glucose intolerance: NAGOYA HEART study. Hypertension. 2012;59:580–6.
77. Matsushita K, Muramatsu T, Kondo T, Maeda K, Shintani S, Murohara T, et al. Rationale and design of the NAGOYA HEART study: comparison between valsartan and amlodipine regarding morbidity and mortality in patients with hypertension and glucose intolerance. J Cardiol. 2010;56:111–7.
78. SPRINT Research Group, Wright JT Jr, Williamson JD, Whelton PK, Snyder JK, Sink KM, et al. A randomized trial of intensive versus standard blood-pressure control. N Engl J Med. 2015;373:2103–16.
79. Kjeldsen SE, Lund-Johansen P, Nilsson PM, Mancia G. Unattended blood pressure measurements in the systolic blood pressure intervention trial: implications for entry and achieved blood pressure values compared with other trials. Hypertension. 2016;67:808–12.
80. Drawz PE, Pajewski NM, Bates JT, Bello NA, Cushman WC, Dwyer JP, et al. Effect of intensive versus standard clinic-based hypertension management on ambulatory blood pressure: results from the SPRINT (Systolic Blood Pressure Intervention Trial) ambulatory blood pressure study. Hypertension. 2017;69:42–50.
81. Lonn E, Bosch J, Pogue J, Avezum A, Chazova I, Dans A, et al. Novel approaches in primary cardiovascular disease prevention: the HOPE-3 trial rationale, design, and Participants' baseline characteristics. Can J Cardiol. 2016;32:311–8.
82. Lonn EM, Bosch J, López-Jaramillo P, Zhu J, Liu L, Pais P, et al. Blood-pressure lowering in intermediate-risk persons without cardiovascular disease. N Engl J Med. 2016;374:2009–20.
83. Grim CE, Li J, Grim CM. Poor retention of blood pressure measurement knowledge and practice by medical students (abstract). Am J Hypertens. 1999;12:150A.
84. Graves JW, Sheps SG. Does evidence-based medicine suggest that physicians should not be measuring blood pressure in the hypertensive patient? Am J Hypertens. 2004;17:354–60.
85. Myers MG. The great myth of office blood pressure measurement. J Hypertens. 2012;39:1894–8.
86. Andreadis EA, Agaliotis GD, Angelopoulos ET, Tsakanikas AP, Chaveles IA, Mousoulis GP. Automated office blood pressure and 2h ambulatory measurements are equally associated with left ventricular mass index. Am J Hypertens. 2011;24:661–6.
87. Filipovský J, Seidlerová J, Kratochvíl Z, Karnosová P, Hronová M, Mayer O Jr. Automated compared to manual office blood pressure and to home blood

pressure in hypertensive patients. Blood Press. 2016;25:228–34.

88. Myers MG, Godwin M, Dawes M, Kiss A, Tobe SW, Kaczorowski J. Measurement of blood pressure in the office: recognizing the problem and proposing the solution. Hypertension. 2010;55:195–200.
89. Mancia G, Fagard R, Narkiewicz K, Redon J, Zanchetti A, Böhm M, et al. 2013 ESH/ESC guidelines for the management of arterial hypertension: the task force for the management of arterial hypertension of the European Society of Hypertension (ESH) and of the European Society of Cardiology (ESC). Eur Heart J. 2013;34:2159–219.
90. Stergiou GS, Parati G, Asmar R, O'Brien E. European Society of Hypertension Working Group on blood pressure monitoring. Requirements for professional office blood pressure monitors. J Hypertens. 2012;30:537–42.
91. Medaval. The standard for medical device evaluation. Blood pressure monitors. www.medaval.org. Assessed 4 Nov 2015.
92. Stergiou GS, Kollias A, Destounis A, Tzamouranis D. Automated blood pressure measurement in atrial fibrillation: a systematic review and meta-analysis. J Hypertens. 2012;30:2074–82.
93. Feig PU, Roy S, Cody RJ. Antihypertensive drug development: current challenges and future opportunities. J Am Soc Hypertens. 2010;4:163–73.
94. Stergiou GS, Parati G, Vlachopoulos C, Achimastos A, Andreadis E, Asmar R, et al. Methodology and technology for peripheral and central blood pressure and blood pressure variability measurement: current status and future directions - Position statement of the European Society of Hypertension Working Group on blood pressure monitoring and cardiovascular variability. J Hypertens. 2016;34:1665–77.
95. Myers MG, Tobe SW, McKay D, Bolli P, Hemmelgarn BR, McAlister FA. New algorithm for the diagnosis of hypertension. Am J Hypertens. 2005;18:1369–74.
96. National Institute for Health and Clinical Excellence. Hypertension, NICE clinical guidelines 127. London, UK: National Clinical Guidelines Centre; 2011.
97. Myers MG, Kaczorowski J, Paterson JM, Dolovich L, Tu K. Thresholds for diagnosing hypertension based on automated office blood pressure measurements and cardiovascular risk. Hypertension. 2015;66:489–95.
98. Li Y, Staessen JA, Lu L, Li LH, Wang GL, Wang JG. Is isolated nocturnal hypertension a novel clinical entity? Findings from a Chinese population study. Hypertension. 2007;50:333–9.
99. O'Brien E, Parati G, Stergiou G, Asmar R, Beilin L, Bilo G, et al. European Society of Hypertension position paper on ambulatory blood pressure monitoring. J Hypertens. 2013;31:1731–68.
100. Parati G, Stergiou GS, Asmar R, Bilo G, de Leeuw P, Imai Y, et al. European Society of Hypertension guidelines for blood pressure monitoring at home: a summary report of the second international consensus conference on home blood pressure monitoring. J Hypertens. 2008;26:1505–26.

Part IV

Pioneers in Hypertension Research

The Life and the Major Scientific Contributions of Irvine Page

15

Emmanuel A. Andreadis
and Charalampia V. Geladari

It is universally acknowledged that Irvine Heinly Page was one of the most acclaimed physicians of his times. He is still considered to be a pioneer researcher in the field of Hypertension since his scientific contributions are tremendous and have positively impacted the lives of thousands of hypertensives around the world [1]. We truly feel that it is necessary for a young scientist engaged in hypertension research to be aware of his life and works, as he can be an excellent role model for many to follow, and his work, a great fountain of inspiration to researchers, worldwide. It is an honor to write this chapter-tribute to him, yet a difficult venture, since we have not met him ever in person, and have never interacted with him personally. We guess that not many are blessed with such a gift to enjoy the great satisfaction derived from the interaction with such a mentor and personality.

Dr. Irvine Page was born in Indianapolis, in Indiana, at the dawn of the Twenteeth Century, in 1901. His father, Lafayette Page, was a respectable physician in the topical community, and this surely influenced his decision to become a doctor. His brother was a lawyer, and his sister, Ruth Page, was an accomplished ballet dancer, who died in 1991. Irvine Page himself was not devoid of music education since as a teenager he played the banjo and he wanted also to become a professional musician. This asset helped him to gain financial support in college as he directed a dance band and nicely supplemented his family's backing, while he enrolled in the Cornell University. He graduated in 1921 when he earned a degree in Chemistry. Afterwards, he worked for a period of 1 year with the great Elliot Joslin on Insulin, which was then, newly-discovered. Biochemistry was indeed a fascinating field for the young Page, and he enrolled in Cornell Medical College, having being attracted by James Sumner, a distinguished biochemist and a Nobel Prize Winner for his work on crystallizing urease. There, the Dean of Medicine, having recognized his exceptional talent in Biochemistry, persuaded him to enroll in Medical School and pursue a career as a physician scientist [1, 2].

After having received his medical degree from Cornell University, he trained as an Intern for 2 years at the Bellevue Hospital and the

E. A. Andreadis (✉)
Hypertension and Cardiovascular Disease Prevention Center, Evangelismos General Hospital, Athens, Greece

Fourth Internal Medicine Department, Evangelismos State General Hospital, Athens, Greece

C. V. Geladari
Fourth Internal Medicine Department, Evangelismos State General Hospital, Athens, Greece

Department of Medicine, Division of Cardiology, Beth Israel Deaconess Medical Center, Harvard Medical School, Boston, MA, USA

V. Papademetriou et al. (eds.), *Management of Hypertension*,
https://doi.org/10.1007/978-3-319-92946-0_15

Presbyterian Hospital, in New York City. However, his passion for Biochemistry was not suppressed by his love for medicine and his patients. Therefore, when in 1928, was invited to join the Kaiser Wilhelm Institute of Psychiatry in Munich, he accepted the invitation and moved on to establish a new department of brain chemistry there. He soon met and married his wife, Beatrice Allen, who – as his sister – was a dancer. Dr. Irvine Page had done an exceptional work at the Kaiser Wilhelm Institute and no similar department existed anywhere in the world at that time, a fact that establishes Dr. Page as an innovator [3].

Under the threat of the Second World War and the rise of Hitler's Empire, he decided to return in the United States of America, to find a shelter for his family and continue his scientific activities in his homeland. Yet, no position was offered to him to work there. And then, he had a godsent stroke of luck. Dr. Donald Van Slyke, a renowned Dutch American Biochemist, while visiting Munich with his family, called Page in the middle of the night to treat his daughter's finger infection. His daughter's infection was treated successfully and Dr. Irvine Page was surprisingly offered aposition to work at the Rockefeller Institute in New York City. Dr. Page worked there with Dr. Donald Van Slyke, from 1931 to 1937. That was it! His work on hypertension research had already begun. His interest in the field, however, had started 2 months prior to leaving Europe, when he visited Frankfurt to work with Frans Volhard and his two assistants, Bohn and Hessel, who studied hypertension and its related mechanisms [4].

At that time, hypertension was considered to be essential for the perfusion of vital organs, such as the brain, heart, and the kidneys, thus termed essential ("essentielle hypertonie"). At the Rockefeller Institute, Dr. Irvine Page made his first important observation; using colloidal sulfur injections, he lowered blood pressure, and he found that despite this fact, kidney function was well maintained, a finding contradictory to the existing belief.

After having completed his stay at the Rockefeller Institute, he moved on to work in Indianapolis City Hospital from 1937 to 1945, along with Arthur Corcoran, Kenneth Kohlstaedt and Oscar Helmer. In 1940, he published a paper about a crystalline pressor substance resulting from the reaction between renin and renin-activator, which he termed "angiotonin". One month later, Braun-Menendez et al., from Buenos Aires, published a similar work, where they termed the pressor substance causing renal hypertension, "hypertensin". As we all know, this pressor substance is now called "angiotensin", as Dr. Page and Braun-Menendez agreed some years later.

In 1945, Dr. Irvine Page moved to Cleveland Clinic where he made his most legendary contributions in the hypertension field. He lead his scientific team there successfully for the next 21 years working on hypertension and heart disease. During his leadership years, serotonin was discovered, angiotensin and angiotensin inhibitors were synthesized, nitroprusside was first used in humans, the interaction of the sympathetic nervous system and angiotensin was described, and the diagnosis and treatment of renovascular hypertension were developed. Dr. Page alsowas the first to describe the famous "mosaic theory" of hypertension.

The mosaic theory of hypertension – definitely his greatest contribution in the field –isa combination of individual and interacting mechanisms including different parameters (biochemical, disturbances of the nervous system, hormonal perturbations and structural defects in arteries and organs) that underline the pathophysiology of this complex disease. Interestingly, it has been showed that as molecular events occur in the brain, the kidney and the vasculature the response to these events depends on target tissue. Consequently, an increase neuronal firing is produced in the central nervous system, vasoconstriction and vascular remodeling in peripheral vessels occur, and sodium reabsorption in the distal renal tubule increases. Furthermore, it has been clear that genetics and environmental factors contribute to oxidant generation and inflammation. In other words, it is suggested that patients with hypertension differ among themselves due to genetic predisposition. Moreover, salt content of the diet has shown to be crucial, as environmental factor and stress trace metals could work as an additional risk factor. Anatomical factors have also been implicated as a main principle of the Mosaic Theory [1, 2].

After the recognition of the Mosaic Theory to the field of Hypertension and Cardiovascular Disease Research the Irvine Page Award has been established in order to help researchers to produce respectable results in the complex field of the pathophysiology of hypertension. He also notified the importance of prevention of heart disease suggesting that 'It is vastly more important to prevent atherosclerosis than to repair the damage after it has been done" [1, 2]. His Mosaic Theory provided an outline to study the various hypertension "forces" at a molecular and cellular level, has greatly aided our understanding of this complex and devastating condition. Today, 67 years after the development of the Theory, Page's words are confirmed "Rather the mosaic concept is intended to provide a logical and orderly way of thinking about all forms of hypertension as a subject for research and as a means of analyzing the problem in patients" [4].

Apart from being an appreciated and distinguished scientist, Dr. Irvine Page was also a great organizer and leader. He is known for organizing American Foundation for High Blood Pressure, which later became the Council of High Blood Pressure Research of the American Heart Association [4, 5]. In addition, he was a founding member of the Institute of Medicine of the National Academy of Sciences, whereas he has also been president of the American Heart Association, the American Society for Clinical Pharmacology and Therapeutics, and the Society for Experimental Biology and Medicine [5].

Dr. Irvine Page had his first heart attack in 1967, at the age of 66 years. He also had failing health for many years after a stroke, and he died from heart attack at the age of 90 in June 1991. Undoubtedly, Dr. Irvine Page contributed greatly to the understanding of hypertension, and its complex mechanisms, during his almost 60 years of scientific career, starting from publishing his first scientific paper in 1935 to the publication of a great manuscript entitled "Hypertension Mechanisms", in 1987. He will definitely be remembered as the physician-scientist who altered the course of the investigation and treatment of high blood pressure, and influenced through his studies the lives of many hypertensives around the world, having earned at the same time sincere and lasting appreciation from his peers.

References

1. Harrison DG. The mosaic theory revisited: common molecular mechanisms coordinating diverse organ and cellular events in hypertension. J Am Soc Hypertens. 2013;7:68–74.
2. Page IH. Brief commentary. The mosaic theory 32 years later. Hypertension. 1982;4:117.
3. Dustan HP. In: Dustan HP, editor. Irvine Heinly page, 1901–1991, A Biographical memoir v.68. Washington, DC: National Academy of Sciences; 1995.
4. Frohlich ED, Dustan HP, Bumpus FM, Irvine H. Page: 1901–1991. The celebration of a leader. Hypertension. 1991;18:443–5.
5. Gifford R. Profiles in cardiology: Irvine H. Page. Clin Cardiol. 1987;10:68–9.

16 Neurogenic Mechanisms in Pre-hypertension and Pharmacologic Approaches to the Prevention and Treatment of Hypertension: Highlights of Professor Stevo Julius' Scientific Contributions

Brent M. Egan

Stevo Julius, MD, ScD, has served as Professor of Medicine at the University of Michigan Medical Center for more than 50 years where he continues as Professor Emeritus. During that time, he has made numerous original and important scientific contributions. His initial research centered on defining personality characteristics and autonomic mechanisms in the hemodynamic profile of individuals with borderline hypertension or pre-hypertension [1, 2]. Dr. Julius' early work was instrumental in defining a key primary role for the sympathetic nervous system in borderline and established hypertension [3–5].

In the middle phase of his scientific career, Dr. Julius and colleagues documented a key primary role for the sympathetic nervous system in the pathogenesis of hyperinsulinemia, insulin resistance, and the cardiometabolic syndrome [6–9]. All of the cardiometabolic phenomena were associated with increased heart rate a marker of neurogenic activation. While an extensive body of research documents that excess caloric intake and obesity can drive the cardiometabolic syndrome [10], Dr. Julius demonstrated that elevated blood pressure was already present in young, normal weight children of hypertensive parents [8]. Excess weight gain and further elevation of blood pressure as well as multiple features of the cardiometabolic syndrome followed this early 'pre-hypertensive' phase. Collectively, these data suggest that sympathetic activation with elevated blood pressure can precede the cardiometabolic syndrome.

During the latter part of his still active career, Professor Julius has worked with longtime colleagues on pharmacological interventions for the prevention and treatment of hypertension [11–14]. The rational and provocative interpretation of the data from these trials has often challenged existing paradigms and stimulated critical thinking to enhance our understanding of hypertension-related risk and its mitigation. This review highlights several of Dr. Julius' original scientific contributions and the many clinically insightful and relevant applications of that work.

Borderline Hypertension – The Early Years

Personality characteristics associated with pre-hypertension and hypertension In 1964, Harburg and Julius obtained blood pressures on 800 male undergraduate students at the University of

B. M. Egan (✉)
University of South Carolina School of Medicine – Greenville, Care Coordination Institute, Greenville, SC, USA
e-mail: began@ccihealth.org

V. Papademetriou et al. (eds.), *Management of Hypertension*, https://doi.org/10.1007/978-3-319-92946-0_16

Michigan who were waiting in line to register for classes. From this group, 74 white men were selected for having systolic blood pressure BP, mmHg) values either in the upper or lower end of the distribution [1]. Students were classified as having high or low systolic BP according to their paired casual (screening and first follow-up visit), usual (self-measured home BP). Of 21 persons with a high paired casual SBP >140, 16 also had repeated home SBP readings >131. Among this group, 11 had high home BP readings, defined as sustained hypertension. The BP patterns of these young men were then related with self-ratings on the Cattell 16 Personality Factor Questionnaire.

Sustained elevation of systolic BP in male college students was associated with 'submissiveness' and 'sensitivity' as defined by Cattell's Questionnaire. Subjects with 'high paired casual' systolic BP values described themselves as motivated to obtain social contacts, but in a 'sensitive' and 'anxious' manner. Subjects who were later selected for having a single high systolic BP on first entering the physician's office (second casual reading) tended more frequently to yield in an argument and then afterwards to change their private opinions toward agreement with partners who had an initially low systolic BP [1].

A subsequent study in 1986 by Professor Julius and coworkers utilized advances in questionnaire methodology to more thoroughly dissect personality characteristics of young college males with elevated BP in the screening, clinic and home environments [2]. The questionnaires included Spielberger's State-Trait Personality Inventory, the Anger Expression Scale, and the State Anger Reaction Scale1 [15]. As with the previous study [1], BP measurements were obtained on students waiting to register for their next semester classes. Undergraduate men in the upper end of the BP distribution were recalled to complete the questionnaires and to undergo self-measured home BP measurements. Two groups were identified. One group maintained high BP at home, and the second group had normal BP at home. Of interest, the group that maintained high BP at home reported greater intensity of anger and suppressed their anger to a greater extent than the group whose BP was normal at home.

The findings in this 1986 report were consistent with Alexander's original work and hypothesis [16] that inhibition of angry or hostile impulses can increase systemic BP. Moreover, the hypertensive personality has a long-term conflict between the need for passive dependence and the need for expressing hostile impulses. According to Alexander, it is this long-term conflict which can lead to sustained elevation of arterial BP or hypertension, evident among young men in the 1986 report [2].

Linkage of anger to sympathetic activation and parasympathetic withdrawal Marci, et al. studied autonomic and prefrontal cortex responses to autobiographical recall of emotions [17]. Of emotions studied, anger was the only one to show a significant increase in sympathetic activity, accompanied by a significant decrease in cardiac parasympathetic or vagal tone as measured by the high frequency component of heart rate variability. While the study by Marci and colleagues is not the first to show that anger induces sympathetic activation, it is amongst the clearest to show a reciprocal and concomitant reduction of cardiac vagal tone.

The role of sympathetic activation and parasympathetic inhibition in the hyperkinetic hemodynamic profile of borderline hypertension Dr. Julius and colleagues published a series of papers on the hemodynamics of borderline hypertension in the prestigious American Heart Association Journal, Circulation in 1971. One report captured their work on sequential autonomic blockade of β-adrenoceptors with the non-selective blocker propranolol followed by parasympathetic inhibition using atropine [3]. Both autonomic blocking agents were administered intravenously at doses known to fully block the respective systems.

At baseline, individuals with hyperkinetic borderline hypertension had higher values than nomortensive controls for cardiac output and heart rate (Fig. 16.1). β-adrenoceptor blockade led to a larger fall of cardiac output and heart rate among individuals with hyperkinetic borderline hypertension. These data were consis-

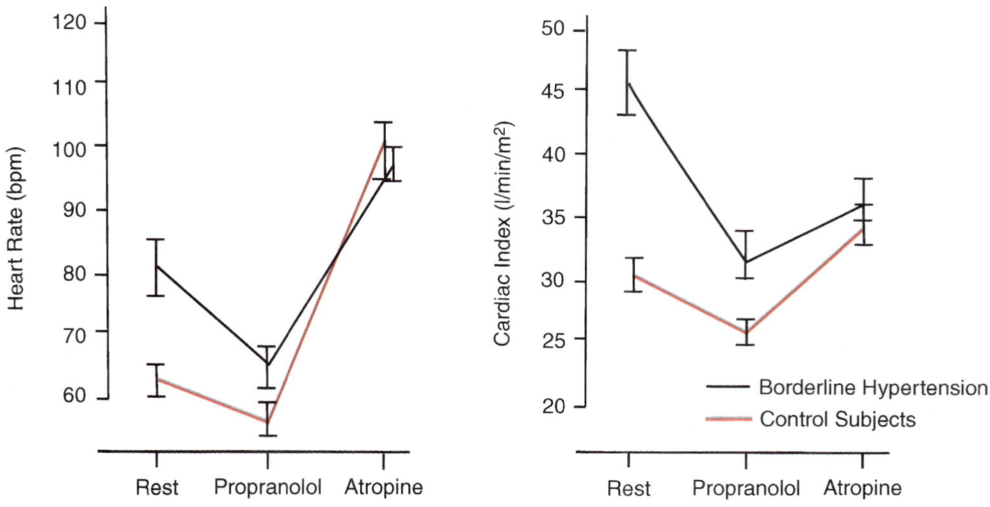

Adapted from Julius S, et al: Circulation 1971[3]

Fig. 16.1 At baseline, heart rate and cardiac index are higher in hyperkinetic borderline hypertensives than age- and sex-matched normal controls. After propranolol, heart rate and cardiac index decline more in the hyperkinetic than normal group, yet values remain higher in the former. With addition of atropine, heart rate and cardiac index increase less in the hyperkinetic than in the control group and significant between group differences were abolished

tent with increased cardiac beta-adrenergic tone in the hyperkinetic group. Yet, cardiac output and heart rate remained significantly higher in the hyperkinetic borderline hypertensive group than in the normal controls. When atropine was administered while continuing beta-adrenergic blockade with propranolol, cardiac output and heart rate increased less in subjects with hyperkinetic borderline hypertension than in normal controls. The responses to atropine indicate that cardiac parasympathetic tone is lower in hyperkinetic borderline hypertension than in normal controls.

Only after total cardiac autonomic blockade with both propranolol and atropine were the differences in cardiac output and heart rate no longer significantly different between the group with hyperkinetic borderline hypertension and healthy controls. These data indicate that the hyperkinetic state of borderline hypertension reflects a reciprocal autonomic abnormality characterized both by increased sympathetic and reduced parasympathetic tone.

Transition from hyperkinetic borderline hypertension to normokinetic borderline and established essential hypertension Research on borderline or pre-hypertension consistently identifies a hyperkinetic subset of young individuals with elevated cardiac output and a fast heart rate. Faster heart rates, even within the range of 60–100 beats/min, which are considered normal, are a strong predictor of future essential hypertension [18], and many hyperkinetic subjects appear to develop classical established hypertension [19]. However, the hyperkinetic state is much less common in adults with hypertension. Thus, transition from the hyperkinetic borderline hypertension to normokinetic, high-resistance hypertension almost certainly occurs, which is supported by data from sequential hemodynamic studies [19].

In fact, Julius and colleagues provided further evidence that individuals with borderline hypertension and normal cardiac output may represent a later phase of the prior hyperkinetic state. More specifically, baseline heart rate was elevated less among individuals with borderline hypertension and normal cardiac output than in prior studies of the hyperkinetic subset with borderline hypertension. Following cardiac autonomic blockade with intravenous propranolol and atropine, their cardiac output was lower than normal controls [20]. Heart rate responses to the β-agonist isoproterenol were less in borderline hypertensives with normal cardiac output than in demographically matched normotensive controls. The borderline blood pressure elevation in subjects with normokinetic borderline hypertensive was maintained by an elevated vascular resistance. Compared to normokinetic group with borderline hypertension, the higher blood pressure in established hypertension reflects a further increase of vascular resistance as a normal cardiac out is maintained.

Of note, while hypertension in obesity was identified as a state of high cardiac output and normal vascular resistance, vascular resistance is elevated when compared to obese, demographically matched normal controls [21, 22]. The Ann Arbor group documented that forearm vasodilator responses to regional infusion of phentolamine were greater in overweight and obese than in leaner subjects, despite higher baseline flows with normal resistance in the obese group [23]. The inappropriately normal vascular resistance in obese subjects with elevated blood pressure is maintained by enhanced vascular alpha-adrenergic tone similar to the increased vascular α-adrenergic tone similar to that observed in neurogenic, high-renin hypertension [4, 5].

Mechanisms underlying the hemodynamic transition from hyperkinetic borderline hypertension to normokinetic hypertension AUTOREGULATION. Dr. Arthur Guyton and colleagues demonstrated that volume expansion leads to increased cardiac output and tissue perfusion in excess of metabolic demands [24]. When this occurs, most organ systems increase vascular resistance to re-establish the balance between metabolic demands and supply, which raises arterial blood pressure. The phenomenon of matching blood flow to metabolic demands by varying vascular resistance is termed 'autoregulation' [25].

Basis for an alternative explanation to autoregulation for the hemodynamic transition from hyperkinetic borderline to established hypertension with normal cardiac output Studies in borderline hypertension provided two important pieces of evidence contrary to autoregulation as the mechanism for the hemodynamic transition. First, plasma volume was lower and not higher among borderline hypertensives than normal controls, when adjusted for body weight or when compared in weight-matched individuals with borderline hypertensive to healthy controls [26]. Second, in subjects with hyperkinetic borderline hypertension, higher cardiac output occurred together with greater total body oxygen consumption [27]. In fact, the regression line for cardiac output versus total body oxygen consumption was the same in subjects with borderline hypertension and demographically matched normal controls. The stimulus for autoregulation, based on whole body studies, was not apparent in hyperkinetic borderline hypertensives.

Neurogenic and vascular transformation An alternative explanation for the hemodynamic transition from hyperkinetic borderline to normokinetic borderline and essential hypertension: Focus on decreased β-adrenergic sensitivity, cardiovascular remodeling and increased vascular α-adrenergic tone.

Cardiac changes Sustained increases in cardiac sympathetic drive lead to decreased chronotropic and inotropic responses to β_1-adrenooceptor activation [20, 28, 29]. Furthermore, a decline in left ventricular compliance may contribute to lower stroke volume in patients with normokinetic mild hypertension [20, 30]. More specifically, Julius and colleagues documented that stroke volume in patients with mild hypertension was lower than in normotensive controls following cardiac autonomic blockade with propranolol and atropine. Stroke volume following cardiac autonomic blockade becomes largely dependent on end- diastolic volume. In these studies, cardiopulmonary blood volume was similar in hypertensive adults and normotensive controls, which suggests similar levels of preload [20, 30].

A stiffer, less compliant left ventricular in hypertensives could lead to lower ventricular volume end-diastole and a reduced stroke volume [28]. Decreased cardiac compliance, in turn, most likely reflects early cardiac restructuring in response to longstanding mild blood pressure elevation. Julius and coworker proposed that the combination of down-regulation of cardiac β_1-adrenergic receptors with decreased chronotropic and inotropic responses to sympathetic drive together with decreased cardiac compliance and stroke volume contribute to the normalization of cardiac output in established hypertension [31].

Vascular changes Concurrent structural vascular remodeling supports the progressive rise in vascular resistance. Sustained blood pressure elevation leads to remodeling of the arterial wall. Increased sympathetic stimulation is also well-documented vascular trophic factor [32, 33]. Thus, individuals with neurogenic borderline and established hypertension appear especially prone to cardiac and vascular remodeling. While medial smooth muscle hypertrophy with an increase in muscle wall mass can occur, the predominant change may reflect remodeling of the wall mass around a small vascular lumen based on anatomical studies in Denmark and physiologic studies in Ann Arbor [34, 35]. With either true hypertrophy with an increased vascular wall mass or remodeling of the vascular media with a normal wall mass surrounding a small lumen, the vascular wall:lumen ratio increases. In this setting, minimum vascular resistance is higher and vasoconstrictor responses are non-specifically amplified. Folkow and colleagues were the pioneers in showing how an increased wall:lumen ratio contributes to hypertension by augmenting vascular resistance and responses to vasoactive stimuli [36]. Relevant to hypertension, Flkow demonstrated that an increased wall:lumen ratio leads to a non-specific amplification of vasoconstrictor responses with a steeper slope and greater maximum vascular resistance.

Subsequent studies by Dr. Julius and colleagues in relatively young subjects with Stage 1 hypertension compared to demographically and weight-matched normotensive controls were consistent with vascular remodeling as a non-specific amplifier of arterial resistance in response to different vasoconstrictors (Fig. 16.2) [37]. Folkow's criteria for vascular remodeling as an amplifier of resistance responses were met in the Stage 1 hypertensive compared to matched controls including: (i) minimum forearm vascular resistance, an index of vascular remodeling (ii)

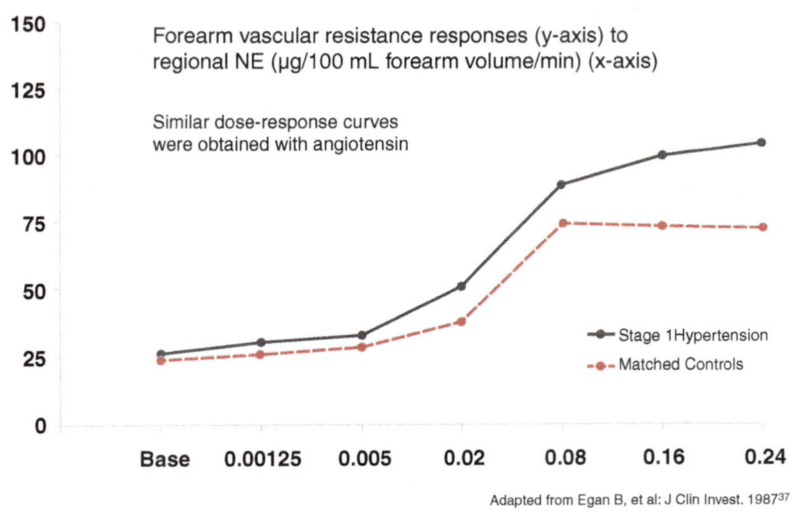

Fig. 16.2 Baseline forearm vascular resistance was slightly higher in Stage 1 hypertensives than matched normal controls. Note forearm resistance responses between the two groups diverge progressively with increasing doses of regional norepinephrine. Maximum forearm responses were also greater in hypertensives than in matched normotensive controls. Forearm vascular resistance responses to a graded regional infusion of norepinephrine (NE) are shown in Stage 1 hypertensive men and age-, sex-, race- and weight-matched normotensive controls. Note the steeper slope and greater maximum forearm resistance responses to NE in the Stage 1 hypertensive group

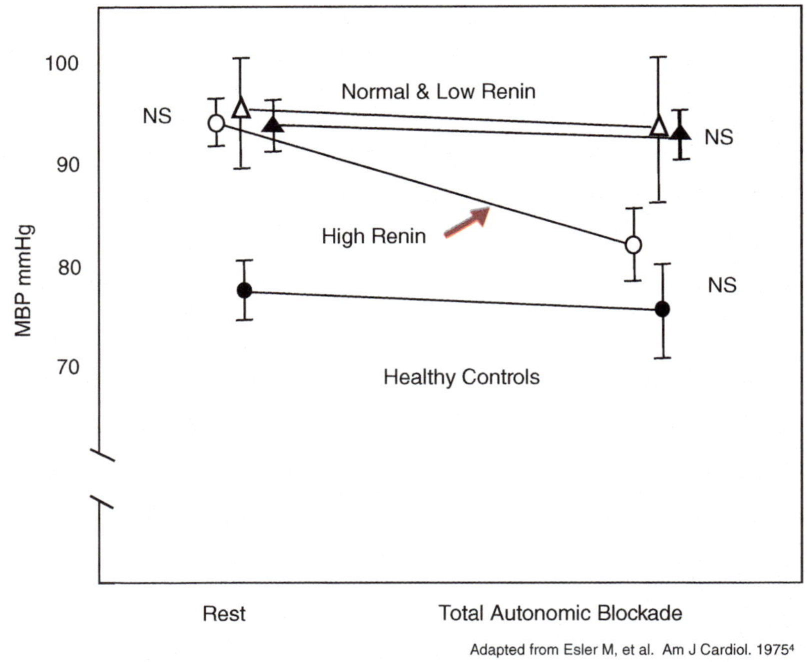

Fig. 16.3 Three groups of subjects with borderline hypertension were studied. The 3 groups included subjects with low renin (closed triangles), normal renin (open triangles) and high renin (open circles) borderline hypertension. All 3 groups with borderline hypertension had higher mean blood pressure (MBP, mmHg) at rest than healthy controls. Following total autonomic blockade with propranolol, atropine, and phentolamine, MBP fell only in the high renin group and was no longer significantly greater than MBP in normal controls (closed circles)

vascular sensitivity to both vasoconstrictors, as estimated by the concentration required to induce 30% of the maximal vasoconstrictor response, was similar (iii) forearm vasoconstrictor responses to both norepinephrine and angiotensin were characterized by a steeper slope and (iv) greater maximum resistance responses. Forearm vascular responses to both vasoconstrictors were also directly related to the minimum vascular resistance, a measure of vascular remodeling. Moreover, the vasodilator response to phentolamine was significantly greater in subjects with

Stage 1 hypertension than in controls indicating greater vascular alpha-tone. The latter finding coincides with earlier studies by Drs. Esler, Julius and colleagues described next.

Neurogenic borderline and established essential hypertension The investigative team then documented that adding systemic α-adrenergic blockade with phentolamine to cardiac autonomic blockade with propranolol and atropine normalized arterial blood pressure in approximately one-third of subjects with borderline hypertension (Fig. 16.3) [4, 5].

These subjects were characterized by high-renin values, which likely reflected increased sympathetic drive to β_1-receptors on the juxtaglomerular cells, which stimulate renin secretion. The fact that acute and total autonomic blockade normalized blood pressure by reducing vascular resistance suggested to the authors that angiotensin probably did not play a critical role in the elevated blood pressure of borderline hypertensive subjects with high plasma renin values.

The investigators subsequently extended their observations on high-renin and neurogenic hypertension to adults with established essential hypertension [5]. Subsequent studies using more contemporary methodologies including muscle sympathetic nerve activity and norepinephrine turnover documented sympathetic overactivity is present in a substantial proportion of adults with essential hypertension including those who are obese [38, 39].

Renal norepinephrine spillover as increased in obese hypertensives and normotensives with increased cardiac norepinephrine spillover in obese hypertensives. The increased renal sympathetic activity likely supports the volume expansion with obesity and in obesity hypertension, while increased sympathetic drive to other organs including the heart appears to contribute to the elevated blood pressure. One might postulate that the increased systemic blood pressure should suppress renal and cardiac sympathetic activity in the hypertensive obese subset, which would support evidence by Guyton and colleagues on the critical importance of factors intrinsic and extrinsic to the kidney that increase sodium-volume retention required to sustain hypertension [24, 25].

Sympathetic activation and the cardiometabolic syndrome In a population-based community sample in Tecumseh, MI, Dr. Julius and colleagues demonstrated that heart rate, a marker of sympathetic activation, correlated with several metabolic features of the cardiometabolic syndrome among young adults in the early phase of hypertension (Fig. 16.4) [40].

The relationship between heart rate and hyperinsulinemia was especially strong. The hyperinsulinemia most likely represents a compensatory response to insulin resistance as identified by the inverse relationship with HDL-cholesterol and direct link with hypertriglyceridemia.

Skeletal muscle is a key target organ for insulin action [41]. Resistance to insulin-mediated glucose disposal, a dominant feature of the cardiometabolic syndrome, is exacerbated by increased vascular alpha-adrenergic tone [42–45], which is a key feature of neurogenic hypertension. [4, 5] Drs. Jamerson and Julius demonstrated that insulin-mediated glucose disposal in the human forearm was acutely reduced in response to thigh-cuff inflation, which pools blood in the lower extremities, thereby unloading cardiopulmonary mechanoreceptors and inducing reflex forearm vasoconstriction [44]. In fact, reflex neurogenic vasoconstriction induced a greater degree of forearm insulin resistance than an intra-arterial norepinephrine infusion, which reduced forearm blood flow to the same extent as thigh cuff inflation [45]. Thus, reflex neurogenic vasoconstriction reduced glucose utilization by mechanisms other than or in addition to reduced blood flow (Fig. 16.5) [45].

The authors cited studies indicating that reflex neurogenic vasoconstriction reduces the number of open capillaries in skeletal muscle.

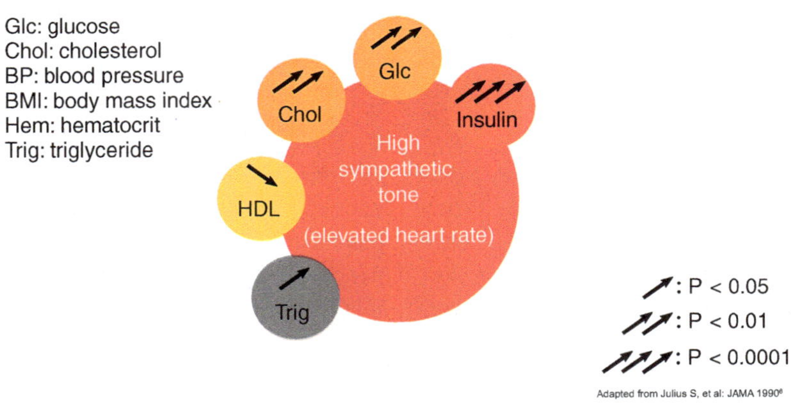

Fig. 16.4 Among young adults in Tecumseh, Michigan, Dr. Julius and colleagues documented that resting heart rate was highly correlated with plasma insulin, strongly correlated with fasting glucose (Glc) and total cholesterol (Chol), and modestly yet significantly with high-density lipoprotein cholesterol (HDL) and trigyclerides (Trig). Three arrows denotes significance at p < 0.001, two arrows p < 0.01, and a single arrow p < p0.05. Arrows pointing up and to the right indicate a positive association between heart rate and metabolic variables, whereas the arrow pointing down and to the left indicates a negative association

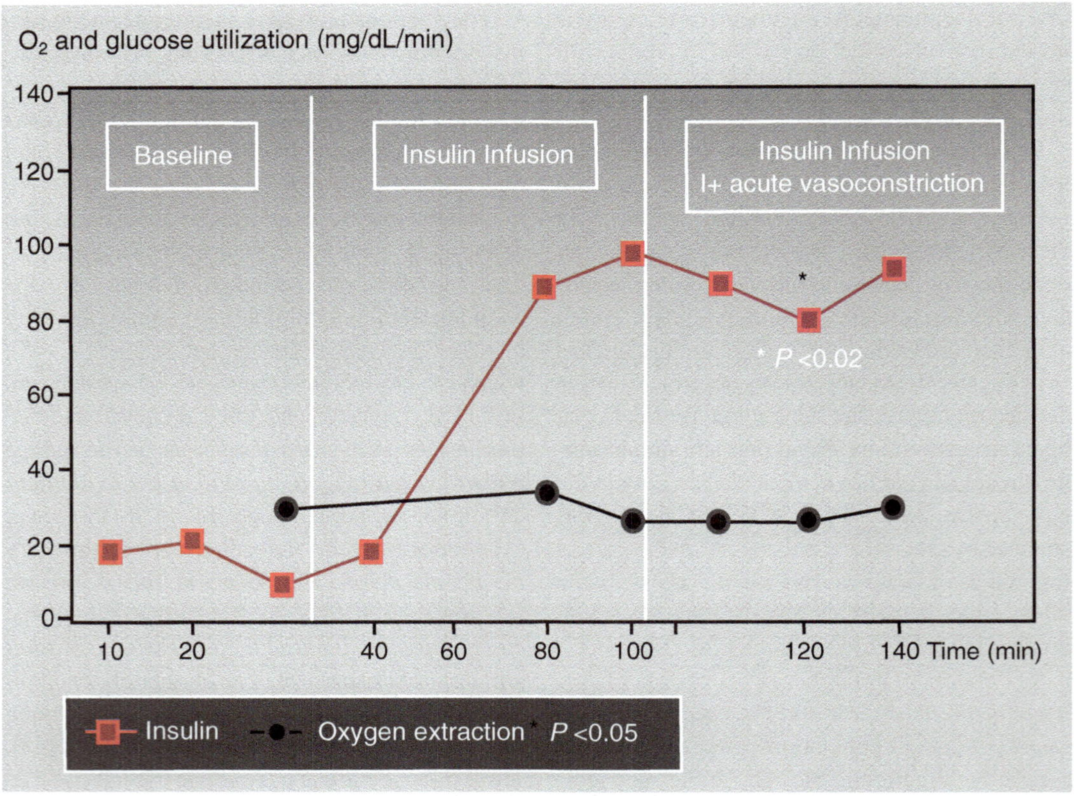

Adapted from K Jamerson, et al: Hypertension 1993[9]

Fig. 16.5 After a 30-min baseline period, insulin was infused regionally to raise forearm insulin ~100 uU/mL for 90 min. Glucose utilization after 40–60 min of regional insulin rose 4–five fold from baseline values. Thigh cuff inflation (beginning 60 min after the regional insulin infusion and continuing during thigh cuff inflation) minutes reduced forearm blood flow 19% and glucose utilization fell 23%, $p < 0.02$ [44]

Moreover, capillary density in skeletal muscle is a major determinant of insulin-mediated glucose disposal in this tissue [46]. Their experimental data suggested that neurogenically-mediated vasoconstriction [44, 45], observed in high-renin patients with borderline and established essential hypertension [4, 5], significantly diminishes insulin-mediated glucose disposal in skeletal muscle. This notion is consistent with studies showing that selective α_1-adrenoceptor antagonists improve insulin-mediate glucose disposal in hypertensive patients to a greater extent than renin-angiotensin system blockers [42, 43].

Clinical importance of neurogenic effects on cardiometabolic variables Effective antihypertensive therapy reduces stroke more than myocardial infarction [47, 48]. One potential explanation for the differential benefit of antihypertensive therapy is that hypertension is frequently associated with multiple other cardiovascular risk factors that raise the risk for myocardial infarction more than the risk for stroke. In fact, increased sympathetic tone may be involved in the genesis of multiple, pressure-independent coronary risk factors in hypertension [31].

Hypertension is frequently associated with hyperinsulinemia and insulin resistance [49]. Insulin resistance is frequently accompanied by a complex atherogenic dyslipidemia characterized by increased triglycerides, reduced HDL-cholesterol, and an increased number of dense

LDL-cholesterol particles [50]. Julius and colleagues provided evidence that these cardiometabolic risk factors are related to increased sympathetic drive [40, 44]. They previously reported that increased sympathetic drive is associated with a relative resting tachycardia and elevated hematocrit [3, 26]. All of these factors (overweight/obesity, hyperinsulinemia, insulin resistance, dyslipidemia, tachycardia, higher hematocrit) are established risk factors for coronary heart disease and sudden death [31, 50–53].

Increased sympathetic drive and obesity: β-adrenoceptor down-regulation and thermogenesis Julius and colleagues documented that hyperkinetic borderline hypertension was characterized by increased cardiac output, which was matched to heightened oxygen consumptions [3, 27]. However, as noted previously, persistent excess sympathetic drive leads to desensitization or down-regulation of β-adrenoceptors. The Ann Arbor group in collaboration with Italian colleagues explored the connection between down-regulation of cardiac and thermogenic responses to the β-adrenoceptor agonist isoproterenol [54]. Subjects for this study included hypertensive adults and normal controls of comparable age but with lower body mass indices. The investigators documented that baseline heart rate was higher in the hypertensive group but that the responses of heart rate and oxygen consumption to isoproterenol were blunted in the hypertensive group. In fact, the chronotropic and thermogenic responses to isoproterenol were inversely related to urinary norepinephrine, an index of sympathetic drive.

Repeated neurogenic pressor episodes and future hypertension A long-standing hypothesis posits that repeated neurogenic pressor episodes lead to sustained hypertension by inducing cardiovascular remodeling and renal injury [31]. Dr. Julius and colleagues described a reproducible hypertensive response to modest compression of both hind limbs in dogs using a fitted suit inflated to 30 mmHg [55]. While the inflation produced no discernible discomfort, systolic blood pressure rose approximately 30 mmHg 60–90 min after suit inflation and was maintained for the duration of 6-h hind limb compression. Heart rate also rose approximately 15 beats/min during hind limb compression. Over 9 weeks, 6 h of daily hind limb compression did not raise resting systolic blood pressure or heart rate but resulted in a 25%–30% increase in left ventricular muscle mass. Thus, repeated neurogenic elevations of blood pressure sufficient to induce significant cardiac remodeling did not lead to sustained hypertension. While these experiments do not disprove the hypothesis that repeated neurogenic pressor episodes lead to sustained hypertension, the findings, nevertheless, raise questions.

In related studies, Julius and coworkers showed that the pressor responses to hind limb compression could be abolished by combined α- and β-adrenoceptor blockade but not by individual blockade of α- or β-adrenoceptors. In fact, in the presence of α-adrenoceptor blockade, dogs experienced the same hypertensive response to thigh cuff inflation mediated by a greater rise of cardiac output when neurogenic vasoconstriction was constrained. Conversely, during β-adrenoceptor blockade, the usual pressor response was mediated by a larger rise of vascular resistance when the increase of cardiac output was constrained. These and other observations led Julius and colleagues to consider the 'pressure' seeking properties of the nervous system, which can be satisfied with variable contributions of flow and resistance [54].

Evidence of increased sympathetic tone in human hypertension has also been documented in human platelets. Kjeldsen and co-workers documented increased thromboglobulin, reflecting increased platelet turnover, and plasma epinephrine as well as a correlation between these two variables in hypertensive patients [56]. In subsequent studies in collaboration with the Ann Arbor group, Kjeldsen documented an inverse relationship between platelet noradrenaline, a marker for increased sympathetic drive, and decreased β-adrenoceptor responses [57]. The data suggest that increased sympathetic drive increases platelet turnover. Moreover, platelet norepinephrine, a long-term marker of sympathetic drive, is ele-

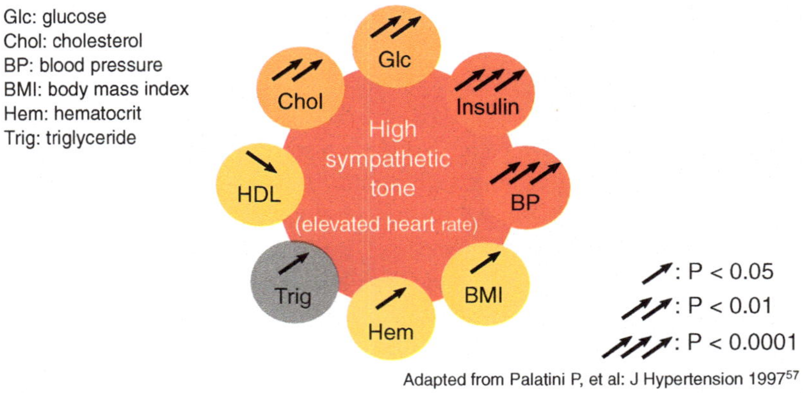

Fig. 16.6 High sympathetic tone as reflected by elevated heart rate

vated in hypertension and is predictive of decreased β-receptor responses. These studies provide novel methodologic confirmation of excess sympathetic drive and down-regulation of β-adrenoceptor responsiveness in hypertensive patients.

Summary of Dr. Julius work on increased sympathetic drive and multiple cardiovascular risk factors As summarized Fig. 16.6 [58], increased sympathetic drive, manifest as a faster heart.

High sympathetic tone as reflected by elevated heart rate, is strongly and positively correlated with blood pressure and hyperinsulinemia as well as glucose, triglycerides, cholesterol, hematocrit, and body mass index, and inversely correlated with HDL-cholesterol. Moreover, suppressed anger appears to underlie the sympathetic activation and parasympathetic withdrawal, which unleash a cluster of risk factors for cardiovascular disease. During the next phase of his productive scientific career, Dr. Julius and colleagues focused efforts on preventing hypertension and its cardiovascular consequences.

Clinical trials to advance knowledge on prevention hypertension and its clinical consequences Trial of Preventing Hypertension (TROPHY) [58]. In the more contemporary phase of his still active career, Professors Julius and colleagues have conducted a landmark trial on preventing hypertension in subjects with pre-hypertension as defined by resting blood pressures in the 130–139/85–89 mmHg range. While blood pressure in this range have been defined as pre-hypertension since 1939 [59], the 2017 Hypertension Guideline developed by the American College of Cardiology and the American Heart Association now defines Stage 1 hypertension by blood pressure values of 130–139/80–89 mmHg [60]. Given this evolution in defining Stage 1 hypertension, TROPHY assumes even greater significance.

In TROPHY, approximately 800 subjects with repeating clinic blood pressure values in the 130–139/85–89 mmHg range were randomized to lifestyle intervention and the angiotensin receptor blocker, candesartan, or to lifestyle and placebo control [11]. After 2 years, candesartan was withdrawn and all subjects were followed for two additional years. As shown in Fig. 16.7, during the first 2 years, more subjects randomized to placebo developed hypertension than those randomized to candesartan, 40.4% vs 13.6%, p < 0.001. Thus, active treatment with candesartan reduced incident hypertension by two-thirds.

At 4 years, among subjects that had taken candesartan the first 2 years, 53.2% of them developed hypertension as compared to 63.0% in the placebo control group, p < 0.001, or a 15.6% relative reduction in incident hypertension [11]. It could be argued that most of the benefit for hypertension prevention was lost when candesartan was withdrawn. However, the 15.6% relative reduction of incident hypertension 2 years after candesartan was withdrawn is comparable to the reduction of incident hypertension seen with

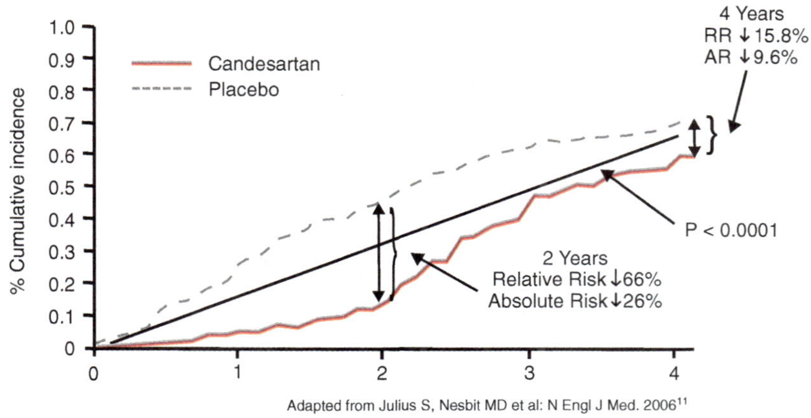

Fig. 16.7 Subjects with BP 130–139/85–89 randomized to candesartan (blue line) developed hypertension at 1/3 the rate of those on placebo during the 1st 2 years. While some 'catch up' occurred in Years 3 and 4 when both groups received placebo, those initially on candesartan had a 15.8% relative reduction of incident hypertension at 4 years

intensive and persistent lifestyle intervention over the same time period.

Given challenges with improving lifestyle patterns in the general population, pharmacotherapy provides a safe alternative for hypertension prevention. In fact, during the four-years of TROPHY, serious adverse events occurred in 5.9% of patients assigned to the placebo group versus 3.5% among those randomized from the active treatment group. With the recent designation of Stage 1 hypertension as blood pressures in the 130–139/80–89 mmHg range, TROPHY is among the studies showing that blood pressure can be safely and effectively lowered in these individuals. More specifically, the 2017 ACC / AHA Hypertension Guideline recommends pharmacotherapy for Stage 1 hypertension when it occurs in conjunction with either clinical cardiovascular disease or a 10-year cardiovascular disease risk ≥10% [59].

Valsartan, amlodipine long-term evaluation (VALUE) study Importance of early blood pressure control [12]. Professor Julius was a lead investigator on this important clinical trial, which generated some important and unexpected insights into preventing cardiovascular events in subjects at high risk. Among the important, unexpected insights, VALUE results indicated that differences in hypertension control during the first 3–6 months of the trial contributed to an excess of cardiovascular events. While conventional wisdom contends that it is important to 'start low' and 'go slow' when treating hypertension in an older, high-risk population, TROPHY suggesting that 'starting too low' with pharmacotherapy, e.g., 80 mg valsartan, and 'going too slow' in up-titrating doses and adding other classes of antihypertensive medications can lead to serious clinical cardiovascular events. Thus, it is important to balance the adverse effects of more rapid (aggressive) hypertension control with the benefit of fewer cardiovascular events.

Importance of the number of antihypertensive medications [13]. Another important and somewhat unexpected finding of VALUE was that among individuals requiring more than initial monotherapy in an attempt to control their hypertension, there was not a significant difference in clinical outcomes between those who did and did not attain hypertension control. The conventional wisdom is that the principal benefit of treating hypertension is mediated by blood pressure reduction, irrespective of the means by which control is attained. This iconoclastic finding in VALUE has been supported by a number of studies showing that blood pressure control among individuals with treatment resistant hypertension leads to less than expected benefits of blood pres-

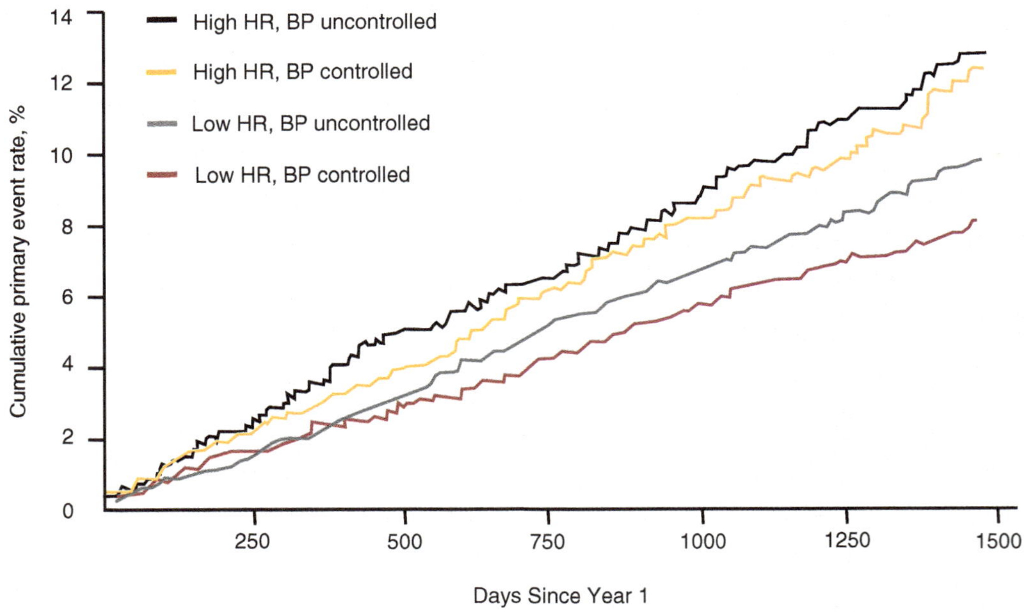

Fig. 16.8 Individuals in the upper quintile of resting heart rate (HR, ≥80 bpm) had more primary cardiovascular events than those with uncontrolled hypertension but resting HR in the lower four quintiles (<80 bpm). In multivariable hazards regression, among individuals with controlled hypertension those with faster heart rates had 53% more cardiovascular events (HR 1.53 [95% CI 1.26–1.85])

sure reduction. Individuals requiring more medications to achieve hypertension control may well be a higher-risk subset with greater degrees of insulin resistance and target organ damage [60]. Nevertheless, data that they do not attain more of the expected benefits of blood pressure reduction will hopefully lead to insights that improve their clinical management and outcomes.

Importance of heart rate in treated hypertensive patients. Heart rate is long recognized as a cardiovascular risk factor [31, 58]. Heart rate reduction with β-blockers is linked to improved clinical outcomes in patients with coronary heart disease or with heart failure with reduced ejection fraction [61, 62]. Yet, the importance of heart rate as a predictor of outcomes in a high-risk group of treated hypertensive patients not selected specifically for coronary heart disease or chronic heart failure has not registered as a significant clinical topic prior to a re-analysis of VALUE trial data (Fig. 16.8) [14].

In this insightful analysis, Dr. Julius and coworkers showed that both blood pressure and heart rate significantly impacted the primary outcome of fatal and non-fatal heart disease and stroke. Within both the uncontrolled and the controlled subgroups of hypertensive patients in VALUE, those with resting heart rate of 80 bpm and higher had worse outcomes than those with lower resting heart rate values.

In summary, more than 50 years of research by Professor Julius and colleagues has documented a key role of high levels of anger and especially suppressed anger and elevated blood pressure. Evidence indicates that anger activates the sympathetic nervous system, while reduce parasympathetic tone. The Ann Arbor group showed that this reciprocal dysfunction of the two limbs of the autonomic nervous system underlies the hyperkinetic borderline hypertension and may be operative in neurogenic, high-renin hypertension. Dr. Julius and coworkers also documented a role for sympathetic activation in cardiometabolic risk and the cardiovascular continuum. In the most recent phase of research, attention has focused on national and multi-national studies on the prevention and treatment of hypertension, which have yielded useful insights that have important implications for hypertension and cardiovascular disease prevention.

References

1. Harburg E, Julius S, McGinn NF, McLeod J, Hoobler SW. Personality traits and behavioral patterns associated with systolic blood pressure in college males. J Chronic Dis. 1964;17:405–14.
2. Schneider R, Egan B, Johnson EH, Drobney H, Julius S. Anger and anxiety in borderline hypertension. Psychosomatic Med. 1986;48:242–8.
3. Julius R, Pascual A, London R. Role of parasympathetic inhibition in the hyperkinetic type of borderline hyper tension. Circulation. 1971;44:413–8.
4. Esler M, Julius S, Randall OS, Ellis CN, Kashima T. Relation of renin status to neurogenic vascular resistance in borderline hypertension. Am J Cardiol. 1075;36:708–15.
5. Esler M, Julius S, Zweifler A, Randall O, Harburg E, Gardiner H, et al. Mild high-renin essential hypertension: neurogenic human hypertension? N Engl J Med. 1977;296:405–11.
6. Julius S, Jamerson K, Mejia A, Krause L, Schork N, Jones K. The association of borderline hypertension with target organ changes and higher coronary risk. Tecumseh Blood Press Stud JAMA. 1990;264:354–8.
7. Julius S, Gudbrandsson T, Jamerson K, Andersson O. The interconnection between sympathetics, microcirculation, and insulin resistance in hypertension. Blood Press. 1992;1:9–19.
8. Julius S, Jamerson K. Sympathetics, insulin resistance and coronary risk in hypertension: the 'chicken-and-egg' question. J Hypertens. 1994;12:495–502.
9. Jamerson K, Julius S, Gudbrandsson T, Andersson O, Brant DO. Reflex sympathetic activation induces acute insulin resistance in the human forearm. Hypertension. 1993;21:618–23.
10. Wilson PWF, Meigs JB. Cardiometabolic risk: a Framingham perspective. Internat J Obes. 2008;32:S17–20.
11. Julius S, Nesbitt SD, Egan BM, Weber MA, Michelson EL, Kaciroti N, et al. Feasibility of treating prehypertension with an angiotensin-receptor blocker. N Engl J Med. 2006;354:1685–97.
12. Julius S, Kjeldsen SE, Weber M, Brunner HR, Ekman S, Hannson L, et al. Outcomes in hypertensive patients at high cardiovascular risk treated with regimens based on valsartan or amlodipine: The VALUE randomized trial. Lancet. 2004;363:2022–31.
13. Weber MA, Julius S, Kjedlsen SE, et al. Cardiovascular outcomes in hypertensive patients comparing single-agent therapy with combination therapy. J Hypertens. 2012;30:2213–22.
14. Julius S, Palatini P, Kjeldsen SE, Zanchetti A, Weber MA, McInnes GT, et al. Usefulness of heart rate to predict future cardiac events in treated patients with high-risk systemic hypertension. Am J Cardiol. 2012;109:685–92.
15. Spielberger CD, Johnson EH, Russell SF, Crane RJ, Jacobs GA, Worden TJ. The experience and expression of anger: construction and validation of an anger expression scale. In: Chesney MA, Rosenman RH, editors. Anger and hostility in cardiovascular and behavioral disorders. New York: Hemisphere/McGraw; 1985. p. 5–30.
16. Alexander F. Emotional factors in essential hypertension: presentation of a tentative hypothesis. Psychosom Med. 1939;1:175–9.
17. Marci CD, Glick DM, Loh R, Dougherty DD. Autonomic and prefrontal cortex responses to autobiographical recall of emotions. Cogn Affect Behav Neurosci. 2007;7:243–50.
18. Levy RL, White PD, Stroud WD. Transient tachycardia: prognostic significance alone and in association with transient hypertension. JAMA. 1945;129:585–8.
19. Lund-Johansen P. Hemodynamic alterations in early essential hypertension: recent advances. In: Gross F, Strassen T, editors. Mild hypertension: recent advances. New York: Raven Press; 1983. p. 237–49.
20. Julius S, Randall OS, Esler MD, Kashima T, Ellis C, Bennett J. Altered cardiac responsiveness and regulation in the normal cardiac output type of borderline hypertension. Circ Res. 1975;36(6 Suppl 1):199–207.
21. Messerli FH, Ventura HO, Resisin E, Dreslinski GR, Dunn FG, MacPhee AA, et al. Borderline hypertension and obesity: two prehypertensive states with elevated cardiac output. Circulation. 1982;66:55–60.
22. Reisin E, Messerli FG, Ventura HO, Frohlich ED. Renal hemodynamic studies in obesity hypertension. J Hypertens. 1987;5:397–400.
23. Egan BM, Schork NJ, Weder AB. Regional hemodynamic abnormalities in overweight men. Focus on alpha-adrenergic vascular responses. Am J Hypertens. 1989;2(6 Part 1):428–34.
24. Guyton AC, Coleman TG. Quantitative analysis of the pathophysiology of hypertension. Circ Res. 1969;24(5 Suppl):1–19.
25. Guyton AC. Dominant role of the kidneys and accessory role of whole-body autoregulationin the pathogenesis of hypertension. Am J Hypertens. 1989;2:575–85.
26. Julius S, Pascual AV, Reilly K, London R. Abnormalities of plasma volume in borderline hypertension. Arch Intern Med. 1971;127:116–9.
27. Julius S, Conway J. Hemodynamic studies in patients with borderline blood pressure elevation. Circulation. 1968;38:282–8.
28. Cohn JN. Relationship of plasma volume changes to resistance and capacitance vessel effects of sympathomimetic amines and angiotensin in man. Clin Sci. 1966;30:267–78.
29. Kjeldsen SE, Moan A, Petrin J, Weder A, Julius S. Effects of increased arterial epinephrine on insulin,

glucose and phosphate. Blood Press. 1996;5:25–31. 28,29
30. Julius R, Pascual A, Abbrecht P, London R. Effect of beta-adrenergic blockade on plasma volume in human subjects. Proc Soc Exp Biol Med. 1972;140:982–5.
31. Julius S, Majahalme S. The changing face of sympathetic overactivity in hypertension. Ann Med. 2000;32:365–70.
32. Hart MN, Heistad DD, Brody MJ. Effect of chronic hypertension and sympathetic denervation on wall/lumen ratio of cerebral vessels. Hypertension. 1980;2:419–28.
33. Bevan RD, Tsuru H, Bevan JH. Cerebral artery mass in the rabbit is reduced by chronic sympathetic denervation. Stroke. 1983;14:393–6.
34. Mulvany MJ. Small artery remodeling in hypertension. Basic Clin Pharm Toxicol. 2011;110:49–55.
35. Egan BM, Schork N, Panis R, Hinderliter A. Vascular structure enhances regional resistance responses in mild hypertension. J Hypertension. 1988;6(1):41–8.
36. Folkow B. Physiological aspects of primary hypertension. Physiol Rev. 1982;62:347–503.
37. Egan B, Panis R, Hinderliter A, Schork N, Julius S. Mechanism of increased alpha-adrenergic vasoconstriction in human essential hypertension. J Clin Invest. 1987;80:812–7.
38. Anderson EA, Sinkey CA, Lawton WJ, Mark AL. Elevated sympathetic nerve activity in borderline hypertensive humans: evidence from direct intraneural recordings. Hypertension. 1989;14:177–83.
39. Esler M. The sympathetic system and hypertension. Am J Hypertens. 2000;13:99S–105S.
40. Julius S, Jamerson K, Mejia A, Krause L, Schork N, Jones K. The association of borderline hypertension with target orgnai changes and higher coronary risk. Tecumseh Blood Pressure Study. JAMA. 1990;264:354–8.
41. De Fronzo RA, Tripathy D. Skeletal muscle insulin resistancc is the primary defect in type 2 diabetes. Diabetes Care. 2009;32(Suppl 2):S157–63.
42. Pollare T, Lithell H, Selinus I, Berne C. Application of prazosin is associated with an increase of insulin sensitivity in obese patients with hypertension. Diabetologia. 1988;31:415–20.
43. Berne C, Pollare T, Lithell H. Effects of antihypertensive treatment on insulin sensitivity with special reference to ACE inhibitors. Diabetes Care. 1991;14. [Suppl 4:39–47.
44. Jamerson KA, Julius S, Gadbrandsson T, Andersson O, Brant DO. Reflex sympathetic activation induces acute insulin resistance in the human forearm. Hypertension. 1993;21:618–23.
45. Jamerson KA, Smith SD, Amerena JV, Grant E, Julius S. Vasoconstriction with norepinrphrine causes less forearm insulin resistance than a reflex sympathetic vasoconstriction. Hypertension. 1994;23(past 2):1006–11.
46. Lillioja S, Young AA, Culter CL, Ivy JL, Abbott WG, Zawadzki JK, et al. Skeletal muscle capillary density and fiber type are possible determinants of in vivo insulin resistance in man. J Clin Invest. 1987;80:415–24.
47. MacMahon S, Peto R, Cutler J, Collins R, Sorlie P, Neaton J, et al. Blood pressure, stroke, and coronary heart disease. Part I, Prolonged differences in blood pressure: prospective observational studies corrected for the regression dilution bias. Lancet. 1990;335:765–74.
48. Willey JZ, Moon YP, Kahn E, Rodriguez CJ, Rundek T, Cheung K, et al. Population attributable risks of hypertension and diabetes for cardiovascular disease and stroke in the Northern Manhattan Study. J Am Heart Assoc. 2014;3:e001106. https://doi.org/10.1161/JAHA.114.001106.
49. Hall JE, Brands MW, Zappe DH, Alonso Galicia M. Insulin resistance, hyperinsulinemia, and hypertension: causes, consequences, or merely correlations? Proc Soc Exp Biol Med. 1994;208: 317–29.
50. Howard BV. Insulin resistance and lipid metabolism. Am J Cardiol. 1990;84(Suppl 1A):28J–32J.
51. Pyorala K, Savolainen E, Kaukola S, Haapakoski J. Plasma insulin as a coronary heart disease risk factor: relationship to the other risk factors and predictive value during 9 ½ year follow-up of the Helsinki Policemen Study. Actu Med Stand Suppl. 1985;701:38–52.
52. Ducimetiere P, Eschwege E, Papoz L, Richard JL, Claude JR, Rosselin G. Relationship of plasma insulin levels to the incidence of myocardial infarction and coronary heart disease mortality in a middle-aged population. Diabetologia. 1980;19:205–10.
53. P P, Benetos A, Grassi G, Julius S, Kjeldsen SE, Mancia G, et al. Identification and management of the hypertensive patient with elevated heart rate: statement of a European Society of Hypertension Consensus Meeting. J Hypertens. 2006;24:603–10.
54. Valentini M, Julius S, Palatini P, Brook RD, Bard RL, Bisognano JD, et al. Attenuation of haemodynamic, metabolic and energy expenditure responses to isoproterenol in patients with hypertension. J Hypertens. 2004;22:1999–2006.
55. Julius S, Li Y, Brant D, Krause L, Buda AJ. Neurogenic pressor episodes fail to cause hypertension, but do induce cardiac hypertrophy. Hypertension. 1989;13:422–9.
56. Kjeldsen SE, Gjesdal K, Eide I, Aakesson I, Amundsen R, Foss OP, et al. Increased beta-thromboglobulin in essential hypertension: interactions between arterial plasma adrenaline, platelet function and blood lipids. Actu Med Scund. 1983;213:369–73.
57. Kjeldsen SE, Zweifler AM, Petrin J, Wder AB, Julius S. Sympathetic nervous system involvement in essential hypertension: increased platelet noradrenaline coincides with decreased β-adrenoreceptor responsiveness. Blood Press. 1994;3:164–71.
58. Palatini P, Julius S. Heart rate and the cardiovascular risk. J Hypertension. 1997;15:3–17.
59. Aronow WS, Casey DE, Collins KJ, et al. 2017 ACC / AHA / AAPA / ABC / ACPM / AGS / APhA / ASH

/ ASPC / NMA / PCNA guideline for the prevention, detection, evaluation, and management of high blood pressure in adults. Hypertension. 2018;71:1269–324.
60. Rao A, Pandya V, Whaley-Connell A. Obesity and insulin resistance in resistant hypertension: implications for the kidney. Adv Chron Kid Dis. 2015;22:211–7.
61. Kotecha D, Flather MD, Altman DG, et al. Heart rate and rhythm and the benefit of beta-blockers in patients with heart failure. J Am Coll Cardiol. 2017;69:2885–96.
62. Gheorghiade M, Goldstein S. β-blockers in the post-myocardial infarction patient. Circulation. 2002;106:394–8.

Part V

Future Perspectives in Cardiovascular Research

New Frontiers in Cardiovascular Research: Microfluidic Modeling of Cardiovascular Diseases and Applications for Hypertension Research

17

Iason T. Papademetriou

General Overview: Microfluidic Organs on a Chip

Although a relatively new field, *in vitro* modeling of tissues and organs is advancing considerably through the use of microfluidic platforms. In contrast to traditional, macroscale cell culture, which consists of monolayers of cells grown in 2 dimensions, microfluidic platforms enable cells to be cultured in microscale channels which can have complex geometries defined by the user, precise exposure to fluid flow, creation of chemical gradients, and concomitant exposure to mechanical stimuli (Fig. 17.1). These functionalities enable numerous features of the tissue microenvironment to be recreated in order to better represent *in vivo* physiology. To date, several microfluidics organs on a chip (μOOC) have been created, including lung [1], liver [2], gut [3], kidney [4, 5], bone [6], brain, [7], heart [8] and blood vessels [9]. μOOC incorporate biological components (e.g. cells, biopolymers, biochemicals) with biophysical components (e.g. fluid flow, tissue geometry) of the tissue microenvironment which were previously difficult to replicate *in vitro*. μOOC are also being linked together to create "body on a chip" systems which facilitate exchange of metabolites between organs, and can be used for drug pharmacokinetic and toxicology studies [10]. μOOC also offer the more general advantages of microfluidic platforms which include monitoring dynamic cellular interactions in real time, lower cost due to reduced reagent volumes and cells, and higher throughput compared with macroscale cell culture.

There is considerable reason to be optimistic that mechanistic insights gained from using μOOC to investigate disease pathophysiology, pharmacokinetics, and pharmacology studies will accelerate drug discovery and development. This is an area of dire need, as the clinical translation of pharmaceuticals has a high failure rate which generally has not improved over the last several decades despite an increase in investment [11]. The development of μOOC in the long term may supplement or replace animal studies and provide complementary data for clinical trials [12].

Microfluidic Organs-on-Chip Relevant to Cardiovascular Diseases

Several μOOC have been developed which are relevant to understanding the basic science of cardiovascular diseases (CVDs), and for aiding development of therapeutics for prevention, diagnosis, or treatment of CVDs. Thus far, μOOC of blood vessels and vascular networks, heart, and

I. T. Papademetriou (✉)
Department of Mechanical Engineering, Boston University, Boston, MA, USA
e-mail: jpapad@bu.edu

V. Papademetriou et al. (eds.), *Management of Hypertension*,
https://doi.org/10.1007/978-3-319-92946-0_17

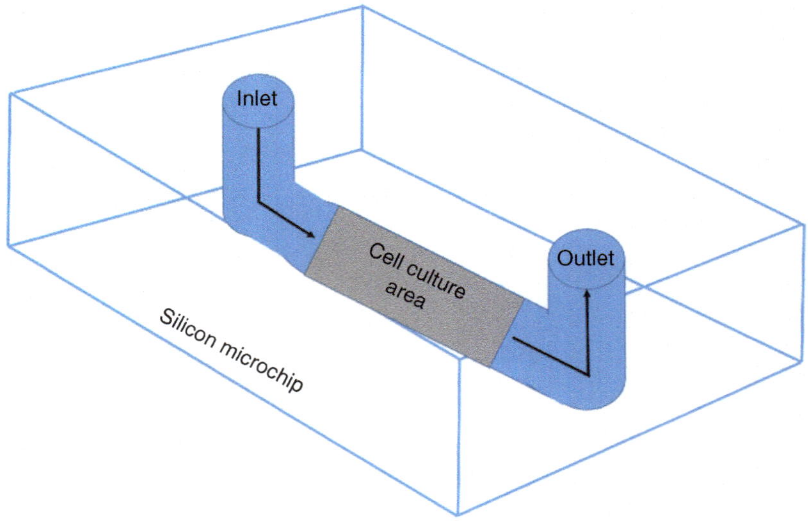

Fig. 17.1 A simple microfluidic cell culture platform. A channel with at least 1 submillimeter dimension is fabricated in a silicone microchip. Cells are cultured in the microchannel and exposed to biochemical and/or biomechanical stimuli (e.g. flow) to aid differentiation into the tissue of interest

kidney have been developed [4, 5, 8, 9]. These μOOC can be used for studies relevant to many CVDs, including hypertension, heart failure, myocardial infarction, arrhythmia, coronary artery disease, thrombosis, and cardiomyopathies. μOOC can considerably improve drug development of CVDs for several reasons (summarized in [13], and described briefly here): While animal models of CVDs often model certain pathophysiological components or lesions present in CVDs, the results from these models often do not translate to results in humans. μOOC which reflect a quasi *in vivo* environment using human cells may provide results more reflective of responses in humans. Second, drug responses can be highly individualized (e.g. species dependence, human-to-human variation). Studies in rodents, for example, would not have predicted that thalidomide would cause limb defects in humans [14]. CVD treatments may be improved by patient stratification. Stratifying drug responses according to patient subgroups could be done using μOOC created with stem cells derived from individual patients. Third, in comparison with clinical trials, μOOC would likely be faster, less expensive, and allow analysis of the mechanism of the response at the organ, cellular, or subcellular level. This section summarizes the main biophysical properties which can currently be recreated by μOOC of blood vessels and heart, and highlights results relevant to CVDs.

Blood Vessels and Vascular Networks

Endothelial cells (ECs) lining the lumen of blood vessels are highly sensitive to biochemical and mechanical signaling from the environment, and the endothelial phenotype adapts accordingly. These adaptations occur via activation of the endothelium which can be physiological or pathophysiological. Examples of physiological adaptations include regulation of vascular tone, vessel formation/regression, endothelial permeability, and other various functional changes related to the immune system, thromboresistance, and healthy body function. On the other hand, pathophysiological changes to the endothelium are an important mechanism underlying CVDs such as atherosclerosis, thrombosis and hypertension. Additionally, hemodynamics involves biophysical phenomena such as Rouleaux formation and sedimentation which are lacking in static cell cultures. Since processes occurring in blood vessels are highly dynamic and rely on biophysical stimuli from the endothelial microenvironment to mediate endothelial adaptations, μOOC may aid understanding of CVDs and provide an improved platform for drug development (Fig. 17.2).

Microchannel Geometry

Microchannels used to create biomimetic blood vessels can be fabricated with diameters

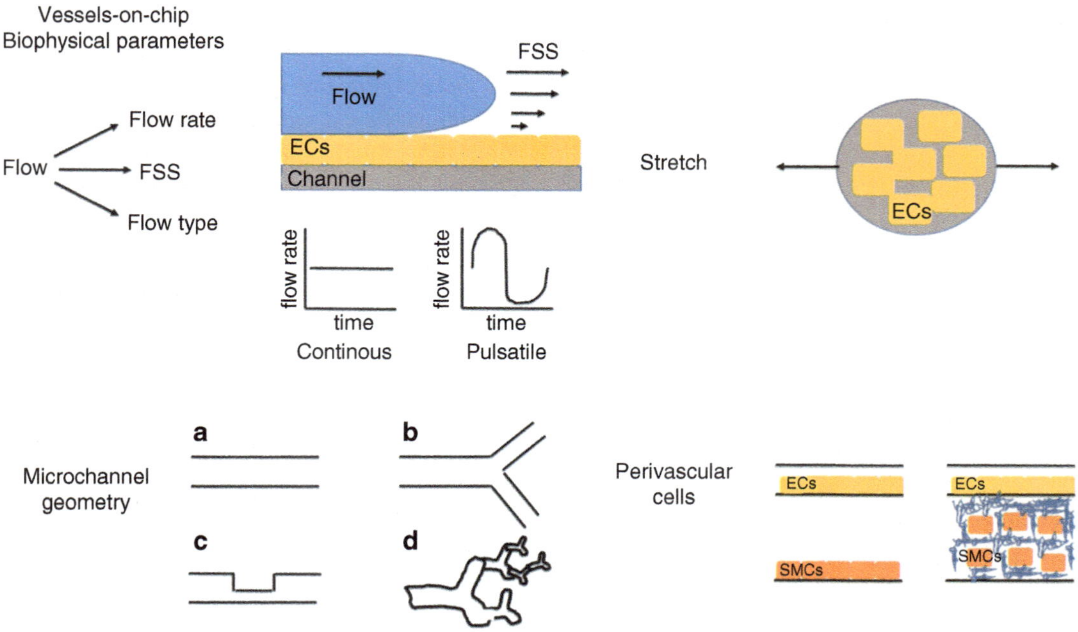

Fig. 17.2 Examples of biophysical parameters for Vessels-on-chip. Flow rate, FSS, and type of flow (e.g. pulsatile vs. continuous) can be used to recreate hemodynamic conditions. Microchannel geometries relevant to vasculature include (**a**) straight channel (**b**) bifurcation (**c**) stenosis (**d**) vascular network. Some Vessels-on-chip enable exposure to cyclic stretch in the presence or absence of concomitant FSS. Perivascular cells (e.g. SMCs) cultured as e) 2-dimensional monolayers or f) in 3-dimensional matrix (e.g. hydrogels) can be incorporated to better mimic the tissue microenvironment

(generally 100–1000 microns) which match that of most native blood vessels. This microchannel diameter range ensures laminar flow which is characteristic of flow in native blood vessels. Another byproduct of the microchannel geometry is that the volume of fluid in microchannels is much smaller than macroscale cell cultures. Microchannels can therefore be used to create a culture platform with a reduced ratio of fluid to cells which more closely approximates fluid-to-cell ratios present *in vivo*. Wang and colleagues, [15], designed such a system which minimized the ratio of culture medium to blood-brain barrier ECs and incorporated flow which was in range of physiological values for blood residence time in human brain. Their device is the first microfluidic model of the blood-brain barrier which achieves barrier tightness in the range reported *in vivo*.

The geometry of blood vessels is related to blood flow properties such as apparent viscosity (due to the fahreus-lindqvuist effect) and fluid shear stress (FSS). Microchannels can be designed with geometries of interest (e.g. stenosis, bifurcations in the case of CVDs) to simulate hemodynamic conditions. Microchannels can also be fabricated with multiple compartments which segregate cell types while allowing intercellular communication. For example, two-compartment systems have been designed which enable co-culture of endothelialized microchannels with perivascular cells [5, 15]. Microchannel geometry can be used to expose ECs to chemical gradients which simulate conditions *in vivo*. This can be accomplished using multiple approaches. For example, a chemical gradient parallel to the microchannel can be established by introducing the chemical on one side of the channel. Similarly, in a two-compartment system, a chemical gradient perpendicular to the microchannel can be established by adding the agent to one of the compartments. Microfluidic vascular networks have also been created to more closely approximate the complex geometry of vasculature *in vivo* [16]. More than endothelialized microchannels, these vascular networks better represent the 3 dimensional geometry of native blood vessels, and can be designed to incorporate multiple segments of the vascular tree in a single system (e.g. from artery to capillary). For example, Moya et al. developed capillary networks which anastamose with fluidic microchannels to enable perfusion at physiological flow and shear rates [16].

Flow

Microfluidics enables precise control of flow parameters (e.g. flow rate, FSS, pulsatile/continuous laminar flows) which can be used to simulate hemodynamics in physiological or pathophysiological conditions. Flow adds a convective component to transport of substances from the blood stream, and affects the rheological properties of blood. Flow rates for blood vessels *in vivo* range from less than 1 cm/s in capillaries to 40–50 cm/s in the aorta, and this range is achievable in microfluidic devices. Simulating physiological flow rates *in vitro* can help to recreate the transport of metabolites and signaling molecules present *in vivo*. A microfluidic blood-brain barrier model, for example, was designed with flow which simulated the blood residence time of human brain blood vessels, and successfully recreated the tightness of the human blood-brain barrier [15]. FSS is a mechanical stress parallel to the direction of flow imparted on endothelium by blood flow. FSS is sensed by the endothelium via a variety of mechanosensitive elements (e.g. endothelial glycocalyx, platelet-endothelial cell adhesion molecule 1, ion channels) which initiate a biological response that changes EC mechanical properties, and can also alter the local extracellular matrix or neighboring cells (e.g. smooth muscle cells (SMC), pericytes) [17, 18]. FSS has been demonstrated to alter EC morphology, activate cell signaling pathways, induce actin cytoskeletal rearrangement, and alter endothelial permeability [19]. FSS ranges from ~3 dyne/cm^2 in capillaries to greater than 100 dyne/cm^2 in arteries, and this range can be achieved with microfluidic devices. Laminar flow occurs in most cases of physiological blood flow and is produced in microfluidic devices due to the microscale diameter of the channels. Pulsatile laminar flow occurs more often in large arteries due to the contraction of the heart, while continuous laminar flow is more characteristic of smaller arteries, capillaries, and the venous system. Pulsatile flow can exert different effects than continuous flow. For example, erythrocyte adhesion to ECs was found to be enhanced by pulsatile flow relative to continuous flow [20]. In addition to flow applied to the lumen of endothelialized microchannels, flow can also be applied abluminally to mimic interstitial flow. Interstitial flow was recently shown to improve the differentiation of microfluidic vascular networks [21]. Chin et al. used pulsatile flow in a blood vessel on a chip system to examine the effect of heart rate, shear stress, and hyperglycemia on production of reactive oxygen species (ROS) [22]. The authors found pulsatile flow increased production of ROS relative to continuous flow. In hyperglycemia, pulsatile flow increased ROS production relative to static condition. These results suggest that pulsatile flow helps recapitulate *in vitro* the effects of exercise and hyperglycemia on ROS production by endothelium. A separate study examined the adhesion of monocytes to endothelium activated with inflammatory cytokine in the presence of flow using endothelialized microchannels prepared with ECs derived from human induced pluripotent stem cells (hiPSCs, [23]). hiPSC-differentiated ECs displayed an endothelial phenotype in the presence of flow, and monocyte adhesion was enhanced in activated vs unactivated conditions. The use of hiPSCs in the model is an important step towards demonstrating the feasibility of using patient-derived stem cells in μOOC.

Cyclic Stretch

Cardiac contractions result in the generation of pulsatile blood flow in the larger segments of the arterial circulation. Pulsatile flow exerts cyclic stretch on ECs and SMCs. As in the case of FSS, cyclic stretch has been found to influence endothelial phenotype. For example, cyclic stretch has been found to induce rearrangement of the actin cytoskeleton [24, 25], and regulate endothelial permeability [26, 27]. Combined exposure of

FSS and cyclic stretch was found to enhance actin realignment relative to FSS alone [25]. Combined exposure to FSS and cyclic stretch enabled ECs to adhere more efficiently to cultured SMCs than static incubation in a microfluidic device [25], supporting the role of mechanical stimuli in interactions between ECs and SMCs. Interestingly, cyclic stretch was also shown to stimulate convective transport in the perivascular space which is retrograde to the direction of luminal fluid flow [27]. This result provides evidence for a mechanism by which interstitial fluid and metabolites are filtered from the brain, and is an interesting example of how the incorporation of mechanical stimuli in microfluidic models can provide insight into the function of the tissue microenvironment. A recent study by Sinha et al. investigated the effect of cyclic stretch and FSS where the applied stretch is anisotropic and not perpendicular to the direction of flow [28] as occurs in tortuous (i.e. not straight) vessels. The authors also pointed out that changes in shape and mechanical properties of the vascular wall make anisotropic, non-perpendicular orientations of cyclic stretch and FSS relevant to modeling atherosclerosis, aneurysms, and hypertension. As expected, when cyclic stretch was applied alone, ECs aligned perpendicular to the direction of stretch, and when FSS was applied alone, ECs oriented parallel to the direction of FSS. Interestingly, when cyclic stretch was applied at a non-perpendicular angle to FSS, FSS and cyclic stretch appeared to have a competitive effect on EC alignment. At a FSS of 0.55 Pa, FSS dominated over cyclic stretch and ECs aligned in the direction of flow. At 0.08 Pa of FSS, cyclic stretch determined the direction of EC alignment. This work showed that concomitant and complex biomechanical stimuli can produce unique effects on EC phenotype which may provide new insights for CVDs.

Incorporation of Perivascular Cells

Intercellular interactions between endothelium and perivascular cells (e.g. SMCs, pericytes) contribute to the physiological function of blood vessels and to mechanisms of disease. The incorporation of these cell types is therefore important for the creation of physiologically relevant engineered blood vessels. SMCs are located in the perivascular space of larger vessels (e.g. arteries, arterioles). EC-SMC interactions regulate a variety of events related to vascular function such as vasoconstriction/dilatation, platelet aggregation, and neutrophil adhesion [29]. Intercellular communication between ECs and SMCs is facilitated biochemically via signaling molecules such as nitric oxide, prostacyclin and hydrogen peroxide, as well as electrically via myoendothelial gap junctions (see [29] for review). Changes in SMC phenotype are associated with disease states. For example, SMC proliferation is correlated with hypertension and atherosclerosis. Caudal arteries in hypertensive rats were found to have increased amounts of myoendothelial gap junctions, suggesting that EC-SMC interactions may be increased during hypertension [30]. Pericytes are primarily found in the microcirculation and at present can be broadly defined as any microvascular periendothelial mesenchymal cell [31]. Pericytes interact with endothelial cells to regulate the barrier function of capillaries, capillary diameter, and turnover of ECs [31]. Pericytes can be correlated with disease development. For example, pericyte loss in retinal microvessels is considered a morphological indication of diabetic retinopathy [32]. As can be seen from this brief synopsis, there is a rich rationale for incorporating perivascular cells into platforms of microfluidic engineered blood vessels.

Heart-on-Chip

Engineered *in vitro* myocardium has been developed to further understanding of cardiac physiology and CVDs. The myocardium contracts as a result of cardiomyocyte (CM) depolarization which is initiated by electrical stimulation from the sinoatrial node and conducted through the atria and ventricles. CMs are elongated and anisotropic, connecting together at their ends via formation on intercellular junctions to form cardiac fibers which constitute the major component of myocardial tissue. Thus, numerous biophysical stimuli contribute to the physiological function of the heart which can be recreated with heart-on-chip platforms. These platforms can be outfitted with electrodes to stimulate CM [33], as well as cantilevers to enable recording of CM contractile force [34].

Engineering a Quasi-*In Vivo* Microenvironment

Heart on a chip platforms expose CM to a quasi *in vivo* microenvironment via incorporation of biophysical stimuli such as electrical stimulation, geometries or substrate patterning which establishes CM anisotropy and elasticity [34–36], compartmentalization of microvessels and CM, fluid flow, cyclic stretch, or incorporation of additional cells present in myocardium such as fibroblasts, ECs, and SMCs. It is important that substrates used for culture of CM have appropriate elasticity, as matrix elasticity affects CM functions (e.g. action potential length, calcium influx [37]). Culture of CM in an anisotropic geometry stimulates CM activity. CM anisotropy can be accomplished by culture on micropatterned extracellular matrix [34, 36], confinement of CM [8], or culture on topographically-patterned substrate [33]. Electrical stimulation can enhance expression of gap junction and sarcomere proteins [33, 38]) and enables maturation of CM derived from human PSCs [39]. Application of cyclic stretch to confined, hydrogel suspended CM resulted in a marked increase in formation of junction complexes compared with static culture [40]. As a result, CM cultured under cyclic stretch exhibited improved differentiation into cardiac tissue and better mechanical and electrical coupling [40]. Physiological elasticity can be obtained by culture of CM on micropatterned biological substrates such as fibronectin [34] or hydrogels [35, 37]. Compartmentalization of CM and microvessels with continuous fluid flow in the vascular compartment enables simulation of nutrient/metabolite exchange between myocardium and microvessels. Mathur et al. used an array of micropillars to separate flow in vascular channels from CM [8]. With this setup, transport occurred exclusively via diffusion, while shielding CM from FSS. In another study, flow, CM anisotropy, and electrical stimulation were established in a perfusable cardiac microtissue which was designed to mimic native cardiac bundles [39]. Perfusion and concurrent electrical stimulation lowered the excitation threshold for cardiac contractility and enhanced maximum beating frequency [39].

Modeling CVDs with Heart-on-Chip Devices

Disease modeling with heart-on-chip devices has been established with insults which produce cardiomyopathy, such as ischemia-reperfusion [41], ischemia [42], cyclic stretch overload [43], as well as the use of diseased cells derived from patients with Barth's syndrome cardiomyopathy [44]. Ischemia-reperfusion produced membrane depolarization and apoptosis in CM after ischemia, and the rate of apoptosis accelerated after reperfusion [41]. One advantage of this system was that it provided a facile method to determine the kinetics of CM apoptosis relative to animal models [41]. A separate study documented cell shrinkage, cytoskeletal disintegration, membrane depolarization, and activation of caspase 3 in CM after exposure to ischemia [42]. Exposure to pathological cyclic stretch has also been investigated in an engineered heart-on-chip device [43]. Cyclic stretch induced pathological remodeling, including decreased α- to β-myosin heavy chain ratios, and changes to CM shape and sarcomere alignment. Peak systolic stress was reduced and calcium transients were similar to those reported for failing CM. Heart on a chip fabricated with human cells derived from iPSCs [38] is expected to improve the translatability of results to humans, and enable studies related to personalized medicine. For example, patient-derived iPSCs and heart-on-chip technology was used to model and test therapies for Barth's syndrome cardiomyopathy [44].

Harnessing Microfluidic Organs on Chip for Hypertension Research

As described in section "Microfluidic Organs–on–chip relevant to cardiovascular diseases", numerous platforms are currently available which can be utilized to inform the basic science of cardiac physiology and CVDs, as well as aid drug development for CVDs. The following section highlights some of the applications of μOOC for hypertension research.

Endothelial Dysfunction and Hypertension

Endothelial dysfunction is a defined pathophysiological state of the endothelium which impairs vascular function, and is pro-thrombotic, pro-inflammatory, and pro-constrictive [45]. Endothelial dysfunction is associated with hypertension, although the relationship is complex and currently unclear. Upregulation of inflammatory and vasoconstrictive factors in endothelium increases vascular tone and systemic tone, and results in sodium retention by the kidneys [46]. The downstream effects of these changes are postulated to result in hypertension. μOOC present an opportunity to investigate this relationship. For example, blood vessel μOOC may be used to examine the effect of changes in sodium/potassium, hormones (e.g. angiotensin II), fluid volume, or albumin levels on blood pressure and endothelial phenotype. μOOC have been outfitted with pressure sensors suitable for monitoring pressure within fluidic microchannels, and pressures within the physiological range have been achieved [47]. The results could be compared in activated endothelium (e.g. via stimulation by inflammatory cytokines), and in unactivated endothelium. Such an experiment would provide insight into the contribution of endothelial dysfunction to the development of hypertension. This type of study is not possible with static cell cultures, and the analysis in animal models would likely be more difficult due to the added complexity of the native *in vivo* environment. The role of hemodynamic conditions (e.g. continuous vs pulsatile flow, flow rate, FSS, cyclic stretch) could be investigated in a similar fashion.

Blood vessels on a chip could also be used to test the efficacy and toxicity of antihypertensives which act on the vasculature. Kidney μOOC could be used to test antihypertensives acting on the kidney (e.g. SGLT2 inhibitors which control reabsorption of glucose). Multiple μOOC linked together could be used to investigate systemic regulation of blood pressure. For example, kidney, lung, blood vessels, and brain could be used to examine blood pressure regulation by the renin-angiotensin system (RAS). Such a setup could potentially recreate the inter-organ endocrine signaling present in RAS, and would aid in decoupling the contribution of individual organs or tissues. Individualized μOOC fabricated using stem cells derived from peripheral blood of patients [48] could allow assessment of hypertension development and responsivness to antihypertensives which is specific to a patients genetic background. A protocol which enables differentiation of stem cells to SMCs would be needed to incorporate patient-derived SMCs into the device.

Endothelial Dysfunction and Atherosclerosis

The association between endothelial dysfunction and atherosclerosis is also complex, although considerably more well defined than with hypertension. Endothelial dysfunction and changes in blood flow result in vascular permeability that enables accumulation and modification of lipids in the subendothelial space [49]. This encourages the recruitment of monocytes to endothelium and transmigration to the subendothelial space. Monocytes differentiate into macrophages which subsequently develop into foam cells due to the internalization of lipids. Foam cells accelerate inflammation and initiate the formation of the atherosclerotic lesion. Chemokines and growth factors subsequently induce proliferation of SMCs into the intima, leading to formation of a fibromuscular plaque. Although this constitutes merely the early stages of atherosclerosis, there are multiple points where the relationship between endothelial dysfunction and biophysical events (e.g. monocyte recruitment, transmigration) can be investigated (Fig. 17.3). Importantly, the blood vessel microenvironment plays a role in atherosclerosis development, as vessel bifurcations and low FSS are characteristic of

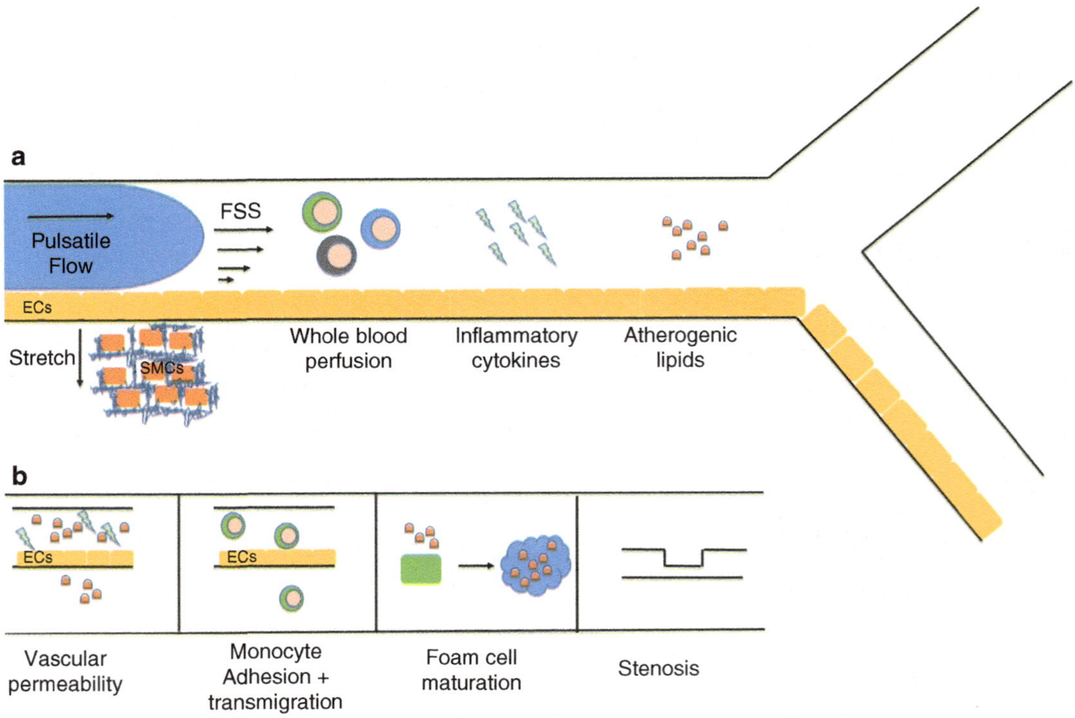

Fig. 17.3 Vessel-on-chip for modeling early stages of atherosclerosis. (**a**) Endothelialized microchannels exposed to pulsatile flow, FSS, cyclic stretch, and co-cultured with 3-dimensional SMCs in a bifurcated geometry. Perfusion with whole blood, inflammatory cytokines, and atherogenic lipids could be used to model early stages of atherosclerosis. (**b**) Examples of biophysical events which could be investigated using vessel-on-chip technology

atheroprone sites. Stenosis resulting from atherosclerosis results in hemodynamic changes which may contribute to the disease progression. Intercellular exchange of metabolites, hormones, and other biochemicals occurs between endothelium and perivascular cells. Vessels-on-chip could allow these biophysical parameters to be incorporated simultaneously or in isolation, potentially enabling the effect of each cue to be decoupled from other parameters. μOOC modeling atherosclerosis have been developed [50–52]. Recently, vessel-on-chip incorporated a pneumatic channel in order to tune stenosis of an endothelialized microchannel [52]. The device incorporated fluid flow at low FSS and whole blood perfusion to examine leukocyte endothelial interactions at various levels of stenosis [52]. μOOC modeling of atherosclerosis using patient specific cells appears possible currently, as peripheral blood drawn from patients can be used to generate ECs from stem cells [48]. Whole blood from the patient could be used as well, particularly for studies examining monocyte recruitment to the vessel wall.

References

1. Huh D, Leslie DC, Matthews BD, Fraser JP, Jurek S, Hamilton GA, et al. A human disease model of drug toxicity-induced pulmonary edema in a lung-on-a-chip microdevice. Sci Transl Med. 2012;4(159):159ra47.
2. Lee PJ, Hung PJ, Lee LP. An artificial liver sinusoid with a microfluidic endothelial-like barrier for primary hepatocyte culture. Biotechnol Bioeng. 2007;97(5):1340–6.
3. Kim HJ, Huh D, Hamilton G, Ingber DE. Human gut-on-a-chip inhabited by microbial flora that experiences intestinal peristalsis-like motions and flow. Lab Chip. 2012;12(12):2165–74.
4. Jang KJ, Suh KY. A multi-layer microfluidic device for efficient culture and analysis of renal tubular cells. Lab Chip. 2010;10(1):36–42.

5. Vedula EM, Alonso JL, Arnaout MA, Charest JL. A microfluidic renal proximal tubule with active reabsorptive function. PLoS One. 2017;12(10):e0184330.
6. Jusoh N, Oh S, Kim S, Kim J, Jeon NL. Microfluidic vascularized bone tissue model with hydroxyapatite-incorporated extracellular matrix. Lab Chip. 2015;15(20):3984–8.
7. Kilic O, Pamies D, Lavell E, Schiapparelli P, Feng Y, Hartung T, et al. Brain-on-a-chip model enables analysis of human neuronal differentiation and chemotaxis. Lab Chip. 2016;16(21):4152–62.
8. Mathur A, Loskill P, Shao K, Huebsch N, Hong S, Marcus SG, et al. Human iPSC-based cardiac microphysiological system for drug screening applications. Sci Rep. 2015;5:8883.
9. Smith Q, Gerecht S. Going with the flow: microfluidic platforms in vascular tissue engineering. Curr Opin Chem Eng. 2014;3:42–50.
10. Prantil-Baun R, Novak R, Das D, Somayaji MR, Przekwas A, Ingber DE. Physiologically based pharmacokinetic and Pharmacodynamic analysis enabled by microfluidically linked organs-on-chips. Annu Rev Pharmacol Toxicol. 2018;58:37–64.
11. Scannell JW, Blanckley A, Boldon H, Warrington B. Diagnosing the decline in pharmaceutical R&D efficiency. Nat Rev Drug Discov. 2012;11(3):191–200.
12. Sackmann EK, Fulton AL, Beebe DJ. The present and future role of microfluidics in biomedical research. Nature. 2014;507(7491):181–9.
13. Ribas J, Sadeghi H, Manbachi A, Leijten J, Brinegar K, Zhang YS, et al. Cardiovascular organ-on-a-chip platforms for drug discovery and development. Appl In Vitro Toxicol. 2016;2(2):82–96.
14. Barnard ND, Kaufman SR. Animal research is wasteful and misleading. Sci Am. 1997;276(2):80–2.
15. Wang YI, Abaci HE, Shuler ML. Microfluidic blood-brain barrier model provides in vivo-like barrier properties for drug permeability screening. Biotechnol Bioeng. 2017;114(1):184–94.
16. Moya ML, Hsu YH, Lee AP, Hughes CC, George SC. In vitro perfused human capillary networks. Tissue Eng Part C Methods. 2013;19(9):730–7.
17. Baeyens N, Bandyopadhyay C, Coon BG, Yun S, Schwartz MA. Endothelial fluid shear stress sensing in vascular health and disease. J Clin Invest. 2016;126(3):821–8.
18. Polacheck WJ, Li R, Uzel SG, Kamm RD. Microfluidic platforms for mechanobiology. Lab Chip. 2013;13(12):2252–67.
19. Tarbell JM. Shear stress and the endothelial transport barrier. Cardiovasc Res. 2010;87(2):320–30.
20. White J, Lancelot M, Sarnaik S, Hines P. Increased erythrocyte adhesion to VCAM-1 during pulsatile flow: application of a microfluidic flow adhesion bioassay. Clin Hemorheol Microcirc. 2015;60(2):201–13.
21. Hsu YH, Moya ML, Abiri P, Hughes CC, George SC, Lee AP. Full range physiological mass transport control in 3D tissue cultures. Lab Chip. 2013;13(1):81–9.
22. Chin LK, Yu JQ, Fu Y, Yu T, Liu AQ, Luo KQ. Production of reactive oxygen species in endothelial cells under different pulsatile shear stresses and glucose concentrations. Lab Chip. 2011;11(11):1856–63.
23. Wang L, Xiang M, Liu Y, Sun N, Lu M, Shi Y, et al. Human induced pluripotent stem cells derived endothelial cells mimicking vascular inflammatory response under flow. Biomicrofluidics. 2016;10(1):014106.
24. Punchard MA, Stenson-Cox C, O'Cearbhaill ED, Lyons E, Gundy S, Murphy L, et al. Endothelial cell response to biomechanical forces under simulated vascular loading conditions. J Biomech. 2007;40(14):3146–54.
25. Zheng W, Jiang B, Wang D, Zhang W, Wang Z, Jiang X. A microfluidic flow-stretch chip for investigating blood vessel biomechanics. Lab Chip. 2012;12(18):3441–50.
26. Collins NT, Cummins PM, Colgan OC, Ferguson G, Birney YA, Murphy RP, et al. Cyclic strain-mediated regulation of vascular endothelial occludin and ZO-1: influence on intercellular tight junction assembly and function. Arterioscler Thromb Vasc Biol. 2006;26(1):62–8.
27. Partyka PP, Godsey GA, Galie JR, Kosciuk MC, Acharya NK, Nagele RG, et al. c. Biomaterials. 2017;115:30–9.
28. Sinha R, Le Gac S, Verdonschot N, van den Berg A, Koopman B, Rouwkema J. Endothelial cell alignment as a result of anisotropic strain and flow induced shear stress combinations. Sci Rep. 2016;6:29510.
29. Triggle CR, Samuel SM, Ravishankar S, Marei I, Arunachalam G, Ding H. The endothelium: influencing vascular smooth muscle in many ways. Can J Physiol Pharmacol. 2012;90(6):713–38.
30. Sandow SL, Bramich NJ, Bandi HP, Rummery NM, Hill CE. Structure, function, and endothelium-derived hyperpolarizing factor in the caudal artery of the SHR and WKY rat. Arterioscler Thromb Vasc Biol. 2003;23(5):822–8.
31. Armulik A, Genove G, Betsholtz C. Pericytes: developmental, physiological, and pathological perspectives, problems, and promises. Dev Cell. 2011;21(2):193–215.
32. Pfister F, Przybyt E, Harmsen MC, Hammes HP. Pericytes in the eye. Pflugers Arch. 2013;465(6):789–96.
33. Heidi AHT, Cui B, Chu ZE, Veres T, Radisic M. Cell culture chips for simultaneous application of topographical and electrical cues enhance phenotype of cardiomyocytes. Lab Chip. 2009;9(4):564–75.
34. Sheehy SP, Grosberg A, Qin P, Behm DJ, Ferrier JP, Eagleson MA, et al. Toward improved myocardial maturity in an organ-on-chip platform with immature cardiac myocytes. Exp Biol Med (Maywood). 2017;242(17):1643–56.
35. Annabi N, Selimovic S, Acevedo Cox JP, Ribas J, Afshar Bakooshli M, Heintze D, et al. Hydrogel-coated microfluidic channels for cardiomyocyte culture. Lab Chip. 2013;13(18):3569–77.
36. Feinberg AW, Feigel A, Shevkoplyas SS, Sheehy S, Whitesides GM, Parker KK. Muscular thin films for

building actuators and powering devices. Science. 2007;317(5843):1366–70.
37. Boothe SD, Myers JD, Pok S, Sun J, Xi Y, Nieto RM, et al. The effect of substrate stiffness on Cardiomyocyte action potentials. Cell Biochem Biophys. 2016;74(4):527–35.
38. Ruan JL, Tulloch NL, Razumova MV, Saiget M, Muskheli V, Pabon L, et al. Mechanical stress conditioning and electrical stimulation promote contractility and force maturation of induced pluripotent stem cell-derived human cardiac tissue. Circulation. 2016;134(20):1557–67.
39. Xiao Y, Zhang B, Liu H, Miklas JW, Gagliardi M, Pahnke A, et al. Microfabricated perfusable cardiac biowire: a platform that mimics native cardiac bundle. Lab Chip. 2014;14(5):869–82.
40. Marsano A, Conficconi C, Lemme M, Occhetta P, Gaudiello E, Votta E, et al. Beating heart on a chip: a novel microfluidic platform to generate functional 3D cardiac microtissues. Lab Chip. 2016;16(3):599–610.
41. Khanal G, Chung K, Solis-Wever X, Johnson B, Pappas D. Ischemia/reperfusion injury of primary porcine cardiomyocytes in a low-shear microfluidic culture and analysis device. Analyst. 2011;136(17):3519–26.
42. Ren L, Liu W, Wang Y, Wang JC, Tu Q, Xu J, et al. Investigation of hypoxia-induced myocardial injury dynamics in a tissue interface mimicking microfluidic device. Anal Chem. 2013;85(1):235–44.
43. McCain ML, Sheehy SP, Grosberg A, Goss JA, Parker KK. Recapitulating maladaptive, multiscale remodeling of failing myocardium on a chip. Proc Natl Acad Sci U S A. 2013;110(24):9770–5.
44. Wang G, McCain ML, Yang L, He A, Pasqualini FS, Agarwal A, et al. Modeling the mitochondrial cardiomyopathy of Barth syndrome with induced pluripotent stem cell and heart-on-chip technologies. Nat Med. 2014;20(6):616–23.
45. Dharmashankar K, Widlansky ME. Vascular endothelial function and hypertension: insights and directions. Curr Hypertens Rep. 2010;12(6):448–55.
46. Brandes RP. Endothelial dysfunction and hypertension. Hypertension. 2014;64(5):924–8.
47. Chen Y, Chan HN, Michael SA, Shen Y, Chen Y, Tian Q, et al. A microfluidic circulatory system integrated with capillary-assisted pressure sensors. Lab Chip. 2017;17(4):653–62.
48. Simara P, Tesarova L, Rehakova D, Farkas S, Salingova B, Kutalkova K, et al. Reprogramming of adult peripheral blood cells into human induced pluripotent stem cells as a safe and accessible source of endothelial cells. Stem Cells Dev. 2018;27(1):10–22.
49. Gimbrone MA Jr, Garcia-Cardena G. Endothelial cell dysfunction and the pathobiology of atherosclerosis. Circ Res. 2016;118(4):620–36.
50. Estrada R, Giridharan GA, Nguyen MD, Prabhu SD, Sethu P. Microfluidic endothelial cell culture model to replicate disturbed flow conditions seen in atherosclerosis susceptible regions. Biomicrofluidics. 2011;5(3):32006–3200611.
51. Kim Y, Lobatto ME, Kawahara T, Lee Chung B, Mieszawska AJ, Sanchez-Gaytan BL, et al. Probing nanoparticle translocation across the permeable endothelium in experimental atherosclerosis. Proc Natl Acad Sci U S A. 2014;111(3):1078–83.
52. Menon NV, Tay HM, Pang KT, Dalan R, Wong SC, Wang X, et al. A tunable microfluidic 3D stenosis model to study leukocyte-endothelial interactions in atherosclerosis. APL Bioeng. 2018;2(1) https://doi.org/10.1063/1.4993762.

Printed by Printforce, the Netherlands